Viral Encephalitis in Humans

Viral Encephalitis in Humans

by

John Booss

National Director of Neurology, Department of Veterans Affairs, VA Connecticut, West Haven, and Professor of Neurology and of Laboratory Medicine, Yale University School of Medicine, New Haven, Connecticut

Margaret M. Esiri

Professor of Neuropathology, Department of Clinical Neurology, University of Oxford, and Honorary Consultant Neuropathologist, Oxford Radcliffe NHS Trust, Oxford, United Kingdom

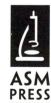

ASM PRESS

WASHINGTON, D.C.

Copyright ©   2003 ASM Press
American Society for Microbiology
1752 N Street, N.W.
Washington, DC 20036-2904

Library of Congress Cataloging-in-Publication Data

Booss, John.
   Viral encephalitis in humans / by John Booss, Margaret M. Esiri.
      p. ; cm.
Includes bibliographical references and index.
   ISBN 1-55581-240-6
   1. Encephalitis.   2. Virus diseases.
   [DNLM: 1. Encephalitis, Viral–diagnosis.   2. Encephalitis,
Viral–therapy.   3. Encephalitis Viruses–pathogenicity.   WL 351 B724v
2003]   I. Esiri, Margaret M.   II. Title.

RC390.B66   2003
616.8'32–dc21   2003000069

All Rights Reserved
Printed in the United States of America

10   9   8   7   6   5   4   3   2   1

Address editorial correspondence to: ASM Press, 1752 N St., N.W., Washington, DC 20036-2904, U.S.A.

Send orders to: ASM Press, P.O. Box 605, Herndon, VA 20172, U.S.A.
Phone: 800-546-2416; 703-661-1593
Fax: 703-661-1501
Email: books@asmusa.org
Online: www.asmpress.org

Contents

Preface

Our purpose is to assist the clinician who has responsibility for the diagnosis and management of viral encephalitis. The tasks of that clinician on confronting a case of viral encephalitis are both complex and urgent. The potential viral causes of infection are myriad, and the clinical expressions of those infections are diverse and often overlapping. Much of the information about the viral causes of encephalitis in other texts is arranged by viral taxonomy, that is, according to the physical-chemical characteristics of families of viruses. Such a presentation, however, makes the assumption that the cause of the encephalitis is known.

In our view, a more useful organization of information for the clinician is based on clinical and epidemiological information available at the time of presentation of the patient. This includes disease tempo, whether an acute, subacute, or chronic process; epidemiologic data, whether the case is sporadic or potentially epidemic in nature; and the temporal profile, whether an infectious process or a parainfectious immune-mediated encephalomyelitis. The structure of the book derives from those types of clinical data; that is, sections are devoted to encephalitides which are acute sporadic, acute epidemic, parainfectious immune mediated, and subacute or chronic. Within each type of encephalitis, further clinical and epidemiologic data help narrow the spectrum of viral agents to focus the laboratory evaluation and select therapeutic intervention.

The reader will find that the discussions in this book are rooted in neuropathological descriptions and pathogenesis concepts. This is no mere academic exercise. Rather, it reflects our strongly held belief that an understanding of pathogenesis facilitates the diagnostic process as well as being central to therapeutic intervention. For example, the direct lytic infection of herpes simplex encephalitis demands prompt antiviral therapy, the perivenous demyelination in parainfectious encephalomyelitis suggests immune-based interventions, and the brain stem localization of several infections such as West Nile virus raises the potential need for rapid intervention with assisted respiration. Continued investigation into the pathogenesis of the AIDS dementia complex is necessary if we are to prevent or reverse this illness.

Since the publication of our first book, *Viral Encephalitis: Pathology, Diagnosis and Management*, in 1986, the world has experienced a dramatic spread of some then-recognized forms of encephalitis such as those associated with AIDS, West Nile virus infection, enterovirus-71, and Japanese encephalitis. New forms of viral encephalitis have appeared such as that due to Nipah virus. The threat of the use of smallpox virus as a weapon raises the specter of neurological complications of both the disease itself and its vaccination. These changes constitute major challenges to the medical community. In addition, rapid advances in molecular virology, imaging technology, and molecular pharmacology have resulted in an abundance of new data on the various types of encephalitis. These scientific and technological advances, coupled with the changes in the global viral disease spectrum, have prompted the publication of a new book, considerably larger and considerably more heavily referenced than our first book on the topic. We trust that the reader will perceive the collaborative style of this volume, as perspectives from pathology and clinical neurology have reciprocally informed its production.

As with our first book on viral encephalitis, the preparation of this new volume has benefited from the enormous patience and support of J.B.'s family, and it is to them, Mary Ann, Christine, and Dave, that he dedicates this volume.

Acknowledgments

Critical evaluation of the manuscript has been crucial for this book. Those who have reviewed chapters include Seth Love, Marie Landry, Dave Ferguson, Frank Bia, Don Mayo, Rick Tenser, Alex Tselis, Burk Jubelt, Nick Karabatsos, Christina Marra, Bruce Cohen, Bob McKendall, and Jung Kim. Each has improved our efforts, and we thank them. Deficiencies which remain are, of course, our responsibility.

Conversations with others, casual or focused, have served to modify important points. Alex Tselis has discussed numerous topics. At a greater remove but fundamentally important are those students, teachers, and colleagues who have helped shape our understanding. Special recognition should go to the relatives of those who have died who have agreed to autopsies that have provided knowledge about the pathology of encephalitis.

M.M.E. is grateful to Joanna Wilkenson for help in preparing the manuscript. It has been a great pleasure to once again work with Deborah Beauvais in preparing the manuscript, and we owe much to her consistency and ability. M.M.E. would like to acknowledge the help from the Medical Informatics Department of the Medical Sciences Division of Oxford University. J.B. is grateful to Gordon Sze for advice and consultation with respect to figures for MRI. He is grateful, too, to Geri Mancini of the Yale Radiology Digital Service.

Appreciation should be extended to the Encephalitis Support Group in the United Kingdom and to Elaine Dowell, the National Coordinator of that group, who expressed concern to M.M.E. that the first book had become outdated and suggested that an updated book would be useful.

Finally, it is a pleasure to acknowledge the support and understanding of our editors at ASM Press, Greg Payne and Eleanor Tupper. Collectively, they gracefully negotiated our delays, strongly supported the transatlantic interdisciplinary nature of the undertaking, and improved the organization of the book.

INTRODUCTION

1

Pathological Features of Encephalitis in Humans

This chapter aims to provide an overview of the pathology of human encephalitis. We describe procedures that are of value in examining central nervous system (CNS) tissues from cases of suspected encephalitis, and histopathological features common to most forms of viral encephalitis. We also discuss factors that confer specificity in the case of particular viral infections of the CNS, such as selectivity with regard to a host cell type that a virus may show, the character of the immune response, and the tempo of the disease.

SOURCES OF INFORMATION ON THE PATHOLOGY OF ENCEPHALITIS

Knowledge about the pathology of encephalitis is based primarily on the study of human biopsy and autopsy material. Understanding of the pathological processes involved has also been immensely extended by experimental studies in animals. These studies have been of two main types: viruses that cause human disease have been administered to animals that are not their natural hosts, and naturally occurring viral diseases of animals have been studied in a search for parallels to human disease. The association of a virus with its natural host species is generally a very close and specific one, and it is therefore only with caution that findings in animals can be applied to humans. However, these studies furnish almost the only evidence that can be obtained on the events that occur during the incubation period of a disease, that interval between the time of entry of a virus into its host and the onset of clinical disease. Furthermore, by manipulating the genetic makeup of animals or of the infecting virus, a vast amount has been learned recently about virulence factors in viruses and the role of host genes, e.g., those coding for cytokines in protection from, or exacerbation of, damage in viral encephalitis. While these insights have as yet resulted in little knowledge that is directly applicable to human disease, there is little doubt that they will do so in time. Cell culture is another technique of major importance to the understanding of viral encephalitis. Most of the pathological descriptions in this book will be based on examination of human material, but animal studies will be referred to when these offer particular illumination that is relevant to the pathogenesis of human diseases. This chapter gives an overview of the pathology of human encephalitis. More detailed pathology of individual human diseases will be given in the appropriate succeeding chapters.

Many of the observations relating to the pathology of human encephalitis are based on examination of the brain at autopsy. Inflammatory changes in the brain were described in isolated reports during the 19th century. However, it was with the abrupt appearance during World War I of the epidemic of encephalitis lethargica, with its high mortality rate, that the first detailed pathology of series of cases was described.

It is important to realize that the evidence provided by autopsy examination is limited. First, in any individual case, the disease process can be studied at only one time. Serial observations, such as those made available by sequential biopsy techniques, are not obtainable in this disease. To some extent, this drawback can be overcome by studying large numbers of cases in which death has occurred at differing stages of the disease. However, evidence of the earliest pathological changes is hard to come by, for patients do not die until the pathology is relatively advanced. Information from magnetic resonance imaging (MRI) and computerized tomography (CT) scanning is providing useful supplementary evidence about the earlier stages of encephalitis. Second,

autopsy material provides information only about the most severe forms of diseases that are not uniformly fatal. This includes most forms of encephalitis, for it is only with rabies virus infection that the mortality rate approaches 100%. Milder forms of encephalitis, from which recovery with or without residual morbidity generally occurs, rarely become available for pathological study.

Examination of biopsy specimens affords valuable information, particularly on ultrastructural aspects of a disease, because the material is better preserved and more free from unwanted artifacts when it is immediately immersed in fixative than when it is removed after the inevitable delays that attend autopsy examination. Biopsy samples suffer, however, from the disadvantage that they are very small and may not have been taken from the part of the brain most likely to yield the greatest information on the pathological changes present. Every effort must be made to extract as much information as possible from a biopsy sample. This will generally

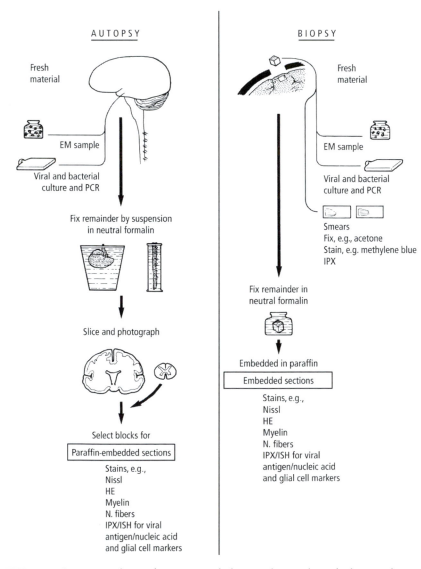

FIGURE 1.1 Summary chart of recommended procedures when dealing with autopsy or biopsy specimens from a case of suspected encephalitis. IPX, immunoperoxidase; ISH, in situ hybridization; EM, electron microscopy; HE, hematoxylin and eosin.

involve dividing it to provide samples for routine fixation for light microscopy, electron microscopy, viral and bacterial culture, and PCR techniques for detection of pathogens. These techniques are briefly described in Fig. 1.1.

NAKED-EYE EXAMINATION OF THE BRAIN AND ROUTINE LIGHT MICROSCOPY

Naked-eye examination and light microscopy are the classical techniques of pathological examination that formed the basis of the early studies of encephalitis. Although they are so routine and well established, they are not always carried out to best advantage. Autopsy examination of some forms of encephalitis, including hazard group 4 (CDC/NIH Biosafety Level 4) biological agents, is not permitted in a hospital or public mortuary in most countries. These include tick-borne encephalitides, Venezuelan equine encephalomyelitis, simian virus B, monkey pox virus, and mopeia virus infections (COSHH, 1999; Advisory Committee on Dangerous Pathogens website [http://www.doh.gov.uk/acdp]; Centers for Disease Control and Prevention, 1999). Human immunodeficiency virus (HIV) infection, rabies, and prion diseases are classified in the United Kingdom in hazard group 3, and autopsies on such cases can be undertaken if published recommendations are followed (Advisory Committee on Dangerous Pathogens, 1998, 1995a, 1995b, 1994; Centers for Disease Control and Prevention, 2002; Ironside and Bell, 1996).

Satisfactory naked-eye examination of the brain requires that the brain be removed from the skull with care to ensure that no artifactual tears are produced. These are easily caused when the brain is swollen or softened, particularly in the upper brain stem, if the cerebral hemispheres are not adequately supported while the brain stem and cerebellum are extracted from the posterior fossa. If insufficient cerebrospinal fluid (CSF) was obtained during life for all necessary investigations, a further sample can be taken at the time of autopsy, along with an additional sample of serum to allow corrections to be made for possible blood contamination of the CSF. CSF can be conveniently obtained with a plastic pipette from the prepontine cistern before removal of the brain. Similarly, a throat swab and sample of large bowel contents should be taken if adequate specimens were not taken during life for viral culture. If possible, the spinal cord and at least a few dorsal root ganglia should be removed together with the brain.

After the brain is removed with full aseptic precautions, it should be placed in a dish and weighed, and its external surface should be carefully examined. Small specimens for viral culture and PCR and, in some instances, electron microscopy should be taken from selected regions that appear inflamed, congested, or slightly softened. Such specimens are likely to be more rewarding than those from frankly necrotic, liquefied areas of the brain. If there is no naked-eye abnormality, as is frequently the case, these fresh samples for special study are best taken from the part of the brain that might be expected from the clinical history and examination, or from MRI and CT scan appearances, to be the most involved. Thus, if a hemiparesis and/or focal epilepsy was clinically apparent, specimens should be taken from the appropriate cerebral hemisphere; if brain stem signs were present,

and were not considered to be simply a reflection of brain swelling and herniation, regions of the brain stem should be sampled; and so on. Direct consultation with the clinician concerned can make all the difference between success and failure in carrying out these investigations, and as the techniques involved are time-consuming and expensive, time and effort spent in the judicious selection of specimens is well worthwhile.

After the necessary fresh samples have been taken, the brain should be suspended in a large container of fixative and left for at least 3 weeks before being sectioned (Fig. 1.1).

After fixation, the brain stem is separated from the cerebral hemispheres, the cerebrum is sectioned at 1-cm intervals either in the coronal or horizontal plane, and the sections are scrutinized for macroscopic pathology. The brain stem and cerebellum are sliced at smaller intervals. In many instances, there are no specific changes to be seen on naked-eye inspection. The brain may show a variable amount of edema, with narrowing of the lateral and third ventricles, and flattening of cortical gyri. Congestion frequently occurs, and sometimes petechial hemorrhages are present. Meninges are usually only mildly opaque in the acute stages of encephalitis but may be toughened and thickened over areas of chronic damage. More severe swelling and softening will be apparent, particularly in the temporal lobes in acute encephalitis caused by herpes simplex virus (see chapter 4).

Photography can be conveniently carried out before and after slicing the brain. Blocks for light microscopic examination are then selected and should be taken from relatively normal as well as abnormal areas, because microscopic changes are frequently found in areas that appear normal to naked-eye examination and may present an earlier stage of the disease process.

Blocks for light microscopy should be taken for embedding in paraffin wax, and a variety of staining techniques should be employed. Those that are particularly helpful are Nissl (a good cell stain), stains for myelin and nerve fibers, and immunostaining for glial cells. Glial cell immunostaining involves, for example, using well-established antibodies to CD68 for microglia and macrophages; glial fibrillary acidic protein (GFAP) for astrocytes; leukocyte common antigen, CD3, -4, and -8, and B-cell antigens for lymphocytes; and immunoglobulins for plasma cells (Fig. 1.2 and 1.3). An

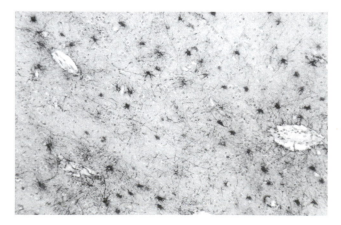

FIGURE 1.2 Astrocytic reaction in white matter demonstrated by GFAP immunostaining in a case of HIV encephalitis.

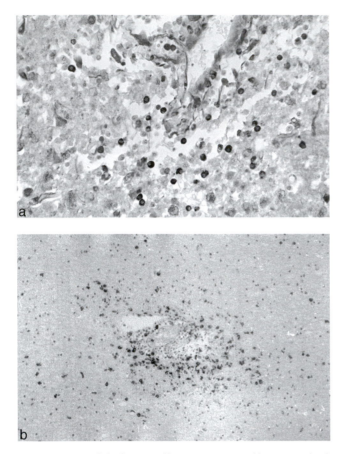

FIGURE 1.3 (a) Plasma cells immunostained by an antibody to immunoglobulin G in a case of herpes simplex encephalitis. (b) Macrophages immunostained by an antibody to CD68 surrounding a small vein in acute hemorrhage leukoencephalitis.

antibody to carbonic anhydrase isoenzyme II detects reactive oligodendrocytes (Morris et al., 1994). Antibody to β-amyloid precursor protein is useful for detecting recently damaged axons (Sherriff et al., 1994). Paraffin sections can be used to search for viral antigens using the immunoperoxidase technique with any recommended pretreatments, such as autoclaving, and for viral RNA or DNA by using in situ hybridization (see below).

In cases of suspected Creutzfeldt-Jakob disease (CJD), embedded material is used for light microscopy with preembedding exposure of the fixed tissue to formic acid (see chapter 15). This procedure substantially reduces infectivity of prions. The recommendations of the Advisory Committee on Dangerous Pathogens (1998) (Ironside and Bell, 1996) from the United Kingdom and of the Centers for Disease Control and Prevention and the Department of Health and Human Services in the United States (Centers for Disease Control and Prevention, 2002) should be followed in dealing with material from such cases. Dissecting instruments should either be disposed of by incineration, if disposable, or be sterilized in a 10% hypochlorite solution or 1 N NaOH. Dissecting surfaces should be exposed for 2 h to the same solution. Gloves should be worn and care should be taken to avoid cuts with a microtome knife. Thus, an

experienced technician should perform the section cutting. The knife itself, if not disposable, should be chemically sterilized and autoclaved after use (single cycle at 134°C [207 KPa, 30 lb/in^2] for 18 min). It is reassuring to note that no excess risk of developing CJD relates to laboratory technical or mortuary work, nor to pathologists, even though special precautions have been taken for only about the last 25 years (Brown et al., 1982).

The preparation of smears may be useful, particularly in the evaluation of biopsy material, when a rapid diagnosis is required. A small fragment of the biopsy is smeared thinly on a clean glass slide, air dried, fixed, and stained with methylene blue or a similar stain or with the immunoperoxidase technique. Sections stained with methylene blue take only a few minutes to prepare, and the immunoperoxidase technique using an antibody to herpes simplex virus takes less than one-half hour. A positive result provides rapid confirmation of the diagnosis; a negative result does not exclude the diagnosis because of the possibility of sampling error, and it is necessary to await viral culture and other investigations before a definitive answer can be obtained.

IMMUNOCYTOCHEMISTRY

A variety of techniques is available to search in histological material for specific viral antigens. Immunofluorescence was the first of these to be developed and has been in routine use for many years. This was followed by the development of immunocytochemical techniques, which have considerably extended the scope of these investigations. These techniques rely, like immunofluorescence, on the use of highly specific antisera that bind to the antigens being sought in the tissue section or smear. The sites of antibody binding are detected by means of a histochemical reaction, usually the reaction of peroxidase with diaminobenzidine, instead of a fluorescent marker. The techniques have several advantages over immunofluorescence (Sternberger, 1979): they are more sensitive and can therefore detect smaller quantities of antigen; they circumvent the problem of autofluorescence; they do not require the use of a fluorescence microscope; and the preparations do not fade rapidly. The techniques can be used for electron microscopy, and, best of all, as a result of the enhanced sensitivity, most viral antigens can be detected after formalin fixation, presumably because a sufficient number of unaltered antigenic sites remain. Microwave or autoclave pretreatment of sections often enhances antigenicity (Brown, 1998). The following viruses have all been detected using the immunoperoxidase technique on routinely processed formalin-fixed, paraffin-embedded material, sometimes years after processing (Fig. 1.4): herpes simplex virus (Benjamin and Ray, 1975; Budka and Popow-Kraupp, 1981; Esiri, 1982; Kumanishi and Hirano, 1978; Lohler, 1982), varicella-zoster virus (Horten et al., 1981), Epstein-Barr virus (Hummel et al., 1995), rabies virus (Atenasiu, 1973; Budka and Popow-Kraupp, 1981 Mrak and Young, 1994), human T-cell leukemia virus type 1 (Moore et al., 1989), HIV (Kure et al., 1990), measles virus (Budka et al., 1982; Esiri et al., 1982; Kumanishi and Seichii, 1979), papovavirus (Itoyama et al., 1982), cytomegalovirus (Lohler, 1982), influenza A virus (Lohler, 1982; Reinacher et al., 1983), and

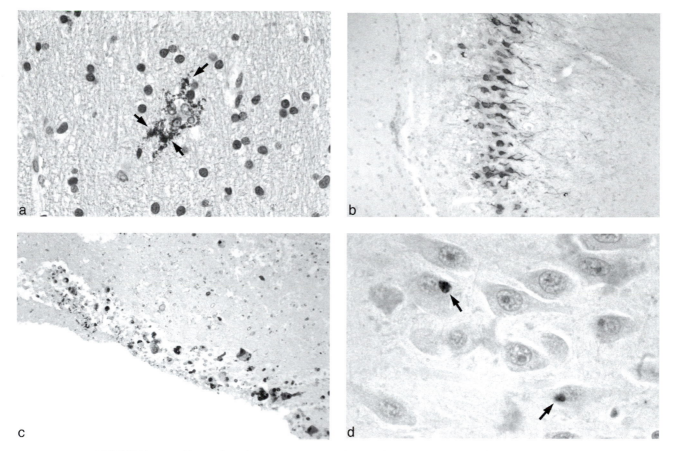

FIGURE 1.4 Examples of immunostaining for viral antigens in formalin-fixed paraffin-embedded tissue. (a) HIV in the processes of a multinucleated macrophage in HIV encephalitis (arrows). (b) Herpes simplex virus in the hippocampus in herpes simplex encephalitis. (c) Cytomegalovirus in ependymal and subependymal cells in a case of necrotizing ventriculo-encephalitis with AIDS. (d) Rabies virus in negri bodies of hippocampal neurons (arrows). (Courtesy of G. Gosztonyi.)

enterovirus 71 (Wong et al., 1999). Protease-resistant prion protein can also be detected in this way in cases of suspected CJD (Bell et al., 1997). Such a procedure is clearly a safer as well as a more convenient means of searching for viral antigens, and the tissue architecture is better preserved than in cryostat sections.

PCR

PCR is a technique that has contributed greatly over the last few years to the diagnosis of viral encephalitis, particularly when applied to CSF. It has, for example, largely replaced brain biopsy for the diagnosis of herpes simplex encephalitis. The technique relies on the in vitro synthesis of millions of copies of a specific nucleic acid sequence possibly derived from only a few original copies of that sequence in the starting material (DeBiasi and Tyler, 1999). It makes use of a heat-stable DNA-synthesizing enzyme, DNA polymerase, to synthesize DNA fragments on oligonucleotide primers specifically designed to bind to complementary nucleic acids in homogenized brain tissue as well as CSF. The main caveats to its use are that because of its extreme sensitivity,

precautions must be observed to avoid false positives from contamination and that genuine positive results must be interpreted with caution because PCR can detect latent or low-grade persistent infection as well as active disease (Kleinschmidt-DeMasters et al., 2001).

IN SITU HYBRIDIZATION

The technique of in situ hybridization uses a labeled probe complementary to a nucleic acid sequence that is specific for a virus-coded gene to detect the presence of the virus in a tissue section (Gosztonyi and Terborg, 1992). It is thus somewhat analogous to immunocytochemistry in which labeled antibody can be used to detect viral protein in a tissue section. In situ hybridization may be used to detect, in particular, viruses for which sensitive antibody reagents are not readily available, e.g., JC virus (Fig. 1.5) and measles virus. The sensitivity of in situ hybridization can be extended by employing rounds of PCR to amplify the nucleic acid signal, but this carries a significantly added risk of nonspecific reactions and artifacts (Long et al., 1993; Walker et al., 1995).

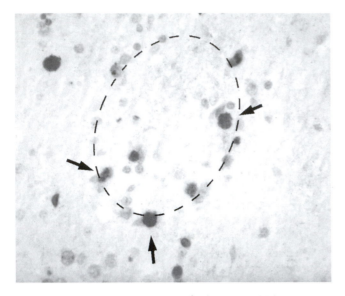

FIGURE 1.5 Demonstration of JC virus DNA using in situ hybridization in a case of progressive multifocal leukoencephalopathy. The positively reacting nuclei (arrows) mainly surround a small focus of demyelination indicated by the dashed line.

ELECTRON MICROSCOPY

Thin-section transmission microscopy is the form of electron microscopy most commonly used to examine biopsy and autopsy samples from cases of encephalitis. The visualization of viruslike particles using this technique was instrumental in initially demonstrating the viral nature of two diseases, subacute sclerosing panencephalitis and progressive multifocal leukoencephalopathy (Bouteille et al., 1965; Zu Rhein and Chou, 1965).

The chief value of electron microscopy lies in the demonstration of distinctive virus structure, as in encephalitis due to herpes simplex virus, rabies virus, or adenovirus. Virions can be detected in autopsy as well as biopsy samples because their structure is not significantly degraded after death of the patient. However, because of the very small size of the samples that can be examined in this way, it is a relatively insensitive technique for demonstrating the presence of virus. This problem can to some extent be overcome, either by selecting for ultrastructural examination only those blocks that can be shown, using the immunoperoxidase technique at the light microscope level on $1\text{-}\mu$m sections, to contain viral antigen, or by using the negative staining technique. In this technique, a homogenate is made of the fresh or frozen tissue to be sampled; this is then centrifuged at intermediate speed and the supernatant is examined for viral particles after negative staining (Dayan and Almeida, 1975). The technique is more likely than thin-section electron microscopy to detect viral particles if there are only small numbers present in the tissue, particularly if antibody to the suspected virus is added to the brain suspension. The virus is clumped by the antibody and becomes easier to spot. Even if these maneuvers are employed, the technique of negative staining remains relatively insensitive, and the procedure necessitates the loss of all tissue structure, so that no information

is obtained on the type of cell harboring the virus. On the other hand, valuable information can be obtained on the substructure of the virus particles. This can be of great value in characterizing the virus and in distinguishing those particles that are truly viruses from those components of brain ultrastructure that superficially resemble viruses and that have sometimes been mistakenly assumed in transmission electron micrographs to be viruses.

PATHOLOGICAL FEATURES COMMON TO MOST FORMS OF VIRAL ENCEPHALITIS

Although the types of virus that may produce encephalitis are diverse, there is considerable uniformity in the pathology they produce, at least in the mature nervous system of an immunocompetent host. In many cases, this will enable a shrewd guess as to the nature of the illness, even in the absence of supportive clinical or virological evidence. There are some well-known diseases, including encephalitis lethargica (see chapter 10), in which no viral agent has been identified, but in which such an etiology is suspected on pathological grounds. Those features common to many forms of viral encephalitis are described below, followed by an account of some of the features that are restricted to specific viral infections.

Cell Death

Virus infection of brain cells, as of cells elsewhere in the body, is followed by alterations in the cells' metabolism which, in lytic infections, lead to the death of the host cells. Cell lysis affords an opportunity for new virus particles to be released to infect other cells. Simultaneously, a general inflammatory response, with the development of edema, and an immune response both evolve. The extent, rate, and selectivity of cell death vary considerably, but it is always evident. Degenerate features that are recognizable microscopically are swelling and cloudiness, or shrinkage with eosinophilia of neuronal cytoplasm and pyknosis of nuclei. This is followed by loss of staining properties of the cell, giving it a faint "ghost" appearance. At this stage, a macrophage reaction is frequently present, with a small cluster of microglial cells and a few lymphocytes surrounding the remnant of the neuron. Microglial cells are distinguishable in routinely stained sections by the presence of their elongated, or comma-shaped, slightly irregular nuclei.

The whole configuration of dead neuron and surrounding cells is termed "neuronophagia" (Fig. 1.6). In an acute lytic process, many such figures will be seen, for example, in the anterior horns of the spinal cord in acute poliomyelitis. In a more slowly evolving disease, they will only occasionally be seen, for example, in the late stages of subacute sclerosing panencephalitis. The microglial cells, sometimes admixed with a few astrocytes and lymphocytes, remain at the site after the neuron remnant has disappeared. These foci of reactive cells are termed glial stars, nodules, clusters, or knots. Animal studies indicate that it takes no more than a few days for a dead cell to disappear under these conditions, but some residual glial cells remain for months or years. Glial cells and neurons undergo cell lysis in some virus infections,

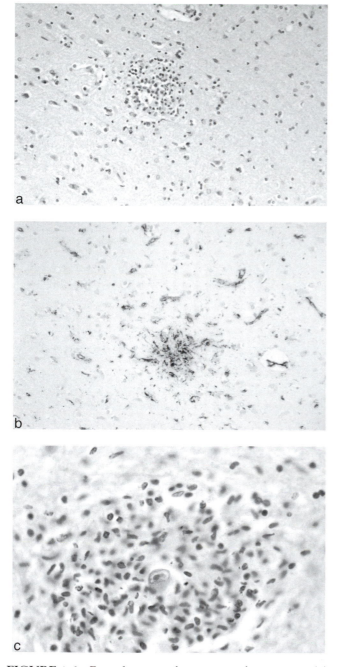

FIGURE 1.6 Foci of neuronophagia seen at low power in (a) and (b) and at higher power in (c). In (c), there is a central degenerate neuron in the dentate nucleus of the cerebellum. The neuron contains an intranuclear inclusion body suggestive of cytomegalovirus infection. Sample was collected from a patient with encephalitis with microglial nodules following renal transplantation. Panels (a) and (c) hematoxylin and eosin stain; (b) immunostain for macrophages using *Ricinus communis* agglutinin.

but the process is less conspicuous in glial cells than in neurons. Although in some cases of encephalitis cell death occurs on a relatively small scale and is appreciable only on microscopic examination, in other cases the damage to cells can be massive and lead to areas of necrosis that are easily

visible to the naked eye. This is especially the case in herpes simplex encephalitis, in which the extent of the necrosis of the temporal lobes resembles infarction. In this instance, the bilateral distribution of the lesions and the fact that the areas of necrosis do not coincide with arterial territories should alert the pathologist to the encephalitic nature of the lesions.

In contrast to viral killing of cells by lysis, or necrosis, in which cell membranes are rendered permeable and rupture with release of cytoplasmic contents, viruses may kill cells via apoptosis, a form of programmed cell death involving host cell mechanisms. In apoptotic cell death, the plasma membrane integrity is preserved until relatively late in the process, when blebs appear. Meanwhile, the nuclear chromatin condenses and is cleaved by endonucleases. This process is a common mechanism of cell death in nervous system development, probably in some neurodegenerative diseases and in some virus infections. It does not usually produce much inflammation. Apoptosis can be inferred in tissue sections from the detection of the enzymes involved, including caspases, proapoptotic members of the Bcl-2 family of molecules, products of cleavage of DNA repair enzymes such as poly(ADP-ribose) polymerase (PARP), and detection of endonuclease-cleaved chromosomal DNA using the terminal deoxynucleotidyltransferase-mediated dUTP-biotin nick end labeling method (Duriez and Shah, 1997; Simbulan-Rosenthal et al., 1998).

Experimental studies of apoptosis in viral encephalitis suggest that many viruses can trigger apoptotic mechanisms in host cells through a variety of pathways, some of which impair the normal protective action of the protein Bcl-2 (Griffin and Hardwick, 1997; Levine et al., 1993). Other mechanisms include direct action of a viral protein, e.g., E1A protein of adenovirus (Rao et al., 1992), or upregulation of the proapoptotic Fas ligand that interacts with Fas (CD95), a member of the tumor necrosis factor (TNF) receptor family. The latter is a mechanism possibly employed by HIV (Westendorp et al., 1995). Greater susceptibility of immature neurons to apoptosis may contribute to the more devastating effect on the young seen in some forms of CNS infection (Lewis et al., 1996).

Whether apoptosis is in the interest of the virus or the host is debatable and relates to a number of variables such as the productivity of the virus, the life span of infected cells, and the density of connections between cells (Krakauer, 2000). In general, apoptosis is viewed as favorable to the host ("altruistic cell suicide"), and it is of interest that many viruses have also evolved antiapoptotic strategies. However, in the case of postmitotic neurons, any advantage that apoptosis has for ridding the host of the virus must be weighed against the loss of irreplaceable neurons (Allsopp and Fazakerley, 2000).

Cell Alterations

Many viruses inflict sufficiently severe damage to cause death of the host cell. Some also seem capable of producing other structural alterations in the cell that do not necessarily result directly in cell death. One example of such a change is the development of neurofibrillary tangles—abnormal cytoplasmic aggregates of paired helical filaments. These

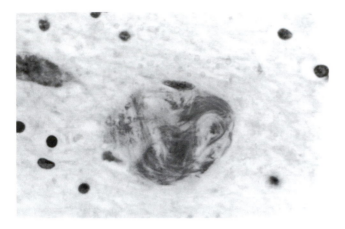

FIGURE 1.7 Neurofibrillary tangle in a substantia nigra neuron from a case of postencephalitic parkinsonism. Congo red stain.

have been described in cortical neurons in long-standing cases of subacute sclerosing panencephalitis (Gutewa and Osetowska, 1961; Mandybur et al., 1977; Paula-Barbosa et al., 1979) and herpes simplex encephalitis and in the pigmented cells of the substantia nigra in postencephalitic parkinsonism (Hallervorden, 1935) (Fig. 1.7). The bizarre astrocytes seen in the brain in progressive multifocal leukoencephalopathy (Fig. 1.8) (see chapter 10) may also be considered to be in this category. In some instances, there are no detectable structural changes, but functions such as maintenance of synaptic plasticity and cognitive function are impaired (de la Torre et al., 1996).

Inflammation

Within a few days, an inflammatory reaction develops at the site of infection, reflecting an immune reaction to foreign antigens. The tissue becomes edematous, producing a spongy appearance, and inflammatory cells accumulate in and around the walls of venules. As with inflammation elsewhere, there is in acute infection an initial outpouring of

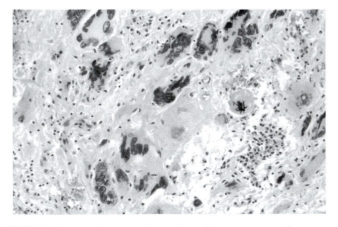

FIGURE 1.8 Bizarre multinucleated astrocytes in the cerebellum of a young man with progressive multifocal leukoencephalopathy complicating a severe congenital immunodeficiency syndrome. Hematoxylin and eosin stain.

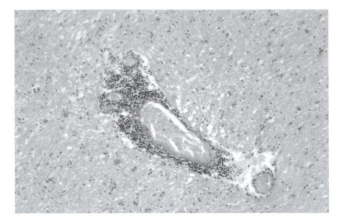

FIGURE 1.9 Typical perivascular cuffs of mononuclear inflammatory cells surrounding a small vein in a case of brain stem encephalitis resembling encephalitis lethargica.

neutrophil polymorphs, but after a day or two, these are largely replaced by mononuclear cells, macrophages, lymphocytes, and increasingly after the first week, plasma cells.

In the second and third weeks of an acute infection, the "cuffs" of inflammatory cells in the perivascular spaces are several cells thick and mitotic figures may be seen among them (Fig. 1.9). Macrophages migrate from these cuffs into the surrounding parenchyma, where they may supplement locally activated microglial cells, enlarge, develop elongated processes and swollen cytoplasm, and show enhanced lysosomal activity (Fig. 1.3b). Many engulf degenerate products of myelin so that they stain positively for myelin and later for neutral fat. Although B lymphocytes remain within perivascular spaces, T lymphocytes and plasma cells extend from perivascular spaces into surrounding parenchyma (Fig. 1.3 and 1.10). The lymphocytes and plasma cells, like the macrophages, persist in large numbers for several weeks after the disappearance of detectable virus, and more scanty lymphocytic cuffing, occupying relatively expanded perivascular spaces, may be seen months or even years after the acute infection has subsided. Inflammatory cells, particularly macrophages, accompany any destructive process in the CNS.

The relative preponderance of lymphocytes and plasma cells in the inflammatory infiltrate is characteristic of encephalitis, reflecting the presence of an immune response to foreign antigens. However, relatively few of the inflammatory cells are likely to be T cells specifically directed against viral antigens; the majority of infiltrating cells in inflammatory CNS disease are nonspecific in nature (Ransohoff, 1999). A similar inflammatory reaction will also be seen at the edge of an abscess or in some protozoal infections of the brain, and this may give rise to diagnostic difficulty, particularly in the interpretation of biopsies.

Role of Cytokines and Chemokines

The signal for entry of inflammatory cells into the relatively protected environment of the CNS is provided by release of chemokines, a family of chemoattractant cytokines that are relatively short-lived in their actions, operate over short distances, and mediate their effects via G-protein-coupled

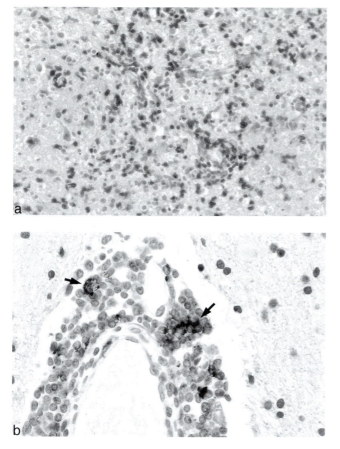

FIGURE 1.10 (a) CD68⁺ cells extending into parenchyma from small veins in a case of brain stem encephalitis. In contrast, (b) immunostained B cells (arrows) remain in perivascular spaces. Both panels counterstained with hematoxylin.

receptors (Adams and Lloyd, 1997; Lawson, 1995; Williams and Hickey, 1996). Both cytokines and chemokines exert their effects by binding to receptors. Chemokines are divided into two main subclasses, the α and β chemokines. Broadly speaking, the α chemokines attract neutrophils and the β chemokines attract monocytes.

The resident microglia of the CNS are the first cells to respond to invasion of a foreign antigen by upregulating expression of major histocompatibility complex (MHC) class II antigens on their surface and releasing proinflammatory chemokines and cytokines such as interleukin-1 and tumor necrosis factor alpha (TNF-α). This response of local microglia represents a relatively primitive response that lacks the specificity contributed by antigen-specific T cells that later enter from the blood. Nevertheless, it can constitute the predominant response, as demonstrated in an animal model of cytomegalovirus encephalitis (Booss et al., 1989).

Microglial cells also react to neuronal damage by upregulating MHC class II antigens (Neumann, 2001). The chemokines and other cytokines released help to lower the blood-brain barrier to entry of white blood cells and high-molecular-weight proteins such as immunoglobulins and complement. Matrix metalloproteinase enzymes, some of which are constitutively produced by CNS cells as

proenzymes and others of which are produced under the influence of cytokines and tissue injury, play a major role in facilitating opening of the blood-brain barrier (Rosenberg, 1999). Other processes also needed to transfer cells from blood to brain include alterations in leukocyte and endothelial cell surface molecules favoring adhesion of leukocytes. These involve selectins, integrins, and members of the immunoglobulin superfamily of molecules expressed on endothelial cells. Target cell-specific chemoattractant molecules, the majority of them chemokines, play critical roles in controlling leukocyte migration (Springer, 1994; von Andrian and Mackay, 2000). In some cases, viruses themselves have genes coding for chemokine-like molecules or their receptors and can thus influence host responses to their presence (Mathur et al., 1992). On the other hand, some chemokines can effectively inhibit viral infection of normally permissive cells. This has been shown for chemokines that use the receptor CCR5 and HIV infection (see chapter 12).

Glial Reaction

Along with development of inflammation, an astrocytic reaction is seen at the site of virus-induced damage, and this occurs more diffusely in edematous areas. This is a nonspecific reaction that occurs whenever degeneration takes place in the CNS, but its distribution in patches is particularly characteristic of encephalitis. Reactive astrocytic change is well visualized with immunostaining using an antibody to GFAP (Fig. 1.2). The cell body and nucleus enlarge, the nucleus adopts an eccentric position at the margin of the cell body, and the processes of the cell enlarge and extend. Sometimes binucleate forms are seen. Weeks and months later, dense glial fibrillary material is laid down in the processes and forms the basis of tough glial scarring that persists for years.

Inclusion Bodies

Many inclusion bodies that occur in neurons and glial cells have no known connection with viral infections, and viral infections of the brain are not always associated with the presence of inclusion bodies. Nevertheless, some forms of viral encephalitis are associated with the presence of inclusion bodies that are of some diagnostic value. For example, rabies infection is often accompanied by the development of cytoplasmic bodies called Lyssa and Negri bodies. These are most easily detected in hippocampal or cortical pyramidal neurons, Purkinje cells of the cerebellum, and other large neurons. They consist of hyaline eosinophilic bodies, one or several of which may be seen in the cytoplasm adjacent to the nucleus (Fig. 1.11a). In the early stages of herpes encephalitis, round or oval eosinophilic inclusion bodies, which are larger than a nucleolus and tend to be surrounded by a clear halo of nucleoplasm (Cowdry type A inclusion), may be seen in neuron and glial nuclei. Similar inclusion bodies are seen in neuron and oligodendrocyte nuclei in subacute sclerosing panencephalitis and immunosuppressive measles encephalitis (Fig. 1.11b). When present, these inclusion bodies often contain viral components, either nucleoprotein or other virus-coded material.

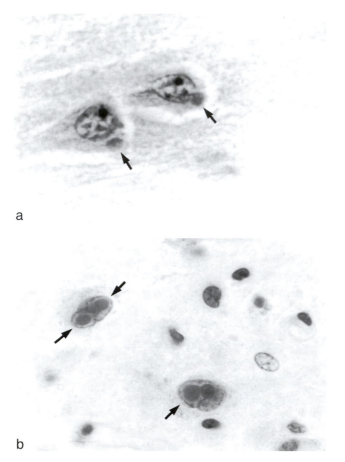

a

b

FIGURE 1.11   (a) Negri bodies (arrows) in the cytoplasm of cortical pyramidal neurons in rabies. (b) Cowdry type A inclusion bodies (arrows) in neuronal nuclei in a case of immunosuppressive measles encephalitis. Both panels, hematoxylin and eosin stain.

PATHOLOGICAL FEATURES RESTRICTED TO CERTAIN FORMS OF ENCEPHALITIS

There are four main features that can confer specificity on the pathology of particular forms of encephalitis: first, the mode of entry of a virus into the nervous system; second, the selectivity with respect to host cell type that a virus may display once it has reached the nervous system; third, the tempo of the disease process; and fourth, the relative contribution of the immune response to the overall pathology. The first two factors help to determine the topographical sites of damage, which provides an important distinguishing feature of some forms of encephalitis (Fig. 1.12).

Mode of Entry of Viruses into the Nervous System

The variety of viruses that may be pathogens in the brain is very great. Some of these viruses rarely infect humans, and when they do, their pathological effects are largely confined to the nervous system; an example is rabies virus. However, many of them are ubiquitous viruses encountered by the vast majority of the population. Yet encephalitis, at least in a recognizable clinical form, is uncommon. The reasons for its

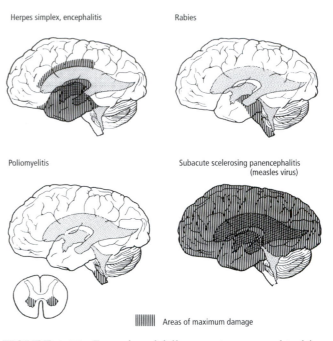

Herpes simplex, encephalitis   Rabies

Poliomyelitis   Subacute sclerosing panencephalitis (measles virus)

|||||||| Areas of maximum damage

FIGURE 1.12   Examples of differences in topographical location of damage found in different forms of viral encephalitis (ventricular system stippled).

development in only a tiny fraction of the population exposed to these viruses are poorly understood. Nevertheless, some of the factors responsible may be surmised from observations in humans and from experimental evidence in animals.

For direct virally inflicted damage to occur, a virus must first gain access to the nervous system. Historically, the first recognized route was passage along nerves, as proposed by Morgagni in 1769 in relation to rabies infection. He noted that paresthesiae at the site of the bite that afforded entry of the rabies agent preceded the development of more widespread neurological symptoms. This led him to suggest that the agent was carried along nerves. This was confirmed by experimental observations at the end of the 19th and beginning of the 20th centuries. Herpes B virus (*Herpesvirus simiae*) infection in humans is also associated with paresthesiae or clinical signs related to the segmental level of the bite that transmits the virus, suggesting neural spread of the virus to the nervous system. Herpes simplex virus may also reach the brain by traveling along nerves. Spread along olfactory nerves has been suspected in transmission of rabies in bat-infested caves. Poliomyelitis virus shows a clear ability in experimental infection to travel along nerves.

The rate of movement of viruses along nerves in experimental infections suggests that the mechanisms involved are fast retrograde and anterograde transport systems that operate normally in nerves (Grafstein and Forman, 1980). This has been shown for herpes simplex virus (Kristensson et al., 1974), poliovirus (Bodian and Howe, 1941; Jubelt et al., 1980), and rabies virus (Gosztonyi, 1979; Murphy et al., 1973). Drugs that influence the cytoskeleton, thought to be involved in these transport mechanisms, interfere with such viral transport in nerves.

Most other viruses reach the nervous system via the bloodstream. They reach the blood after initial replication at sites related to their points of entry into the body (e.g., gastrointestinal tract-related lymphoid tissue for enteroviruses, muscle and subcutaneous tissue for togaviruses). Many protective mechanisms operate to inactivate these viruses and prevent their spread to the CNS. Only when these mechanisms fail will the opportunity arise for CNS disease to develop. Phagocytic cells at the initial site of entry of the virus, and cells of the reticuloendothelial system, such as the Kupffer cells of the liver, may phagocytose and inactivate a virus before or after it reaches the bloodstream. Interferon is produced by cells infected at the entry site and limits susceptibility of neighboring cells to infection. Immune responses involving both cellular and humoral immunity are mounted at the time of entry of the virus into the body and help to prevent the virus from reaching the brain. Finally, the anatomical configuration of brain blood capillaries, with their tight junctions and close relationship to astrocytic end feet, comprises the blood-brain barrier and acts as a further deterrent along the route a virus must take from blood to brain.

Experimental studies have indicated different mechanisms of transport across the blood-brain barrier for different viruses. Some viruses appear capable of initially infecting endothelial cells in the brain (for example, poliomyelitis virus [Blinzinger et al., 1969] and Sindbis virus, one of the togavirus group [Johnson, 1965]). Others infect glia surrounding small vessels without any evidence of endothelial cell infection (for example, experimental arbovirus infection in mice [Murphy and Whitfield, 1970]). Some viruses appear to traverse the endothelium within infected leukocytes or in pinocytotic vesicles (Brightman, 1968; Liou and Hsu, 1998; Pathak and Webb, 1974; Summers et al., 1978). HIV is one of the viruses thought to enter the brain in infected leukocytes. The blood-CSF barrier differs from the blood-brain barrier in ways that may facilitate movement of viruses into the CSF, and this may well be the route taken by the viruses that cause aseptic meningitis. The capillaries here are more freely permeable, and fenestrations occur in the endothelium. Furthermore, the choroid plexus cells themselves may become infected with some viruses (e.g., mumps virus [Wolinsky et al., 1976]), thereby enhancing seeding of virus into the CSF.

Some viruses, particularly under conditions of infection by small infective doses, may use a combination of vascular and neural routes to reach the CNS. For example, intraperitoneal infection of hamsters with the arbovirus that causes St. Louis encephalitis resulted in a brief period of viremia, followed by a rising infectivity titer in the olfactory neuroepithelium and then in olfactory bulbs and brain. Virus particles were demonstrable in olfactory axons, and encephalitis was considered to result from centripetal spread of virus from infected olfactory epithelial cells to which virus had gained entry through lack of a blood-brain barrier (Monath et al., 1983). Similarly, intravenous inoculation of herpes simplex virus in mice resulted in infection of sensory ganglia, which also lack any barrier equivalent to the blood-brain barrier, and subsequent spread of virus to adjacent areas of the CNS (Anderson and Field, 1983). In the first of these two experimental models, direct spread of virus from blood to brain was considered unimportant, and in the second it was unproven.

The possibility of a similarly indirect route of entry to the CNS by viruses that show a viremic phase in human infection should not be dismissed. For example, some puzzling aspects of human infection with poliovirus, such as the tendency for paralysis to affect recently injected muscle, would be best explained by enhanced leakage of virus from blood to muscle at the site of minor trauma and subsequent neural spread from muscle to spinal cord (Wyatt, 1982).

It is clear that viruses causing encephalitis differ with respect to the sites at which they make their initial entry into the CNS. This in turn may be expected to influence the manner in which the disease presents and the topographic distribution of the lesions (Fig. 1.12). Viruses that enter the brain directly from the blood are widely disseminated from the start because there are multiple entry sites scattered throughout the brain. On the other hand, herpes simplex virus produces an anatomically discrete, though extensive, focus of damage centered on the temporal lobes and the limbic system, a distribution of damage that is probably determined by a neural route of entry into the brain. However, while topographical localization may be an important clue to the causative virus in a case of encephalitis, it is rarely absolutely specific by itself.

Selective Vulnerability of Cells of the CNS

Other considerations apply in determining the distribution and type of damage produced by viruses once they reach the brain. Of particular importance is the differing vulnerability of the diverse cell types present within the brain to infection by a particular virus (Johnson, 1980). This in turn probably depends mainly on whether or not the cell possesses surface receptors that enable the virus to be absorbed on the cell membrane and taken into the cell. For example, susceptibility of oligodendrocytes to lytic damage by the JC papovavirus that causes progressive multifocal leukoencephalopathy is responsible for the typical demyelinated foci that characterize this disease. HIV, the retrovirus that causes AIDS, enters cells through binding of its surface protein gp120 to the CD4 molecule expressed on T-helper lymphocytes and macrophages. This interaction requires a coreceptor from among the family of chemokine receptors (CXCR4 or CCR5). The main type of cell harboring HIV in the CNS is the macrophage (see chapter 12). Although not a virus, the agent of prion diseases also needs to gain entry to neurons via a surface receptor, probably the laminin receptor precursor (Gauczynski et al., 2001). It appears to travel from neuron to neuron across synapses, which presumably also entails receptor-mediated entry to the postsynaptic cell. Herpes simplex virus uses the low-density-lipoprotein receptor, in conjunction with heparan sulfate proteoglycan, as its receptor for entry into neurons. This receptor is also used to transfer lipoprotein into cells (Mahley and Rall, 2000). The receptor is present on all neurons, so its distribution cannot explain the anatomical specificity of herpes simplex encephalitis which, as seen above, is more likely related to the anatomical route by which the virus reaches the brain.

Tempo of the Disease Process

Another important determinant of the pathology is the tempo of the disease process. An acute infection with a highly lytic virus such as herpes simplex virus type 1 produces an acutely inflamed brain with prominent congestion, edema, focal hemorrhage, and severe inflammation. A more slowly evolving disease such as subacute sclerosing panencephalitis, caused by slower spreading and insidious but widespread infection by measles virus of neurons and oligodendroglia, produces gradual loss of both neurons and myelin and eventually a gliotic, atrophic, and chronically inflamed brain.

Role of the Immune Response

The appearance of the characteristic inflammatory infiltrate in encephalitis is dependent on the presence of an intact immune response. The relative contributions of cellular and humoral immunity, both in eliminating virus and in contributing to the damage produced, remain relatively ill-defined in human encephalitis. There is, however, little doubt of their importance. Activated macrophages in particular can bring a formidable array of toxic mechanisms to bear at the site of infection: secreted proteolytic enzymes, free radicals, cytokines, and eicosanoids. Macrophage products, in turn, can interact with astrocytes to inhibit their uptake of glutamate, thus promoting opportunities for glutamate to exert neuro- and gliotoxic effects.

Cytokines such as gamma interferon and TNF-α also enhance potentially toxic nitric oxide production by astrocytes (Chao et al., 1996; Lee et al., 1993). Secreted cytokines also have the potential to interfere with normal neurotropic functions, as has been shown by interaction of TNF-α and insulinlike growth factor 1 in cultures of cerebellar granule cells (Venters et al., 1999). Cytotoxic T cells are of particular importance in eliminating virus-infected cells. However, inflammatory cells have also recently been recognized to produce neurotropic substances, notably brain-derived neurotropic factor, which may exert local neuroprotective effects in inflammatory diseases (Kerschensteiner et al., 1999).

Vascular damage resembling that produced in a hypersensitivity reaction, probably related to the deposition of immune complexes, is sometimes a prominent feature of the pathology of herpes simplex type 1 encephalitis and of the more fulminating hemorrhagic forms of perivenous (parainfectious) encephalitis. This is associated with fibrinoid necrosis of small blood vessels, exudation of plasma proteins, and multiple small hemorrhages caused by leakage of red blood cells through damaged endothelium (Fig. 1.13). Fibrin thrombi may be present in these vessels (Haymaker et al., 1958). In the nonhemorrhagic form of perivenous encephalitis, there is intense perivascular cuffing with mononuclear inflammatory cells associated with immediately surrounding sleeves of demyelination (Fig. 1.14 and 1.15). Neurons are not damaged in this condition, and the cause of the disease is thought to be an immune-mediated attack directed towards myelin or oligodendrocytes (see chapter 7). Genetic factors are probably important in determining susceptibility to this type of attack (Lebon et al., 1986; Piyasirisilp et al., 1999) and also in modifying

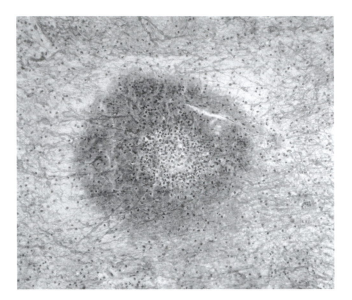

FIGURE 1.13   Acute hemorrhagic leukoencephalitis showing a small vein at the center surrounded by leukocytes. Beyond these, there is a zone of red blood cells and demyelinated white matter parenchyma. Luxol fast blue stain.

neurovirulence in experimental viral infections (Knobler et al., 1982; Johnson et al., 2000).

It is unclear whether defective cell-mediated immune responses to measles virus may play a supportive role in enabling measles virus to persist in the nervous system and cause subacute sclerosing panencephalitis. In contrast, very high levels of circulating antibody to some components of measles virus are found in this disease. The virtual absence of an effective immune response in some cases of progressive multifocal leukoencephalopathy dramatically modifies the pathology of this disease. Inflammation may be absent from the brain, and the viral nature of this disease was not confirmed until virus particles were detected by electron microscopy in the brain. Progressive multifocal leukoencephalopathy usually develops in patients with an

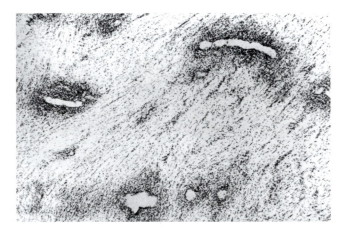

FIGURE 1.14   Cerebral white matter from a case of perivenous encephalitis. Venules are surrounded by an intense inflammatory cell infiltrate. Nissl stain.

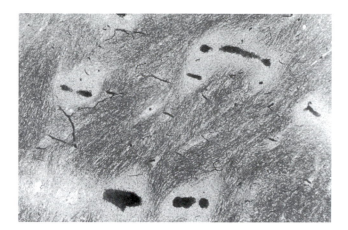

FIGURE 1.15 Adjacent section to that shown in Fig. 1.14, stained for myelin and showing perivenous myelin pallor. Weil's stain.

additional disease associated with immunosuppression, such as Hodgkin's disease or other lymphoma or sarcoidosis, but above all, AIDS (see chapter 12).

Another disease whose pathology is quite unlike the characteristic appearance of a viral encephalitis is CJD (see chapter 15). This disease is caused by a transmissible agent that consists of an abnormal structural configuration of a host-encoded protein, prion protein, which does not evoke an immune response. Hence, there is little or no inflammatory response in the brain.

The CNS, being remote from the immune system, provides a potential sheltered site in which viruses can survive unchecked, particularly if systemic immunity is depressed. This may afford an opportunity for viruses to cooperate in the production of disease. For example, human herpesvirus 6 has been found in brains of healthy subjects and in those of subjects with AIDS, but in particularly high concentration in lesions of progressive multifocal leukoencephalopathy and multiple sclerosis, raising the possibility that it may contribute to the pathogenesis of these diseases (Blumberg et al., 2000). Clinicians and pathologists need to be aware of the occurrence of atypical infections of the brain in which the expected pathological features are greatly modified or absent in patients with altered immune responses. Examples of such conditions are AIDS, progressive multifocal leukoencephalopathy, and immunosuppressive measles encephalitis, which has been most frequently described in children with leukemia (Breitfeld et al., 1973) (see chapter 13). This last differs pathologically from subacute sclerosing panencephalitis chiefly in the paucity of inflammation, the presence of multinucleate giant cells, probably derived from infected glial cells, and the absence of features associated with chronicity of infection.

Unequivocal evidence for the importance of intact immune responses in determining the nature of the histopathological lesions produced in viral encephalitis has emerged from studies in animals. By manipulating the immune apparatus—for example, by inducing immunosuppression with X-irradiation or administration of immunosuppressive drugs—typically inflammatory diseases, such as those produced by the togaviruses in rodents, are converted to noninflammatory degenerative or encephalopathic diseases (Grcevic and Vince, 1976; Webb and Hall, 1972; Zlotnik et al., 1970). Some viral infections (for example, that causing the severe inflammatory disease lymphocytic choriomeningitis in normal, adult, previously uninfected mice) are converted to ostensibly asymptomatic infections by elimination of the immune response to the virus. This is the case if infection is encountered in utero, as occurs in natural maternal infection, when fetuses are subsequently tolerant of the virus (Buchmeier et al., 1980; Berger et al., 2000).

In such model systems, there is now considerable interest in searching for more subtle influences that the presence of the virus may exert. For example, expression of molecules such as neurotransmitter receptors on the surface of cells may be modified (Glasgow, 1979) or synthesis of enzymes may be depressed (Oldstone et al., 1977); possible involvement of such mechanisms in human diseases of the CNS has hardly begun to be explored.

COMPLICATIONS AND SEQUELAE

Secondary changes frequently occur and confound the damage produced by the virus and the immune response in encephalitis. The most common of these is edema, which can cause potentially fatal herniations. These may involve the cingulate gyrus herniating beneath the falx, the unci herniating through the tentorial notch (see Fig. 4.1), or the cerebellar tonsils herniating through the foramen magnum (Fig. 1.16). Vascular events are also common and may be associated with such herniations as, for example, when blood flow in one or both posterior cerebral arteries is interrupted by an uncal hernia, resulting in posterior cerebral artery territory infarction. Generalized hypoxia is also commonly found, sometimes related to the development of epileptic seizures, respiratory depression, or bronchopneumonia. Small foci of rarefaction necrosis are a common late feature of arbovirus encephalitis and may be due to alterations in blood flow in small vessels, with or without edema. Sagittal sinus thrombosis with consequent cerebral venous infarction (Fig. 1.17) is another complication of encephalitis; it was a common complication of encephalitis lethargica (Buzzard and Greenfield, 1919).

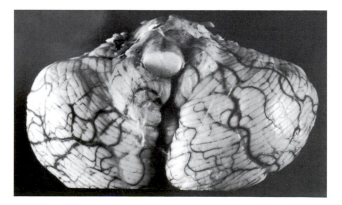

FIGURE 1.16 Cerebellar tonsillar herniation, particularly marked on the right side (left side in photograph).

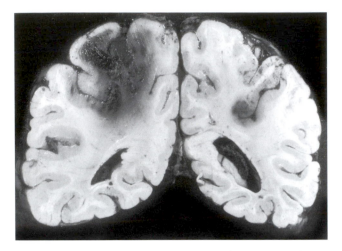

FIGURE 1.17   Venous infarction secondary to sagittal sinus thrombosis in a case of encephalitis of undiagnosed cause.

Late sequelae of encephalitis include the development of atrophy, which may be either focal or generalized, depending on the nature of the encephalitis. This will be evidenced by, for example, shrunken temporal cortical gyri after herpes simplex encephalitis; loss of pigmented cells in the substantia nigra after encephalitis lethargica; and enlargement of the ventricles, diffuse gliosis, and shrinkage of the white matter, either from direct involvement of the white matter in the encephalitic process, as in subacute sclerosing panencephalitis, or as a consequence of secondary Wallerian degeneration. Long-standing epilepsy, a common sequel in survivors of encephalitis, may result in evidence of repeated head injuries (old contusions) and cerebellar Purkinje cell loss. These late secondary sequelae may make the unraveling of pathological events almost impossible unless a detailed clinical account of the original illness is available.

THE NEED FOR AUTOPSIES

In recent decades, the autopsy rates in most hospitals have dropped dramatically. There are few conditions for which the autopsy is more important than viral encephalitis. The opportunity that an autopsy affords to examine brain tissue with the microscope is still an essential part of maintaining awareness of how novel viral infections may affect the brain. The past few years have seen descriptions of several such infections: Nipah virus encephalitis (see chapter 10), enterovirus 71 encephalitis (see chapter 10), parvovirus B19 meningoencephalitis (see chapter 5), and variant CJD (see chapter 15). Only a little earlier, the first descriptions of HIV encephalitis (see chapter 12) appeared. Viruses will continue to evolve, develop neurovirulence, and affect the brain in unpredictable ways. We need to foster understanding of the need for autopsies in cases of suspected viral encephalitis as a means to understanding these diseases better and ultimately to help treat and prevent them.

REFERENCES

Adams, D. H., and A. R. Lloyd. 1997. Chemokines: leucocyte recruitment and activation cytokines. *Lancet* **349:**490–495.

Advisory Committee on Dangerous Pathogens. 1994. Precautions for work with human and animal transmissible spongiform encephalopathies. H.M. Stationery Office, London, United Kingdom.

Advisory Committee on Dangerous Pathogens. 1995a. *Protection against Blood-Borne Infections in the Workplace: HIV and Hepatitis.* H.M. Stationery Office, London, United Kingdom.

Advisory Committee on Dangerous Pathogens. 1995b. *Categorisation of Biological Agents According to Hazard and Categories of Containment.* H.M. Stationery Office, London, United Kingdom.

Advisory Committee on Dangerous Pathogens. 1998. *Transmissible Spongiform Encephalopathy Agents: Safe Working and the Prevention of Infection.* H.M. Stationery Office, London, United Kingdom.

Allsopp, T. E., and J. K. Fazakerley. 2000. Altruistic cell suicide and the specialized case of the virus-infected nervous system. *Trends Neurosci.* **23:**284–290.

Anderson, J. R., and H. J. Field. 1983. The distribution of herpes simplex type 1 antigen in mouse central nervous system after different routes of inoculation. *J. Neurol. Sci.* **60:**181–195.

Atenasiu, P. 1973. *Laboratory Techniques in Rabies,* p. 338. In M. M. Kaplan and H. Koprowski (ed.), WHO Monograph Series. World Health Organization, Geneva, Switzerland.

Bell, J. E., S. M. Gentleman, J. W. Ironside, L. McCardle, P. L. Lantos, L. Doey, J. Lowe, J. Fergusson, P. Luthert, S. McQuaid, and I. V. Allen. 1997. Prion protein immunocytochemistry—UK five centre consensus report. *Neuropathol. Appl. Neurobiol.* **23:**26–35.

Benjamin, D. R., and C. G. Ray. 1975. Use of immunoperoxidase on brain tissue for the rapid diagnosis of herpes encephalitis. *Am. J. Clin. Pathol.* **64:**472–476.

Berger, D. P., D. Homann, and M. B. A. Oldstone. 2000. Immunocytotherapy of persistent viral infection, p. 289–295. In P. K. Peterson and J. Remington (ed.), *New Concepts in the Immunopathogenesis of CNS Infections.* Blackwell Science, Oxford, United Kingdom.

Blinzinger, K., J. Simon, D. Magrath, and L. Boulger. 1969. Poliovirus crystals within the endoplasmic reticulum of endothelial and mononuclear cells in the monkey spinal cord. *Science* **163:**1336–1337.

Blumberg, B. M., D. J. Mock, J. M. Powers, M. Ito, J. G. Assouline, J. V. Baker, B. Chen, and A. D. Goodman. 2000. The HHV6 paradox: ubiquitous commensal or insidious pathogen? A two-step in situ PCR approach. *J. Clin. Virol.* **16:**159–178.

Bodian, D., and H. A. Howe. 1941. The rate of progression of poliomyelitis virus in nerves. *Bull. Johns Hopkins Hosp.* **69:**79–85.

Booss, J., P. R. Dann, B. P. Griffith, and J. H. Kim. 1989. Host defense response to cytomegalovirus in the central nervous system. Predominance of the monocyte. *Am. J. Pathol.* **134:**71–78.

Bouteille, M., R. Houdart, and G. Delarue. 1965. Ultrastructural arguments in favor of the histogenetic oneness of astrocytomas, glioblastoma multiforme and oligodendrogliomas. *Rev. Neurol.* (Paris) **112:**69–71.

Breitfeld, V., Y. Hashida, F. E. Sherman, K. Odagiri, and E. J. Yunis. 1973. Fatal measles infection in children with leukemia. *Lab. Invest.* **28:**279–291.

Brightman, M. W. 1968. The intracerebral movement of proteins injected into blood and cerebrospinal fluid of mice. *Prog. Brain Res.* **29:**19–40.

Brown, C. 1998. Antigen retrieval methods for immunohistochemistry. *Toxicol. Pathol.* **26:**830–831.

Brown, P., C. J. Gibbs, Jr., H. L. Amyx, D. T. Kingsbury, R. G. Rohwer, M. P. Sulima, and D. C. Gajdusek. 1982. Chemical disinfection of Creutzfeldt-Jakob disease virus. *N. Engl. J. Med.* **306:**1279–1282.

Buchmeier, M. J., R. M. Welsh, F. J. Dutko, and M. B. Oldstone. 1980. The virology and immunobiology of lymphocytic choriomeningitis virus infection. *Adv. Immunol.* **30:**275–331.

Budka, H., and T. Popow-Kraupp. 1981. Rabies and herpes simplex virus encephalitis. An immunohistological study on site and distribution of viral antigens. *Virchows Arch. A. Pathol. Anat. Histol.* **390:**353–364.

Budka, H., H. Lassmann, and T. Popow-Kraupp. 1982. Measles virus antigen in panencephalitis. An immunomorphological study stressing dendritic involvement in SSPE. *Acta Neuropathol.* **56:**52–62.

Buzzard, E. F., and J. G. Greenfield. 1919. Lethargic encephalitis; its sequelae and morbid anatomy. *Brain* **42:**305–388.

Centers for Disease Control and Prevention. 1999. *Biological Safety Level 4 Agents. Biosafety in Microbiological and Biomedical Laboratories,* 4th ed. Centers for Disease Control and Prevention and National Institutes of Health, U.S. Department of Health and Human Services. U.S. Government Printing Office, Washington, D.C.

Centers for Disease Control and Prevention. 2002. *Draft Guidelines for Disinfection and Sterilization in Health Care Facilities.* Centers for Disease Control and Prevention, Atlanta, Ga.

Chao, C. C., S. Hu, W. S. Sheng, D. Bu, M. I. Bukrinsky, and P. K. Peterson. 1996. Cytokine-stimulated astrocytes damage human neurons via a nitric oxide mechanism. *Glia* **16:**276–284.

COSHH. 1999. Regulations on control of substances hazardous to health. H. M. Stationery Office, London, United Kingdom.

Dayan, A. D., and J. D. Almeida. 1975. The morphologist's contribution to the study of viral encephalitis, p. 32–55. *In* L. S. Illis (ed.), *Viral Diseases of the Nervous System.* Baillière Tindall, London, United Kingdom.

DeBiasi, R. L., and K. L. Tyler. 1999. Polymerase chain reaction in the diagnosis and management of central nervous system infections. *Arch. Neurol.* **56:**1215–1219.

de la Torre, J. C., M. Mallory, M. Brot, L. Gold, G. Koob, M. B. Oldstone, and E. Masliah. 1996. Viral persistence in neurons alters synaptic plasticity and cognitive functions without destruction of brain cells. *Virology* **220:**508–515.

Duriez, P. J., and G. M. Shah. 1997. Cleavage of poly(ADP-ribose) polymerase: a sensitive parameter to study cell death. *Biochem. Cell Biol.* **75:**337–349.

Esiri, M. M. 1982. Herpes simplex encephalitis. An immunohistological study of the distribution of viral antigen within the brain. *J. Neurol. Sci.* **54:**209–226.

Esiri, M. M., D. R. Oppenheimer, B. Brownell, and M. Haire. 1982. Distribution of measles antigen and immunoglobulin-containing cells in the CNS in subacute sclerosing panencephalitis (SSPE) and atypical measles encephalitis. *J. Neurol. Sci.* **53:**29–43.

Gauczynski, S., J. M. Peyrin, S. Haik, C. Leucht, C. Hundt, R. Rieger, S. Krasemann, J. P. Deslys, D. Dormont, C. I. Lasmezas, and S. Weiss. 2001. The 37-kDa/67-kDa laminin receptor acts as the cell-surface receptor for the cellular prion protein. *EMBO J.* **20:**5863–5875.

Glasgow, L. A. 1979. Biology and pathogenesis of viral infections, p. 39–76. *In* G. J. Galasso, T. C. Merigan, and R. A. Buchanan (ed.), *Viral Agents and Viral Diseases in Man.* Raven Press, New York, N.Y.

Gosztonyi, G. 1979. Possible mechanisms of spread of fixed rabies virus along neural pathways, p. 323–345. *In* P. A. Bachmann (ed.), *Proc. 4th Munich Symposium on Microbiology. (Mechanisms of Viral Pathogenesis and Virulence.).*

Gosztonyi, G., and M. Terborg. 1992. In situ hybridization

histochemistry in the diagnosis of viral infections of the central nervous system. *Acta Histochem. Suppl.* **42:**123–130.

Grafstein, B., and D. S. Forman. 1980. Intracellular transport in neurons. *Physiol. Rev.* **60:**1167–1283.

Grcevic, N., and V. Vince. 1976. p. 127–149. *In* Vesenjak-Hirjan (ed.), *Tick-Borne Encephalitis in Croatia (Yugoslavia).* Jugoslavenska Akademige 327, Zagreb, Yugoslavia.

Griffin, D. E., and J. M. Hardwick. 1997. Regulators of apoptosis on the road to persistent alphavirus infection. *Annu. Rev. Microbiol.* **51:**565–592.

Gutewa, J., and E. Osetowska. 1961. A chronic form of subacute sclerosing panencephalitis (a case with a history of 5 years); clinical and pathological study, p. 386–404. *In* L. van Bogaert, J. Radermecker, J. Hozay, and A. Lowenthal (ed.), *Encephalitides.* Elsevier, Amsterdam, The Netherlands.

Hallervorden, J. 1935. Anatomische Untersungen zur Pathogenese des postencephalitischen Parkinsonismus. *D.Z. Nervenheilk* **136:**68–77.

Haymaker, W., M. G. Smith, L. van Bogaert, and C. de Chenar. 1958. Pathology of viral disease in man characterised by nuclear inclusions, p. 95–104. *In* W. S. Field and R. L. Blattner (ed.), *Viral Encephalitis.* Charles C. Thomas Co., Springfield, Ill.

Horten, B., R. W. Price, and D. Jimenez. 1981. Multifocal varicella-zoster virus leukoencephalitis temporally remote from herpes zoster. *Ann. Neurol.* **9:**251–266.

Hummel, M., I. Anagnostopoulos, P. Korbjuhn, and H. Stein. 1995. Epstein-Barr virus in B-cell non-Hodgkin's lymphomas: unexpected infection patterns and different infection incidence in low- and high-grade types. *J. Pathol.* **175:**263–271.

Ironside, J. W., and J. E. Bell. 1996. The 'high-risk' neuropathological autopsy in AIDS and Creutzfeldt-Jakob disease: principles and practice. *Neuropathol. Appl. Neurobiol.* **22:**388–393.

Itoyama, Y., H. D. Webster, N. H. Sternberger, E. P. Richardson, Jr., D. L. Walker, R. H. Quarles, and B. L. Padgett. 1982. Distribution of papovavirus, myelin-associated glycoprotein, and myelin basic protein in progressive multifocal leukoencephalopathy lesions. *Ann. Neurol.* **11:**396–407.

Johnson, A. J., M. Rodriquez, and L. R. Pease. 2000. Class I major histocompatibility molecules play a critical role in resistance to Theiler's virus infection, p. 296–316. *In* P. K. Peterson and J. S. Remington (eds.), *New Concepts in the Pathogenesis of CNS Infections.* Blackwell Science, Oxford, United Kingdom.

Johnson, R. T. 1965. Virus invasion of the central nervous system. A study of Sindbis virus infection in the mouse using immunofluorescent antibody. *Am. J. Pathol.* **46:**929–943.

Johnson, R. T. 1980. Selective vulnerability of neural cells to viral infections. *Brain* **103:**447–472.

Jubelt, B., G. Gallez-Hawkins, O. Narayan, and R. T. Johnson. 1980. Pathogenesis of human poliovirus infection in mice. I. Clinical and pathological studies. *J. Neuropathol. Exp. Neurol.* **39:**138–148.

Kerschensteiner, M., E. Gallmeier, L. Behrens, V. V. Leal, T. Misgeld, W. E. Klinkert, R. Kolbeck, E. Hoppe, R. L. Oropeza-Wekerle, I. Bartke, C. Stadelmann, H. Lassmann, H. Wekerle, and R. Hohlfeld. 1999. Activated human T cells, B cells, and monocytes produce brain-derived neurotrophic factor in vitro and in inflammatory brain lesions: a neuroprotective role of inflammation? *J. Exp. Med.* **189:**865–870.

Kleinschmidt-DeMasters, M. D., R. L. DeBiasi, and K. L. Tyler. 2001. Polymerase chain reaction as a diagnostic adjunct in herpes virus infections of the nervous system. *Brain Pathol.* **11:**452–464.

Knobler, R. L., L. A. Tunison, P. W. Lampert, and M. B. Oldstone. 1982. Selected mutants of mouse hepatitis virus type 4 (JHM strain) induce different CNS diseases. Pathobiology of disease induced by wild type and mutants ts8 and ts15 in BALB/c and SJL/J mice. *Am. J. Pathol.* **109:**157–168.

Krakauer, D. C. 2000. Evolving cell death in the virus-infected nervous system. *Trends Neurosci.* **23:**611–612.

Kristensson, K., E. Lycke, and J. Sjostrand. 1974. Spread of herpes simplex virus in peripheral nerves. *Acta Neuropathol.* **17:**44–53.

Kumanishi, T., and A. Hirano. 1978. An immunoperoxidase study on herpes simplex virus encephalitis. *J. Neuropathol. Exp. Neurol.* **37:**790–795.

Kumanishi, T., and I. Seichii. 1979. SSPE: immunohistochemical demonstration of measles virus antigen(s) in paraffin sections. *Acta Neuropathol.* (Berlin) **48:**161–163.

Kure, K., W. D. Lyman, K. M. Weidenheim, and D. W. Dickson. 1990. Cellular localization of an HIV-1 antigen in subacute AIDS encephalitis using an improved double-labeling immunohistochemical method. *Am. J. Pathol.* **136:**1085–1092.

Lawson, L. J. 1995. Leukocyte migration into the central nervous system, p. 27–60. *In* N. Rothwell (ed.), *Immune Responses in the Nervous System.* Bios, Oxford, United Kingdom.

Lebon, P., G. Ponsot, J. Gony, and J. Hors. 1986. HLA antigens in acute measles encephalitis. *Tissue Antigens* **27:**75–77.

Lee, S. C., D. W. Dickson, W. Liu, and C. F. Brosnan. 1993. Induction of nitric oxide synthase activity in human astrocytes by interleukin-1 beta and interferon-gamma. *J. Neuroimmunol.* **46:**19–24.

Levine, B., Q. Huang, J. T. Isaacs, J. C. Reed, D. E. Griffin, and J. M. Hardwick. 1993. Conversion of lytic to persistent alphavirus infection by the bcl-2 cellular oncogene. *Nature* **361:**739–742.

Lewis, J., S. L. Wesselingh, D. E. Griffin, and J. M. Hardwick. 1996. Alphavirus-induced apoptosis in mouse brains correlates with neurovirulence. *J. Virol.* **70:**1828–1835.

Liou, M. L., and C. Y. Hsu. 1998. Japanese encephalitis virus is transported across the cerebral blood vessels by endocytosis in mouse brain. *Cell Tissue Res.* **293:**389–394.

Lohler, J. 1982. Virus infections of the central nervous system. Demonstration of viral antigens in paraffin-embedded autopsy material by the PAP technic (Sternberger). *Acta Histochem. Suppl.* **25:**107–111.

Long, A. A., P. Komminoth, E. Lee, and H. J. Wolfe. 1993. Comparison of indirect and direct in-situ polymerase chain reaction in cell preparations and tissue sections. Detection of viral DNA, gene rearrangements and chromosomal translocations. *Histochemistry* **99:**151–162.

Mahley, R. W., and S. C. Rall, Jr. 2000. Apolipoprotein E: far more than a lipid transport protein. *Annu. Rev. Genomics Hum. Genet.* **1:**507–537.

Mandybur, T. I., A. S. Nagpaul, Z. Pappas, and W. J. Niklowitz. 1977. Alzheimer neurofibrillary change in subacute sclerosing panencephalitis. *Ann. Neurol.* **1:**103–107.

Mathur, A., N. Khanna, and U. C. Chaturvedi. 1992. Breakdown of blood-brain barrier by virus-induced cytokine during Japanese encephalitis virus infection. *Int. J. Exp. Pathol.* **73:**603–611.

Monath, T. P., C. B. Cropp, and A. K. Harrison. 1983. Mode of entry of a neurotropic arbovirus into the central nervous system. Reinvestigation of an old controversy. *Lab. Invest.* **48:**399–410.

Moore, G. R., U. Traugott, L. C. Scheinberg, and C. S. Raine. 1989. Tropical spastic paraparesis: a model of virus-induced, cytotoxic T-cell-mediated demyelination? *Ann. Neurol.* **26:**523–530.

Morris, C. S., M. M. Esiri, T. J. Sprinkle, and N. Gregson. 1994. Oligodendrocyte reactions and cell proliferation markers in human demyelinating diseases. *Neuropathol. Appl. Neurobiol.* **20:**272–281.

Mrak, R. E., and L. Young. 1994. Rabies encephalitis in humans: pathology, pathogenesis and pathophysiology. *J. Neuropathol. Exp. Neurol.* **53:**1–10.

Murphy, F. A., and S. G. Whitfield. 1970. Eastern equine encephalitis virus infection: electron microscopic studies of mouse central nervous system. *Exp. Mol. Pathol.* **13:**131–146.

Murphy, F. A., S. P. Bauer, A. K. Harrison, and W. C. Winn, Jr. 1973. Comparative pathogenesis of rabies and rabies-like viruses. Viral infection and transit from inoculation site to the central nervous system. *Lab. Invest.* **28:**361–376.

Neumann, H. 2001. Control of glial immune function by neurons. *Glia* **36:**191–199.

Oldstone, M. B., J. Holmstoen, and R. M. Welsh, Jr. 1977. Alterations of acetylcholine enzymes in neuroblastoma cells persistently infected with lymphocytic choriomeningitis virus. *J. Cell Physiol.* **91:**459–472.

Pathak, S., and H. E. Webb. 1974. Possible mechanisms for the transport of Semliki forest virus into and within mouse brain. An electron-microscopic study. *J. Neurol. Sci.* **23:**175–184.

Paula-Barbosa, M. M., R. Brito, C. A. Silva, R. Faria, and C. Cruz. 1979. Neurofibrillary changes in the cerebral cortex of a patient with subacute sclerosing panencephalitis (SSPE). *Acta Neuropathol.* (Berlin) **48:**157–160.

Piyasirisilp, S., B. J. Schmeckpeper, D. Chandanayingyong, T. Hemachudha, and D. E. Griffin. 1999. Association of HLA and T-cell receptor gene polymorphisms with Semple rabies vaccine-induced autoimmune encephalomyelitis. *Ann. Neurol.* **45:**595–600.

Ransohoff, R. M. 1999. Chemokines and central nervous system inflammation, p. 413–436. *In* R. R. Ruffolo, G. Z. Fenerstein, A. J. Hunter, and G. Poste (ed.), *Inflammatory Cells and Mediators in CNS Diseases.* Harwood, Taylor & Francis Group, London, United Kingdom.

Rao, L., M. Debbas, P. Sabbatini, D. Hockenbery, S. Korsmeyer, and E. White. 1992. The adenovirus E1A proteins induce apoptosis, which is inhibited by the E1B 19-kDa and Bcl-2 proteins. *Proc. Natl. Acad. Sci. USA* **89:**7742–7746.

Reinacher, M., J. Bonin, O. Narayan, and C. Scholtissek. 1983. Pathogenesis of neurovirulent influenza A virus infection in mice. Route of entry of virus into brain determines infection of different populations of cells. *Lab. Invest.* **49:**686–692.

Rosenberg, G. 1999. Cytokines and matrix metalloproteinases in inflammation of the blood brain barrier, p. 413–436. *In* R. R. Ruffolo, G. Z. Fenerstein, A. J. Hunter, and G. Poste (ed.), *Inflammatory Cells and Mediators in CNS Diseases.* Harwood, Taylor & Francis Group, London, United Kingdom.

Sherriff, F. E., L. R. Bridges, and S. Sivaloganathan. 1994. Early detection of axonal injury after human head trauma using immunocytochemistry for beta-amyloid precursor protein. *Acta Neuropathol.* **87:**55–62.

Simbulan-Rosenthal, C. M., D. S. Rosenthal, S. Iyer, A. H. Boulares, and M. E. Smulson. 1998. Transient poly(ADP-ribosyl)ation of nuclear proteins and role of poly(ADP-ribose) polymerase in the early stages of apoptosis. *J. Biol. Chem.* **273:**13703–13712.

Springer, T. A. 1994. Traffic signals for lymphocyte recirculation and leukocyte emigration: the multistep paradigm. *Cell* **76:**301–314.

Sternberger, L. A. 1979. *Immunocytochemistry*, 2nd ed. John Wiley, New York, N.Y.

Summers, B. A., H. A. Greisen, and M. J. Appel. 1978. Possible initiation of viral encephalomyelitis in dogs by migrating lymphocytes infected with distemper virus. *Lancet* **ii:**187–189.

Venters, H. D., Q. Tang, Q. Liu, R. W. VanHoy, R. Dantzer, and K. W. Kelley. 1999. A new mechanism of neurodegeneration: a proinflammatory cytokine inhibits receptor signaling by a survival peptide. *Proc. Natl. Acad. Sci. USA* **96:**9879–9884.

von Andrian, U. H., and C. R. Mackay. 2000. T-cell function and migration. Two sides of the same coin. *N. Engl. J. Med.* **343:**1020–1034.

Walker, F., C. Bedel, O. Boucher, M. C. Dauge, C. Vissuzaine, and F. Potet. 1995. In situ gene amplification on tissue sections (in situ PCR). A new technique for pathologists. *Ann. Pathol.* **15:**459–465.

Webb, H. E., and J. G. Hall. 1972. An assessment of the role of the allergic response in the pathogenesis viral diseases. *Symp. Soc. Gen. Microbiol.* **22:**383.

Westendorp, M. O., R. Frank, C. Ochsenbauer, K. Stricker, J. Dhein, H. Walczak, K. M. Debatin, and P. H. Krammer. 1995. Sensitization of T cells to CD95–mediated apoptosis by HIV-1 Tat and gp120. *Nature* **375:**497–500.

Williams, K. C., and W. F. Hickey. 1996. Traffic of lymphocytes into the CNS during inflammation and HIV infection, p. 31–55. *In* R. W. Price and J. J. Sidris (ed.), *The Cellular Basis of Central Nervous System HIV-1 Infection and the AIDS Dementia Complex.* Haworth Medical Press, New York, N.Y.

Wolinsky, J. S., T. Klassen, and J. R. Baringer. 1976. Persistence of neuroadapted mumps virus in brains of newborn hamsters after intraperitoneal inoculation. *J. Infect. Dis.* **133:**260–267.

Wong, K. T., K. B. Chua, and S. K. Lam. 1999. Immunohistochemical detection of infected neurons as a rapid diagnosis of enterovirus 71 encephalomyelitis. *Ann. Neurol.* **45:**271–272.

Wyatt, H. V. 1982. Any questions? *Tropical Doctor* **12:**218.

Zlotnik, I., C. E. Smith, D. P. Grant, and S. Peacock. 1970. The effect of immunosuppression on viral encephalitis, with special reference to cyclophosphamide. *Br. J. Exp. Pathol.* **51:**434–439.

Zu Rhein, G. M., and S. M. Chou. 1965. Particles resembling papovaviruses in human cerebral demyelinating disease. *Science* **148:**1477–1479.

Diagnostic Evaluation

The diagnosis of encephalitis is suggested when brain dysfunction is accompanied by evidence of central nervous system (CNS) inflammation. Not infrequently, patients with encephalitis have a brief prodrome of fever, malaise, headache, and nausea. This may be followed by confusion and delirium, which in turn gives way to stupor and a progressive decline of consciousness. Seizures, focal motor signs, and aphasia are commonly observed. In some cases, psychological disturbance may be a prominent early feature. Nuchal rigidity is present in some cases, but cerebrospinal fluid (CSF) pleocytosis is present in almost all. There are many other conditions, however, that can produce a similar clinical picture and that may require radically different therapy. Hence, the first task of the clinician in evaluating a patient with suspected encephalitis is to exclude other conditions that may masquerade as encephalitis (see Table 2.1).

DIFFERENTIATION OF ENCEPHALITIS FROM OTHER CONDITIONS

Encephalopathy
In the elderly, infection of other organ systems such as the lungs or gastrointestinal tract may be followed by fluid and electrolyte imbalance, reduced oxygenation of the blood, and impaired caloric intake. These in turn may produce an encephalopathy associated with confusion, agitation, somnolence, and disorientation. In some cases the appearance may be strikingly similar to a diffuse encephalitis. However, evidence of inflammation of the CNS is absent and the cerebral symptoms recede on correction of the systemic factors and treatment of the infection. Children may also demonstrate signs of encephalopathy during high fevers associated with infections. Agitation, visual hallucinations and distortions, and fearfulness occur. However, these episodes are usually brief in duration and do not of themselves indicate infection of the CNS. Thus systemic infections, particularly in the young and elderly, may be associated with toxic-metabolic encephalopathies that must be differentiated from infection of the brain itself. Nonfebrile causes of encephalopathy are extensive and must be systematically considered (see Table 8.1). Absence of a pleocytosis in the CSF and improvement with resolution of the systemic disease are characteristic.

TABLE 2.1 Steps in evaluating suspected viral encephalitis

1. Exclude alternative diagnoses of an infectious and noninfectious nature
2. Using clinical and epidemiologic features, determine the type of encephalitis (Table 2.2)
3. Based on the type of encephalitis, select the appropriate diagnostic virology studies to determine the infecting virus (Table 2.4 and specific chapters)
4. Initiate management and antiviral therapy based first on a presumptive diagnosis, followed subsequently by confirmed diagnosis (chapter 3 and specific chapters)

Focal CNS Disease

Encephalitis may also be mimicked by focal noninflammatory cerebral disease with secondary infection elsewhere in the body. For example, patients immobilized by stroke or brain tumor are at risk for several infections such as pneumonia or urinary tract infection. The resulting clinical exam may be virtually indistinguishable from encephalitis complicated by remote infection. Usually the temporal sequence of events and paucity of evidence for CNS inflammation allow these conditions to be distinguished from encephalitis. Still more difficult to evaluate clinically are those occasional patients with a cryptic brain tumor who first demonstrate cerebral signs with the advent of an unrelated systemic infection. The correct diagnosis is usually suggested by neuroimaging.

Multifocal and Diffuse CNS Disease

Under certain circumstances several other intracranial conditions may resemble encephalitis. Subarachnoid hemorrhage induces a pleocytosis in the CSF. It can produce focal and diffuse cerebral dysfunction in a progressive fashion by direct parenchymal damage, vasospasm, and hydrocephalus. Usually the clinical onset distinguishes the conditions. However, when a stuporous or comatose patient is unable to relate the onset, the issue may not be resolved until neuroradiographic demonstration of an aneurysm. Similarly, the history and analysis of neuroimaging study usually result in the accurate diagnosis of subdural hematoma. On occasion, progressive obtundation, in the absence of a history of head trauma, and in association with minimal or moderate abnormalities of the CSF, may suggest subacute encephalitis. The diagnosis of subdural hematoma in such cases may require a tenacious suspicion. Migraine headache with CSF pleocytosis may present a difficult diagnostic challenge (Fig. 2.1). Yet another condition to be considered is vasculitis. In the presence of a known systemic vasculitis, the diagnosis is readily suggested. However, in those rare cases in which the vasculitis starts in the brain, or is restricted to the brain, the differentiation from encephalitis may be difficult. The diagnosis may be suggested by neuroimaging. In other cases, however, the diagnosis may be less clear and meningeal-cortical biopsy may be required.

Other CNS Infections

High on the list of conditions to be distinguished from viral encephalitis are CNS infections associated with other classes of infectious agents. Accurate diagnosis is urgent, as such infections will usually be treatable. Chronic meningitis due to opportunistic or partially treated bacterial, tuberculosis,

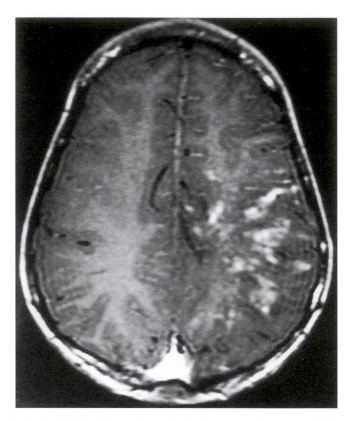

FIGURE 2.1 First task, exclude alternative diagnoses. MRI of a 4-year-old boy with a history of headache and the acute onset of hemiplegia. CSF revealed a pleocytosis with polymorphonuclear predominance. Axial MRI (T1 weighted with gadolinium) revealed areas of enhancement in parietal occipital lobes. The clinical profile, CSF, and MRI would have been compatible with infection of the brain; however, a full evaluation revealed a migraine syndrome (Goldstein et al., 1990). Courtesy Gordon Sze, Yale University School of Medicine.

or fungal infection may induce parenchymal damage and can be confused with encephalitis. Thorough culturing of the CSF, PCR, and testing for antigens and antibodies are required. A significantly reduced CSF glucose is highly suggestive of a nonviral process but is not invariably present with other infections and is occasionally found in some viral infections of the CNS such as mumps, lymphocytic choriomeningitis, or zoster. Bacterial cerebritis and early abscess formation may not be distinguishable from viral encephalitis by examination and CSF culture or by imaging and may require biopsy in order to isolate an organism. On occasion, subdural empyema may present signs, symptoms, and test results compatible with encephalitis. Venous sinus thrombosis may complicate intracranial infections, develop in the face of infections elsewhere, or occur apparently spontaneously.

The infection most regularly confused with encephalitis is viral aseptic meningitis. While in many cases the disease is clearly restricted to the meninges, other cases present difficult clinical patterns. In fact, many infections involve both the meninges and the brain parenchyma. These cases need to be distinguished from those in which clinical signs result from secondary mechanisms. Various symptoms may occur in the presence of increased intracranial pressure, altered cerebral metabolism, and the toxic products of host-virus interaction. In a few cases with CSF pleocytosis, we have observed transient symptoms compatible with focal cerebral ischemia.

TYPES OF ENCEPHALITIS: KEY INITIAL QUESTIONS

Definition of the specific etiology of a case of encephalitis is important for several reasons. First, by identifying the etiologic agent or mechanism, the patient is spared therapies and diagnostic maneuvers directed at other potential etiologies. Second, the clinician is able to be more specific in the projection of the possible course and outcome of the illness. Third, the information is of public health importance. For example, identification of cases of arbovirus encephalitis may result in public health intervention to control the vector. The information is also useful to other clinicians attempting to evaluate similar cases in the region. Most important, however, is the use of antiviral therapy. Prompt antiviral therapy for herpes simplex encephalitis (HSE), for example, is necessary to reduce mortality and improve outcomes. Varicella-zoster virus (VZV), cytomegalovirus (CMV), human immunodeficiency virus (HIV), and many enteroviruses are other examples for which specific antiviral compounds are available. As the molecular mechanisms of viral replication are specifically defined, the opportunity for producing selective antiviral agents is created. The number of specific antiviral agents available for clinical use is continuing to expand. Increased numbers of antiviral agents, each directed at specific viruses or groups of viruses, greatly sharpen the need for accurate and rapid virological diagnosis.

Hence, the second task of the clinician evaluating a patient with suspected viral encephalitis is to determine the type of encephalitis. There are three key questions to be determined: tempo of illness; clustering of cases; and phases, that is, whether there is an association with a preceding systemic viral illness or antigen challenge.

Tempo of Illness

The temporal profile of encephalitis can range from acute to chronic. Fulminant acute presentations such as can be seen with eastern equine encephalitis or acute hemorrhagic leukoencephalopathy require rapid therapeutic intervention. Raised intracranial pressure, mass effect, recurrent seizures, and need for mechanical respiration require emergent intervention and intensive care unit management. Diagnostic evaluation proceeds in parallel with efforts to control the effects of a fulminant encephalitis. At the other end of the spectrum, the insidious onset of symptoms and signs over weeks to months can characterize chronic processes as diverse as the cognitive impairments in HIV/AIDS and the dementing disorder Creutzfeldt-Jakob disease (CJD). Many encephalitides develop acutely over a few days and have often run their active course by 2 to 3 weeks. HSE fits this temporal pattern, as do many cases of arbovirus encephalitis. Thus, it is diagnostically useful to categorize encephalitis as acute or subacute/chronic.

Case Clusters, Outbreaks, and Epidemics

The aggregation of similar cases, ranging from pairs to hundreds of persons, is a marker for transmission of illness and therefore the types of agents that might be responsible. Human-to-human transmission, as with influenza and the enteroviruses, insect-to-human transmission as in the arboviral diseases, and animal-to-human transmission, such as in Nipah virus encephalitis, are mechanisms that underlie aggregates of cases generally termed epidemic. Encephalitis itself may be epidemic, as in arboviral infections such as West Nile fever, or CNS complications may occur as occasional components of epidemics in which other organs are the principal target, such as influenza. In either case the illness is characterized as epidemic, in contrast to sporadic.

When considered in conjunction with the tempo of the illness, encephalitis falls into certain categories, including acute sporadic, acute epidemic, subacute/chronic sporadic, and subacute/chronic epidemic. To reiterate, different viruses and processes will be found in different categories. As examples, HSE is the most important acute sporadic encephalitis, and the AIDS dementia complex is the most common chronic epidemic encephalitis.

Phases

Careful history documentation from someone close to the patient can be extremely helpful to determine if there were separable phases to the illness. This is particularly so for acute encephalitis. Thus, a biphasic illness in which systemic illness preceded and was clearly separated by a few days to a few weeks from the CNS component characterizes the immune-mediated illness called acute disseminated encephalomyelitis (ADEM). Worldwide, the most common cause of postviral encephalomyelitis is likely to be measles virus. In developed nations in which childhood immunizations are widely implemented, nonspecific febrile illnesses and respiratory or gastrointestinal illnesses are the most common precedents. Vaccination can also trigger an ADEM. With vaccination for smallpox lately reinstituted, the potential for postvaccinial ADEM has reemerged. Virological, histopathological, and experimental evidence suggests that postinfectious or postimmunization illnesses are immune mediated. Hence, the category is termed acute para- (or post)-infectious encephalomyelitis. As the term ADEM implies, the spinal cord as well as the brain can be involved. The peripheral nervous system can sometimes be involved as well. Multifocal CNS white matter involvement seen by neuroimaging is a useful clue. Whether or not transient or abortive infection of the cerebrovascular endothelium triggers the process in certain cases is an emerging question in pathogenesis.

Considerable caution must be exercised in concluding that a biphasic illness has occurred with separable systemic and CNS phases. Thus HSE and other types of encephalitis can have a prodrome of malaise and nonspecific complaints prior to the emergence of encephalitis. Usually the prodrome leads directly into the encephalitis and is not clearly separable by the patient or his or her close associates. Certain arboviral infections such as Colorado tick fever or the Central European form of tick-borne encephalitis may have biphasic disease patterns, with so-called "saddleback" fever elevations. Locality and season are critical to sorting out these illnesses. Enteroviruses too are frequently characterized by biphasic illness in which CNS symptoms may be associated with fever, rash, and myalgias.

CLINICAL CLASSIFICATION OF ENCEPHALITIS

Consideration of the questions of acute versus subacute/chronic, sporadic versus epidemic, and infectious versus parainfectious allows one to focus on the most likely processes and viral agents in each category (Table 2.2). Further questions, such as season of year, geographic region, or exposure to insect-borne or animal-transmitted viruses, allow further discrimination of the agents and processes to be evaluated by laboratory examination. Brief consideration of each of the categories follows.

Acute Sporadic Encephalitis

In the absence of case clustering, epidemic infection, or a preceding systemic infection, viruses which produce sporadic encephalitis are considered. Chief among these, because of its severity and because of the availability of specific antiviral treatment, is HSE. It often presents with characteristic clinical and neurodiagnostic features implicating the frontal-temporal region of the brain. However, several other viruses are associated with apparently sporadic cases of encephalitis. Some of these infections may be recognized by the association of a systemic illness such as mumps or infectious mononucleosis. A crucial distinction is exposure to

TABLE 2.2   Clinical classification of encephalitis

Acute sporadic
    Brain only, HSV
    With systemic illness, e.g., adenovirus, EBV, mumps, HHV-6
    From animals, e.g., rabies, lymphocytic choriomeningitis,
        B virus of monkeys
Acute parainfectious/postvaccinial
    Following childhood exanthems such as measles, chicken pox,
        or rubella, nonspecific "viral" syndromes, and following
        vaccinations, including smallpox:
            Encephalopathy, including Reye's syndrome
            ADEM
            Acute hemorrhagic leukoencephalopathy (Hurst)
            Vasculitis/vasculopathy
Acute epidemic
    Human-to-human transmission, e.g., influenza, enteroviruses
    Insect-to-human transmission, e.g., Japanese encephalitis,
        West Nile fever, St. Louis encephalitis, La Crosse virus,
        eastern equine encephalitis
    Animal-to-human transmission, e.g., Nipah virus
    Unknown type of transmission, e.g., von Economo's encephalitis
Subacute and chronic
    Epidemic, e.g., HIV
    Immunocompromised host, e.g., PML, CMV, VZV,
        immunosuppressive (or inclusion-bearing) measles,
        EBV, HHV-6
    Immunocompetent host, e.g., SSPE, progressive rubella
        panencephalitis, VZV
    Prion disorders, e.g., sporadic CJD, vCJD

animals. Most obvious in this category is the bite of an infected animal to transmit rabies. However, other viruses which can cause encephalitis may also be transmitted by exposure to animals or their excretions, such as rodent-transmitted lymphocytic choriomeningitis virus or B-virus infection following exposure to monkeys or their tissues.

Acute Epidemic Encephalitis

The season of the year in temperate climates is a crucial issue. For example, in the United States in the summer and fall, one may expect to encounter yearly outbreaks of enterovirus infection and the possibility of arboviral infection. Climatic factors that facilitate the proliferation of the vector may predispose to increased arboviral activity. Region is another key for the arboviruses. In the United States, the upper Midwest experiences yearly outbreaks of La Crosse virus encephalitis, whereas the East Coast and Gulf Coast states are at risk for eastern equine encephalitis. West Nile fever spread rapidly southward and reached the West Coast of the United States in 2002 following its introduction into New York City in 1999. Other epidemic infections have other routes of transmission, for example, the fecal-oral route in enteroviral infections. Whereas the presence of the vector is an adequate explanation for the seasonal activity of arboviral infections, the summer-fall activity of enteroviral infections in temperate climates has not been adequately explained. With the global eradication program for polio, enterovirus 71 is emerging as a damaging CNS pathogen. Influenza is epidemic in the winter and early spring in temperate climates. Occasional cases of CNS complications have been reported in association with influenza and other respiratory illnesses.

Acute Parainfectious or Postvaccination Encephalitis

The CNS may suffer as a consequence of the host response to a preceding systemic viral infection. These complications are termed "parainfectious." The mechanisms are felt to be principally immunological in nature and to resemble experimental allergic encephalomyelitis. Several clinical clues to this category of encephalitis can be sought. A history of a specific systemic infection such as measles, or a nonspecific febrile illness, or an immunization usually within the preceding month, followed by an asymptomatic period prior to CNS symptoms, is often described. The presence of dysfunction of multiple discrete loci in the nervous system is also helpful. Signs of spinal cord and/or peripheral nerve involvement in association with encephalitis support a diagnosis of parainfectious encephalomyelitis. Neuroimaging, particularly magnetic resonance imaging (MRI), may demonstrate multifocal disease. Thus the temporal profile and the distribution of loci of dysfunction in the nervous system are keys to the diagnosis of this type of encephalitis.

Subacute and Chronic Encephalitis

In contrast to the rapid, sometimes explosive onset of an acute viral encephalitis, the subacute and slow viral processes are often insidious in onset. These are a heterogeneous group of conditions in which the duration of disease may be measured in weeks to months and years, symptoms are restricted to the CNS, and the outcome is often fatal. It is useful to further subdivide the subacute and chronic category of encephalitides into those that occur in immunocompromised or immunocompetent hosts. Thus HIV is an epidemic chronic immunosuppressing illness that produces a chronic encephalitis, the AIDS dementia complex. Other chronic and subacute encephalitides occur in HIV and in other immunosuppressing illnesses or treatments such as progressive multifocal leukoencephalopathy (PML) or CMV encephalitis. In immunocompetent hosts, an unusual host-virus interaction can produce a defective measles infection of the brain, subacute sclerosing panencephalitis (SSPE). Although they are a different category of illness altogether, involving aberrant protein folding and aggregation rather than viral replication, we include consideration of the prion disorders such as CJD in the chronic category. This is because of their transmissibility under certain circumstances and because the workup of these disorders will often include consideration of chronic viral encephalitis.

DIAGNOSTIC EVALUATION OF ENCEPHALITIS

The examination and laboratory evaluation of a case of encephalitis is an exercise in both clinical neurology and diagnostic virology. The double process must be carried throughout the whole of the evaluation: history taking, physical examination, and laboratory studies. The neurological history, examination, and diagnostic studies can determine the anatomic location of dysfunction in the nervous system, distinguish encephalitis from other categories of disease, and sometimes suggest the specific viral etiology. However, it remains for the diagnostic virology studies to prove the etiologic agent. Five categories of information are required during an evaluation of neurovirological disease: clinical, epidemiological, and neurodiagnostic information, demonstration of the virus, and demonstration of an antibody response to the virus. Virologically oriented studies must proceed in stride with the clinical neurological studies.

Clinical Evaluation

Key to obtaining a good virological history is the assistance of a person living with the patient. This is obviously necessary when the patient's consciousness is impaired but is also necessary in assessing a fully conscious patient. We attempt to obtain a full vaccination and viral disease history. The latter is facilitated by reviewing a list of viruses while asking about diseases and symptomatology. Such a list is useful because it is a rare clinician who can retain in memory the long list of viruses during clinical questioning. The examples in Table 2.2 can serve as a starting point.

The importance of the general physical examination in encephalitis cannot be overemphasized. The observation of skin or mucous membrane lesions greatly narrows the list of likely agents and provides a source for viral isolation. The presence of tonsil hypertrophy, lymphadenopathy, or splenic enlargement is evidence for a systemic lymphoid response. Attention to each body region and organ system may also give clues to the presence of a virus infection in which the dominating feature is encephalitis. Evidence for upper respiratory, myocardial and pericardial, pulmonary,

and gastrointestinal diseases will each limit the spectrum of likely viral agents. The presence of nuchal rigidity requires careful examination. Apparent meningeal irritation can be mimicked by generalized myalgia in which the neck muscles are particularly involved. In elderly patients the presence of osteoarthritis as a limiting feature of neck flexion may be sought by determining if head rotation is also limited. Neurological causes of nuchal rigidity include not only inflammation of the meninges but also rostrocaudal herniation of the cerebellar tonsils in the presence of increased intracranial pressure.

Three general comments about the neurological examination are in order. First, it must cover the peripheral nervous system and spinal cord in addition to the brain. Evidence for concurrent involvement of the peripheral nervous system with the brain often puts the disease into the category of a parainfectious encephalomyelitis. West Nile virus is an exception; it can cause a brain stem encephalitis combined with a peripheral axonopathy. Similar comments apply to the demonstration of simultaneous spinal cord and brain involvement, usually implying a postinfectious process. Certain exceptions exist such as bulbar-spinal polio, tick-borne encephalitis with cervical spinal cord involvement, and West Nile virus, which can produce encephalitis and anterior horn cell disease.

The second general comment is the need for serial examinations. The observation of sequential development of separate foci of dysfunction in the peripheral and central nervous systems suggests a parainfectious process. In contrast, the evolution of signs implicating the frontal-temporal region strongly suggests HSE. Careful serial examinations are also required for management of increasing intracranial pressure. Although progressive decline of consciousness has many potential causes in viral encephalitis, the most dangerous are cerebral swelling with pressure on the brain stem and viral involvement of the brain stem itself. Progression of cerebral symptoms may result from spreading viral infection of brain cells, progressive demyelination, vascular complications, and cerebral edema. Hence, serial observations are required for management.

The third general comment is that clinical neuroanatomic localization is quite useful to suggest the investigation of certain specific viruses and syndromes (Table 2.3).

Epidemiological Data

By its nature, the epidemiological investigation overlaps both the clinical and the laboratory portions of the workup. Thus, in addition to the history of viral disease in the patient, exposure to infectious diseases at home, at work, and during travel are important. Travel brings with it exposure to infectious agents that may not be prevalent in the home region. Certain persons, such as teachers of young children, as well as schoolchildren themselves, are constantly exposed to viral infections in the community. In addition, certain age groups are more likely than others to suffer particular infections. For example, schoolchildren are most likely to demonstrate the symptoms of La Crosse virus encephalitis. Exposure to infected animals or insects can occur in several situations. Construction workers, picnickers, and others involved with the outdoors for occupation or recreation may be at risk to

TABLE 2.3 Neuroanatomic localization of encephalitis: examples of syndromes and infections

Massive bilateral cortical involvement
   Eastern equine encephalitis
Temporal lobe
   HSV
   Numerous other viruses, such as La Crosse virus encephalitis
Unilateral or bilateral massive white matter disease
   Acute hemorrhagic leukoencephalopathy
Multifocal white matter disease
   ADEM
   PML
   Multifocal VZV encephalopathy
   CMV
   HIV leukoencephalitis
Ventriculitis/ependymitis
   CMV
Diffuse bilateral subcortical involvement
   HIV
Deep gray matter
   Many arboviruses, including Japanese, St. Louis, eastern equine and western equine encephalitis
   CJD, vCJD
   ADEM
Brain stem
   Polio
   Enterovirus 71
   Nipah virus
   West Nile virus
   Bickerstaff's encephalitis
   ADEM
   HSV
   PML
   Miller Fisher syndrome
   VZV
   Rabies virus
Cerebellum
   ADEM
   VZV
   EBV
   PML
   HIV
   Numerous other viruses
Spinal cord
   ADEM
   Polio
   Enteroviruses, as a group
   Enterovirus 70
   CMV
   VZV
   HSV
   HIV
   Human T-cell lymphotropic virus type 1
   Certain arboviruses, such as tick-borne encephalitis and West Nile virus

encephalitis-bearing mosquitoes or ticks, depending on the region. Various domestic and wild animals, particularly bats in the United States, transmit rabies through infected saliva. Exposure to rodents and their excretions raises the possibility of infection with lymphocytic choriomeningitis virus. Finally, although consideration of the season and of the region allows certain predictions concerning viral activity to

be made, the local health department laboratories should be contacted with regard to current virus activity in the community.

Neurodiagnostic Studies

General laboratory studies and neurodiagnostic studies contribute to the differentiation of encephalitis from other processes, help to diagnose the specific type of encephalitis, and aid in management. For example, chest X rays, electrocardiograms, liver function tests, and urinalysis can each demonstrate clinically unsuspected organ dysfunction, revealing more about the infection or its complications. The peripheral white blood cell count may show leukocytosis or leukopenia in various viral infections or in various stages of one infection. The differential white blood cell count may show the presence of atypical lymphocytes.

CSF

Thorough examination of the CSF is crucial. In the presence of signs of increased intracranial pressure and no evidence of meningeal irritation, computerized tomography (CT) scanning on an emergent basis prior to initial lumbar puncture protects against the possibility of herniation from shift of a space-occupying lesion. In the presence of signs of fever and meningeal irritation, no time should be lost in performing the lumbar puncture to diagnose a treatable bacterial meningitis requiring immediate therapy. Thought should therefore be given to the sequence of the lumbar puncture and the CT scan, but both should be completed promptly. At the start of a viral meningoencephalitis, the pleocytosis may be principally polymorphonuclear. Although the presence of a normal glucose level will mitigate against a bacterial infection, reexamination of the CSF should be performed within 24 h, close attention should be paid to CSF culture for bacteria, and antibiotic coverage may be required until bacterial meningitis is ruled out. In some cases of viral encephalitis, the CSF continues to demonstrate a predominance of polymorphonuclear cells. In most cases of encephalitis, however, mononuclear cells predominate. In rare cases, no cells will be found. The presence of red blood cells and xanthochromia bespeaks a significant degree of parenchymal destruction. Although this observation has been used as an indication of HSE, not all cases of HSE demonstrate it, and conversely, other types of encephalitis may show it as well. A disproportionate number of red blood cells to white blood cells must raise the possibility that the primary cerebral event was bleeding rather than encephalitis. Alternatively, the presence of significant numbers of red cells and/or polymorphonuclear white cells should raise the consideration of acute hemorrhagic leukoencephalopathy (Hurst). A serum glucose sample should be taken at the time of lumbar puncture. The CSF glucose is usually about two-thirds of that in the serum. On rare occasions the CSF glucose will be reduced in the presence of a viral meningoencephalitis.

Locally produced immunoglobulin appears in the CSF, contributing to the protein level, sometimes resulting in oligoclonal bands of immunoglobulin and producing a measurable immune-specific antibody response. Local production of antibody within the CNS implies presence of the antigen except under circumstances of nonspecific immune activation. The presence of oligoclonal bands has been emphasized in multiple sclerosis and in SSPE. However, they may be found in many prolonged infections of the nervous system. Specificity of diagnosis can often be achieved by measuring CSF antibody. If one can demonstrate that antibody against a specific virus is locally produced, not simply derived from the serum, it strongly implicates that virus. Comparison of CSF and serum immunoglobulin G (IgG) or CSF and serum levels of an uninvolved marker antibody is used to exclude serum contamination of CSF (see below). In addition to a CSF sample taken for viral antibody, others should be taken for virus isolation and PCR. CSF PCR has become the diagnostic modality of choice in many viral infections. It has replaced cerebral biopsy in the diagnosis of HSE.

Neuroimaging

The CT scan is useful in the exclusion of other diseases and sometimes suggests the type of encephalitis. CT scanning may demonstrate abnormalities in the frontal-temporal region, supporting the diagnosis of HSE. However, the MRI is more useful in excluding other processes, localizing the encephalitis, and suggesting the nature of the viral infection. Multifocal white matter abnormalities can be seen in parainfectious encephalomyelitis, deep gray matter abnormalities are observed in the arboviral encephalitides, and mesial temporal-inferofrontal localization of disease can indicate herpes simplex virus (HSV) encephalitis. Brain MRI in AIDS can suggest a spectrum of disease processes. Specific abnormalities on MRI are useful in the documentation of the prion disorders, sporadic CJD and variant CJD (vCJD). Thus the MRI can provide very useful information in all categories of viral encephalitis. Taken in combination with CSF PCR and antibody studies and serum IgM enzyme-linked immunosorbent assay (ELISA), the MRI is an essential component of the diagnostic workup of encephalitis.

EEG

In general, the electroencephalogram (EEG) is quite sensitive to changes brought about by encephalitis. It is usually abnormal in cases of encephalitis, although when the disease is confined to the cerebellum or the brain stem, it may be normal. In some instances the EEG can support a specific etiologic diagnosis. Thus lateralized abnormalities occur in a high percentage of cases of HSE, and the presence of periodic lateralized epileptiform discharges provides even greater support. Unfortunately, a significant percentage of cases that are not proven to be caused by HSV also have lateralized EEG abnormalities, and other conditions such as vascular disease, which can resemble HSE, can produce periodic lateralized epileptiform discharges. Paroxysmal bursts of abnormal high-amplitude activity and burst suppression are diagnostically useful in both SSPE and CJD.

Evoked potential studies can be useful in some cases of encephalitis in defining loci of dysfunction and in following the evolution of the disease. Abnormalities in the visual evoked potential study reflecting optic nerve or chiasm dysfunction may occur in multiple sclerosis and in ADEM and would not be expected in an encephalitis limited to the brain. Auditory evoked potential studies are useful in defining abnormal function of the brain stem and may be useful when clinical signs of cerebral dysfunction obscure brain stem signs. They are clearly useful to help define brain stem encephalitis and loci of dysfunction in disseminated encephalomyelitis. The somatosensory evoked potentials are also useful in the elucidation of scattered lesions. Evoked potential studies have also been useful in the prediction of outcome of Reye's syndrome.

DIAGNOSTIC VIROLOGY AND SEROLOGY

General

The third task of the clinician, which is at the heart of the workup of encephalitis, is the selection of assays to determine the specific infecting virus or to demonstrate the absence of replicating virus in an immune-mediated parainfectious process. The need for rapid viral diagnosis is propelled by the increasing number of specific antivirals available for treatment. Dramatic advances in the diagnosis and treatment of acute viral diseases have revolutionized patient care. In respiratory diseases, for example, the development of new antivirals to treat influenza and the consequent need to make a diagnosis promptly have resulted in the development of antigen identification assay kits. These may be applied at the point of care, such as in the emergency department or physician's office, allowing the initiation of immediate antiviral therapy in appropriately diagnosed patients. Sampling respiratory infections is, however, considerably more direct than is sampling of CNS infections.

The evolution of diagnostic virology has resulted in several types of technology that may be variably available in different settings. Although the original techniques of isolation of agents in eggs and animals were cumbersome and time-consuming, they offered the advantage of amplifying a broad range of agents. The development of tissue cultures proved more efficient and widely adaptable. Primary, continuous, transformed, and genetically modified cell lines serve a variety of diagnostic purposes. The application of polyclonal and monoclonal antibodies increases the speed and specificity of diagnosis and supplements traditional cell culture techniques of determining cytopathic effect, hemadsorption, and viral interference. Antigen detection and nucleic acid detection by PCR and reverse transcriptase PCR can be applied directly to tissue or fluid samples, greatly accelerating the rapidity of viral diagnosis.

Techniques to identify antibody responses have also resulted in acceleration of viral diagnosis, particularly to achieve a presumptive diagnosis. Traditional serological techniques have been dependent on the demonstration of a fourfold increase in antibody, usually requiring 2 to 3 weeks to develop between the collection of acute- and chronic-phase samples. In practice, the convalescent-phase sample is often not collected. The development of IgM capture methodology coupled with detection systems such as IgM ELISA allows the presumptive identification and treatment of viral infection in the early stages of clinical disease.

A brief word on diagnosis by CSF antibody is in order. Except in circumstances of polyclonal stimulation, such as in multiple sclerosis, the demonstration of locally produced specific antibody strongly suggests the presence of the antigen, and therefore a diagnosis. Furthermore, demonstration of locally produced antibody in CSF compared to serum often does not require acute and convalescent samples. In some CNS infections, CSF antibody may appear before serum antibody. The crucial point is to demonstrate local production, rather than transudation from serum, because breakdown of the blood-brain barrier commonly occurs with CNS inflammation. A rough indication of breakdown is the level of CSF albumin. It is a much smaller molecule than Ig, and normal levels in the CSF imply relative integrity of the blood-brain barrier. In the presence of a normal level of CSF albumin, a CSF-to-serum ratio of 1:20 may serve as a rough cutoff point for locally produced antibody.

More accurate determination of locally produced antibody depends on the ratio of antibody to the virus of interest in serum and CSF, compared with the CSF and serum ratio of antibodies to an unrelated antigen. Alternatively, the comparison can be to total Ig levels of the appropriate class. A ratio of ratios can be established:

$$\frac{\text{Antibody against the agent: CSF/serum}}{\text{Antibody against an uninvolved agent: CSF/serum}}$$

Preferential antibody production in CNS is demonstrated when the ratio is significantly greater than unity. The actual cutoff value chosen will depend on the experience of the individual laboratory.

Examples of Laboratory Diagnosis

PCR and IgM capture methodologies have transformed the diagnosis of encephalitis (Table 2.4). Previously, brain biopsy was the "gold standard" for the diagnosis of HSE. PCR on CSF has supplanted brain biopsy for the diagnosis of HSE. The diagnosis of arboviral encephalitis has traditionally depended on the development of fourfold elevations in specific antibody, usually after the acute infection had run its course. Now, however, the application of IgM capture techniques allows a presumptive diagnosis during the acute infection. Diagnosis of enteroviral infections of the CNS, principally aseptic meningitis, but also encephalitis, had been dependent on isolation of virus from CSF. Diagnosis is now considerably speeded up by PCR or nucleic acid sequence-based amplification (NASBA) on CSF, and in some cases, such as in congenital hypogammaglobulinemic-associated chronic CNS infection, such tests are more sensitive. The diagnosis of encephalitis in immunocompromised patients benefits from the application of multiplex PCR, in which several *Herpesvirus* family viruses such as HSV, CMV, Epstein-Barr virus (EBV), human herpesvirus 6 (HHV-6), and VZV can be identified, in addition to standard CSF PCR to identify JC virus as the cause of PML. It must be emphasized that highly sensitive diagnostic methods such as PCR require fastidious technique to exclude contamination. They can also present interpretive challenges on occasion, when an agent is identified that does not match the clinical circumstances. Expert laboratory consultation is essential.

TABLE 2.4 Specimens to be considered in evaluating a case of viral encephalitis

CSF
    Virus isolation, PCR, NASBA, antigen detection
    IgM capture ELISA
    CSF/serum ratios of suspect virus to reference virus antibody
      or Ig
Blood/serum/plasma
    Virus isolation, PCR, NASBA, antigen detection
    IgM capture ELISA antibodies
    Acute and convalescent antibodies
Saliva
    PCR
    Virus isolation
    Antibodies
Lesion and skin samples
    Lesion samples for virus isolation, immunohistology, and antigen
      demonstration
    Mucous membrane specimens for virus isolation, antigen
      detection, electron microscopy (EM)
    Nuchal skin biopsy with hair follicles, (rabies)
Urine, throat swab, and stool samples
    Virus isolation, antigen detection, PCR, EM

The diagnosis and management of HIV infection is a highly specialized area. Diagnosis by antibody includes an initial screening ELISA followed by Western blot confirmation. Early infection, the acute retroviral syndrome, or seroconversion illness is characterized by initially negative antibody studies but positive plasma HIV RNA or positive HIV p24 antigen. Infection and the potential clinical course can be evaluated by measurement of the viral set point, the established viral load in the absence of antiretroviral therapy. Initiation of therapy and change of therapy are dependent on regular monitoring of clinical manifestations, the level of circulating CD4 T cells as a proxy for virus effect on host, and HIV RNA load in plasma. Because of the remarkable capacity of HIV to escape control by antiretroviral drugs via mutation, genotype and phenotype analyses are applied to help select the antiretroviral agent regimen. Evidence for HIV in the CSF can be found early in the course of illness, in the absence of CNS signs. Whether or not CSF studies can serve as a proxy measurement to assess the "sanctuary" status of virus in CNS under conditions of systemic viral control requires further investigation.

More than one diagnostic technique will be required in certain infections. For example, both CSF PCR and CSF-to-serum antibody ratio should be assayed in suspected VZV infections of the CNS. Such methodology is particularly important with the recognition that VZV infection of the CNS can occur in the absence of vesicles (zoster sine herpete) or be temporally remote from an identifiable zoster rash. Rabies virus identification is a good example of the application of multiple technologies. The presence of CSF antibodies makes the diagnosis, even in persons who have received pre- or postexposure prophylaxis. However, serum antibody, PCR on saliva, antigen detection on nuchal skin biopsies, and histopathological observation of Negri bodies can each be used. The non-infectious diseases-oriented clinician will likely require consultative guidance. The adoption of a structured approach to the diagnosis of encephalitis will facilitate the choice of appropriate assays.

ENCEPHALITIS OF UNDETERMINED ETIOLOGY

Advances in public health implementation of vaccination, vector control, secure and intact housing, and canine control have, somewhat paradoxically, made the diagnosis of the etiology of encephalitis more complex. The childhood exanthems, acute flaccid paralysis, and hydrophobia/aerophobia are each clinically recognizable as aids to the diagnosis of an infection of the CNS. The spectrum of encephalitis under control of these conditions shifts to viruses with less clear clinical and epidemiologic manifestations. The application of molecular technology may limit the spectrum of diagnostic methods used. At present, molecular diagnostic technologies have a narrow spectrum; that is, they identify only those agents specifically targeted. Many viral infections still require cell culture or animal inoculation for isolation and identification. In these days of managed care and cost containment, a full spectrum of diagnostic technology is unlikely to be applied to all cases of acute encephalitis.

Even under the best of diagnostic circumstances, a significant proportion of cases of encephalitis will remain etiologically undetermined. In a landmark study, which remains in many respects a gold standard of diagnostic investigation, Meyer et al. (1960) were able to identify the etiology of encephalitis in 100 of 139 cases (72%). The diagnostic laboratory evaluation was tailored by a review of the case history, clinical findings, season, and other epidemiologic information. A wide range of laboratory procedures was employed, including numerous serologic assays and cell culture, animal, and embryonated egg isolation systems. Only those cases with sufficient clinical specimens and clinical history were included for analysis. Yet even under these idealized circumstances, 28% of cases remained etiologically undetermined. The diagnostic issue is complicated by the capacity of several processes or viral agents to present similar clinical pictures. In the prospective controlled trial in the United States of therapy of HSE, requiring cerebral biopsy, somewhat over half of the biopsies, 113 of 202, yielded HSV (Whitley et al., 1982). Alternative diagnoses were determined or strongly suggested in 35 of the biopsies, and other evidence of HSE was present in 4. Yet despite the clinical presentations, biopsies, and other evidence, 50 of 202, or roughly 25%, remained undiagnosed.

Significant percentages of acute encephalitis have remained undiagnosed in case series recently reported from several continents. In Toronto, Ontario, Canada, Kolski et al. (1998) were able to make a confirmed or probable etiologic diagnosis in 40% of cases of childhood encephalitis and to suggest a possible diagnosis in a further 26% of cases. In Sweden, Studahl et al. (1998) determined an etiologic agent in 52% of cases of acute viral encephalitis in adults. In Thailand, Chokephaibulkit et al. (2001) were able to identify the viral agents in 26 of 40 children (56%), with arboviral agents (dengue virus and Japanese encephalitis virus) constituting 14 of the 26 positives. Each of these studies was prospective in nature, yet 35 to 48% of cases of encephalitis remained etiologically undetermined.

SUMMARY

To summarize, the crucial task for the clinician confronted with an individual with encephalitis is to maximize the likelihood of making a specific etiologic diagnosis for individual therapy and for public health reasons. The first requirement is that a systematic approach to diagnosis be undertaken, such as we have advocated in our 1986 text and here, relying on clinical and epidemiological features or alternative approaches such as those of Cinque et al. (1996) or Davis (2000). The clinicians, epidemiologists, neuroradiologists, the diagnostic virology laboratory, and the neuropathologist must cooperate closely. The range of potential etiologic candidates will determine which diagnostic samples should be obtained at what times and which assays should be employed. Finally, one must be alert to the possibility of a new agent emerging, such as Nipah virus; the appearance of an epidemic virus in a new location, such as West Nile virus in North America; or an unusual CNS complication of a virus not usually associated with encephalitis, such as adenovirus.

REFERENCES

Chokephaibulkit, K., P. Kankirawatana, S. Apintanapong, V. Pongthapisit, S. Yoksian, and U. Kositanont. 2001. Viral etiologies of encephalitis in Thai children. *Pediatr. Infect. Dis. J.* **20:**216–218.

Cinque, P., G. M. Cleator, T. Weber, P. Monteyne, C. J. Sindic, and A. M. van Loon, for The EU Concerted Action on Virus Meningitis and Encephalitis. 1996. The role of laboratory investigation in the diagnosis and management of patients with suspected herpes simplex encephalitis: a consensus report. *J. Neurol. Neurosurg. Psychiatr.* **61:**339–345.

Davis, L. 2000. Diagnosis and treatment of acute encephalitis. *Neurologist* **6:**145–159.

Goldstein, J. M., B. A. Shaywitz, G. Sze, and S. Nallainathan. 1990. Migraine associated with focal cerebral edema, cerebrospinal fluid pleocytosis, and progressive cerebellar ataxia: MRI documentation. *Neurology* **40:**1284–1287.

Kolski, H., E.-L. Ford-Jones, S. Richardson, M. Petric, S. Nelson, F. Jamieson, S. Blaser, R. Gold, H. Otsubo, H. Heurter, and D. MacGregor. 1998. Etiology of acute childhood encephalitis at the Hospital for Sick Children, Toronto, 1994–1995. *Clin. Infect. Dis.* **26:**398–409.

Meyer, H. M., Jr., R. T. Johnson, I. P. Crawford, H. E. Dascomb, and N. G. Rogers. 1960. Central nervous system syndromes of viral etiology. A study of 713 cases. *Am. J. Med.* **129:**334–347.

Studahl, M., T. Bergstrom, and L. Hagberg. 1998. Acute viral encephalitis in adults—a prospective study. *Scand. J. Infect. Dis.* **30:**215–220.

Whitley, R. J., S.-J. Soong, C. Linneman, Jr., C. Liu, G. Pazin, C.A. Alford, and the National Institute of Allergy and Infectious Diseases Collaborative Antiviral Study Group. 1982. Herpes simplex encephalitis. Clinical assessment. *JAMA* **247:**317–320.

Further Reading

Flint, S. J., L. W. Enquist, R. M. Krug, V. R. Racaniello, and A. M. Skalka (ed.). 2000. Virus cultivation, detection, and genetics, p. 24–56. *Principles of Virology: Molecular Biology, Pathogenesis, and Control.* ASM Press, Washington, D.C.

Hsiung, G. D., C. Y. Fong, and M. L. Landry. 1994. *Hsiung's Diagnostic Virology*, 4th ed. Yale University Press, New Haven, Conn.

Lennette, E. H., and T. F. Smith. 1999. *Laboratory Diagnosis of Viral Infections*. Marcel Dekker, New York, N.Y.

Neal, J. B. 1942. *Encephalitis. A Clinical Study*. Grune and Stratton, New York, N.Y.

Richman, D. D., R. J. Whitley, and F. G. Hayden (ed.). 2002. *Clinical Virology*, 2nd ed. ASM Press, Washington, D.C.

Rivers, T. M. 1948. *Viral and Rickettsial Infections of Man*. J.B. Lippincott, Philadelphia, Pa.

Specter, S., R. L. Hodinka, and S.A. Young. 2000. *Clinical Virology Manual*. ASM Press, Washington, D.C.

Storch, G. A. 2000. *Essentials of Diagnostic Virology*. Churchill-Livingstone, New York, N.Y.

Storch, G. A. 2001. Diagnostic virology, p. 495–531. *In* D. M. Knipe, P. M. Howley, D. E. Griffin, R. A. Lamb, M. A. Martin, B. Roizman, and S. E. Straus (ed.), *Fields Virology*, 4th ed. Lippincott Williams and Wilkins, Philadelphia, Pa.

3

Management Decisions in Acute Encephalitis

COMMON MANAGEMENT ISSUES

Rapidly progressing encephalitis may confront the clinician with urgent problems in management at the time of presentation or soon thereafter. For example, a steadily declining level of consciousness may reflect rising intracranial pressure (ICP), which requires prompt attention. Intervention to control increased ICP or some other urgent problem may be initiated before the specific cause of an encephalitis has been discovered. Many management problems are common to various forms of encephalitis, as discussed in this chapter. The specific management issues and therapies directed at the individual causes of encephalitis are discussed in the appropriate chapters.

The treatment of viral encephalitis has benefited from developments in four areas in recent years. First, the number of antiviral and immunomodulating therapies has multiplied (Anonymous, 2002; Centers for Disease Control and Prevention, 2002 [http://www.HIVATIS.org]; Redington and Tyler, 2002; Yen et al., 2002; Samuel, 2001) (Appendix to this chapter). Antivirals are often targeted to specific molecular functions such as reverse transcriptase in human immunodeficiency virus (HIV). Experience with plasmapheresis, intravenous (i.v.) immunoglobulin (Ig), and high-dose i.v. pulse steroids has been gained in addition to standard steroid therapy. Second, technologies for rapid and sensitive virus diagnosis have emerged, including point of care diagnostic kits, IgM capture methodologies to facilitate presumptive diagnosis based on an early single sample, and most dramatically, cerebrospinal fluid (CSF) PCR identification of infectious agents. CSF PCR has replaced cerebral biopsy in the diagnosis of herpes simplex encephalitis (HSE). Multiplex PCR can be used, for example, with the immunocompromised patient to seek any of several likely viral suspects. In some diseases, quantitative PCR on CSF can be used to track the effectiveness of therapy. Third, dramatic improvements in imaging technology, particularly magnetic resonance imaging (MRI), have increased the capacity to track the evolution and response to treatment of central nervous system (CNS) infections and immune-mediated disorders. Fourth, the development of neurointensive care units with advances in physiological monitoring and the subspecialty of acute care-intensivist neurology have improved the management of severe encephalitis complicated by respiratory compromise, impaired cerebral perfusion, raised ICP, and control of intractable seizures. The patient's clinician must provide guidance to the intensivist with respect to anticipated complications of the suspected infection or process.

TABLE 3.1   Management issues common to many types of encephalitis

Reversal of cause (see the Appendix to this chapter and text
    sections)
        Antiviral therapy
        Immunomodulating therapy
Control of direct complications
        Maintenance of respiration
        Maintenance of cerebral perfusion
        Control of ICP
        Management of fluid and electrolyte balance
        Control of seizures
Prevention of secondary complications
        Decubiti
        Corneal abrasions
        Contractures
        Infections: pneumonia, urinary tract, sepsis
        Deep vein thrombosis, pulmonary embolism
        Gastrointestinal hemorrhage

Acute management of viral encephalitis falls into three categories (Table 3.1). First, therapy for the specific etiology attempts to interrupt the primary pathogenesis. For encephalitis due to virus replication in the brain, this means use of an antiviral agent. The number of antivirals for which specific therapy is available has burgeoned. Attempts to interfere with immune-mediated pathogenic mechanisms in parainfectious encephalomyelitis by immunomodulating therapy are etiologically directed. The therapies specific for various types of encephalitis are discussed for each virus. A checklist for review of therapies is provided as an appendix to this chapter. The second category is the management of the acute manifestations of encephalitis. These include assisted respiration, raised ICP, fluid and electrolytic imbalance, and seizures. Third is the prevention of acute and chronic complications such as superimposed bacterial infection resulting in pneumonia, urinary tract infection, decubiti and sepsis, and the prevention of deep vein thrombosis. Anticoagulation to treat an established deep vein thrombosis can be catastrophic in encephalitis with a hemorrhagic component. Early initiation of physical therapy should be undertaken. It is unacceptable to see a patient who has been otherwise expertly managed through the life-threatening acute stage of encephalitis left with disabling limb contractures.

ANTIVIRAL AND IMMUNOMODULATING THERAPY

Prompt intervention is required to interrupt the pathogenic process in the many types of encephalitis to preserve brain tissue and allow restitution of function. In certain infections and processes, the need is particularly urgent. In HSE, for example, delay in the institution of antiviral therapy is associated with a deterioration of consciousness and poor outcomes. In certain immune-mediated encephalopathies, such as acute hemorrhagic leukoencephalopathy, rampant cerebral swelling poses a threat to life, and urgent measures to control edema, reduce ICP, and blunt an immunopathological process are required.

With the further development of antiviral treatments and rapid virus diagnosis assays, the clinical approach to the treatment of encephalitis is shifting, as is appropriate, from symptomatic treatment to pathogenetically specific interventions. Clinicians now need to treat viral infections of the nervous system that range in diagnostic security from potential, through presumptive, to proven. As a consequence, "empiric coverage" with certain antivirals is a common practice. In these circumstances it is imperative that a structured approach to virus diagnosis, as described in chapter 2, be applied to selection of therapy (Appendix to this chapter).

The clinician confronting the need to intervene in cases of acute encephalitis has two areas of ambiguity. First, any given patient will present varying degrees of uncertainty about the nature of the encephalitis. Second, except in certain infections, notably systemic HIV and herpes simplex virus (HSV), efficacy data is lacking. The justification for treatment rests more often on theoretical considerations, such as immunomodulating therapy in the parainfectious processes, in vitro virus susceptibility data (as yet untranslated into robust clinical trials, such as ribavirin or alpha interferon in certain arboviral infections), and conflicting results from small uncontrolled clinical series. The clinician must be prepared to deal with a fair amount of uncertainty when making initial decisions about treatment. The uncertainty reinforces the need for a structured approach to diagnosis and treatment decisions.

THERAPY BY TYPE OF ENCEPHALITIS

Acute Sporadic

For acute sporadic encephalitis, most clinicians think first of HSE and will often include "coverage" with acyclovir. That is particularly justified when clinical and/or imaging and/or electroencephalogram (EEG) data suggest a frontotemporal localization. Careful monitoring of renal function and continued etiologic workup pending results of the CSF PCR are required. Repeat CSF PCR may be necessary to make the diagnosis or confirm a negative initial result (Weil et al., 2002).

Acute Parainfectious

In many cases of acute parainfectious encephalitis, the therapeutic decision concerns immunomodulating/immunosuppressive therapy. Intervention is most readily justified in patients in whom CNS dysfunction was preceded in the previous few days to weeks by a systemic infection that cleared or by immunization and in whom there is MRI evidence of multifocal white matter disease. Intervention is most urgent when the clinical exam and neuroimaging suggest hemispheral swelling, as in acute hemorrhagic leukoencephalopathy, or diffuse swelling, which can be associated with the encephalopathies following or in conjunction with acute systemic infection, which is often nonspecific, respiratory, or gastrointestinal in nature. High-dose pulse steroid treatment is often the first treatment selected in these circumstances; i.v. Ig, plasmapheresis, and/or repeat pulse steroid treatment are used in those patients that fail to respond sufficiently. To these treatments may be added active immunosuppressive therapy in certain selected cases. Interventions to measure and control dangerously raised ICP may be urgent (see below).

Acute Epidemic

For acute epidemic encephalitis, the clinician will have the advantage of season, location, and clinical profile to sort out the CNS complications of respiratory, enterovirus, and arbovirus infections. The clinician may have the further advantage of knowing if an outbreak is under way. Intervention will be determined by the temporal profile and likely pathogenic agent. Thus, an acute encephalopathy following an influenzalike illness may merit treatment with steroids, whereas such an illness in the context of the acute respiratory illness may justify use of an anti-influenza virus therapy. The latter strategy is bolstered by a positive CSF PCR, if obtainable. In enterovirus "season," encephalitic complications of an otherwise typical aseptic meningitis would merit CSF PCR or nucleic acid sequence-based amplification (NASBA) for enteroviruses and compassionate-use treatment with pleconaril. In the case of arbovirus encephalitis, alpha interferon has been shown to be effective in vitro against West Nile fever virus; a clinical trial was approved as of summer 2002. In vitro data have also demonstrated reduction of viral replication for La Crosse virus and West Nile fever virus by ribavirin.

Subacute/Chronic

Certain encephalitides that commonly present with a subacute/chronic temporal profile can also present acutely. It is diagnostically useful when they occur in the context of a known immunosuppressing illness such as HIV/AIDS or therapeutic immunosuppression for organ transplantation. The presence or proximity in time of clinical clues such as the lesions of zoster or cytomegalovirus (CMV) infection elsewhere in the body are useful to initiate specific antiviral treatment of a presumptive infection. Clues may be found on MRI, such as the distinctive appearance of varicella-zoster virus (VZV) multifocal leukoencephalopathy in immunocompromised patients (Weaver et al., 1999) (Fig. 9.3).

Checklist Review

It is useful to systematically review potentially treatable viral causes of encephalitis. A representative checklist is presented at the end of this chapter. Several caveats must be noted. First, the list is not intended to recommend therapy; rather, it is intended to assist the clinician in considering therapeutic options. The treatments for most types of encephalitis have not been subjected to randomized controlled clinical trials. In many instances, as previously noted, the rationale is only suggestive, based on pathogenesis concepts, in vitro data, conflicting anecdotal reports, or small clinical series. The clinician should consult the relevant chapter to determine the basis and evidence on which various therapies can be considered.

CLINICAL EVALUATION FOR ACUTE MANAGEMENT

Maintenance of vital functions and preservation of neural function are clear goals in the patient with encephalitis. Several decisions may need to be made in the course of management: transfer to an intensive care unit (ICU) for monitoring, endotracheal intubation or tracheostomy and assisted ventilation, the placement of an ICP monitoring device,

TABLE 3.2 Brain stem functions to be evaluated in coma (McNealy and Plum, 1962)

Level of consciousness
Pupillary responses
Respiratory pattern
Oculovestibular responses
    Doll's eye movements
    Ice-water caloric stimulation
Motor responses
    To noxious stimuli
    Plantar responses
    Tone

therapy to reduce ICP, management of intractable seizures, and maintenance of fluid and electrolyte balance. Implementation is dependent on the evolution of the clinical examination supplemented by neuroimaging and physiological monitoring devices.

Crucial in the clinical evaluation for management is an evaluation of brain stem function and the risks to brain stem function. Dysfunction of the brain stem in encephalitis comes about through pressure from swollen hemispheres and/or through a direct effect of virus replication or the immune response on the brain stem itself. During the acute stages of encephalitis, compromise of brain stem functions is apt to be progressive, but the rate of progress and the possibility of stabilization are not predictable. Therefore, serial reproducible clinical, imaging, and physiological examinations are required to follow the course. One of the simplest methods is to assess the response to increasing intensity of stimulation. As consciousness declines, purposeful attempts to avoid a noxious stimulus are followed by ominous signs of decorticate and decerebrate posturing.

McNealy and Plum (1962) employed a simple but reproducible examination (Table 3.2) to assess the lateral and central herniation syndromes in patients with supratentorial mass lesions. The Glasgow Coma Scale (GCS) was developed to facilitate standardized evaluation of progressive neurological dysfunction (Table 3.3). Use of scores in the GCS

TABLE 3.3 GCS scores from each of the three areas are summed for an overall GCS score (Jennett et al., 1977)

Response to stimuli	Score
Motor responses	
Obeys command	6
Localizes stimulus	5
Withdraws from stimulus	4
Abnormal flexion to stimulus	3
Extensor response to stimulus	2
No response	1
Verbal responses	
Oriented	5
Confused conversation	4
Inappropriate words	3
Incomprehensible sounds	2
No response	1
Eye opening	
Spontaneous	4
To speech	3
To pain	2
No response	1

allowed comparisons of the head trauma experience at medical centers in different countries (Jennett et al., 1977). Both the McNealy-Plum and the GCS examinations are useful in following the course of encephalitis. However, it should be recognized that encephalitis with brain stem involvement does not reproduce the progressive clinical patterns of cerebral hemispheral swelling. Serial imaging for evidence of focal mass effect and generalized cerebral swelling amplifies clinical observations. Evoked physiological responses, such as the brain stem auditory-evoked response, provide further monitoring capacity. In patients with evidence of rapidly progressive intracranial swelling, the decision to institute intensive monitoring and support is easily made. In others, however, serial clinical and computerized tomography evaluations will be necessary to determine whether the disease has stabilized or is progressing in a manner requiring intensive monitoring and support.

ACUTE MANAGEMENT DECISIONS

Decisions involved in management of acute encephalitis cover a wide range of facility, nursing, and therapeutic options (Table 3.4).

ICU Management

The patient with acute encephalitis requires frequent neurological evaluation to guide therapeutic intervention. The progression of neurological deterioration in such a patient may be smoothly progressive or irregular. Acute deterioration can result from rapid cerebral swelling, focal brain stem involvement, infarction, venous thrombosis, cerebral shift, hemorrhage, and seizures. Therefore, placement of a patient with encephalitis in an ICU for continuous observation is usually required. In particular, patients with progressive impairment of consciousness require ICU management. Explicit problem-focused nursing care in an ICU setting will allow prompt identification of progression and superimposed processes, improving long-term outcomes (e.g., Krywanio, 1991).

Assisted Respiration

The question of endotracheal intubation and respiratory support requires constant consideration. The rationale for intubation includes both protective and therapeutic considerations. Most obviously, respiratory support is required

TABLE 3.4 Management decisions in acute encephalitis

Location of care—required intensity of observation and
   intervention:
      Standard nursing unit
      ICU
Antiviral agents
Immunomodulating agents
Fluid and electrolyte management
ICP monitoring and therapy
Seizure monitoring and treatment, including non-motor
   status epilepticus
Assisted respiration, intubation, tracheostomy
Hemodynamics, cerebral perfusion, cerebral oxygenation:
   measurement and control

TABLE 3.5 Examples of brain stem compromise in encephalitis

Extrinsic pressure on brain stem from swollen hemispheres
   HSV
   Eastern equine encephalitis
   Reye's and other fulminant encephalopathies
   Acute hemorrhagic leukoencephalitis
Intrinsic involvement of brain stem
   Enteroviruses
      Poliovirus
      Enterovirus 71
   West Nile fever virus
   Nipah virus
   Acute disseminated encephalomyelitis (ADEM)

in the event of compromise of the medullary centers for respiration. However, even partial compromise of oxygen delivery will exacerbate cerebral damage and can be countered by mechanical ventilation. Certain viruses and syndromes have a greater predilection than others to cause respiratory compromise (Table 3.5). Intubation and respirator use facilitate several other therapeutic measures, including controlled hyperventilation and seizure management (Table 3.6).

ICP Monitoring

A third management decision concerns the placement of an ICP monitoring device (Wijdicks, 1997; Vespa and Bleck, 2000). The value of these devices lies in the continuous measurement of ICP, allowing the calculation of cerebral perfusion pressure. In turn, this allows rapid therapeutic intervention when the pressures pass critical points. An ICP monitoring device may be placed because of imaging evidence of cerebral swelling and progressive obtundation that have not responded to attempts to control them. Absolute criteria are difficult to establish because of the unpredictability of stabilization and reversal of the underlying encephalitis. If intracranial swelling is progressive in the face of initial attempts at control, intracranial monitoring is clearly indicated. The danger in such cases is in waiting too long, with subsequent tissue damage. The choice of which device to use is dependent on the local surgical experience, with certain caveats. Contraindications exist for passing monitoring devices through or placing them in parenchyma in patients with bleeding/coagulation defects or a hemorrhagic component in the brain. Placement of a ventricular catheter can be extremely difficult when the ventricles are collapsed; this can require several passes through inflamed tissue.

TABLE 3.6 Rationale for endotracheal intubation and controlled ventilation in encephalitis

Maintenance of optimal oxygenation
Controlled hypocarbia
Prophylaxis against sudden compromise of medullary centers for
   respiration
      By transmitted pressure
      By encephalitic involvement of the brain stem
Facilitation of anticonvulsant therapy of refractory seizures
Required for barbiturate coma therapy

REDUCTION OF RAISED ICP

There are several mechanisms by which viruses cause injury to the brain. Direct viral cytopathic effect and the induction of apoptosis are two principal mechanisms of neural cell death. Mediators of host defense can result in activation of cytotoxic mechanisms, antibody and complement-mediated cytotoxicity, cell-mediated cytotoxicity, and the destructive effects of cytokines. These mechanisms bring in their wake local edema and a breakdown of the blood-brain barrier. Viruses can attack the cerebrovasculature itself, disrupting vasoregulatory mechanisms, injuring the endothelium, and weakening vessel walls. Antigen-antibody complexes and complement activation to cause vasculitis are other mechanisms that can injure the blood-brain barrier. As a consequence of these mechanisms working separately and in concert, local edema is amplified and a generalized breakdown in the blood-brain barrier can occur. For reasons that are poorly understood, each of these mechanisms may have a limited duration and intensity and produce only limited transient effect, if any, on ICP. In other instances, however, such as in HSE, massive local swelling may produce a shift of intracranial contents and a lateral herniation syndrome. Other instances may be associated with massive diffuse swelling, such as in an acute encephalopathy associated with a childhood respiratory illness, overwhelming the compensatory mechanisms and producing a central herniation syndrome.

The raised ICP associated with certain viral infections can reduce cerebral perfusion pressure to the point that widespread ischemic brain injury results. It is crucial to the good outcome of the patient's illness that the risk of raised ICP be repeatedly assessed. Neurological ICUs can provide the capacity to measure ICP and several hemodynamic, blood gas, and physiological variables. These multiple measurements determine when intervention is necessary, the beneficial effects of intervention, and possible deleterious rebound effects of interventions. The integration of the measurements and control of intervention is best handled by a specially trained intensivist.

Several general measures can reduce episodes of raised ICP (Wijdicks, 1997). These include maintenance of adequate oxygen, often by assisted respiration, reduction of fever, maintenance of blood pressure, control of seizures, and proper head elevation, which is often best at 30°. Agitation may present a dilemma because it can be a component of encephalitis, alternating with or preceding depression of consciousness. Episodes of agitation can elevate ICP, and short-acting medication should be used cautiously for control.

Cerebral perfusion pressure must be maintained at 70 mm Hg or above (Vespa and Bleck, 2000). Cerebral perfusion pressure represents the difference between the mean arterial pressure and ICP; its usual range is 70 to 100 mm Hg. The normal ICP waveforms change with increased ICP. Additionally, an upward trend of pressure and the appearance of plateau (A) waves of several minutes in duration and over 50 mm Hg of increase indicate a deteriorating situation (Wijdicks, 1997).

Recommendations for interventions have changed as the field has evolved. Normovolemia, not fluid restriction,

TABLE 3.7 Fluid and electrolyte issues in encephalitis

Control of cerebral edema
Maintenance of cerebral perfusion
Syndrome of inappropriate antidiuretic hormone secretion
Adrenalitis
    CMV
Renal impairment
    Acyclovir therapy
    St. Louis encephalitis virus

is advised (Wijdicks, 1997). Fluid and electrolyte balance are of fundamental importance in the management of encephalitis (Table 3.7). Hyperventilation to reduce pastial CO_2 pressure and thereby reduce cerebral blood flow is very effective. However, the risk of rebound blood flow and the long-term effects of overuse of hyperventilation are concerns (Wijdicks, 1997). Osmotic therapy, such as mannitol, is an extremely effective rapid intervention. Rebound of ICP is also a concern with osmotic intervention. Nonetheless, osmotic therapy, hyperventilation, and optimizing head position are the principal interventions to reduce ICP in encephalitis (Barnett et al., 1988). Drainage of CSF from a ventricular catheter may not be an alternative when ventricles have been reduced to slits. High-dose steroids are often used in the hope that they will blunt the immune reponse underlying some parainfectious encephalopathies and stabilize the blood-brain barrier. They may also blunt cytokine-induced neurotoxicity to some degree (Aiba et al., 2001). However, the effectiveness of that intervention has not been tested in a large randomized controlled trial of encephalopathy/encephalitis. Barbiturate coma, which is difficult to manage, can be attempted in experienced medical centers in cases where other interventions have failed. Surgical decompression of injured tissue is sometimes attempted if medical efforts to reduce ICP are insufficient and if there is a reasonable expectation of good quality of life on survival. Hemicraniectomy has been reported as an aggressive treatment approach (Schwab et al., 1997).

CONTROL OF SEIZURES

Seizures during acute encephalitis can significantly complicate the evaluation of the progress of the underlying disease. Thus if a patient with encephalitis first comes to medical attention following a seizure, recovery from the postictal state can be misinterpreted as improvement of the encephalitis. Conversely, prolonged depression of consciousness following a seizure in a patient under observation for encephalitis can result in an exaggerated sense of deterioration. Motor seizures will be associated wih elevations of ICP. Nonmotor seizures, particularly nonmotor status epilepticus, can cloud the evaluation of the course of encephalitis. Use of antiepileptic drugs that significantly cloud consciousness can further obscure the evaluation. Hence prompt and decisive therapy of seizures, with frequent EEG monitoring, is essential (Fig. 3.1).

Seizure activity in the presence of raised ICP and cerebral swelling produces several destructive effects and must

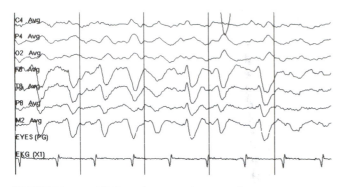

FIGURE 3.1 EEG evaluation of impaired consciousness in a 61-year-old man with alteration of mental status following cerebrovascular accident. EEG tracings from right hemisphere demonstrate rhythmic spike and slow wave activity with nonconvulsive status epilepticus. (Courtesy of Huned Patwa, Yale University School of Medicine.)

be controlled. Increased metabolic activity results in local acidosis, vasodilation, and increased cerebral blood flow. In addition, central venous pressure is significantly increased. Muscular contractions in seizures increase intrathoracic pressure, with increased transmitted venous pressure to the brain. Each of these changes exacerbates cerebral swelling and increases the risk of shift and brain herniation.

Management of seizures is facilitated by endotracheal intubation and mechanical ventilation, thereby allowing delivery of drugs that may cause respiratory suppression. Treatment of intractable seizures in encephalitis may require very high levels of anticonvulsants. Monitoring of serum levels of anticonvulsants is needed to assess the therapeutic response. Anesthetic levels of medication may be required if standard i.v. therapies such as phenytoin, benzodiazepines, and phenobarbital fail. Intractable seizures, with the resulting increase of ICP, are a reason to consider neuromuscular paralysis of the comatose patient. Because barbiturates and neuromuscular paralysis significantly reduce the information available by clinical examination, monitoring by EEG and evoked-potential stimulation is useful.

MANAGEMENT IN THE RECOVERY PERIOD

In the immediate recovery period, bacterial superinfection, decubiti, and pulmonary embolism must be carefully guarded against. Deep vein thrombosis as a prelude to pulmonary embolism must be particularly avoided. Thus the prolonged bed rest and immobility imposed by the illness and sedative medication are significant risk factors. Regularized bedside passive and active range-of-motion exercises should be instituted as soon as feasible. There is no convenient rule of thumb to decide when anticoagulants can be safely administered in cases where tissue breakdown or a hemorrhagic component occurs. Prevention is crucial.

An assessment of motor function must be made in order to plan physical therapy. Early and consistent rehabilitation efforts are paramount to prevent the development of contractures. The progress of a bed-bound patient to a

wheelchair, walking frame, crutches, walking stick, and finally to unaided ambulation requires continual therapy and assessment. Similarly, the use of various splints and braces will evolve as the patient improves or stabilizes. The need for anticonvulsant medication should also be periodically reviewed.

Cognitive function, intelligence, memory, and speech function (Marshall, 1982) should be tested prior to discharge to a rehabilitative setting, and plans for therapy should be established. Repeat testing at 6 months and 1 year should give evidence of the progress and ultimate outlook. Altered behavior and personality often bring difficult emotional problems for families and therapeutic problems for medical staff. At worst, they can produce dangerously aggressive behavior and verbal abusiveness, requiring use of major tranquilizing medication. Not infrequently it will result in "sundowning," or increased activity in the hours of darkness. Although mild nighttime sedation often suffices, care should be exercised to guard against paradoxical responses to such medication. In children and adolescents, careful attention should be paid to the appropriate level of education. Too rapid a return to standard schooling may impose further stresses on a recovering intellect. However, the capacity for significant improvement in children months after encephalitis is sometimes remarkable. Regularized testing and assessment at 3-month intervals would seem appropriate for children.

Various disabilities may develop in the recovery or postrecovery periods. The postencephalitic parkinsonism that developed in many patients weeks or months following von Economo's encephalitis lethargica is well known. Postencephalitic behavioral disorders have long been recognized (Bender, 1942). They may occur de novo in the recovery period or be recognized as the patient regains other functions. While some behavioral disorders are permanent, many gradually disappear. The incidence of seizures following encephalitis is greatest in those in whom seizures occurred during the acute illness. Annegers et al. (1988) found a cumulative risk of 10% at 5 years for those who had had seizures in the acute period; cumulative risk increased to 22% by 20 years. In contrast, the risk was 10% at 20 years for those without seizures in the acute period.

There is great variation in outcomes of various types of encephalitis (Tselis and Booss, 2000). There is also great variation in both the degree and speed of recovery in survivors. We have observed very ill patients reverse course rapidly during the acute phase and be well on the way to recovery within a day or two. At the other end of the spectrum are the patients who demonstrate very little immediate recovery after stabilization and who require prolonged convalescent care or permanent institutionalization.

Some patients who leave the acute-care hospital with major defects may significantly improve over several months to a year or more. For example, we have observed an 8-year-old girl who experienced an encephalitis of undiagnosed etiology and left the acute-care hospital with significant motor and language defects and seizures. At the follow-up examination at 10 weeks, the seizures had stopped, but she was aphasic and had little use of her right hand. At the 5-month visit, however, her neurological examination was altogether normal, including motor and speech functions.

Remarkable recovery after prolonged periods can also occur in adults. A 28-year-old man left the acute-care facility with global aphasia and severe dementia and required total care. Little improvement was noted in a long-term-care facility until 6 months later; marked improvement was described in the 10th month. He was verbally fluent and capable of discharge to home.

Both of these cases demonstrate the capacity of some patients for long-term recovery in the face of apparently devastating disease. Therefore, a long-term management plan and scheduled follow-up evaluations are crucial. The plan must take into account the setting in which care is provided as well as the type of rehabilitation offered. Some patients are able to return home after acute-care hospitalization with only moderate household assistance. For others, however, transfer to a rehabilitation facility, convalescent hospital, or chronic-care hospital may be required. Regularly scheduled

follow-up visits are needed to assess progress, adjust treatment, and manage late-developing sequelae.

APPENDIX

ENCEPHALITIS TREATMENT CHECKLIST ARRANGED BY CLINICAL CLASSIFICATION

This list does not constitute a series of recommendations and is not exhaustive, but it is intended to orient the clinician to potential interventions. In a few instances, such as HSE, systemic HIV infection, and Japanese encephalitis, controlled trials have been conducted. In other instances, such as immunomodulating therapy in parainfectious encephalomyelitis, therapy is based on pathogenesis concepts but without large controlled clinical trials. In many instances, however, interventions are based on small uncontrolled clinical trials with conflicting data. The reader is referred to the text for descriptions of the evidence.

Encephalitis/agent[a]	Interventions to consider	Chapter
Acute sporadic		
HSV	Acyclovir	4
HHV-6	Foscarnet, ganciclovir	5
B virus of monkeys	Acyclovir, foscarnet, ganciclovir	6
Rabies prophylaxis	Wound care, antiserum, vaccine	6
Acute parainfectious		
Encephalopathy	i.v. pulse steroids	8
ADEM	i.v. pulse steroids	
	i.v. Ig	
	Plasmapheresis	
Postvaccination ADEM or encephalopathy	Immunomodulatory therapy as above	8
VZV in immunocompetent or immunocompromised		
Encephalitis	Acyclovir and steroid	9
Herpes zoster ophthalmicus and delayed contralateral hemiplegia	Acyclovir and steroid	9
Vasculitis/vasculopathy	Acyclovir and steroid	
Myelitis	Acyclovir and steroid	9
Brain stem	Acyclovir and steroid	9
Multifocal VZV leukoencephalopathy	Acyclovir and steroid	13
Adult cerebellitis	Acyclovir and steroid	9
Acute epidemic, nonarbovirus		
Postinfluenzal ADEM	Immunomodulatory therapy as above	8, 10
Enteroviruses	Pleconaril	10
Nipah virus	Ribavirin	10
Acute epidemic, arbovirus		
West Nile fever	Alpha interferon	11
La Crosse virus	Ribavirin	11
Rift Valley fever	Ribavirin	11
Chronic epidemic		
HIV	Four classes of antiretroviral therapy	12
Subacute/chronic in immunocompromised		
PML	Immune reconstitution such as highly active antiretroviral therapy in HIV. Consider cidofovir, topotecan, or alpha interferon	13
CMV	Foscarnet, ganciclovir, cidofovir	13
Enteroviruses	Pleconaril, specific Ig	13

(Continued on next page)

APPENDIX: Encephalitis treatment checklist arranged by clinical classification (*Continued*)

Encephalitis/agent[a]	Interventions to consider	Chapter
Immunosuppressive (or inclusion-bearing) measles	Ribavirin	13
VZV	Acyclovir	9
HHV-6	Foscarnet, ganciclovir	13
Subacute/chronic in immunocompetent		
Subacute sclerosing encephalitis	Alpha interferon, intraventricular	14
	Isoprinosine, orally	
	Ribavirin, i.v.	
Progressive rubella encephalitis	Plasmapheresis	14
HTLV-1-associated myelopathy/tropical spastic paraparesis	Steroid in rapidly evolving cases or following transfusion	14
	In chronic cases, alpha interferon, anti-Tac antibody, lamivudine	14
Rasmussen's encephalitis	Plasmapheresis	14
	Antiviral if CSF PCR or biopsy evidence of virus	
	Hemispherectomy	
Prion disorders		
CJD, vCJD	Various interventions, local protocols under way	15

[a] HHV-6, human herpesvirus 6; PML, progressive multifocal leukoencephalopathy; HTLV-1, human T-cell leukemia virus type 1; CJD, Creutzfeldt-Jakob disease; vCJD, variant CJD.

REFERENCES

Aiba, H., M. Mochizuki, M. Kimura, and H. Hojo. 2001. Predictive value of serum interleukin-6 level in influenza virus-associated encephalopathy. *Neurology* **57:**295–299.

Annegers, J. F., W. A. Hanser, E. Beghi, A. Nicolosi, and L. T. Kurland. 1988. The risk of unprovoked seizures after encephalitis and meningitis. *Neurology* **38:**1407–1410.

Anonymous. 2002. Drugs for non-HIV viral infections. *Med. Letter* **44:**9–16.

Barnett, G. H., A. H. Ropper, and J. Romeo. 1988. Intracranial pressure and outcome in adult encephalitis. *J. Neurosurg.* **68:**585–588.

Bender, L. 1942. Post-encephalitic behavior disorders in childhood, p. 361–384. *In* J. B. Neal (ed.), *Encephalitis. A Clinical Study.* Grune and Stratton, New York, N.Y.

Centers for Disease Control and Prevention. 2002. Guidelines for using anti-retroviral agents among HIV infected adults and adolescents: recommendations of the Panel on Clinical Practices for Treatment of HIV. *Morb. Mortal. Wkly. Rep.* **51(RR7):** 1–56 plus inside covers.

Jennett, B., G. Teasdale, S. Galbraith, J. Pickard, H. Grant, R. Braakman, C. Avezaat, A. Mass, J. Minderhoud, C. J. Vecht, J. Heiden, R. Small, W. Caton, and T. Kurze. 1977. Severe head injuries in three countries. *J. Neurol. Neurosurg. Psychiatr.* **40:**291–298.

Krywanio, M. L. 1991. Varicella encephalitis. *J. Neurosci. Nursing* **23:**363–368.

Marshall, R. C. 1982. Language and speech recovery in a case of viral encephalitis. *Brain Lang.* **17:**316–326.

McNealy, D. E., and F. Plum. 1962. Brain stem dysfunction with supratentorial mass lesions. *Arch. Neurol.* **7:**10–32.

Redington, J. J., and K. L. Tyler. 2002. Viral infections of the nervous system, 2002. Update on diagnosis and treatment. *Arch. Neurol.* **59:**712–718.

Samuel, C. E. 2001. Antiviral actions of interferons. *Clin. Microbiol. Rev.* **14:**778–809.

Schwab, S., E. Junger, M. Spranger, A. Dorfler, F. Albert, H. H. Steiner, and W. Hacke. 1997. An aggressive treatment approach in severe encephalitis. *Neurology* **48:**412–417.

Tselis, A. C., and J. Booss. 2000. Viral encephalitis, p. 237–256. *In* R. W. Evans, D. S. Baskin, and F. M. Yatsu (ed.), *Prognosis of Neurological Disorders.* Oxford University Press, New York, N.Y.

Vespa, P. M., and T. P. Bleck. 2000. Principles of neurointensive care, p. 917–930. *In* W. G. Bradley, R. B. Daroff, G. M. Fenichel, and C. D. Marsden (ed.), *Neurology in Clinical Practice*, 3rd ed. Butterworth Heineman, Boston, Mass.

Weaver, S., M. K. Rosenblum, and L. M. DeAngelis. 1999. Herpes varicella zoster encephalitis in immunocompromised patients. *Neurology* **52:**193–195.

Weil, A. A., C. A. Glaser, Z. Amad, and B. Forghani. 2002. Patients with suspected herpes simplex encephalitis: rethinking an initial negative polymerase chain result. *Clin. Infect. Dis.* **34:**1154–1157.

Wijdicks, E. F. M. 1997. *The Clinical Practice of Critical Care Neurology.* Lippincott-Raven Publishers, Philadelphia, Pa.

Yen, P. G., S. M. Hammer, C. C. J. Carpenter, D. A. Cooper, M. A. Fischl, J. M. Gatell, B. G. Gazzaard, M. S. Hirsch, D. M. Jacobsen, D. A. Katzenstein, J. S. G. Montaner, D. D. Richman, M. S. Saag, M. Schechter, R. T. Schooley, M. A. Thompson, S. Vella, and P. A. Volberding. 2002. Anti-retroviral treatment for adult HIV infection in 2002. Updated recommendations of the International AIDS Society-USA Panel. *JAMA* **288:**222–235.

ACUTE SPORADIC ENCEPHALITIS

Herpes Simplex Encephalitis

INTRODUCTION AND CLASSIFICATION OF ACUTE SPORADIC ENCEPHALITIS

When confronted with a case of apparent sporadic encephalitis, most clinicians focus on the possibility of herpes simplex encephalitis (HSE). The evaluation will be expedited, and antiviral therapy will often be started promptly before the deterioration of consciousness. This is appropriate because one of the most important prognostic indicators for the outcome of HSE is the level of consciousness. On the other hand, the initiation of antiviral therapy may carry with it the presumption that the diagnosis has been accepted and further workup for etiology may be discontinued. This is unfortunate because there are numerous causes of encephalitis that can be diagnosed if the clinician selects the proper assays for the diagnostic virology laboratory (e.g., Bia et al. [1980]).

Once the clinician has started the process of ruling out other infectious causes such as meningitis and abscess, noninfectious causes such as stroke, primary or metastatic tumors, and metabolic encephalopathy must also be considered. When encephalitis is included in the differential diagnosis, the various types of encephalitis—subacute and chronic versus acute; epidemic versus sporadic; and infectious versus postinfectious—must be evaluated by the history, physical examination, and laboratory evaluations as reviewed in chapter 2.

Further evaluation of the multiple potential viruses that can cause sporadic infectious encephalitis is greatly facilitated by a systematic diagnostic process (Booss and Esiri, 1986; Cinque et al., 1996; Davis, 2000). The approach that we prefer distinguishes encephalitides that can infect other organs as well as the central nervous system (CNS), those for which there is an animal reservoir or insect vector, and HSE, which under most circumstances is restricted to the brain (Table 4.1). Exceptions occur in immunocompromised patients and in herpes simplex virus (HSV) infections in the neonate, which are often disseminated.

Attention to the course of the illness is diagnostically useful. Prompt recovery from depressed consciousness, for example, can occur in virus-triggered diffuse encephalopathy. Focality or multifocality may emerge over time in the clinical exam and/or in neuroimaging. Such changes in the clinical course and exam will suggest a different or narrowed spectrum of etiologies.

TABLE 4.1 Types of acute sporadic encephalitis and
location of discussion in this volume

Encephalitis alone
  HSV—this chapter
Encephalitis with systemic disease—chapter 5
  Exanthematous diseases
    Parvovirus B-19
    Human herpesvirus 6
    Considered elsewhere in this volume
      Measles—chapters 7 and 8
      Rubella—chapters 7 and 8
      Chicken pox, zoster—chapter 9
      Enteroviruses—chapter 10
  Mumps virus
  Epstein-Barr virus
  Adenovirus
  Respiratory diseases—chapter 10
  Gastroenteritis
    Rotavirus
  Hepatitis viruses
Encephalitis viruses with animal reservoirs—chapter 6
  Sporadic arboviruses—chapter 11
  Lymphocytic choriomeningitis virus
  Rabies virus
  B virus of monkeys
  Nipah virus—chapter 10

HSV

HSV is one of a large group, the herpesviruses, that are characterized by their similar morphology, large DNA genomes, and tendency to persist in their natural hosts. The virus particles measure 120 to 300 nm in diameter and contain double-stranded DNA, which encodes at least 77 genes. The tegument surrounding the capsid consists of a bilayered membrane containing antigenic glycoproteins and lipid (Roizman, 1982; Wildy et al., 1982; Whitley, 1996). Natural infection with HSV is confined to humans. Two types of HSV, types 1 and 2 (HSV-1 and HSV-2), have been distinguished; these differ slightly in antigenic, physical, chemical, and biological properties and in the lesions they produce in humans. They share approximately 50% DNA identity.

The type 1 virus usually causes a stomatitis on primary infection. This is usually asymptomatic and gives rise to systemic antibody formation. Serological studies indicate that up to 90% of the adult population has been exposed to this virus (Nahmias and Roizman, 1973). Following primary infection, the virus is thought to travel centripetally along branches of the trigeminal nerve and produce a latent infection of the trigeminal ganglion. Latent infection can be demonstrated by explantation of ganglion tissue and maintenance in tissue culture or by detection of HSV DNA by PCR. By these techniques, up to 90% of humans can be shown to yield HSV-1 from trigeminal ganglia (Bastian et al., 1972; Baringer and Swoveland, 1973; Plummer, 1973; Rodda et al., 1973), and the virus is occasionally recoverable from other ganglia (Warren et al., 1978).

In about 20% of the population, primary infection is followed at intervals by the recrudescence of vesicular eruptions (cold sores), usually in the region of the lips. These appear under the poorly understood influence of diverse factors such as fever, exposure to strong sunlight, or, in females, menstruation. Virus can be recovered from these recurrent lesions and is also quite commonly shed from the oral cavity even in the absence of overt lesions. Recrudescent lesions in territory supplied by the trigeminal nerve are almost the rule following surgical section of the proximal trigeminal root in patients with trigeminal neuralgia. This was noted by Cushing as early as 1904 and occurred in 90% of a series of patients studied by Carton (1953). Reactivation also occurs with other types of surgical manipulation of the trigeminal root and ganglion, such as microvascular decompression (Tenser, 1998). It requires the presence of an intact nerve supply between the trigeminal ganglion and the skin.

Experimental infection of laboratory animals with HSV-1 has been studied from the 1920s to the present time. These studies have shown that the virus travels along axons and that latency in ganglia is maintained within neurons (Cook et al., 1974; McLennan and Darby, 1980). During latency, infectious virus is not recoverable but a latency-associated RNA transcript is detectable, which does not code for a known protein but can facilitate reactivation (Wagner and Bloom, 1997).

Infection with type 2 virus is generally venereal. It produces vesicular eruptions on genital mucosa and neighboring skin. Primary infection can occur at birth during passage through an infected birth canal, but most primary infections occur with the onset of sexual maturity in teenagers or young adults. The type 2 virus is recoverable from sacral sensory ganglia at autopsy in 10 to 15% of subjects sampled (Baringer, 1974). Recrudescent lesions due to the type 2 virus occur intermittently, as with type 1 virus, and are often associated with painful dysasthesia referable to the affected nerve root and sometimes give rise to recurrent aseptic meningitis (Kleinschmidt-DeMasters and Gilden, 2001; Love and Wiley, 2002). Very rarely, HSV-2 is the cause of acute encephalitis or transverse myelitis (Aurelius et al., 1993; Nakajima et al., 1998).

HISTORICAL CONSIDERATIONS

HSV-1 is so ubiquitous that only towards the middle of the last century did it begin to be accepted that it can occasionally cause a severe form of encephalitis. Skepticism regarding a role for HSV in the etiology of encephalitis had been generated earlier when Levaditti et al. (1922) claimed that HSV was the cause of encephalitis lethargica, a claim that could not subsequently be substantiated (Flexner, 1923). However, Smith et al. (1941) reported isolation of HSV from the brain of an infant with severe acute encephalitis, and Haymaker (1949) described three cases of acute sporadic encephalitis in adults in which HSV was cultured from the brain. Many subsequent reports have confirmed HSV-1 as the usual cause of acute necrotizing encephalitis.

Precise figures on the incidence of encephalitis caused by HSV are difficult to obtain because the diagnosis tends to be confirmed only in specialized medical centers. Nahmias and Dowdle (1968) estimated a figure of one case per million population per year in the United States. Longson (1975) gave a similar figure of 50 cases a year in the United Kingdom, and Skoldenberg et al. (1984) gave an estimated incidence of 2.3 cases per million inhabitants per year in Sweden. Although these figures indicate that HSE is an uncommon disease, its high mortality rate (about 70% in untreated cases) makes it the most common cause of fatal sporadic encephalitis (Meyer et al., 1960; Rappel et al., 1971; Baringer, 1978). Morbidity is also high, with serious neurological sequelae remaining in about 50% of untreated survivors (Whitley et al., 1981), though this figure has been much reduced by treatment with acyclovir since the 1980s.

Although there are studies of HSV-1 mutants that have genes capable of modulating neurovirulence and neuroinvasiveness (Izumi and Stevens, 1990; Stevens, 1993; Chou et al., 1990), there is no evidence for person-to-person transmission of encephalitis by a neurovirulent strain of HSV. Two independent spatial-temporal clusters of HSE were investigated to determine if a single virus caused each cluster (Hammer et al., 1980; Landry et al., 1983). In both instances, endonuclease mapping of the viral isolates demonstrated the viruses within the cluster to be different. That is, separation of genome fragments by gel electrophoresis revealed each isolate to have a separate pattern. Although such data does not rule out the possibility of a neurovirulent sequence located within fragments of various sizes, the rarity of spatial-temporal clusters argues against such a sequence.

PATHOLOGY OF HSE

Naked-Eye Appearance of the Brain

In most cases of HSE, the naked-eye appearance of the brain is quite distinctive, whether the patient dies at a relatively acute stage of the disease or months or years later. Most of the patients included in autopsy studies (Haymaker, 1949; Haymaker et al., 1958; Drachman and Adams, 1962; Hughes, 1969; Kleihues, 1969; Adams and Miller, 1973) have died in week 2 to 6 following the onset of neurological symptoms. In these cases, the brain shows acute inflammation, congestion, and softening centered on the temporal lobes (Fig. 4.1). Both temporal lobes are invariably affected but one often much more severely so than the other, and there may be only one visibly affected on naked-eye examination. The meninges overlying the temporal and inferior frontal lobes may appear slightly cloudy and congested. At times the areas affected extend from the temporal lobes into neighboring inferior frontal lobes (orbital gyri) and parietal and occipital lobes. Upon slicing the brain, the involvement of deeper areas is apparent. This can include the temporal lobes, particularly their anterior parts, the unci, amygdaloid nuclei, hippocampi, and insulae and parahippocampal, posterior orbital, fusiform, and cingulate gyri (Fig. 4.2). In acute cases in these areas there is swelling, congestion, and frequently petechial or larger hemorrhages.

After 2 weeks or so, these changes proceed to frank necrosis and liquefaction (Fig. 4.3). The edema extends beyond the areas immediately involved, and the asymmetry of the process results in midline shift and subfalcine herniation. Uncal herniation is frequently bilateral but asymmetrical in severity. Hemorrhages in the upper brain stem and acute hemorrhagic infarction in the posterior cerebral arterial territory may be evident as a consequence of uncal herniation.

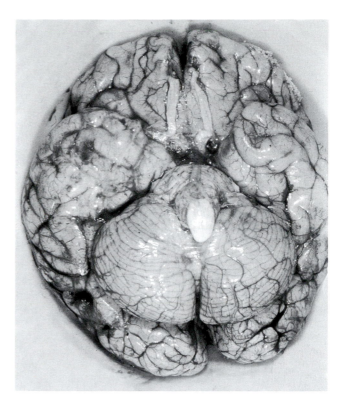

FIGURE 4.1 Appearance of undersurface of the brain in acute HSE. There are swelling, petechial hemorrhages, and necrosis of the temporal lobes, more marked on the right (left in picture).

Microscopic Appearances

Microscopic examination generally reveals intense destructive and inflammatory changes in the areas affected. However, at the earliest stage, as seen in patients who died or were subjected to biopsy in the first week after onset of neurological illness, the histological changes are not dramatic

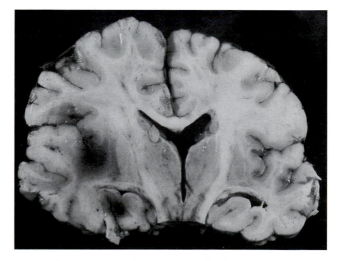

FIGURE 4.2 Coronal slice across the brain from a case of acute HSE (14 days' duration) showing hemorrhage and swelling of the left temporal lobe and insula.

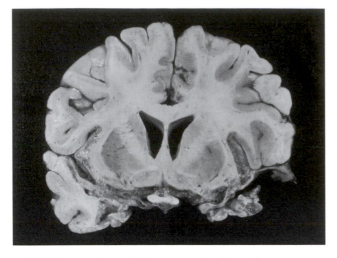

FIGURE 4.3 Coronal slice across the brain from a case in which symptoms of HSE commenced 6 weeks before death. Liquefaction necrosis is evident in both temporal lobes, worse on the right than the left. The insula is affected bilaterally and the cingulate gyrus is affected on the right.

and may be nonspecific. There is congestion of the capillaries and other small vessels in the cerebral cortex and subcortical white matter, often with petechial hemorrhages and acute shrinkage and eosinophilia of neurons, possibly with some foci of neuronophagia (Fig. 4.4). Edema may be evident from the spongy state of the cortex, seen as multiple rounded empty spaces. Edema is sometimes laminar in distribution in the cortex (Fig. 4.5). Astrocytes and microglia invariably show early change with swelling of the cell body, but this becomes more evident in the second and third weeks.

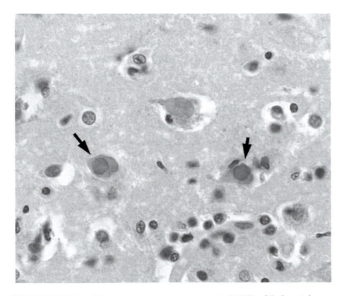

FIGURE 4.4 Microscopic appearance in HSE of 5 days' duration. There is evidence of early inflammation and eosinophilic neurons containing nuclear inclusion bodies (arrows). Hematoxylin and eosin stain.

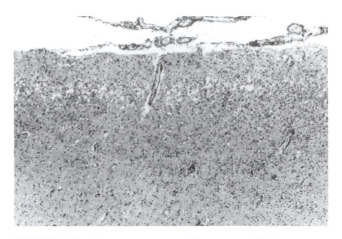

FIGURE 4.5 Low-power view of the temporal lobe cortex in a case of HSE of 14 days' duration. Inflammation is seen in the meninges and cortex, and edema is prominent in layer 2 of the cortex. Hematoxylin and eosin stain.

A useful diagnostic feature in a few cases is the presence of intranuclear inclusion bodies (Cowdry type A inclusions). These have an eosinophilic, homogeneous appearance, and they are frequently surrounded by a clear unstained zone beyond which lies a rim of marginated chromatin. Cowdry type A inclusions are more likely to be seen in the first week than later, but their absence does not exclude the diagnosis. Use of Bouin's fixative is said to improve their visualization. They are particularly numerous in immunosuppressed subjects with human immunodeficiency virus (HIV) infection (Tan et al., 1993).

Perivascular inflammation is present in gray and white matter and in the meninges, particularly in sulci adjacent to involved cortex. The infiltrate at this stage is relatively scant—one or two cell layers in width in perivascular spaces—and consists of lymphocytes, a few macrophages, and occasional plasma cells (Fig. 1.3a). Neutrophil polymorphs are also frequently present in perivascular cuffs and in parenchyma where neurons are acutely degenerate.

The immunoperoxidase technique is useful for demonstrating HSV antigens on sections of paraffin-embedded material or on smears (Benjamin and Ray, 1975; Kumanishi and Hirano, 1978). With this technique many of the shrunken, eosinophilic cortical neurons, including those containing inclusion bodies, will be found to contain viral antigen (Fig. 4.6). This may be present in both cytoplasm and nucleus of neurons and glial cells (astrocytes, oligodendrocytes, and, rarely, ependymal cells). Inclusion bodies themselves stain positively for viral antigen. Neurons and glial cells sometimes contain viral antigen when inflammation is scant or even absent and when appearances in a small biopsy sample might be interpreted as those of a different process, such as hypoxia, or as nondiagnostic. When HSE is suspected clinically, it is therefore important to search for viral antigen, even if the characteristic features of encephalitis are not present, particularly if the biopsy is taken during the first week of the course of the disease.

In the second and third weeks of the disease the congestion and edema persist and petechial or larger hemorrhages

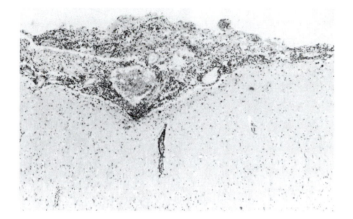

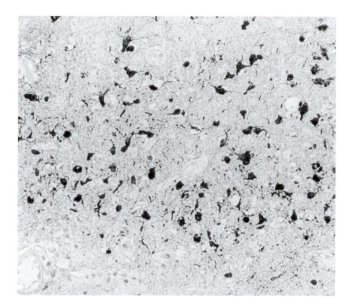

FIGURE 4.6 Cortical neurons intensely stained for HSV antigen in acute encephalitis. Counterstained with hematoxylin.

may be present. These suggest the development of endothelial damage, and indeed fibrinoid necrosis or fibrin thrombi are sometimes noted in small vessels (Haymaker et al., 1958). Acute neuronal degeneration is still present. Some authors have suggested on the basis of the endothelial damage and the presence of fibrin thrombi in small vessels, together with the neuronal change, which may be morphologically indistinguishable from "acute ischemic change," that much of the damage that occurs in HSE is due to secondary vascular pathology. However, the abundance of viral antigen, which can be demonstrated using the immunoperoxidase technique, often in neurons displaying features of acute ischemic change, suggests that virus-mediated damage is the more important process in the intense necrosis that occurs (Esiri, 1982). This view also accords with the highly lytic effects of the virus in tissue culture and with the observation of extensive and characteristic necrosis in cases of HIV with HSV-1 encephalitis, despite a paucity of inflammation (Tan et al., 1993; Chrétien et al., 1996). All of the neurons and many of the glial elements in the most affected areas are killed. The inflammatory reaction mounts so that in the second and third weeks the perivascular cuffs in the cortex and white matter are several cells thick. Inflammatory cells are present in large numbers in the parenchyma and meninges (Fig. 4.7). Macrophages fill the necrotic areas, as they do in an acute infarct, and there is a well marked astrocytosis around the necrotic areas. The lymphocytic and plasma cell infiltrate is far more abundant than in an infarct but can resemble that seen around an abscess (Fig. 4.8). Viral antigen is still frequently demonstrable during the second week but is less abundant during the third week and disappears completely at the end of the third week (Esiri, 1982). The factors responsible for the disappearance of viral antigen are not known, but presumably the mounting immunological response plays a major part. Sites containing the most

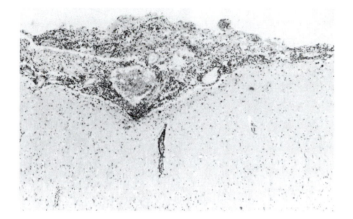

FIGURE 4.7 Low-power view of temporal cortex in HSE (16 days' duration) showing heavy meningeal inflammatory infiltrate. Hematoxylin and eosin stain.

abundant viral antigen are illustrated diagrammatically in Fig. 4.9.

Invariably, the pathological changes seen microscopically extend beyond the areas that are abnormal to naked-eye inspection. Sometimes microscopic damage involves all of the temporal lobe and adjacent parts of the frontal, parietal, and occipital lobes. Other parts of the brain are usually spared, including the lateral and superior parts of the frontal lobes, the basal ganglia (apart from the claustrum and inferior margins of the caudate, putamen, and globus pallidus, where they lie adjacent to more severely damaged structures), the superior aspects of the parietal and occipital lobes, and the pons, medulla, and cerebellum. Even in these areas there are frequently perivascular cuffs of inflammatory cells.

In contrast to the characteristic pattern of HSV-1 encephalitis described here, the virus may on exception cause a primary brain stem encephalitis (Tyler et al., 1995; Ellison and Hanson, 1977; Roman-Campos and Toro, 1980; Schmidbauer et al., 1989; Rose et al., 1992; Mertens et al., 1993; Sakakibara et al., 1998) or a myelitis (Folpe et al., 1994; Petereit et al., 1996; Shyu et al., 1993).

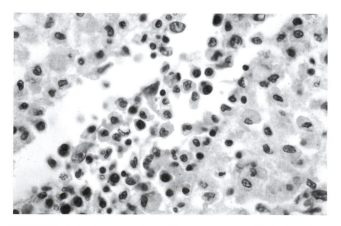

FIGURE 4.8 Perivascular infiltrate in acute HSE (12 days' duration). A few lymphocytes and more frequent plasma cells and macrophages are present. Hematoxylin and eosin stain.

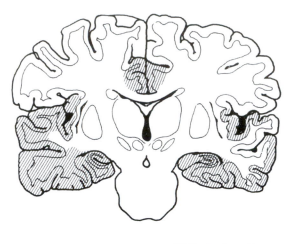

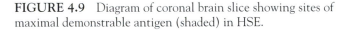

FIGURE 4.9   Diagram of coronal brain slice showing sites of maximal demonstrable antigen (shaded) in HSE.

Although viral antigen disappears about the end of the third week of the illness, the inflammation persists for several more weeks in a severe form and then only gradually subsides, so that some perivascular cuffing with lymphocytes and occasional plasma cells may still be present three or more years later. Marked reactive gliosis and some endothelial proliferation are seen for many weeks and are followed by the development of fibrillary glial scarring. Lipid-filled phagocytes are numerous for several weeks and then gradually diminish over succeeding months. The leptomeninges overlying the

necrotic tissue are initially inflamed and later thickened by collagen deposition. Cysts come to occupy the areas of intense destruction.

The various appearances of the brain years later have been well described by Hierons et al. (1978). They are distinctive chiefly by the pattern of damage remaining, with the temporal poles "being reduced to a collapsed bag of thickened leptomeninges" (Fig. 4.10). Secondary degeneration is seen in the later stages in the fornices and in the cerebral peduncles, where temporopontine fibers in particular are lost. The mammillary bodies, septal nuclei, and parts of the thalamus may also show some evidence of scarring.

Other Pathology

There is no other associated cerebral pathology in most cases of HSE. No increased incidence has been recorded in association with immunosuppression or immunodeficiency, although these states are associated with unusually severe peripheral infections with HSV. We have seen one case in which there was a long history of illness clinically diagnosed as multiple sclerosis and an acute terminal neurological illness that proved to be HSE. The presence of lesions characteristic of both diseases was confirmed at autopsy, and HSV was cultured from the brain. Acute hemorrhagic leukoencephalitis (Martins et al., 1964) and perivenous encephalitis (Koenig et al., 1979) (chapters 7 and 8, respectively) have been described as rare complications of HSE.

Electron Microscopy

Electron microscopy of samples from areas containing viral antigen reveals the characteristic herpes virions (Fig. 4.11).

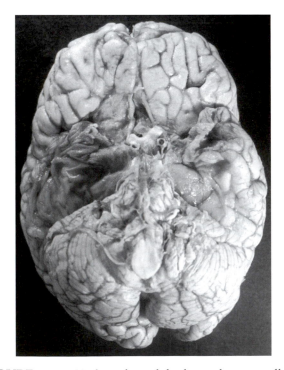

FIGURE 4.10   Undersurface of the brain showing collapse and necrosis of the temporal lobes (the right being the most affected) (on left in figure) from a case of HSE (6 months' survival).

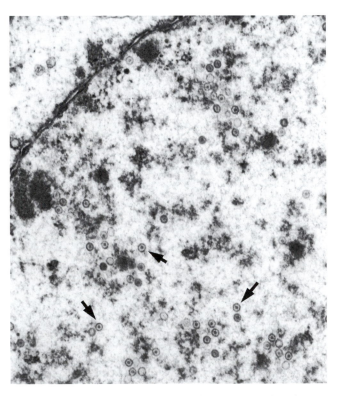

FIGURE 4.11   Electron micrograph of intranuclear herpes virions (arrows) from a biopsy of the temporal lobe in a case of HSE. Uranyl acetate and lead citrate stain; ×25,200.

However, electron microscopy is a relatively insensitive diagnostic procedure. In a series of reported cases it yielded positive results in only 45% of biopsies from which HSV was cultured (Nahmias et al., 1982). Electron microscopic appearances of herpes simplex virions are indistinguishable morphologically from other herpes group viruses. Naked nucleocapsids, some possessing an electron-dense DNA core enclosed in an oval or hexagonal nucleocapsid, are seen in neuronal and glial nuclei and measure approximately 100 nm in diameter. Enveloped particles with an outer membrane derived from host nuclear membrane are seen in neuronal and glial cell cytoplasm and measure 150 to 200 nm in diameter.

Many cases in which latent HSV-1 has been demonstrated in the brain have shown no evidence of neurological disease, and the question arises of how more frequent reactivation of latent virus in the CNS, as occurs peripherally, is avoided. It has been suggested, for example, that nerve growth factor may be protective against reactivation (Steiner and Kennedy, 1995). Conversely, risk factors need to be identified for acute HSV-1.

PATHOLOGY OF ATYPICAL HSV-1 ENCEPHALITIS AND HSV-2 ENCEPHALITIS AND MYELITIS

Occasional cases of acute encephalitis due to HSV-1 show atypical distribution of damage. The brain stem is the most common site of such atypical infection.

HSV-2 produces a broader spectrum of disease. Classically, it was recognized to give rise to a blood-borne widespread necrotizing encephalitis in neonates and was associated with dissemination of the virus to other organs as well. This pattern of spread was thought to follow infection acquired from an infected birth canal. However, in one recent study (Sauerbrei et al., 2000), in addition to being associated with two such cases of infection in newborns, HSV-2 was also associated with focal encephalitis in three adults and with transverse lumbar myelitis in two adults. Others have described brain stem encephalitis and recurrent myelitis due to HSV-2 (Nakajima et al., 1995).

PATHOGENESIS OF HSE

The pathogenesis of encephalitis due to HSV-1 is unclear. The problem is to understand why a virus that establishes a latent infection in the great majority of the population, from which it is periodically reactivated and shed with little or no morbidity, occasionally gives rise to a fulminating encephalitis. It is known that the majority (70%) of patients with HSE possess antibodies to the virus at the outset of the illness, indicating that they have been previously exposed to the virus (Nahmias et al., 1982), and some patients also have a known history of recurrent cold sores. In these patients encephalitis represents a secondary or recurrent infection. DNA restriction enzyme analysis has shown that in a few such cases the virus present in the brain is identical to that recoverable from the oral cavity, but in other cases this is not so (Whitley et al., 1982a). There is no evidence that the virus recoverable from the brain is a particularly neurovirulent strain. In those patients without specific antibody at the start

of the encephalitic illness, this appears to be a primary infection with the virus. No differences in the pathology have been noted between cases in which the encephalitis is a primary versus secondary infection, with the exception of herpes neonatorum, in which the virus involved is usually type 2 and there is a generalized encephalitis.

Recent studies by Itzhaki and colleagues (1997, 1998) and Lin et al. (2001) have suggested that some people may be genetically predisposed to develop symptoms of peripheral HSV infection and to develop HSV-1 encephalitis. These investigators have shown that possession of one or two $\epsilon 4$ alleles of the gene coding for apolipoprotein E is more common in people who suffer from recurrent cold sores (Itzhaki et al., 1997) and that possession of one $\epsilon 2$ allele of this gene is higher in those developing acute HSV-1 encephalitis (Lin et al., 2001). However, another study of a larger number of cases of HSV-1 encephalitis showed no overrepresentation of the $\epsilon 2$ apolipoprotein allele (Nicoll et al., 2001).

It has long been recognized that the damage produced in HSE is largely confined to the limbic system, a group of structures that are closely linked anatomically and functionally. Once virus has reached the limbic system, its spread along known contralateral and ipsilateral connections within it provides an anatomical explanation for the bilaterality of the lesions.

The question remains of how the virus reaches the limbic system. It is known that the virus has a marked tendency to travel along neural pathways. Therefore, the limbic localization of the damage would be best explained if the virus gained entry to the brain along olfactory pathways (Johnson and Mims, 1968). The olfactory bulbs and tracts are not destroyed or severely inflamed in HSE, and early attempts to demonstrate virus there by immunofluorescence were rarely successful (MacCallum, 1973). However, Dinn (1980) and Ojeda (1980) were able to demonstrate viral antigen there in a few cases, and in a larger immunoperoxidase study (Esiri, 1982), viral antigen was found in glial cells of the olfactory tracts in 9 of 15 cases examined at autopsy in the first three weeks after the onset of the illness. There was, however, no way of knowing whether this antigen represented centripetally or centrifugally spreading virus.

Davis and Johnson (1979) suggested that virus may reach the inferior frontal and temporal lobes from the trigeminal ganglion after reactivation there, followed by spread along branches of the trigeminal nerve that supply the leptomeninges. There is as yet no evidence to support this suggestion.

A third possibility is that the virus reactivates inside the brain from a site of latency established earlier, perhaps following asymptomatic entry of virus along the olfactory pathway (Esiri, 1982). This also is a speculative suggestion, but recent animal and human studies using DNA hybridization and PCR techniques demonstrate that latent infection with HSV may occur in the CNS as well as in sensory ganglia (Cook and Stevens, 1976; Sequiera et al., 1979; Cabrera et al., 1980; Fraser et al., 1981; Baringer and Pisani, 1994; Stroop et al., 1984; Drummond et al., 1994; Itzhaki et al., 1993; Jamieson et al., 1992; Bertrand et al., 1993; Gordon et al., 1996; Itabashi et al., 1997). Recently, latent brain infection with HSV-1 has been implicated in reactivation of acute HSV-1 in one young patient treated surgically for mesial temporal sclerosis which developed as a complication of earlier HSV-1 encephalitis, and another case in which HSV DNA was detected, years after acute HSV/encephalitis, in brain tissue removed for treatment of severe epilepsy (Lellouch-Tubiana et al., 2000). Autopsy studies have also detected HSV-1 DNA in the cerebrum or brain stem months to years after acute encephalitis (Nicoll et al., 1993). Sites involved in experimental infections and in human brain have included central olfactory connections. However, a definitive explanation for the intriguing localization of damage in most cases of HSE is still unavailable.

CLINICAL EVALUATION OF HSE

Epidemiology

Demographic analysis of 113 proven cases of HSE collected by the U.S. Collaborative Antiviral Study Group (CASG) of the National Institute of Allergy and Infectious Diseases demonstrated that 86% of the patients were white, 54% were male, and no seasonal trend was apparent (Whitley et al., 1982b). Although there was no decade between 6 months and more than 60 years in which HSE was particularly likely to occur, the isolation of HSV in suspect cases increased after the age of 50. Although HSE can occur in the immunocompromised individual, the usual patient is immunologically impaired. Thus far, no environmental cofactors have been identified that increase the risk of HSE. In a review of our own case material, the presence of an emotional upset before the onset of HSE was noted on occasion; however, this point does not appear to have been systematically studied. Once the acute illness has started, personality changes and emotional instability are often prominent as a consequence of the regions of the brain involved by disease.

Although HSE is a sporadic disease, epidemiological information is crucial when HSE is suspected. If the patient is likely to be suffering from an epidemic infection of a neurotropic virus or, conversely, has sustained a CNS complication of an epidemic nonneurotropic infection, anti-HSV therapy is not indicated. Two types of epidemiological information are necessary. First, local health authorities should be contacted to determine what viruses are prevalent in the region. In summer and early fall, enteroviruses and arboviruses can produce encephalitis. Parainfectious encephalitis can follow many kinds of infection at all times of the year. The second type of information concerns viral illness in the patient's family and contacts. If the patient has had CNS symptoms develop after general systemic symptoms that duplicated those of others, a CNS complication of a transmissible systemic viral infection may have occurred. This point requires a great deal of care, however, for HSE is not infrequently preceded by nonspecific "viral symptoms."

Clinical Presentations

Classic Form

The most commonly recognized neurological presentation of HSE is associated with signs and symptoms that localize to the temporal lobe and/or to the adjacent frontal and parietal lobes (Table 4.2). Personality change, focal motor seizures,

TABLE 4.2 Neurological complications of HSV

Frontotemporal encephalitis
   Classic
      Severe, acute, focal
   Formes frustes
   Stuttering in onset
   Subacute, chronic
Brain stem encephalitis
Myelitis
Sacral radiculomyelitis
Sacral radiculitis with meningitis
Meningitis
   Monophasic
   Recurrent, including Mollaret's meningitis

and dysphasia are often found. Progressive severe neurological deterioration, including impaired consciousness, usually follows over the next few days. There is evidence of a CNS infection with fever and a cerebrospinal fluid (CSF) pleocytosis. In the typical case, the electroencephalogram (EEG) and neuroimaging techniques demonstrate localization in the temporal lobes. The tempo of neurological progression can vary from strokelike rapidity to a more gradual evolution over several days. However, the neurological stage often follows a brief period of nonspecific prodromal illness.

Nonspecific prodromal signs include fever, lassitude, myalgia, gastrointestinal upset, headache, and other "viral syndrome" symptoms, which often last up to 3 to 4 days prior to the encephalitic manifestations. It is extremely important and sometimes difficult to separate the premonitory systemic symptoms in HSE from the antecedent illness associated with a parainfectious encephalomyelitis. The premonitory illness tends to lead directly into the encephalitis without a clear intervening asymptomatic period. Subtle signs of CNS dysfunction may in fact have been present during the premonitory period. Slight changes in behavior, minimal memory impairment, and minimal dysphasia are sometimes recounted by contacts of the patient after the recognition of more obvious neurological dysfunction.

Signs and symptoms of infection may not all be obvious at presentation, but some evidence of infection is usually present. Fever and a CSF pleocytosis are routinely documented within the first stages of the evaluation. In the era before PCR, fever was documented at some point prior to biopsy in all our patients with proven HSE. In the U.S. collaborative study, 92% of patients were found to have fever on presentation, and 97% had a CSF pleocytosis (Whitley et al., 1982b). Patients without CSF abnormalities can be seen in HSE; however, it is unusual for the CSF to remain normal over the course of the illness. Signs of meningeal irritation, for example, stiff neck, may not be present on examination. Changes in the peripheral white blood cell count are not diagnostically useful. Lymph node or splenic enlargement is not found.

The abrupt onset of seizures in the presence of fever often leads quickly to the suspicion of HSE. In the day or so after a seizure, the patient may appear to improve, and appropriate diagnostic and therapeutic maneuvers may therefore be delayed. Thus, although the encephalitis may in fact be progressing, the apparent neurological state may improve as seizures are brought under control. This is a dangerous paradox, for time may be lost in starting appropriate antiviral therapy.

Confusion, disorientation, and loss of short-term memory are nonspecific findings present in many types of encephalopathy and encephalitis. In particular, the elderly may present with confusion in the presence of a non-CNS infection such as pneumonia or a urinary tract infection. Once again, valuable time may be lost if forgetfulness and disorientation are disregarded in an elderly febrile patient. It is crucial to examine such patients for signs of focal neurological defect and to perform an examination of the CSF for evidence of CNS infection. Conversely, personality change can be so severe and abrupt as to mimic an acute psychosis. These patients may present first to psychiatric facilities prior to the demonstration of other neurological dysfunction. In the course of HSE, patients may appear to be responding to hallucinations, often with an anxious or terrified expression. In a patient with a history of alcoholism, such hallucinations may be interpreted as delerium tremens, and diagnostic maneuvers may be delayed. Patients suspected of having delerium tremens should have the CSF examined for signs of infection. As a general rule, personality or behavioral change in a febrile patient should raise the suspicion of HSE.

Dysphasia may be unmistakable and appear with such abruptness as to resemble the effects of a cerebrovascular accident. However, the attempt to demonstrate dysphasia in a confused febrile patient may be sufficiently difficult that it becomes clear only as the illness evolves. In still other cases that do not present with dysphasia and in which obtundation precludes satisfactory examination, dysphasia may not become apparent until the recovery period.

Motor weakness and reflex asymmetry are often seen. The U.S. collaborative study found hemiparesis at presentation in 38% of biopsies in HSV-positive cases (Whitley et al., 1982b). Dense hemiparetic states early in the disease course may follow seizures and apparently improve with time, giving one a false sense of security. Progressive weakness can be seen as the illness progresses, presumably as a result of tissue destruction. Gait instability has been noted in our own case material, and ataxia was reported in 40% of the HSV-positive cases in the U.S. collaborative study (Whitley et al., 1982b). We have not observed visual field loss in our HSV-proven patients, although it was reported in 14% of HSV-positive patients in the U.S. collaborative study. Occipital involvement, though rare, has been reported (Bergey et al., 1982). Presentation with somatic sensory loss appears to be unusual. It is not listed in the table published by the U.S. collaborative study (Whitley et al., 1982b). In one of our patients, sensory loss compatible with vascular disease was followed successively by improvement and then by an HSV-positive encephalitis 3 weeks later. It was not possible to distinguish between a biphasic encephalitis and a cerebrovascular accident followed by encephalitis. While primary involvement of the brain stem can occur with HSV, nuclear cranial nerve defects are rare in the classic form of HSE. However, dysconjugate eye movements, impairment of the abducens nerves secondary to increased intracranial

pressure, unilateral pupillary dilation due to lateral herniation, and facial weakness of the upper motor neuron type are certainly observed. Cranial nerve defects were reported in 32% of the HSV-positive patients in the U.S. collaborative study (Whitley et al., 1982b).

The level of consciousness is an important clinical consideration, and the rate of decline of consciousness is variable. Seizures, postictal depression of consciousness, and the sedative qualities of various anticonvulsant medications can each complicate the clinical evaluation of level of consciousness. Patients who present with an apparent acute psychosis may receive heavy sedation in the attempt to manage combative behavior, thus limiting the assessment of level of consciousness.

Formes Frustes and Atypical HSE

It has long been suspected that milder, less destructive forms of HSE existed; however, the difficulty of proving this effectively prevented documentation. By definition mild and not associated with death, such potential cases did not come to autopsy. In life, they would be insufficiently severe to merit brain biopsy. Except in rare cases, HSV cannot be isolated from the CSF in adult-type HSE, but it can be isolated in neonatal-type HSE. Antibody develops too late, presumably after clearance of clinical symptoms, to allow definition of milder forms. The development of diagnosis by CSF PCR has identified such cases.

Domingues et al. (1997) prospectively evaluated focal, mild, and diffuse encephalitis. Mild encephalitis was defined as either focal or diffuse, but without severe reduction of the level of consciousness, i.e., a Glasgow coma scale (GCS) score above 13 and normal neurological function after therapy. Of 49 prospectively evaluated cases of encephalitis, 12 were characterized as mild, of which 3 were positive for HSV by CSF PCR.

Fodor et al. (1998) reviewed records from a large diagnostic virology laboratory to determine the frequency of mild and atypical cases of HSE. Atypical encephalitis was defined as an acute encephalopathy without focal findings and only mild changes in the level of consciousness or mental status exam. Fodor and colleagues found that 7.6% of over 1,200 samples sent for CSF PCR analysis were positive for HSV. Of these, 52% were from cases of meningitis, 26% were from cases of encephalitis, 17% were from cases of neonatal infection, and 5% could not be categorized because of the absence of clinical information. Of 24 adults with HSV-positive encephalitis, 4 (17%) were identified as atypical. All four had seizures of various types, and clinical exam abnormalities were confined to mental status. Nonetheless, magnetic resonance imaging (MRI) revealed abnormalities in both patients who were tested. HSV-1 and HSV-2 each infected two of these patients. Three of the four patients were immunocompromised. The authors noted that two of the four patients had predominantly unilateral involvement of the nondominant temporal lobe and surrounding tissue and commented that such localization may have a better clinical outcome (Fodor et al., 1998).

In light of the anatomic localization, it is not surprising that impaired new learning and memory are among the neuropsychological sequelae to HSE (Gordon et al., 1990). It might be anticipated that a forme fruste HSE could be restricted to impairment of short-term memory. Young et al. (1992) reported such a case in which profound memory problems were documented in a 37-year-old man whose only other manifestation of encephalitis was recurrent headache and vomiting. Both CSF PCR and intrathecal antibody production were positive for HSV, EEG showed bilateral episodic delta activity, and computerized tomography (CT) of the head revealed a low-density lesion in the right temporal lobe. Acyclovir treatment resulted in slight clinical improvement of mental status as assessed by serial sevens testing. Psychometric testing following therapy revealed impaired visual and verbal memory and impaired delayed recall. Taken together, these reports demonstrate that HSE can present as a mild encephalitis without significant impairment of consciousness but with seizures and/or alterations of mental status on exam, particularly defects in memory functions. Nonetheless, MRI may show focal evidence of encephalitis, and the EEG may demonstrate unilateral or bilateral abnormalities. The key to diagnosis and management of course is prompt performance of CSF PCR for HSV.

On occasion, HSE can have a stuttering evolution or a more prolonged course than is usually associated with acute HSE. The case of Young et al. (1992) described above had an outset of severe bitemporal headache with vomiting that resolved after a few days. The headache reappeared a week later and again resolved. It was only after the patient returned to work and could not remember the names of his coworkers that he sought medical attention. He was only hospitalized 3 weeks after the first headache. The literature also contains reports suggesting that HSE might smolder for months (Sage et al., 1985; Kleinschmidt-DeMasters and Gilden, 2001). While atypical for HSE, HSV should be sought by CSF PCR in any case of subacute or chronic encephalitis that has eluded definition.

Brain Stem

The number of reports of brain stem encephalitis resulting from HSV are so few as to make generalized comments precarious. Tyler et al. (1995) have reviewed the cranial nerve dysfunction previously reported in the literature. Dysfunction extended from the oculomotor complex and included disorders of facial motor and sensation and impairment of cranial nerves IX and XII, in addition to long tract signs of varying severity, ataxia, and incoordination. In an immunohistopathological study of microglial nodules in the brain stem, Schmidbauer et al. (1989) found DNA of HSV by in situ hybridization in brain stem nuclei that were connected to trigeminal, superior cervical, and vagus cranial nerve ganglia previously shown to harbor HSV. DNA of HSV was occasionally found in other locations, including the cerebellum and the cerebrum. No evidence for active replication, in the form of viral proteins, was found. No clinical details beyond the diagnoses were given, hence the clinical relevance of these findings is not clear. The majority of HSV DNA-positive cases had some form of immunocompromise.

Documentation of CNS HSV infection has often been limited, suggesting, but not proving, HSV infection of the brain stem. Material from a case coming to autopsy following clinical signs of a lateral medullary syndrome demonstrated herpesvirus group capsids as well as intranuclear inclusions (Roman-Campos and Toro, 1980). However, more specific characterization among the several members of the herpesvirus group was not achieved. Ataxia, dysarthria, and dysphagia were presenting signs in a patient with elevated CSF anti-HSV antibody who ultimately recovered (Jain and Maheshwari, 1984). Other cases have been reported in which documentation rested on serum antibody changes. For example, Ellison and Hanson (1977) reported on a 10-year-old child who survived multiple cranial nerve involvement, ataxia, hemiparesis, and seizures. HSV was isolated from a tracheal aspirate, and a declining serum titer against HSV was demonstrated at 5 weeks.

If the demonstration of virus, its nucleic acid, or its antigens in CNS or CSF, or the presence of significant antibody in the spinal fluid compared to the serum, is required, fewer cases are acceptably documented. Dayan et al. (1972) reported two cases of brain stem encephalitis due to HSV. A 14-year-old boy with confusion, dysarthria, and fever was found to have palatal weakness. He evolved to demonstrate impaired consciousness, bilateral facial weakness, irregular respirations, extensor spasms, and hemiparesis. The CSF demonstrated a pleocytosis. At autopsy, patchy hemorrhagic infarction and a necrotizing encephalitis of the cerebral hemispheres as well as the brain stem was found. HSV antigen was found in the cortex and in the brain stem. The presence of HSV antigen in the cortex and in the brain stem was demonstrated by indirect immunofluorescence. HSV was isolated from the spinal fluid of both the second case of Dayan et al. (1972) and case 9 of Al-Din et al. (1982). In addition to other signs, each case demonstrated ptosis, gaze paresis, facial weakness, ataxia, and impaired consciousness. Both patients survived, one with partial and the other with complete recovery. The CSF in both cases demonstrated a pleocytosis. That of Dayan et al. (1972) also demonstrated a significant number of red cells and elevated protein. In each case the EEG was bilaterally slow. In one case, CT scan and pneumoencephalography were normal (Al-Din et al., 1982). Hirst et al. (1983) reported downbeat nystagmus and autopsy demonstration of HSV antigen in the brain stem of an immunocompromised patient with significant hemispheral involvement.

The case report of Tyler et al. (1995) was unusual in the documentation of recurrent episodes of HSV brain stem encephalitis as documented by CSF PCR and intrathecal anti-HSV antibody production. Multifocal involvement of the brain stem ranged from the midbrain rostrally to the medulla caudally, with long tract involvement. The patient had recurrent episodes of herpes labialis, suggesting the possibility of centripetal infection of the nervous system from the trigeminal ganglia. Antiviral therapy did not prevent recurrences of brain stem symptoms.

Although a third of patients with hemispheral HSE may demonstrate signs of cranial nerve defects (Whitley et al., 1982b), the clinician is up against a difficult problem with brain stem encephalitis in which frontal-temporal lobe signs are absent or insignificant. There is no strongly suggestive clinical presentation as there is with HSV infection of the hemispheres, or conversely, with the bulbar presentation of polio. CSF PCR for HSV, combined with CSF-to-serum antibody ratio studies in prolonged or recurrent cases, ought to be determined in all cases of brain stem encephalitis. Acute therapy with intravenous (i.v.) acyclovir should be undertaken in positive cases. However, the sensitivity of HSV brain stem encephalitis to antiviral therapy is unknown, as is whether oral suppressive therapy is needed following i.v. therapy.

Aseptic Meningitis, Recurrent (Mollaret's) Meningitis, Radiculitis, Myelitis, and Associated Combined Syndromes

Aseptic Meningitis. The association of genital HSV infection and aseptic meningitis has been recognized since the start of the 20th century (Ravaut and Darré, 1904). Although often due to HSV-2, it may also be associated with HSV-1. Signs of aseptic meningitis have been found in 36% of women and in 13% of men during primary genital infection with HSV-2 (Corey et al., 1983). The meningitis may occur with or without genital lesions (Terni et al., 1971; Skoldenberg et al., 1973). Virus can often be isolated from the CSF (Skoldenberg et al., 1973), and on occasion the CSF glucose is found to be significantly lowered (Morrison et al., 1974). The viral diagnostic assay of choice is CSF PCR for HSV. Of CSF samples testing positive for HSV by PCR in a large university-based diagnostic virology lab, 52% showed meningitis (Fodor et al., 1998). Herpetic proctitis in homosexual men can be associated with aseptic meningitis (Heller et al., 1982) and with sacral radiculomyelopathy (Samarasinghe et al., 1979).

Mollaret's Meningitis. Mollaret's meningitis certainly fits the pattern of a herpes simplex-related illness—that is, recurrent self-limited benign episodes. Steel et al. (1982) reported the isolation of HSV-1 in Mollaret's meningitis. Since that time, HSV-2 has been the most commonly identified cause of Mollaret's meningitis. Jensenius et al. (1998) reported nine cases of Mollaret's meningitis associated with HSV-2 as detected by CSF PCR. They were found in an area of Norway containing about 940,000 inhabitants during a 45-month period. The investigators calculated that a minimum prevalence rate for the geographic region studied would be about 1 per 100,000 inhabitants. Recurrence can involve both meningitis and mucocutaneous symptoms, meningitis alone, or mucocutaneous lesions alone (Aurelius et al., 2002). In cases of frequent recurrence of meningitis, suppression with oral antiherpesvirus medication such as acyclovir or valacyclovir could be considered. A prospective placebo-controlled study is reported to be under way with valacyclovir (Aurelius et al., 2002).

Lumbosacral Radiculomyelopathy. The syndrome of lumbosacral radiculomyelopathy can be seen in association with genital and anogenital HSV infection (Caplan et al., 1977; Oates and Greenhouse, 1978). Homosexual men with herpes proctitis appear to be at high risk for the syndrome (Corey et al., 1983). Sensory changes in lumbar and/or sacral dermatomes include pain, parasthesia, and numbness. In addition, urinary retention, constipation, impaired penile erections, reduced anal tone, and absent bulbocavernosis reflexes may be found. Fever and systemic signs of infection are often

present. Signs of meningitic irritation may be present or absent, and pleocytosis may be found on examination of the CSF (Caplan et al., 1977). CSF PCR for HSV and MRI with gadolinium enhancement for localization are crucial. The syndrome often requires catheterization for acute management; however, dysfunction is usually self-limited.

Myelitis. Ascending myelitis associated with HSV in the CSF, although reported (Klastersky et al., 1972; Wiley et al., 1987), appears to be very rare. The evaluation of radiculomyelitis and myelitis is considerably aided by spinal cord MRI with gadolinium enhancement and CSF PCR. Kuker et al. (1999) described a 48-year-old man without immunocompromise in whom acute HSV-1 radiculomyelitis was diagnosed by CSF PCR and anatomically localized by MRI to the cauda equina, dorsal roots, and low thoracic spinal cord. Administration of acyclovir was associated with clearing of CSF HSV. Myelitis associated with HSV can also be found in immunocompromised patients infected with HIV (Britton et al., 1985). Very rarely, recurrent ascending myelitis can be shown to be associated with HSV (Shyu et al., 1993).

Neurodiagnostic Studies

Virus-specific studies of HSE have been useful to document the associated neurodiagnostic findings in classic HSE. In general such studies are of two types: data from the large collaborative antiviral drug trials and data from smaller groups of patients in whom the diagnosis of HSE was confirmed by CSF PCR (e.g., Domingues et al., 1998). The European Union has produced a consensus report summarizing the value of various neurodiagnostic studies (Cinque et al., 1996). The more recent and smaller, CSF PCR-based studies have expanded the spectrum of HSV-related CNS disease states.

CSF

Elevations of protein and white blood cells are usually found in the CSF at the start of HSE. A median value of 80 mg/dl was found in the U.S. collaborative study; however, it was 40 mg/dl or less in 19% of patients (Whitley et al., 1982b). The content of immunoglobulin G (IgG) may increase significantly by the second week of the illness (Carroll and Booss, 1976). An average of 130 white blood cells per mm^3 were found in CSF early in the illness (Whitley et al., 1982b), with only 4% having four or fewer cells per mm^3. Although the cells are usually mononuclear, they may also be polymorphonuclear. Red blood cells in CSF, while often emphasized (Miller et al., 1966), were fewer than 50/mm^3 in over 50% of HSV-positive cases (Whitley et al., 1982b). Conversely, more than 500 red blood cells per mm^3 were found in the CSF of over 20% of HSV-negative cases. Thus, the presence of red blood cells in CSF is an unreliable indicator of HSE. CSF glucose levels below 50% of the serum value may occur but are unusual in HSE and should raise the suspicion of infection with another agent.

It is crucial that adequate studies be obtained on the CSF from the initial tap because increasingly raised pressure may render subsequent taps perilous. Bacterial, tubercular, fungal, and viral diagnostic samples are required. Isolation of HSV is rare in the CSF in HSE; however, attempts should be made to isolate other viral agents along with the demonstration of HSV by PCR. A sample for antiviral antibody with a paired serum sample should be stored for comparison with a later convalescent-phase CSF and serum pair. Demonstration of local production of antibody against HSV in even one pair of serum-CSF samples supports the diagnosis.

EEG

The EEG has a high degree of sensitivity in focal encephalitis (81% positivity in proven HSE in the U.S. collaborative study), but a low degree of specificity for HSE (59% positivity in HSV-negative focal encephalitis) (Whitley et al., 1982b). Specific EEG characteristics such as periodic lateralizing epileptiform discharges, while suggestive (e.g., Smith et al., 1975), are not limited to HSE. Brick et al. (1990) analyzed preoperative EEGs in patients in whom HSE or another etiology was established by brain biopsy. They found no EEG variables that were specific to HSE when performed within 48 h of presentation for care. The European Union consensus report (Cinque et al., 1996) concluded that the EEG offered "limited diagnostic data," with nonspecific slow wave activity early in the course of the illness—5 to 7 days—and more characteristic features found later. In our own view, serial EEGs remain clinically useful in the differential diagnosis and management of encephalitis (Fig. 4.12).

Imaging Techniques

The sensitivity of the CT scan in demonstrating a localized lesion was 59% in the first 3 days, according to the U.S. collaborative study (Whitley et al., 1982b), and 73% in the first 5 days, according to a Swedish collaborative study (Hindmarsh et al., 1986). In the U.S. study, positive findings included localized edema, mass effect, low-density lesions, contrast enhancement, and hemorrhage. CT-scan localization was found in 22% of HSV-negative patients. The investigators commented that "...overdependence on CT scans will delay diagnosis and subsequent institution of therapy" (Whitley et al., 1982b). In the Swedish study, early changes on CT included low-density lesions in the temporal lobe, often in the region of the insula, which were sometimes small and indistinct (Hindmarsh et al., 1986). Blurring of

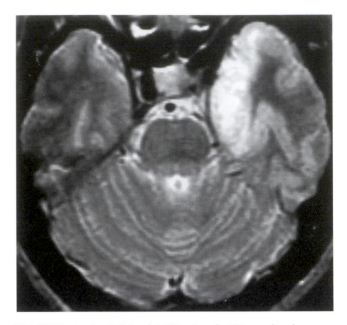

FIGURE 4.13   MRI of HSE. Axial, T2-weighted image, demonstrating mesial temporal lobe hyperintensity on the left. Courtesy of Gordon Sze, Yale University School of Medicine.

the outlines of the sylvian fissure because of edema and compression was also characteristic. In the first 5 days of illness the sensitivity of CT was 73% and specificity was 89% (Hindmarsh et al., 1976). Overall, contrast enhancement was insignificant and hemorrhage was rare and insignificant.

Subsequent to the U.S. and Swedish collaborative studies, MRI has emerged as the diagnostic imaging method of choice (Cinque et al., 1996) (Fig. 4.13). However, no study exists of the magnitude of the collaborative studies. The MRI scans have been judged in the context of CSF PCR results. Domingues et al. (1998) studied 17 patients with focal encephalitis, of whom 9 were positive for HSV by CSF PCR. Overall, MRI was positive in eight of nine of the HSV-positive patients. The lesions presented as high intensity on T2-weighted images and hypointense on T1-weighted images and were localized to the inferomedial region of one or both temporal lobes. Other related regions, such as the external capsule and insular cortex, were also involved. Mass effect was found in three patients. An alternative diagnosis was suggested in three HSV-negative patients—one abscess and two demyelinating disease including acute disseminated encephalomyelitis (ADEM). In the latter cases, the capacity to detect white-matter lesions in ADEM is a major point favoring MRI. Serial studies on a limited scale have demonstrated the evolution of lesions on MRI (Lee et al., 2001). These can include enlargement of the involved cortex, swelling, and hemorrhage, followed in some cases by brain atrophy and encephalomalacia. Disconcertingly, Meyding-Lamadé et al. (1999) reported progressive MRI changes in two patients despite clinical improvement. Careful evaluation will sometimes include repeated MRI exams even after the finding of negative results (Hollinger et al., 2000); hence a positive CSF PCR with a compatible clinical picture merits treatment in the face of negative

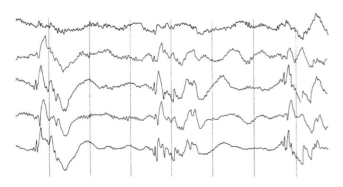

FIGURE 4.12   EEG of a 12-year-old with HSE and new onset of seizures and alteration of mental status. The patient was comatose and on mechanical ventilation at the time of study. EEG demonstrates slowing of background activity and periodic discharges with a frequency of 3 to 4 Hz in the right hemisphere. Courtesy of Huned Patwa, Yale University School of Medicine.

imaging studies. Further, while both the CT and MRI scans can provide evidence of inferofrontal and mesial temporal disease, neither can provide pathognomic evidence for HSE.

Other neuroimaging modalities have been applied to the diagnosis of encephalitis. The U.S. collaborative study found that radioisotopic brain scans provided localization in 50% of HSV-positive patients compared to 14% of negative patients (Whitley et al., 1982b). The abnormalities included unilateral uptake of isotope. Single-photon emission CT using hexamethylpropyleneamine oxime to demonstrate unilateral hyperperfusion has been advocated for diagnostic and prognostic purposes in focal encephalitides (Launes et al., 1997). Unilateral hyperperfusion was found to be an independent predictor of poor outcome. Determination of the type of encephalitis was not uniformly based on diagnostic virological definition of the etiologic agent.

Viral Diagnostic Studies

Except for disseminated herpes in the neonate (see below), isolation of HSV from anywhere other than the brain is not diagnostic of HSE. Even in immunologically impaired adults, peripheral isolation of HSV may not relate to the brain infection. Peripheral changes in antibody titer are of little value in HSE diagnosis. They may rise because of concomitant reactivation of HSV in the oropharynx, or they may fail to rise in HSE. Therefore, acute and chronic CSF and serum pairs should be taken to make the immunological diagnosis of HSE. Because peripheral isolation of HSV is meaningless in HSE and because the immunological response in CSF develops after the acute phase of the disease, brain biopsy was often considered prior to the 1990s. With the development of PCR and the confirmation of its sensitivity and specificity in CSF for HSV, it has become the "gold standard" for the diagnosis of HSE (Kleinschmidt-DeMasters et al., 2001).

Aurelius et al. (1991) applied PCR analysis to CSF from patients in whom HSE had been established by demonstration of HSV or its antigens in brain tissue and/or by intrathecal production of antibody to HSV. Forty-two of 43 patients previously demonstrated to have HSE were positive by PCR analysis of CSF. All controls were negative. Lakeman et al. (1995), using biopsy-confirmed HSV-positive samples from the U.S. collaborative antiviral trial, found positive results on CSF from 53 of 54 patients with biopsy-confirmed HSE. They also found three CSF PCR-positive results from patients in whom brain biopsy failed to yield HSV. By these criteria, the CSF PCR assay had a sensitivity of 96% and a specificity of 94%; positive predictive value was 95% and negative predictive value was 98%. Moreover, the investigators speculated that the three CSF PCR-positive results from patients with negative biopsy results may have been true positives, i.e., PCR might be superior to biopsy.

There are numerous pitfalls in the performance of PCR, including the need for exhaustive controls to exclude external contamination, selection of the appropriate primers, and removal of inhibitors in the CSF. While these are technical matters in the domain of the diagnostic laboratory, it is incumbent on the clinician to use a laboratory with a demonstrated record of diagnostic accuracy.

The advantages of CSF PCR diagnosis of HSE are enormous. For physicians trained subsequent to the development of CSF PCR, the MRI, and the use of acyclovir therapy, it may be difficult to imagine what all the fuss was about in making the diagnosis and initiating therapy in HSE. Suffice it to say that CSF PCR is usually positive at the onset of clinical signs and symptoms, is relatively noninvasive—certainly in comparison to brain biopsy—and remains positive during the first 10 to 14 days of illness, the usual period of acute HSE. These characteristics allow the clinician to initiate antiviral therapy immediately in an HSE suspect, even shortly before obtaining CSF for PCR analysis. Cases have been reported in which the initial CSF PCR was negative, followed by positive results 4 and 7 days later (Weil et al., 2002). Hence, empiric antiviral therapy should be continued in a clinically suspect case, pending the results of follow-up CSF PCR.

CSF Antibody

Development of anti-HSV antibody in the CSF occurs too late to be useful in acute management and therapeutic decisions. However, it is a valuable test in the absence of a diagnostically positive PCR after the first week of illness. Normally, the ratio of serum to CSF antibody titer is at least 200:1 because of the operation of the blood-brain and blood-CSF barriers. Inflammation of the brain or of the leptomeninges will reduce this ratio, but the extent of this reduction can be taken into account by comparing serum and CSF titers for another common virus or for levels of albumin. Excess reduction in the ratio for HSV below that for another common virus indicates the extent of the intrathecal synthesis of antibody to HSV. The titer present in both the serum and the CSF will usually rise during the course of the disease, particularly after the first 5 days, but it will rise comparatively more in the CSF than in the serum. By using two different tests for the presence of antibody in serum and CSF, Nahmias et al. (1982) found that 90% of patients proven by viral culture of biopsy material to have HSE have ratios of serum to CSF antibody of less than 20 by the third week of the illness. This criterion and that of a fourfold rise in CSF titer during the course of the illness are two reliable retrospective indicators of the disease. However, care must be taken by the laboratory to consider cross-reactivity with varicella-zoster virus. The European Union consensus report recommends that measurement of intrathecal antibody production is the assay of choice after 10 to 14 days of illness and when antiviral therapy has been employed for several days (Cinque et al., 1996).

Serial studies on the CSF antibody titers show that high levels persist for a remarkably long time after recovery from encephalitis. Virus-specific IgA and, in some cases, IgM and IgG levels are increased in the CSF for many weeks or months (Cappel et al., 1975; Skoldenberg et al., 1981; Vandvik et al., 1982). Occasionally and inexplicably, a few patients do not show the expected antibody response. For example, we encountered a case of an 80-year-old female with an encephalitic illness lasting 16 days in whom antibody titers to HSV remained less than 1 in 4 in serum and CSF throughout. At autopsy, HSV was cultured from the brain, and abundant viral antigen was demonstrated in both frontal and temporal lobes of the brain, but the inflammatory response was negligible.

Brain Biopsy

With the increased anatomic definition afforded by MRI, the specificity and sensitivity of CSF PCR to identify HSV, and the clinical efficacy and safety of acyclovir treatment when initiated early in the course of the illness, the need to biopsy HSE suspects has dropped off markedly. In more prolonged cases, after 10 to 14 days of illness, the application of assays to measure anti-HSV antibody production in CSF is another relatively noninvasive approach to diagnosis (Cinque et al., 1996). Nonetheless, biopsy must be considered in cases in which clinical, laboratory, and/or imaging studies suggest the possibility of another treatable illness.

THERAPY, COURSE, AND OUTCOMES

Antiviral Therapy

Untreated, the outcome of HSE is devastating—greater than 70% mortality and significant morbidity in a high percentage of survivors (Whitley and Gnann, 2002). Treatment with acyclovir has reduced mortality to about 30% overall (Whitley and Lakeman, 1995). Standard dosing with acyclovir had been 10 mg/kg of body weight every 8 h for 10 days. However, the recognition that significant disabilities were detected in survivors, that recurrence of encephalitis occurred in a variable percentage of survivors following a course of antiviral therapy, and that acute retinal necrosis due to the same strain of HSV (Maertzdorf et al., 2000) could follow antiviral treatment has led to modification of the treatment regimens. Currently recommended therapy for HSE is 10 to 15 mg/kg i.v. acyclovir every 8 h for 14 to 21 days (Whitley and Roizman, 2001). Studies of outcomes of neonatal herpes infections (see below) have demonstrated improved outcomes of neonates with disseminated or CNS HSV infections treated with acyclovir at 20 mg/kg i.v. every 8 h for 21 days when compared to a dose of 15 mg/kg every 8 h for 21 days or to the historical group receiving 10 mg/kg every 8 h for 10 days (Kimberlin et al., 2001b). Reversible neutropenia was detected in a few patients. Hence, twice-weekly absolute neutrophil counts during therapy were recommended, in addition to monitoring the known reversible nephrotoxicity. As pointed out by the European Union concensus report (Cinque et al., 1996), oral suppressive therapy by drugs with good bioavailability following i.v. therapy was under consideration. A study is presently underway by the U.S. CASG.

Therapy should be initiated on presentation of a patient with a temporal-frontal focal encephalitis as soon as emergency imaging studies rule out other focal lesions such as tumor, abscess, stroke, or hemorrhage. The PCR for HSV should be obtained on the first lumbar puncture. However, because CSF PCR can detect HSV even after a few days of treatment, the initiation of therapy should not be delayed if a second tap is required to obtain CSF for the PCR. The urgency of therapy arises from analysis of the prognostic factors that emerged from the U.S. collaborative study—namely, better outcomes were associated with the early initiation of therapy before significant depression of the level

of consciousness (Whitley and Lakeman, 1995). Renal function assays must be closely monitored. Acyclovir therapy can be stopped without harm if another etiology emerges as the cause of the illness.

Course and Outcomes

Development and clinical testing of antiherpes antiviral therapy emerged rapidly in the 1970s and 1980s and continues to the present. The U.S. CASG (e.g., Whitley et al., 1986) and the multicenter Swedish trial group (e.g., Skoldenberg et al., 1984) have produced important data on the diagnosis, natural history, prognostic factors, and outcomes of HSE in addition to establishing the efficacy of antiviral therapy. The more recent development of CSF PCR for diagnosis has allowed the definition of less severe cases of HSE, which, in turn, has resulted in better outcomes (e.g., Domingues et al., 1997).

The course of HSE is variable. The U.S. collaborative study found that the time to biopsy from the start of alteration of consciousness was 4.7 days for lethargy, 4.3 days for semicoma, and 6.5 days for coma (Whitley et al., 1977). Further, the range was 2 to 12 days. Of those who were lethargic, one-third did not progress further in suppression of level of consciousness, one-third progressed to semicoma, and one-third progressed to coma. Conversely, there is ample evidence of reversal of HSE in the absence of antiviral therapy. The need for a large controlled study of the therapy of HSE arose at least in part from the apparent success of various drugs in uncontrolled studies. In light of the failure of these drugs in controlled study, part of the apparent success might have resulted from spontaneous reversals. The course of the illness in the first 2 weeks is crucial. Although significant changes, particularly recurrence, can certainly occur at a later time, stabilization or improvement is often apparent by 2 weeks. Similarly, the period of recovery is extremely variable. Significant clinical recovery can go on for months, particularly in children.

The original report of the use of adenine arabinoside in a double-blind placebo study demonstrated an HSE mortality of 70% in the placebo group (Whitley et al., 1977). In the Swedish collaborative study, mortality was 19% in the acyclovir-treated group (Skoldenberg et al., 1984). The diagnosis of HSE was made by virus isolation and/or antigen detection in the brain or by the demonstration of intrathecal antibody production. At 6 months, 56% of the acyclovir-treated patients had resumed normal life. Further, 4 of 10 patients in semicoma or coma who were treated with acyclovir returned to normal. The U.S. collaborative study, requiring virus isolation from the brain, also demonstrated the superiority of acyclovir therapy (Whitley et al., 1986). Mortality at 1 month was 13%, at 6 months it was 19%, and at 18 months it was 28%. At 6 months in acyclovir-treated survivors, 9% had moderate disability and 38% had mild or no disability. Age and level of consciousness using the GCS were the best prognostic factors. A GCS score of 6 or less portended a bad outcome, either death or severe impairment. Survivors with a GCS score of 10 or greater who were under 30 years of age had the best outcomes.

Despite the marked reduction in mortality brought about by acyclovir therapy, both the U.S. collaborative study and the Swedish multicenter study have demonstrated important long-term sequelae, even in survivors with mild disability. In the Swedish study, long-term follow-up of patients at a single hospital, ranging from 2 to 15 years after onset, found normal neuropsychological functioning in only 1 of 17 HSE survivors (Skoldenberg, 1991). Dementia was found to have developed in 5 of the 17. Intensive neuropsychological testing of four survivors in the mildest outcome category of the U.S. CASG at 1 to 3 years after infection revealed significant dysnomia, reduced verbal intelligence quotients, and impairments of new learning and memory (Gordon et al., 1990). While one patient had had a GCS score of 9 acutely, the others were well above the level predicting a good outcome.

More recent reports that have included cases diagnosed by CSF PCR have had improved mortality results. Only 5.6% of PCR-diagnosed patients died in the series reported by Domingues et al. (1997). McGrath et al. (1997) reported on 42 patients with HSE diagnosed by isolation of HSV from the brain, intrathecal antibody production, or PCR studies on CSF. Seven died, either in the first month or later following severe sequelae. Of the 34 survivors, 5 had severe deficits and all but 1 had neurological symptoms and/or signs. Twenty-nine of the survivors were assessed at various times from 6 months to 11 years following encephalitis. Memory impairment was found in 69%, personality and behavioral abnormalities were found in 45%, and epilepsy was found in 24%. Prognostic factors were in agreement with previous studies. Stupor or coma before treatment was associated with a poor outcome, as was older age. Six of the eight patients who died were over 60 years old. An abnormal CT was found in all 11 patients with a poor outcome and in 14 of 27 patients with a good outcome.

A study by Lahat et al. (1999) confirmed the better outlook in children and the importance of depression of consciousness as a prognostic factor. Of 28 children, 2 died (7%), both of whom had GCS scores less than 6, 10 (36%) had persistent sequelae, and 16 (57%) had no neurological sequelae. Two patients experienced a recurrence within the first week after concluding acyclovir therapy. Sequelae included intelligence quotient scores under 70 in four patients, personality changes in four, speech abnormalities in two, motor skill problems in five, and seizures in four.

In aggregate, these studies demonstrate that although acyclovir has markedly diminished mortality in HSE and the age of the patient and the level of consciousness at initiation of therapy are important prognostic factors, significant sequelae remain, even for those who are able to live independently. Taken together with recurrence of encephalitis, the high frequency of sequelae indicates that continued improvement of antiviral treatment regimens and evaluation of new antiviral compounds is needed.

Recurrent Encephalitis

Recurrence of disease is characteristic of herpetic lesions of the skin and mucosa. More recently, recurrence in the CNS in the form of Mollaret's aseptic meningitis has been shown often to be associated with HSV, particularly type 2 (see above). Rare cases of recurrent brain stem encephalitis (Tyler et al., 1995) and recurrent ascending myelitis (Shyu et al., 1993) due to HSV-1 have been described in which

the initial episodes were treated with courses of steroid but not antiviral medication. Recurrent frontal-temporal HSV encephalitis appears to be restricted to cases in which the initial episode was treated with antiviral medication. Despite the recognition of recurrence in treated HSE for over 2 decades, the roles of renewed viral replication versus an autoaggressive host defense response, or a combination of both, and the best strategies to prevent and treat second episodes of HSE remain open questions.

In an early U.S. collaborative study, 4 of 93 patients had a good response to antiviral therapy, only to have a relapse 1 to 3 months later (Whitley et al., 1981). On second biopsy, HSV was not isolated and electron microscopic evidence for demyelination was not found. Other studies have provided conflicting evidence on the nature of the recurrence. Koenig et al. (1979) were unable to isolate virus in a case of recurrent encephalitis but did find evidence of demyelination. In two other reports, HSV was isolated from biopsy during a second episode of encephalitis following an initial episode 2 months earlier (Davis and McLaren, 1983; Dix et al., 1983). In each instance, the virus was recovered after a prolonged period of cocultivation of brain cells in vitro. Application of CSF PCR has not resolved the issue of renewed viral replication. Dennett et al. (1996) were unsuccessful in attempting to identify HSV DNA in five adult cases of relapsed HSE. Ito et al. (2000) detected HSV DNA in CSF by PCR in two of seven children who suffered relapse. Six of the seven patients suffered relapse within 14 days of completing antiviral therapy, suggesting reactivation of HSV as the pathogenic mechanism. Total acyclovir doses for the initial episodes were lower for the relapsed group than for the nonrelapsed group, but the relapsed group did not have a higher viral load in the initial episode than did the nonrelapsed group. One of the recurrent episodes was associated with isolation of coxsackie A9 virus from the CSF. With a relapse rate of 26%, Ito et al. (2000) suggested that HSE relapse is more common in children than previously recognized. Hargrave and Webb (1998) have found that choreoatherosis is a complication of relapsed HSE in children.

HSV retinitis, which has been described in a few cases following treated HSV encephalitis, may provide indirect evidence for the role of viral replication as a mechanism of recurrent disease. Maertzdorf et al. (2000) described two cases of HSV-1 retinitis following HSE, at 9 months and 10 days, respectively. In each case HSV-1 DNA was identified by PCR in the aqueous humor of the afflicted eye, and in each case the HSV-1 strains in the eye and brain were identical within individuals, although they differed between the cases. In agreement with experimental studies, the investigators suggested that the virus may have reached the eye from the brain via the optic nerve. Thus, early (10 days) and late (9 months) onset of retinitis following encephalitis was associated with evidence for HSV of the same strain in the affected eye as in the brain.

Concerning therapy of recurrent HSV encephalitis, it should be stressed that viral replication and a self-damaging host defense response may exist on a continuum, and both may contribute to CNS injury in any individual case. Hence, it seems reasonable to treat recurrent HSE with both a repeat course of i.v. acyclovir and a course of steroid therapy using a tapering dose. Neither antiviral-resistant mutant virus nor significant superinfection has been shown to be a risk of such a combined therapy. Careful clinical, MRI, and CSF PCR follow-up is strongly urged. The role of follow-up oral antiviral suppressive therapy is under study.

Neonatal Herpes Simplex Infection

Herpes simplex infection of the newborn often involves the nervous system. Untreated, it can have a high mortality rate, particularly in its disseminated form. While congenital and neonatal infections are not a focus of this book, neonatal herpes simplex infection will be summarized here. For more extended discussions, the reader is referred to the review of Arvin and Whitley (2001) and to reports of the U.S. CASG (Kimberlin et al., 2001a, 2001b). Studies from the CASG over 2 decades have shaped our understanding of the biology of maternal transmission, the natural history, and the therapy of herpes neonatorum.

HSV infection of the newborn can reflect intrauterine or postnatal transmission; however, 85 to 90% of infections occur during delivery and are predominantly type 2. Pregnant women with a history of recurrent HSV shedding must be carefully evaluated, particularly at the start of labor. However, the greatest risk for transmission is to the infant whose mother experiences a primary infection at the time of delivery and from whom no passive transfer of antibodies has been received. Rupture of membranes in the presence of genital lesions of HSV-2 is a significant risk factor. Cesarean section is indicated for women with active HSV lesions at the start of labor. The use of fetal scalp monitors must be carefully weighed in light of the risk of electrode placement as a potential site of HSV entry. Viral culturing of the mother and neonate at delivery when the mother has had a history of recurrent genital HSV shedding will assist in management of the neonate.

Hitherto, neonatal herpes infection acquired during delivery had been categorized as localized or disseminated. More recently, the seriousness of CNS complications has been emphasized, so the present classification used by the CASG is HSV localized to skin, eye, and mouth (SEM); CNS involvement with or without SEM involvement; and the disseminated form that involves several organ systems, including CNS in the majority (Kimberlin, 2001a). Each of these forms accounts for roughly one-third of intrapartum-acquired HSV infections. Untreated, SEM infection can progress to include the CNS or disseminate more widely. Cryptic CNS infection can occur in SEM infection, particularly when untreated, such that neurological damage can be found on follow-up. The disseminated form is most apt to appear in the first week postpartum with any of a plethora of signs and symptoms. The CNS form usually presents in the second or third weeks but can appear up to 4 to 6 weeks postpartum, with seizures, irritability, a bulging anterior fontanelle, lethargy, poor feeding, and pyramidal tracts signs.

Viral diagnosis can be achieved by antigen detection in observed lesions or virus isolation from lesions, conjunctivae, stool, urine, CSF, throat, or nasopharynx. CSF PCR and virus isolation are indicated. Antibody does not contribute to the diagnosis because of the usual presence of maternal IgG antibody and the slow development of the IgM response

by the infant. Evaluation of the CNS following clinical exam by lumbar puncture, EEG, and neuroimaging is indicated.

Modifications of treatment with acyclovir have evolved because of the continuing levels of mortality, residual morbidity, and recurrent illness. The recommended duration of treatment has been extended from 10 days to 14 days to 21 days. Recently, higher daily doses than the recommended 10 mg/kg three times a day have been examined by the CASG (Kimberlin, 2001b). It was found that 20 mg/kg three times a day for 21 days produced a statistically significant reduction of mortality in the disseminated form and improved the mortality rate in the CNS form, although the difference did not reach clinical significance. Morbidity in the CNS category remained high, about 70%, in survivors who had received either the standard (historical data) or the high dose. Reversible neutropenia emerged in six patients overall. The investigators concluded that the use of 60 mg/kg/day for 21 days was supported by the data for neonates with disseminated or CNS disease (Kimberlin, 2001b). Serial determinations of absolute neutrophil counts at least twice weekly were recommended. Monitoring of the previously recognized reversible nephrotoxicity is necessary. Suppressive treatment with oral acyclovir or an analog following i.v. therapy remains a research question. For the present, improvement in awareness of neonatal HSV infection will reduce the time before initiation of antiviral-specific therapy and should bring about further improvement of outcomes (Kimberlin, 2001a).

REFERENCES

Adams, H., and D. Miller. 1973. Herpes simplex encephalitis—a clinical and pathological analysis of 22 cases. *Postgrad. Med. J.* **49**:393–397.

Al-Din, A. N., M. Anderson, E. R. Bickerstaff, and I. Harvey. 1982. Brain stem encephalitis and the syndrome of Miller Fisher. A clinical study. *Brain* **105**:481–495.

Arvin, A. M., and R. J. Whitley. 2001. Herpes simplex virus infections, p. 425–446. *In* J. S. Remington and J. O. Klein (ed.), *Infectious Diseases of the Fetus and Newborn Infant*, 5th ed. W. B. Saunders, Philadelphia, Pa.

Aurelius, E., B. Johansson, B., Skoldenberg, A. Staland, and M. Forsgren. 1991. Rapid diagnosis of herpes simplex encephalitis by nested polymerase chain reaction of assay of cerebrospinal fluid. *Lancet* **337**:189–192.

Aurelius, E., B. Johansson, B. Skoldenberg, and M. Forsgren. 1993. Encephalitis in immunocompetent patients due to herpes simplex virus type 1 or 2 as determined by type-specific polymerase chain reaction and antibody assays of cerebrospinal fluid. *J. Med. Virol.* **39**:179–186.

Aurelius, E., M. Gosgren, E. Gille, and B. Skoldenberg. 2002. Neurologic morbidity after herpes simplex virus type 2 meningitis: a retrospective study of 40 patients. *Scand. J. Infect. Dis.* **34**:278–283.

Baringer, J. R. 1974. Recovery of herpes simplex virus from human sacral ganglions. *N. Engl. J. Med.* **291**:828–230.

Baringer, J. R. 1978. Herpes simplex infection of the nervous system, p. 145–159. *In* P. Vinken and G. W. Gruyn (ed.), *Handbook of Clinical Neurology*, vol. 34, part 2. Elsevier, Amsterdam, The Netherlands.

Baringer, J. R., and P. Pisani. 1994. Herpes simplex virus genomes in human nervous system tissue analyzed by polymerase chain reaction. *Ann. Neurol.* **36**:823–829.

Baringer, J. R., and P. Swoveland. 1973. Recovery of herpes simplex virus from human trigeminal ganglions. *N. Engl. J. Med.* **288**:648–650.

Bastian, F. O., A. S. Rabson, C. L. Yee, and T. S. Tralka. 1972. Herpes virus hominis—isolation from human trigeminal ganglion. *Science* **178**:306–307.

Benjamin, D. R., and C. G. Ray. 1975. Use of immunoperoxidase on brain tissue for the rapid diagnosis of herpes encephalitis. *Am. J. Clin. Pathol.* **64**:472–476.

Bergey, G. K., P. K. Coyle, A. Krumholz, and E. Niedermeyer. 1982. Herpes simplex encephalitis with occipital localization. *Arch. Neurol.* **39**:312–313.

Bertrand, P., D. Guillaume, K. Hellauer, D. Dea, J. Lindsay, S. Kogan, S. Gauthier, and J. Poirier. 1993. Distribution of herpes simplex virus type 1 DNA in selected areas of normal and Alzheimer's disease brains: a PCR study. *Neurodegeneration* **2**:201–208.

Bia, F. J., G. F. Thornton, A. J. Main, C. K. Y. Fong, and G. D. Hsiung. 1980. Western equine encephalitis mimicking Herpes simplex encephalitis. *JAMA* **244**:367–369.

Booss, J., and M. M. Esiri. 1986. *Viral Encephalitis: Pathology, Diagnosis, and Management.* Blackwell Scientific Publications, Oxford, United Kingdom.

Booss, J., and J. H. Kim. 1984. Biopsy histopathology in herpes simplex encephalitis and in encephalitis of undefined etiology. *Yale J. Biol. Med.* **57**:751–755.

Brick, J. F., J. E. Brick, J. J. Morgan, and A. R. Gutierrez. 1990. EEG and pathologic findings in patients undergoing brain biopsy for suspected encephalitis. *Electroenceph. Clin. Neurophysiol.* **76**:86–89.

Britton, C. B., R. Mesa-Tejada, C. M. Fenoglio, A. P. Hays, G. G. Garvey, and J. R. Miller. 1985. A new complication of AIDS: thoracic myelitis caused by herpes simplex virus. *Neurology* **37**:1791–1794.

Cabrera, C. V., C. Wohlenberg, H. Openshaw, M. Rey-Mendez, and A. Puga. 1980. Herpes simplex virus-DNA sequences in the CNS of latently infected mice. *Nature* **288**:288–290.

Caplan, L. R., F. J. Kleeman, and S. Berg. 1977. Urinary retention probably secondary to Herpes genitalis. *N. Engl. J. Med.* **297**:920–921.

Cappel, R., L. Thiry, and G. Clinet. 1975. Viral antibodies in the CSF after acute CNS infection. *Arch. Neurol.* **32**:629–631.

Carroll, J. F., and J. Booss. 1976. Cerebrospinal fluid IgG level in herpes simplex encephalitis. *JAMA* **236**:2092–2093.

Carton, C. A. 1953. Effect of previous sensory loss on the appearance of herpes simplex following trigeminal sensory root section. *J. Neurosurg.* **10**:463–468.

Chou, J., E. R. Kern, R. J. Whitley, and B. Roizman. 1990. Mapping of herpes simplex virus-1 neurovirulence to gamma 134.5, a gene nonessential for growth in culture. *Science* **250**:1262–1266.

Chrétien, F., L. Belec, D. A. Hilton, M. Flament-Saillour, F. Guillon, L. Wingertsmann, M. Baudrimont, P. de Truchis, C. Keohane, C. Vital, S. Love, and F. Gray. 1996. Herpes simplex virus type 1 encephalitis in acquired immunodeficiency syndrome. *Neuropathol. Appl. Neurobiol.* **22**:394–404.

Cinque, P., G. M. Cleator, T. Weber, P. Monteyne, C. J. Sindic, and A. M. van Loon for The EU Concerted Action on Virus Meningitis and Encephalitis. 1996. The role of laboratory investigation in the diagnosis and management of patients with suspected herpes simplex encephalitis: a consensus report. *J. Neurol. Neurosurg. Psychiatr.* **61**:339–345.

Cook, M. L., and J. G. Stevens. 1976. Latent herpetic infections following experimental viraemia. *J. Gen. Virol.* **31**:75–80.

Cook, M. L., V. B. Bastone, and J. G. Stevens. 1974. Evidence that neurons harbour latent herpes simplex virus. *Infect. Immun.* **9**:946–951.

Corey, L., H. G. Adams, Z. A. Brown, and K. K. Holmes. 1983. Genital herpes simplex virus infections: clinical manifestations, course, and complications. *Ann. Intern. Med.* **98**:958–972.

Davis, L. E. 2000. Diagnosis and treatment of acute encephalitis. *The Neurologist* **6**:145–159.

Davis, L. E., and R. T. Johnson. 1979. An explanation for the localisation of herpes simplex encephalitis? *Ann. Neurol.* **5**:2–5.

Davis, L. E., and L. C. McLaren. 1983. Relapsing herpes simplex encephalitis following antiviral therapy. *Ann. Neurol.* **13**:192–195.

Dayan, A. D., W. Gooddy, M. J. G. Harrison, and P. Rudge. 1972. Brain stem encephalitis caused by herpesvirus hominis. *Br. Med. J.* **4**:405–406.

Dennett, C., P. E. Klapper, and G. M. Cleator. 1996. Polymerase chain reaction in the investigation of "relapse" following herpes simplex encephalitis. *J. Med. Virol.* **48**:129–132.

Dinn, J. J. 1980. Transolfactory spread of virus in herpes simplex encephalitis. *Br. Med. J.* **2**:1392.

Dix, R. D., J. R. Baringer, H. S. Panitch, S. H. Rosenberg, J. Hagedorn, and J. Whaley. 1983. Recurrent herpes simplex encephalitis: recovery of virus after Ara-A treatment. *Ann. Neurol.* **13**:196–200.

Domingues, R. B., A. M. C. Tsanaclis, C. S. Pannuti, M. S. Mayo, and F. D. Lakeman. 1997. Evaluation of the range of clinical presentations of herpes simplex encephalitis by using polymerase chain reaction assay of cerebrospinal fluid samples. *Clin. Infect. Dis.* **25**:86–91.

Domingues, R. B., M. C. D. Fink, A. M. C. Tsanaclis, C. C. de Castro, G. G. Cerri, M. S. Mayo, and F. D. Lakeman. 1998. Diagnosis of herpes simplex encephalitis by magnetic resonance imaging and polymerase chain reaction assay of cerebrospinal fluid. *J. Neurol. Sci.* **157**:148–153.

Drachman, D. A., and R. D. Adams. 1962. Herpes simplex and acute inclusion body encephalitis. *Arch. Neurol.* **7**:61–79.

Drummond, C. W., R. P. Eglin, and M. M. Esiri. 1994. Herpes simplex virus encephalitis in a mouse model: PCR evidence for CNS latency following acute infection. *J. Neurol. Sci.* **127**:159–163.

Ellison, P. H., and P. A. Hanson. 1977. Herpes simplex. A possible cause of brain-stem encephalitis. *Pediatrics* **59**:240–243.

Esiri, M. M. 1982. Herpes simplex encephalitis: an immunohistological study of the distribution of viral antigen within the brain. *J. Neurol. Sci.* **54**:209–226.

Flexner, S. 1923. Epidemic (lethargic) encephalitis and allied conditions. *JAMA* **81**:1688–1693, 1785–1789.

Fodor, P. A., M. J. Levin, A. Weinberg, E. Sandberg, J. Sylman, and K. L. Tyler. 1998. Atypical herpes simplex virus encephalitis diagnosed by PCR amplification of viral DNA from CSF. *Neurology* **51**:554–559.

Folpe, A., L. W. Lapham, and H. C. Smith. 1994. Herpes simplex myelitis as a cause of acute necrotizing myelitis syndrome. *Neurology* **44**:1955–1957.

Fraser, N. W., W. C. Lawrence, Z. Wroblewska, D. H. Gilden, and H. Koprowski. 1981. Herpes simplex type I DNA in human brain tissue. *Proc. Natl. Acad. Sci. USA* **78**:6461–6465.

Gordon, B., O. A. Selnes, J. Hart, Jr., D. F. Hanley, and R. J. Whitley. 1990. Long-term cognitive sequelae of acyclovir-treated herpes simplex encephalitis. *Arch. Neurol.* **47**:646–647.

Gordon, L., S. McQuaid, and S. L. Cosby. 1996. Detection of herpes simplex virus (types 1 and 2) and human herpes virus 6 DNA in human brain tissues by polymerase chain reaction. *Clin. Diagn. Virol.* **6**:33–40.

Hammer, S. M., T. G. Buchman, L. J. D'Angelo, A. W. Karchmer, B. Roizman, and M. S. Hirsch. 1980. Temporal cluster of herpes sirnplex encephalitis: investigation by restriction endonuclease cleavage of viral DNA. *J. Infect. Dis.* **141:**436–440.

Hargrave, D. R., and D. W. Webb. 1998. Movement disorders in association with herpes simplex encephalitis virus in children: a review. *Devel. Med. Child. Neurol.* **40:**640–642.

Haymaker, W. 1949. Herpes simplex encephalitis in man—with a report of 3 cases. *Neuropath. Exp. Neurol.* **8:**132–154.

Haymaker, W., M. G. Smith, L. van Bogaert, and C. de Chenar. 1958. Pathology of viral disease in man characterized by nuclear inclusions, p. 95–104. *In* W. S. Field and R. Blattner (ed.), *Viral Encephalitis.* Thomas, Springfield, Ill.

Heller, M., R. D. Dix, J. R. Baringer, J. Schachter, and J. E. Conte, Jr. 1982. Herpetic proctitis and meningitis: recovery of two strains of Herpes simplex virus type I from cerebrospinal fluid. *J. Infect. Dis.* **1462:**584–588.

Hierons, R., I. Janota, and J. A. N. Corsellis. 1978. The late effects of necrotising encephalitis of the temporal lobes and limbic area—a clinic-pathological study of 10 cases. *Psychol. Med.* **8:**21–42.

Hindmarsh, T., M. Lindovist, E. Olding-Stenkvist, B. Skoldenberg, and M. Forsgren. 1986. Accuracy of computed tomography in the diagnosis of herpes simplex encephalitis. *Acta Radiol.* Suppl. **369:**192–196.

Hirst, L. W., A. W. Clark, J. S. Wolinsky, D. S. Zee, H. Kaiser, N. R. Miller, P. J. Tutschka, and G. W. Santos. 1983. Downbeat nystagmus. A case report of herpetic brain stem encephalitis. *J. Clin. Neuroophthalmol.* **3:**245–249.

Hollinger, P., L. Matter, and M. Struzenegger. 2000. Normal MRI findings in herpes simplex encephalitis. *J. Neurol.* **247:**799–801.

Hughes, J. T. 1969. Pathology of herpes simplex encephalitis, p. 29–37. *In* C. W. M. Whitty, J. T. Hughes, and F. O. MacCallum (ed.), *Virus Diseases of the Nervous System.* Blackwell Scientific Publications, Oxford, United Kingdom.

Itabashi, S., H. Arai, T. Matsui, S. Higuchi, and H. Sasaki. 1997. Herpes simplex virus and risk of Alzheimer's disease. *Lancet* **349:**1102.

Ito, Y., H. Kimura, Y. Yabata, Y. Ando, T. Murakami, M. Shiomi, and T. Morishima. 2000. Exacerbation of herpes simplex encephalitis after successful treatment with acyclovir. *Clin. Infect. Dis.* **30:**185–187.

Itzhaki, R. F., N. J. Maitland, G. K. Wilcock, C. M. Yates, and G. A. Jamieson. 1993. Detection by polymerase chain reaction of herpes simplex virus type 1 (HSV-1) DNA in brain of aged normals and Alzheimer's disease patients, p. 97–102. *In* B. Corain, K. Iqbal, M. Nicolini, B. Winblad, H. Wisniewski, and P. Zatta (ed.), *Alzheimer's Disease: Advances in Clinical and Basic Research.* Wiley & Sons, New York, N.Y.

Itzhaki, R. F., W. R. Lin, D. Shang, G. K. Wilcock, B. Faragher, and G. A. Jamieson. 1997. Herpes simplex virus type 1 in brain and risk of Alzheimer's disease. *Lancet* **349:**241–244.

Itzhaki, R. F., W. R. Lin, G. K. Wilcock, and B. Faragher. 1998. HSV-1 and risk of Alzheimer's disease. *Lancet* **352:**238.

Izumi, K. M., and J. G. Stevens. 1990. Molecular and biological characterization of a herpes simplex virus type 1 (HSV-1) neuroinvasiveness gene. *J. Exp. Med.* **172:**487–496.

Jain, S., and M. C. Maheshwari. 1984. Herpetic brain-stem encephalitis with features of 'diencephalic epilepsy.' A case report. *Acta Neurol.* (Napoli) **6:**1–4.

Jamieson, G. A., N. J. Maitland, G. K. Wilcock, C. M. Yates, and R. F. Itzhaki. 1992. Herpes simplex virus type 1 DNA is present in specific regions of brain from aged people with and without senile dementia of the Alzheimer type. *J. Pathol.* **167:**365–368.

Jensenius, M., B. Myrvang, G. Storvold, A. Bucher, K. B. Hellum, and A.-L. Bruu. 1998. Herpes virus type 2 DNA detected in cerebrospinal fluid of 9 patients with Mollaret's meningitis. *Acta Neurol. Scand.* **98:**209–212.

Johnson, R. T., and C. A. Mims. 1968. Pathogenesis of viral infections of the nervous system. *N. Engl. J. Med.* **2782:**23–30, 84–92.

Kimberlin, D. W., C.-Y. Lin, R. F. Jacobs, D. A. Powell, L. M. Frenkel, W. C. Gruber, M. Rathmore, J. S. Bradley, P. S. Diaz, M. Kumar, A. A. Arvin, K. Gutierrez, M. Shelton, L. B. Weiner, J. M. Sleasman, T. M. de Sierra, S.-J. Soong, J. Kiell, F. D. Lakeman, F. J. Whitley, and the National Institute of Allergy and Infectious Diseases Collaborative Antiviral Study Group. 2001a. Natural history of neonatal herpes simplex virus infections in the acyclovir era. *Pediatrics* **108:**223–229.

Kimberlin, D. W., C.-Y. Lin, R. F. Jacobs, D. A. Powell, L. Corey, W. C. Gruber, M. Rathore, J. S. Bradley, P. S. Diaz, M. Kumar, A. M. Arvin, K. Gutierrez, M. Shelton, L. B. Weiner, J. W. Sleasman, T. M. de Sierra, S. Weller, S.-J. Soong, J. Kiell, F. D. Lakeman, R. J. Whitley, and the National Institute of Allergy and Infectious Diseases Collaborative Antiviral Study Group. 2001b. Safety and efficacy of high-dose intravenous acyclovir in the management of neonatal herpes simplex virus infections. *Pediatrics* **108:**230–238.

Klastersky, J., R. Cappel, J. M. Snoeck, J. Flament, and L. Thiry. 1972. Ascending myelitis in association with Herpes simplex virus. *N. Engl. J. Med.* **287:**182–184.

Kleihues, P. 1969. Uber das Verteilungsmuster der Encephalitiden vom Herpes simplex-typ. *D. Z. Nervenheilk.* **195:**42–56.

Kleinschmidt-DeMasters, B. K., and D. H. Gilden. 2001. The expanding spectrum of herpesvirus infections of the nervous system. *Brain Pathol.* **11:**440–451.

Kleinschmidt-DeMasters, B. K., R. L. DeBiasi, and K. L. Tyler. 2001. Polymerase chain reaction as a diagnostic adjunct in herpes infections of the nervous system. *Brain Pathol.* **11:**452–464.

Koenig, H., S. G. Rabinowitz, E. Day, and V. Miller. 1979. Post-infectious encephalomyelitis after successful treatment of herpes simplex encephalitis with adenine arabinoside. Ultrastructural observations. *N. Engl. J. Med.* **300:**1089–1093.

Kuker, W., L. Schmade, K. Ritter, and W. Nacimiento. 1999. MRI follow-up of herpes simplex virus (type 1). Radiculomyelitis. *Neurology* **52:**1102–1103.

Kumanishi, R., and A. Hirano. 1978. An immunoperoxidase study of herpes simplex encephalitis. *J. Neuropath. Exp. Neurol.* **37:**790–795.

Lahat, E., J. Barr, G. Barkai, G. Paret, N. Brand, and A. Barzilai. 1999. Long-term neurological outcome of herpes encephalitis. *Arch. Dis. Child.* **80:**69–71.

Lakeman, F. D., R. J. Whitley, and The National Institute of Allergy and Infectious Diseases Collaborative Antiviral Study Group. 1995. Diagnosis of herpes simplex encephalitis: application of polymerase chain reaction to cerebrospinal fluid from brain-biopsied patients and correlation with disease. *J. Infect. Dis.* **171:**857–863.

Landry, M. L., N. Berkovits, W. P. Summers, J. Booss, and G. D. Hsiung. 1983. Herpes simplex encephalitis: analysis of a cluster of cases by restriction endonuclease mapping of virus isolates. *Neurology* **33:**831–835.

Launes, J., J. Sirén, L. Valanne, O. Salonen, P. Nikkinen, A.-M. Seppalainen, and K. Liewendahl. 1997. Unilateral hyperperfusion in brain-perfusion SPECT predicts poor prognosis in acute encephalitis. *Neurology* **48:**1347–1351.

Lee, J. W., I.-O. Kim, W. S. Kim, K. M. Yeon, H.-J. Lee, and Y. S. Hwang. 2001. Herpes simplex encephalitis: MRI findings in two cases confirmed by polymerase chain reaction assay. *Pediatr. Radiol.* **31:**619–623.

Lellouch-Tubiana, A., M. Fohlen, O. Robain, and F. Rozenberg. 2000. Immunocytochemical characterization of long-term persistent immune activation in human brain after herpes simplex encephalitis. *Neuropathol. Appl. Neurobiol.* **26:**285–294.

Levaditti, C., P. Harvier, and P. Nicolarn. 1922. Etude experimentale de l'enciphalitie dite 'lethargique.' *Ann. Inst. Pasteur,* (Paris) **36:**63–148.

Lin, W.-R., M. A. Wozniak, M. M. Esiri, P. Keenerman, and R. F. Itzhaki. 2001. Herpes simplex encephalitis: involvement of apolipoprotein E genotype. *J. Neurol. Neurosurg. Psychiatr.* **70:**117–119.

Longson, M. 1975. The general nature of viral encephalitis in the United Kingdom, p. 19–31. *In* L. S. Illis (ed.), *Viral Diseases of the Nervous System.* Baillière Tindall, London, United Kingdom.

Love, S., and C. A. Wiley. 2002. Viral infections, p. 1–106. *In* D. I. Graham, and P. L. Lantos (ed.), *Greenfield's Neuropathology.* Arnold, London, United Kingdom.

MacCallum, F. O. 1973. Discussion. *Postgrad. Med. J.* **49:**406–409.

Maertzdorf, J., A. Van der Lelij, G. S. Baarsma, A. D. M. E. Osterhaus, and G. M. Verjans. 2000. Herpes virus type 1 (HSV-1)-induced retinitis following herpes simplex encephalitis: indications for brain-to-eye transmission of HSV-1. *Ann. Neurol.* **48:**936–939.

Martins, A. N., L. G. Kempe, and G. J. Hayes. 1964. Acute hemorrhagic leukoencephalitis (Hurst) with concurrent herpes simplex infection. *J. Neurol. Neurosurg. Psychiatr.* **27:**493–501.

McGrath, N., N. E. Anderson, M. C. Croxson, and K. F. Powell. 1997. Herpes simplex encephalitis treated with acyclovir: diagnosis and long-term outcome. *J. Neurol. Neurosurg. Psychiatr.* **63:**321–326.

McLennan, J. L., and G. Darby. 1980. Herpes simplex virus latency: the cellular location of virus in dorsal root ganglia and the fate of the infected cell following virus activation. *J. Gen. Virol.* **51:**233–243.

Mertens, G., M. Ieven, D. Ursi, S. R. Pattyn, J. J. Martin, and P. M. Parizel. 1993. Detection of herpes simplex virus in the cerebrospinal fluid of patients with encephalitis using the polymerase chain reaction. *J. Neurol. Sci.* **118:**213–216.

Meyding-Lamadé, U. K., W. R. Lamadé, B. T. Wildemann, K. Sartor, and W. Hacke. 1999. Herpes simplex virus encephalitis: chronic progressive cerebral magnetic resonance imaging abnormalities in patients despite good clinical recovery. *Clin. Infect. Dis.* **28:**148–149.

Meyer, H. M., Jr., R. T. Johnson, I. P. Crawford, H. E. Dascomb, and N. G. Rogers. 1960. Central nervous system syndromes of viral etiology. A study of 713 cases. *Am. J. Med.* **29:**334–347.

Miller, J. K., F. Hesser, and V. N. Tompkins. 1966. Herpes simplex encephalitis. Report of 20 cases. *Ann. Intern. Med.* **64:**92–103.

Morrison, R. E., M. H. Miller, L. W. Lyon, J. M. Griffiss, and M. S. Artenstein. 1974. Adult meningoencephalitis caused by Herpes virus hominis type 2. *Am. J. Med.* **56:**540–544.

Nahmias, A. J., and W. R. Dowdle. 1968. Antigenic and biologic differences in herpesvirus hominis. *Prog. Med. Virol.* **10:**110–159.

Nahmias, A. J., and B. Roizman. 1973. Infection with herpes simplex viruses 1 and 2. *N. Engl. J. Med.* **289:**667–673, 719–725, 781–789.

Nahmias, A. J., R. J. Whitley, A. X. Visintine, Y. Takei, and C. A. Alford, Jr. 1982. Herpes simplex virus encephalitis: laboratory evaluations and their diagnostic significance. *J. Infect. Dis.* **145:**829–836.

Nakajima, H., D. Furutama, F. Kimura, K. Shinoda, T. Nakagawa, A. Shimizu, and N. Ohsawa. 1995. Herpes simplex virus type 2 infections presenting as brain stem encephalitis and recurrent myelitis. *Intern. Med.* **34:**839–842.

Nakajima, H., D. Furutama, F. Kimura, K. Shinoda, N. Ohsawa, T. Nakagawa, A. Shimizu, and H. Shoji. 1998. Herpes simplex virus myelitis: clinical manifestations and diagnosis by the polymerase chain reaction method. *Eur. Neurol.* **39:**163–167.

Nicoll, J. A., S. Love, and E. Kinrade. 1993. Distribution of herpes simplex virus DNA in the brains of human long-term survivors of encephalitis. *Neurosci. Lett.* **157:**215–218.

Nicoll, S., A. Brass, and H. A. Cubie. 2001. Detection of herpes viruses in clinical samples using real-time PCR. *J. Virol. Methods* **96:**25–31.

Oates, J. K., and P. R. D. H. Greenhouse. 1978. Retention of urine in anogenital herpetic infection. *Lancet* **1:**691–692.

Ojeda, V. J. 1980. Fatal herpes simplex encephalitis with demonstration of virus in the olfactory pathway. *Pathology* **12:**429–437.

Petereit, H. F., S. Bamborschke, and H. Lanfermann. 1996. Acute transverse myelitis caused by herpes simplex virus. *Eur. Neurol.* **36:**52–53.

Plummer, G. 1973. Isolation of herpes viruses from trigeminal ganglia of man, monkeys, and cats. *J. Infect. Dis.* **128:**343–348.

Rappel, M., M. Dubois-Dalcq, S. Sprecher, L. Thiry, A. Lowenthal, S. Pelc, and J. P. Thys. 1971. Diagnosis and treatment of herpes encephalitis—a multidisciplinary approach. *J. Neurol. Sci.* **12:**443–458.

Ravaut, P., and Darré. 1904. Les réactions nerveuses au cours des herpes genitaux. *Ann. Dermatol.* **5:**481–496.

Rodda, S., I. Jack, and D. O. White. 1973. Herpes simplex virus from trigeminal ganglion. *Lancet* **i:**1395–1396.

Roizman, B. 1982. The family herpes viridae: general description, and taxonomy and classification, p. 1–23. *In* B. Roizman (ed.), *The Herpes Viruses,* vol. 1. Plenum Press, New York, N.Y.

Roman-Campos, G., and G. Toro. 1980. Herpetic brain stem encephalitis. *Neurology* **30:**981–985.

Rose, J. W., W. G. Stroop, F. Matsuo, and J. Henkel. 1992. Atypical herpes simplex encephalitis: clinical, virologic, and neuropathologic evaluation. *Neurology* **42:**1809–1812.

Sage, J. I., M. P. Weinstein, and D. C. Miller. 1985. Chronic encephalitis possibly due to herpes simplex virus: two cases. *Neurology* **35:**1470–1472.

Sakakibara, R., T. Hattori, T. Fukutake, M. Mori, T. Yamanishi, and K. Yasuda. 1998. Micturitional disturbance in herpetic brain stem encephalitis; contribution of the pontine micturition centre. *J. Neurol. Neurosurg. Psychiatry* **64:**269–272.

Samarasinghe, P. L., J. K. Oates, and I. P. B. MacLennan. 1979. Herpetic proctitis and sacral radiculomyelopathy—a hazard for homosexual men. *Br. Med. J.* **3:**365–366.

Sauerbrei, A., U. Eichhorn, G. Hottenrott, and P. Wutzler. 2000. Virological diagnosis of herpes simplex encephalitis. *J. Clin. Virol.* **17:**31–36.

Schmidbauer, M., H. Budka, and P. Ambros. 1989. Herpes simplex virus (HSV) DNA in microglial nodular brain stem encephalitis. *J. Neuropathol. Exp. Neurol.* **48:**645–652.

Sequiera, L. W., L. C. Jennings, L. H. Carrasco, M. A. Lord, A. Curry, and R. N. Sutton. 1979. Detection of herpes-simplex viral genome in brain tissue. *Lancet* **2:**609–612.

Shyu, W. C., J. C. Lin, B. C. Chang, H. J. Harn, C. C. Lee, and W. L. Tsao. 1993. Recurrent ascending myelitis: an unusual presentation of herpes simplex virus type 1 infection. *Ann. Neurol.* **34:**625–627.

Skoldenberg, B. 1991. Herpes simplex encephalitis. *Scand. J. Infect. Dis.* **78**(Suppl.)**:**40–46.

Skoldenberg, B., S. Jeansson, and S. Wolontis. 1973. Herpes simplex type 2 in acute aseptic meningitis. *Br. Med. J.* **2:**611.

Skoldenberg, B., K. Kalimo, A. Carlstroin, M. Forsgren, and P. Halonen. 1981. Herpes simplex encephalitis: a serological follow up study. *Acta Neurol. Scand.* **63:**273–285.

Skoldenberg, B., M. Forsgren, K. Alestig, T. Bergstrom, L. Burman, E. Dahlquist, A. Forkman, A. Fryden, K. Lovegren, K. Norlin, R. Norrby, E. Olding-Stenkvist, G. Stiernstedt, I. Uhnoo, and K. DeVahl. 1984. Acyclovir versus vidarabine in herpes simplex encephalitis. Randomized multicenter study in consecutive Swedish patients. *Lancet* ii:707–711.

Smith, J. B., B. F. Westmoreland, T. J. Reagan, and B. A. Sandok. 1975. A distinctive clinical EEG profile in herpes simplex encephalitis. *Mayo Clin. Proc.* **50**:469–474.

Smith, M. G., E. H. Lennette, and H. R. Reames. 1941. Isolation of the virus of herpes simplex and demonstration of intranuclear inclusions in a case of acute encephalitis. *Am. J. Pathol.* **17**:55–68.

Steel, J. G., R. D. Dix, and J. R. Barringer. 1982. Isolation of herpes simplex virus type-1 in recurrent (Mollaret's) meningitis. *Ann. Neurol.* **11**:17–21.

Steiner, I., and P. G. Kennedy. 1993. Molecular biology of herpes simplex virus type 1 latency in the nervous system. *Mol. Neurobiol.* **7**:137–159.

Stevens, J. G. 1993. HSV-1 neuroinvasiveness. *Intervirology* **35**:152–63.

Stroop, W. G., D. Rock, and N. Fraser. 1984. Localisation of herpes simplex virus in the trigeminal and olfactory systems of the mouse central nervous system during acute and latent infection by *in situ* hybridisation. *Lab. Invest.* **51**:27–38.

Tan, S. V., R. J. Guiloff, F. Scaravilli, P. E. Klapper, G. M. Cleator, and B. G. Gazzard. 1993. Herpes simplex type 1 encephalitis in acquired immunodeficiency syndrome. *Ann. Neurol.* **34**:619–622.

Tenser, R. B. 1998. Trigeminal neuralgia. Mechanisms of treatment. *Neurology* **51**:17–19.

Terni, M., P. Caccialanza, E. Cassai, and E. Kieff. 1971. Aseptic meningitis in association with Herpes progenitalis. *N. Engl. J. Med.* **285**:503–504.

Tyler, K. L., D. G. Tedder, L. J. Yamamoto, J. A. Klapper, R. Ashley, K. A. Lichtenstein, and M. J. Levin. 1995. Recurrent brain stem encephalitis associated with herpes simplex virus type 1 DNA in cerebrospinal fluid. *Neurology* **45**:2246–2250.

Vandvik, B., F. Vartdal, and E. Norrby. 1982. Herpes simplex virus encephalitis: intrathecal synthesis of oligoclonal virus-specific IgG, IgA, and IgM antibodies. *J. Neurol.* **228**:25–38.

Wagner, E. K., and D. C. Bloom. 1997. Experimental investigation of herpes simplex virus latency. *Clin. Microbiol. Rev.* **10**:419–443.

Warren, K. G., S. M. Brown, Z. Wroblewska, D. Gilden, H. Koprowski, and J. Subak-Sharpe. 1978. Isolation of latent herpes simplex virus from the superior cervical and vagal ganglions of human beings. *N. Engl. J. Med.* **298**:1068–1069.

Weil, A. A., C. A. Glaser, Z. Amad, and B. Forghani. 2002. Patients with suspected herpes simplex encephalitis: rethinking an initial negative polymerase chain reaction result. *Clin. Infect. Dis.* **34**:1154–1157.

Whitley, R. J. 1996. Herpes simplex virus, p. 2297–2342. *In* B. N. Fields (ed.), *Fields Virology*, 3rd ed. Lippincott-Raven, Philadelphia, Pa.

Whitley, R. J., and J. W. Gnann. 2002. Viral encephalitis: familiar infections and emerging pathogens. *Lancet* **359**:507–514.

Whitley, R. J., and F. Lakeman. 1995. Herpes simplex virus infections of the central nervous system: therapeutic and diagnostic considerations. *Clin. Infect. Dis.* **20**:414–420.

Whitley, R. J., and B. Roizman. 2001. Herpes simplex virus infections. *Lancet* **357**:1513–1518.

Whitley, R. J., S.-J. Soong, R. Dolin, G. J. Galasso, L. T. Ch'ien, C. A. Alford, and the Collaborative Study Group. 1977. Adenine arabinoside therapy of biopsy-proved herpes simplex encephalitis. National Institute of Allergy and Infectious Diseases Collaborative Antiviral Study. *N. Engl. J. Med.* **297**:289–294.

Whitley, R. J., S.-J. Soong, M. S. Hirsch, A. W. Karchmer, R. Dolin, G. Galasso, J. K. Dunnick, C. A. Alford, and the NIAID Collaborative Antiviral Study Group. 1981. Herpes simplex encephalitis. Vidarabine therapy and diagnostic problems. *N. Engl. J. Med.* **304**:313–318.

Whitley, R. J., A. D. Lakeman, A. Nahmias, and B. Roizman. 1982a. DNA restriction enzyme analysis of herpes simplex virus isolates obtained from patients with encephalitis. *N. Engl. J. Med.* **307**:1060–1062.

Whitley, R. J., S.-J. Soong, C. Linneman, Jr., C. Liu, G. Pazin, C. A. Alford, and the National Institute of Allergy and Infectious Diseases Collaborative Antiviral Study Group. 1982b. Herpes simplex encephalitis. Clinical assessment. *JAMA* **247**:317–320.

Whitley, R. J., C. A. Alford, M. S. Hirsch, R. T. Schooley, J. P. Luby, F. Y. Aoki, D. Hanley, A. J. Nahmias, S.-J. Soong, and the NIAID Collaborative Antiviral Study Group. 1986. Vidarabine versus acyclovir therapy in herpes simplex encephalitis. *N. Engl. J. Med.* **314**:144–149.

Wildy, P., H. J. Field, and A. A. Nash. 1982. Classical herpes latency revisited, p. 133–167. *In* B. W. J. Mahy, A. C. Minson, and G. K. Darby (ed.), *Virus Persistence*. Soc. Gen. Microbiol. Symp. 33. Cambridge University Press, Cambridge, United Kingdom.

Wiley, C. A., P. D. Van Patten, P. M. Carpenter, H. C. Powell, and L. J. Thal. 1987. Acute ascending necrotizing myelopathy caused by herpes simplex virus type 2. *Neurology* **37**:1791–1794.

Young, C. A., P. R. D. Humphrey, E. J. Ghadiali, P. E. Klapper, and G. M. Cleator. 1992. Short-term memory impairment in an alert patient as a presentation of herpes simplex encephalitis. *Neurology* **42**:260–261.

Systemic Viral Diseases and Encephalitis

Encephalitis may appear in the context of systemic viral illness or viral infection of another organ system. Consideration of the diagnostic features of the non-central nervous system (CNS) portion of the disease will facilitate an etiologic diagnosis. Diseases of this type may also have a parainfectious immune-mediated pathogenesis. For example, mumps encephalitis sometimes appears early as part of an infectious meningoencephalitis and on other occasions has a timing compatible with a parainfectious process. Nonetheless, the association with clinically recognized mumps facilitates the diagnosis. Sometimes, viruses that are usually associated with systemic illness may present with CNS signs alone. Investigation of the systemic viral illness, fully expressed in the patient's contacts, may provide the clue to an otherwise cryptic encephalitis. Evaluation of the systemic characteristics of the patient's viral illness and of the illnesses among the patient's contacts should therefore be undertaken in each case of encephalitis.

EXANTHEMATOUS DISEASES

Exanthematous diseases were previously labeled numerically from one to six as they were differentiated from other childhood exanthems; now only "fifth" and "sixth" diseases continue to be used in clinical parlance. Viral exanthems associated with encephalitis/encephalopathy are listed in Table 5.1. Second disease was scarlet fever, and fourth disease has not emerged as a separate clinical entity (Frieden and Resnick, 1991). Table 5.1 also lists other exanthems sometimes associated with encephalitis or encephalopathy but does not exhaustively list all viral infections associated on occasion with both a rash and encephalitis or encephalopathy. Bacterial diseases such as Rocky Mountain fever and meningococcal disease (Frieden and Resnick, 1991) are also associated with CNS disease and skin manifestations. Table 5.1 serves as a reminder of the importance of seeking the physical signs of a rash, however faint, or the history of a transient rash, however fleeting, prior to the onset of encephalitis/encephalopathy. Measles and rubella provoke immune-mediated CNS disease and are discussed in chapters 7 and 8 covering para- and postinfectious acute disseminated encephalomyelitis (ADEM). Smallpox (chapter 8) was on occasion followed by an encephalopathy or ADEM. Varicella-zoster virus (VZV) is covered independently in chapter 9. Enteroviral CNS disease usually occurs in the context of summer-fall outbreaks and is discussed in chapter 10, concerning epidemic viral diseases that can be complicated by encephalitis. Erythema infectiosium, or fifth disease, caused by parvovirus B-19, and roseola infantum

TABLE 5.1 Representative viral exanthems and encephalitis/encephalopathy

Disease names	Viruses	Chapter(s)
First disease, measles, rubeola	Rubeola	7 and 8
Third disease, German measles, rubella	Rubella	7 and 8
Fifth disease, erythema infectiosum	Parvovirus B-19	5
Sixth disease, roseloa infantum, exanthem subitum	HHV-6	5
Varicella, chicken pox, zoster	Herpes zoster	9
Enteroviral exanthems	Enteroviruses, coxsackie, echoviruses	10

(exanthem subitum), or sixth disease, caused by human herpesvirus 6 (HHV-6) and, on occasion, by HHV-7, are discussed below.

Erythema Infectiosum, or Fifth Disease, Caused by Parvovirus B-19

Parvoviruses are small DNA viruses (Heegard and Brown, 2002). While a common infection—50% of children have antibody by 15 years of age and over 90% of elderly people have antibody (Brown, 2000)—parvovirus B-19 is a rare cause of encephalitis/encephalopathy. B-19 was discovered during an investigation of anomalous results in lab testing for hepatitis B antigen (Cossart et al., 1975). The discovery of its association with erythema infectiosum came about from the study of an outbreak in north London (Anderson et al., 1983). Targeting erythroid precursors through a virus receptor, blood group P antigen, or globoside, parvovirus B-19 can produce a transient aplastic crisis of red cell production in individuals susceptible to chronic hemolytic anemia. Parvovirus B-19 is also associated with a polyarthropathy, particularly in adults, and hydrops fetalis in the fetus.

The classic facial rash, or "slapped cheeks" rash, occurs in children between the ages of 5 and 15 following an incubation period of about 4 to 14 days after transmission by respiratory droplets (Frieden and Resnick, 1991). The appearance of the facial rash is fiery and abrupt. A few days later, a more generalized reticular rash appears. This rash, often on the extremities, can fluctuate for up to several weeks and is influenced by sunlight, temperature, exercise, and emotion (Frieden and Resnick, 1991). A symmetrical arthritis/anthropathy can be found in adults. Because of the risk to the fetus, prevention of transmission to women of childbearing age, such as in day care centers, schools, and health care settings, is critical.

The association of parvovirus B-19 infection with encephalitis and encephalopathy was not widely reported prior to the association of fifth disease and B-19 in 1983. Balfour et al. (1970) studied 93 patients in an outbreak of erythemia infectiosum in Ohio in 1969; one victim was an 8½-year-old-boy with encephalitis. Bilateral corticospinal tract signs, reduced level of consciousness, and impaired bladder function were reported, corresponding, it would seem, to an encephalomyelitis. CNS dysfunction emerged 5 days after the rash. A moderate lymphocytic pleocytosis was found, and the electroencephalogram (EEG) was diffusely abnormal, with runs of slow activity over the vertex. At 6 weeks, significant recovery had occurred except for slight left-sided weakness with corticospinal tract signs. Hall and Horner (1977) reported a 9-month-old boy whose recovery from encephalitis was not satisfactory; he was left with psychomotor retardation, choreiform movements, and pathological corticospinal tract reflexes. Two cases of serologically confirmed parvovirus B-19 encephalopathy in two 5-year-old girls were reported by Watanabe et al. (1994). One child had convulsions, drowsiness, and an acellular cerebrospinal fluid (CSF), and the other had convulsive status epilepticus and a lymphocytic pleocytosis in the CSF.

More recently, the use of various techniques, including PCR on banked CSF samples, has raised the possibility that parvovirus B-19 meningoencephalitis may be more common than previously appreciated. Barah et al. (2001) found 7 of 162 patients positive from cases of undiagnosed meningoencephalitis in a 1-year period and 15 other positives from other time periods. The ages ranged from 1 day to 5 years; one died and four had neurological sequelae. Abnormal scans (computerized tomography [CT], magnetic resonance imaging [MRI], and ultrasound) were found in patients with neurological sequelae. In follow-up correspondence, Yoto et al. (2001) also reported a retrospective examination of CSF samples by PCR. Three of 744 were found to be positive, two of which were from children with encephalopathy. Recently, Skaff and Labiner (2001) reported a case of parvovirus B-19 encephalitis in a 27-year-old immunocompetent woman with prolonged status epilepticus. Prior to the onset of neurological illness, an erythematous malar rash was documented. The CSF revealed a moderate lymphocytosis. A frontal lobe biopsy at 6 weeks showed chronic minimal leptomeningitis and mild gliosis in the superficial cortex. Remarkable recovery occurred following seizure control, mechanical respiration, supportive therapy, and rehabilitation. Hence, while the role of parvovirus B-19 as an etiology of encephalitis and encephalopathy is not widely appreciated, application of virus-specific assays such as PCR and serology may result in many more cases being recognized.

Aseptic meningitis and stroke have also been reported in connection with parvovirus B-19. The virus is a demonstrated cause, albeit rare, of aseptic meningitis. Tabak et al. (1999) reported that they were able to find only five other cases in the literature in addition to their own. One patient with sickle cell anemia died as a result of an aplastic crisis. The paucity of reported cases may result from a lack of application of specific parvovirus diagnostic assays. Stroke in patients with homozygous sickle cell disease has been reported as a consequence of parvovirus infection, and the importance of the development of a human vaccine has been emphasized (Wierenga et al., 2001). Peripheral nervous system (PNS) manifestations in the form of brachial plexitis have been reported. Staud et al. (1995) reported on a patient who apparently responded to steroid therapy; they found three other case reports in the literature. Numbness and tingling of the extremities of undetermined etiology has also been reported (Faden et al., 1990).

In summary, there are insufficient data to distinguish the encephalitis following parvovirus B-19 infection from other causes of encephalitis. It occurs primarily in children but can occur in adults and is often associated with seizures and depression of the level of consciousness. The CSF may be bland or have a lymphocytic pleocytosis. Neuroimaging may reveal abnormalities, particularly in those destined to have sequelae (Barah et al., 2001). Viral diagnostic studies rely on immunoglobulin M (IgM) and IgG antibody capture enzyme-linked immunosorbent assay (ELISA) or immunofluorescent antibody determinations and CSF PCR. There is no antiviral therapy available for parvovirus B-19 infections. Immune serum globulin has been used in patients with persistent infections due to immunodeficiency disorders to allow restoration of bone marrow function (Naides, 2000). Conversely, steroid therapy may be considered if clinical and neuroimaging features suggest an immune-mediated disorder. Vigorous supportive care is to be encouraged. No vaccine is available.

HHV-6—Exanthem Subitum, Sixth Disease, or Roseola

General

Exanthem subitum, roseola, and sixth disease are synonyms for a brief illness of infants and children characterized by the appearance of a rash following lysis of fever. Clinical descriptions of the illness date back to at least 1809 (E. L. Altschuler, Letter, *Pediatr. Infect. Dis. J.* **19**:902, 2000). While the illness was long suspected to be of viral etiology, the confirming demonstration by Yamanishi et al. (1988) was dependent on the prior isolation and description of a new herpesvirus by Salahuddin et al. (1986). That virus, which came to be called human herpesvirus 6 or HHV-6, was isolated because of the observation of "a small number of short-lived, large refractile cells" in suspension cultures of peripheral blood mononuclear cells from six adult patients with lymphoproliferative disorders, one of whom also had AIDS (Salahuddin et al., 1986). Two years later, Yamanishi et al. (1988) reported the use of the same suspension culture technique to isolate and identify HHV-6 from four 6-month-old infants with exanthem subitum. Children with exanthem subitum can experience the primary infection with HHV-6, whereas patients with immunosuppressive conditions, either disease or therapy induced, reflect the activation from latency of HHV-6. The link to nervous system disease during primary infection was noted in the previously observed association of exanthem subitum with febrile convulsions (e.g., Suga et al., 2000), which can be associated with imaging abnormalities of the brain (Suga et al., 1993). Viral reactivation can be associated with encephalitis or encephalomyelitis in immunocompromised (e.g., Drobyski et al., 1994) and immunocompetent (e.g., McCullers et al., 1995) patients. The observation of HHV-6 in association with multiple sclerosis (MS) plaques (Challoner et al., 1995) has stirred controversy concerning a potential etiologic role of the virus in MS, versus reactivation of a passenger virus.

Pathology and Pathogenesis

HHV-6 is classified as a beta herpesvirus, and its genetic structure resembles those of HHV-7 and cytomegalovirus (CMV). There are two antigenic variants, designated HHV-6A and -B, although many reports do not distinguish between them. Cellular tropisms in vitro differ between the

two; HHV-6B is the variant most frequently associated with encephalitis and shows a readiness to infect cultured oligodendroglia (Albright et al., 1998). The virus is acquired early in life; more than 95% of those over 2 years of age are seropositive (Braun et al., 1997). Primary infection can be nonspecific or unnoticed. The virus can be grown in culture in lymphocytes, monocytes, and bone marrow progenitor cells. Latent infection has been demonstrated in monocytes (Katsafanas et al., 1996; Kondo et al., 1991).

The pathology and pathogenesis of HHV-6 encephalitis are still in the process of being elucidated. Pathological descriptions are mainly in the form of single case reports, and the accounts are of varied patterns of pathology. Most cases have been organ, bone marrow, or stem cell transplant recipients, but a few have been in immunocompetent individuals. To consider the latter cases first, there have been rare fatal cases of HHV-6 encephalitis in immunocompetent children or adults. In one 23-month-old girl, an autopsy showed hemorrhagic encephalitis in the pontine tegmentum and medial thalamus (Ahtiluoto et al., 2000). In a 14-year-old girl with tuberous sclerosis and epilepsy who died unexpectedly, the brain showed intense focal inflammatory changes in and around subependymal tuberous nodules. Immunostaining for HHV-6 was positive in macrophages, astrocytes, lymphocytes, and endothelial cells (Wang et al., 1999). A 19-month-old boy who recovered from an acute encephalopathic illness had high signal lesions on T2-weighted MRI in the left thalamus and pareto-occipital white matter. HHV-6 DNA was found in his CSF (Kamei et al., 1997). A 27-year-old woman with a fatal 11-month-long neurological illness clinically diagnosed as MS also had evidence of HHV-6 in the brain. Prior to the development of this illness she had had a history of seizures, well controlled with medication, for 9 years. At autopsy there were multiple foci of demyelination in corpus callosum, optic nerves, brain stem, and spinal cord. Immunohistochemical staining for HHV-6 revealed widespread virus topographically related to the foci of demyelination (Carrigan et al., 1996). On the same theme, a 10-year-old boy with a severe but nonfatal MS-like illness showed HHV-6 DNA in a biopsied lesion (Poppe et al., 2001); further, in a young woman with a fulminant demyelinating encephalitis, herpesvirus particles were shown by electron microscopy (EM) and HHV-6 antigen and herpesvirus DNA were identified by PCR in a brain biopsy (Novoa et al., 1997). An earlier study also found an association between HHV-6 and MS plaques (Challoner et al., 1995), and a possible relationship between HHV-6 and MS remains a topic of active investigation. An association has also been suggested between epilepsy and HHV-6 DNA, which was detectable by PCR in surgically removed temporal lobe tissue from 6 of 17 subjects (Uesugi et al., 2000). Although HSV-6 DNA has occasionally been found in healthy brain, this is a much higher proportion of positive detection than in healthy brain, although any pathological role of the virus in temporal lobe epilepsy, as in febrile convulsions, remains unclear. In summary, HHV-6 has been implicated in rare cases of acute and subacute encephalitis and other lesions in immunocompetent subjects over a wide age range. It has also been described as causing a chronic myelopathy reminiscent of that seen in human T-cell leukemia virus type 1 infection (MacKenzie et al., 1995).

Among the immunosuppressed population, HHV-6 has also been linked to encephalitic or encephalopathic illnesses, particularly after bone marrow or stem cell transplants. In one case it was considered possible that the bone marrow graft was the source of the infection (Bosi et al., 1998). In a prospective study, HHV-6 DNA was detected in 78% of patients after stem cell transplantation, with maximal amounts of DNA recovered from blood lymphocytes at 4 weeks posttransplant. Three out of 58 patients with HHV-6 DNA developed encephalitis (Ljungman et al., 2000). HHV-6 encephalitis also occurs in AIDS, though relatively infrequently. CSF analysis in 365 AIDS cases revealed HHV-6 DNA in only eight subjects with neurological symptoms (Bossolasco et al., 1999). In immunosuppressed patients, HHV-6 had been described, with JC virus, in lesions of progressive multifocal leukoencephalopathy (Daibata et al., 2001; Ito et al., 2000). As in the immunocompetent cases described, HHV-6 encephalitis in immunosuppressed patients presents with multifocal bilateral lesions in white or gray matter which, on histological examination, show inflammation and necrosis and HHV-6 antigen in neurons, oligodendrocytes, and astrocytes (Tracci et al., 2000; Bosi et al., 1998; Wagner et al., 1997). More subtly, it has been described as the cause of a localized limbic encephalitis based on development of a syndrome of short-term memory loss, insomnia, and electroencephalographic seizure activity in five stem cell transplant recipients, three of whom had HHV-6 DNA in CSF and three of whom had hippocampal sclerosis demonstrated on follow-up MRI or autopsy (Wainwright et al., 2001). Recognition of such manifestations of HHV-6 infection is relatively recent, and demonstration of the full spectrum of its expression is still evolving.

HHV-7, the herpesvirus bearing the greatest similarity to HHV-6, is another ubiquitous virus; antibody is usually acquired by the age of 3 years. Like HHV-6, it is tropic for CD4 lymphocytes, and it too may cause encephalopathic disease, but details of this remain sketchy (Love and Wiley, 2002).

Clinical Manifestations of HHV-6

There are three phases to be considered for the clinical associations of HHV-6: primary infection, latency, and reactivation from latency, often in the context of immunosuppression (Campadelli-Fiume et al., 1999). Primary disease is associated with a few days of high fever, the presence of the classic rash of roseola at defervesence in the minority, inflamed tympanic membranes, upper respiratory infection, or fever of undetermined etiology (Caserta and Hall, 1997). The outcome is benign in most children, but it is a common cause for visits to the emergency department for infants and children, particularly for those between 6 and 12 months of age (Hall et al., 1994). Neurological complications at this stage include febrile convulsions, bulging of the anterior fontanelle, and less frequently, meningoencephalitis. Hall et al. (1994) found that seizures occurred in slightly over 19% of those older than 6 months and that one-third of febrile seizures in children less than 2 years of age who presented to the emergency department were associated with HHV-6. While the majority of the HHV-6-associated febrile seizures are uncomplicated, Suga et al. (1993) found more ominous features in 4 of 21 infants studied, including

TABLE 5.2   Neurological disorders attributed to HHV-6

Febrile convulsions in primary infection in infants
  Exanthem subitum (roseola infantum, sixth disease)
  Fever without rash
Encephalitis
  Immunocompetent
    Children and adults
  Immunocompromised
    Stem cell transplantation
    Bone marrow transplantation
    Organ transplants
    AIDS
White matter disease
  Myelopathy
  Leukoencephalitis
  Encephalomyelitis
  MS (candidate pathogen)

EEG and CT imaging abnormalities. In subsequent studies, Suga et al. (2000) found that HHV-6-associated convulsions could be prolonged and repeated or partial and could be the antecedent for the later emergence of epilepsy.

The second phase is one of clinical latency, in which virus is secreted in saliva by healthy individuals, can be found in some mononuclear cells, and may be relatively dormant in the CNS (Campadelli-Fiume et al., 1999). Secretion of virus in saliva by healthy individuals is thought to be the mechanism of transmission for primary infection of infants and young children. Latency or low-level replication in the CNS may be the basis for the later emergence of clinically apparent CNS illness in immunocompetent or immunocompromised individuals. However, it is also the basis for the dispute concerning the pathogenic importance of the virus in encephalitis, myelitis, and demyelinating disease. In the CNS, is HHV-6 pathogenic or simply a passenger? Caserta et al. (1994) found evidence of HHV-6 in CSF and/or peripheral blood mononuclear cells by PCR after primary infection and observed the importance of the CNS for viral persistence. Luppi et al. (1994) found evidence of HHV-6 by PCR in autopsied brain specimens from 11 of 13 immunocompetent adult patients. One could argue, therefore, that HHV-6 was simply a nonpathogenic bystander in various other CNS illnesses in which it was activated. This is a concern in linking it to MS. Alternatively, it could be argued that under certain circumstances, latency or low-level replication of HHV-6 is changed to an activated state in which it becomes pathogenic.

The third stage emphasized by Campadelli-Fiume et al. (1999) is immunosuppression, in which infection or reactivation can be associated with serious CNS illness (Table 5.2). This includes severe and fatal encephalitis in solid organ, bone marrow, or stem cell transplants. In one case, it was considered possible that the bone marrow graft was the source of the infection (Bosi et al., 1998). In a prospective study, HHV-6 DNA was detected in 78% of patients after stem cell transplantation, with maximal amounts of DNA recovered from blood lymphocytes at 4 weeks posttransplant. Three out of 58 patients with HHV-6 DNA developed encephalitis (Ljungman et al., 2000). Drobyski et al. (1994) described fatal encephalitis in a bone marrow transplant recipient in whom white matter necrosis was found in the deep white matter of the frontal lobe and gray matter necrosis was found in the hippocampal gyrus. Immunohistochemical staining revealed the presence of HHV-6 in both areas. More recently, Wainwright et al. (2001) described a syndrome of limbic encephalitis due to HHV-6 in five patients who had undergone stem cell transplantation. The clinical presentation was characterized by short-term memory impairment, insomnia and confusion associated with temporal lobe seizure activity on EEG. MRI and positron emission tomography studies localized abnormalities to the hippocampal regions. Concern was expressed by the investigators that hippocampal sclerosis could follow. HHV-6 was found in the CSF by PCR and HHV-6 antigens were identified in the hippocampus in an autopsy following death from other causes in one patient. Hence, HHV-6 should be among the viral pathogens considered in any transplant recipient who develops signs of CNS dysfunction.

The role of HHV-6 in CNS disease in human immunodeficiency virus (HIV)/AIDS is difficult to assess. CSF analysis in 365 AIDS cases revealed HHV-6 DNA in eight subjects with neurological symptoms (Bossolasco et al., 1999). Knox et al. (1995) described an infant in whom a fulminant encephalitis developed and in whom immunohistochemical study of postmortem brain tissue revealed widespread HHV-6-infected cells. More ambiguous, however, is the role of HHV-6 CNS infection in adult AIDS. While Knox and Carrigan (1995) reported that HHV-6 infection was associated with areas of demyelination in four of six unselected patients with AIDS, HHV-6 has not received significant clinical attention in HIV-associated CNS illness. Ironically, Kaposi's sarcoma, which is associated with HHV-8, appears to be associated with a lowered risk for AIDS encephalopathy, but a specific role for HHV-8 itself has not been demonstrated (Rezza et al., 1999).

Of significant interest is the demonstration of HHV-6 in association with CNS disease in immunocompetent adults. McCullers et al. (1995) studied two sets of CSF samples from patients previously suspected to have herpes simplex encephalitis (HSE) but that were negative on previous testing. One set was from the U.S. Collaborative Antiviral Study Group (CASG) and was extensively characterized with respect to focal cerebral disease. The other set consisted of samples sent to a university laboratory from patients suspected of having HSE. PCR examination of CSF revealed three positives of 37 samples in the CASG set and six positives of 101 samples in the university set. Hence, HHV-6 was found reproducibly in a low percentage of samples from patients suspected but negative for HSV and almost certainly immunocompetent. CSF in both sets revealed a pleocytosis averaging 81 cells per mm^3. Four of the nine patients had abnormal neuroimaging, one had a low-density parietal lobe lesion on CT, and another had a frontal-temporal lesion on MRI. EEGs were abnormal in seven of the eight tested; five of these abnormalities were focal in nature due to spiking or slowing. Four of the nine HHV-6-positive patients recovered entirely, three had mild to moderate sequelae, one had a severe focal seizure disorder, and one died at 2 months. The last patient's autopsy demonstrated leukoencephalopathy. The possibility of HHV-6 being a nonpathogenic passenger virus

nonspecifically activated by another process must be borne in mind. However, the availability of potentially effective antiviral therapy strengthens the need to seek HHV-6 in encephalitis in immunocompetent as well as immunocompromised patients. Both foscarnet and ganciclovir inhibit HHV-6 replication in vitro, while acyclovir inhibits replication only at high concentrations (Agut et al., 1989). Similarly, both foscarnet (Cole et al., 1998) and gancyclovir (Mookerjee and Vogelsang, 1997) have been reported to successfully treat HHV-6 encephalitis in bone marrow transplant recipients. Diagnostic viral assays will vary depending on the laboratory. However, both CSF PCR and serum and CSF antibody studies may be required to demonstrate active infection.

MacKenzie et al. (1995) described a presumably immunocompetent elderly woman who developed a slowly progressive myelopathy. At autopsy, the entire spinal cord was found to be involved. Chronic inflammation and gliosis were found with myelin loss and microglial proliferation, and perivascular cuffs and gliosis were found in the central gray matter. HHV-6 antibody reactivity was found in the cytoplasm of glial cells, and HHV-6 DNA was found in abnormal spinal cord tissue.

The role of HHV-6 in demyelinating disease is of interest. Novoa et al. (1997) reported a 21-year-old woman with aggressive multifocal demyelinating disease in whom tissue examination revealed HHV-6 by immunohistochemistry and PCR. Carrigan et al. (1996) found widespread immunohistochemical evidence of HHV-6 in the CNS at autopsy of a patient who presented clinically with acute MS symptoms but who was diagnosed pathologically with subacute leukoencephalitis. The association of HHV-6 with MS has received considerable attention since the report of Challoner et al. (1995), in which representational difference analysis of DNA sequences demonstrated HHV-6 in brain samples from persons with MS. It was also found in controls, but only in cases of MS was it found in the nuclei of oligodendrocytes. In numerous subsequent studies the issue of active versus commensal latent infection has been disputed. Knox et al. (2000) presented evidence favoring the pathogenic role of HHV-6 in active systemic infections in the first 10 to 12 years of the illness. Subgroup analysis in antiviral trials in patients with relapsing remitting MS have demonstrated a reduction in the frequency of exacerbations, meriting further study of antiviral therapy (Lycke et al., 1966; Bech et al., 2002). As in the distinction of the role of HHV-6 in encephalitis in immunologically competent patients—pathogenic versus passenger virus—the definition of the role of HHV-6 in MS may hinge on the response to more specifically effective antiviral therapy in large well-designed trials.

MUMPS

Prior to widespread vaccination, mumps was one of the most common causes of aseptic meningitis. Use of the live attenuated mumps virus vaccine in the United States has resulted in a marked reduction of the numbers of cases of mumps and mumps aseptic meningitis and encephalitis. Licensed at the end of 1967, the vaccine is administered in combination with measles and rubella vaccines. The vaccine is 95% effective in inducing protective antibody and, when produced with the Jeryl-Lynn strain, is remarkably free of CNS complications (Center for Disease Control, 1978). Because humans are the only host and because viral latency does not occur, elimination of mumps as a communicable disease is a theoretical possibility and has been achieved in Finland (World Health Organization [WHO], 2001). Until that is universally achieved, however, the complications of hearing loss, orchitis, pancreatitis, meningitis, encephalitis, and myelitis will remain. Large-scale vaccination programs remain to be introduced in most countries in Asia and Africa (WHO, 2001). Insufficient vaccine coverage has resulted in reemergence of outbreaks, with a shift to an older age group (WHO, 2001). The risk of complications increases as the age of incidence increases.

Systemic Disease

Because of its distinctive clinical appearance, mumps, or parotitis epidemica, has been known since the time of Hippocrates (Feldman, 1982). Typically, the disease went through large groups of young susceptible adults such as military recruits in World War I. Now, however, with widespread vaccination, increased urbanization, and increased travel, such outbreaks are rare. The most frequent age range for infection has been 5 to 9 years. Males and females are thought to be equally susceptible to the systemic disease, but males are significantly more susceptible to the development of encephalitis (see below). While the disease can be acquired during any season as an endemic infection in hot climates, the peak incidence in temperate climates is in winter and spring (WHO, 2001). Infection is acquired from infected droplets by the respiratory route. Local replication occurs during an incubation period of about 18 days. Significant viral shedding in the saliva occurs from about 3 days before until 4 days after the appearance of symptoms. Although mumps has a high degree of communicability, as many as one-third of the infections are clinically silent. Clinically inapparent infections can be followed by the whole range of complications of systemic mumps infection.

The disease is usually ushered in with fever, headache, and malaise, followed within a day or two by characteristic swelling of the salivary glands. While bilateral swelling of the parotids occurs most frequently, unilateral swelling occurs in a quarter of the cases. Swelling can also be found in the submandibular or sublingual salivary glands. Swelling and fever tend to subside after a week, to be followed by complete recovery and lasting immunity.

Encephalitis

Pathology

Death from mumps encephalitis is rare, and there are consequently few neuropathological studies. Schwarz et al. (1964) reviewed 19 cases in most of which the changes of "allergic" encephalitis or encephalopathy were described (chapter 7). In one case the findings were different: the brain and meninges showed merely mild generalized cuffing of vessels with lymphocytes and plasma cells, varying degrees of congestion and edema, and scattered microglial nodules (Taylor

TABLE 5.3 Presence of parotitis in mumps encephalitis at time of CNS complications[a]

Determination	Total cases
Mumps encephalitis	51
Parotitis	
Present	24
Absent	27
Parotitis absent at time of CNS complications	36
Sequence	
Parotitis first	11
Simultaneous	4
CNS complications first	9

[a] Azimi et al., 1969.

and Toreson, 1963). One other fatal case with autopsy examination was thought to show both "allergic" changes and those suggestive of viral invasion of the brain. In addition, there was a noncommunicating hydrocephalus, possibly related to inflammatory changes surrounding the aqueduct (Bistrian et al., 1972). Mumps virus was isolated from the CSF in this case. Another fatal case of mumps meningoencephalitis was described after bone marrow transplantation in a child with severe combined immunodeficiency (Bakshi et al., 1996). The virus has not been demonstrated within cells of the CNS in mumps encephalitis, but in mumps meningitis, viral nucleocapsids have been demonstrated in ependymal and choroid plexus cells in an electron microscopic study of the sediment obtained by centrifugation of CSF (Herndon et al., 1974).

Clinical Diagnosis and Management

Estimates of the incidence of encephalitis as a complication in mumps vary from 0.02 to 0.3% of cases (WHO, 2001). This results from at least two factors. First, the great majority of cases of encephalitis are mild and may be difficult to distinguish clearly from aseptic meningitis. Although the onset varies widely, meningoencephalitis often occurs within the first 3 days of glandular swelling. Second, in addition to an early meningoencephalitis, there is a parainfectious encephalitis that often presents in the second week after the start of the systemic illness. CSF pleocytosis, with or without clinical signs, occurs in 40 to 60% of cases of mumps (Gnann, 1997).

Although the age range of highest incidence, 5 to 9 years, is the same as for generalized mumps, there is a marked predilection for males, approximately 3:1, in encephalitis. The onset of the encephalitis is most frequently within the first 3 days of glandular swelling. It may also precede the swelling, follow its disappearance, or appear in the absence of glandular swelling (Table 5.3). Therefore, mumps must be considered in any undiagnosed encephalitis.

Signs of aseptic meningitis predominate in the usual case with headache, stiff neck, vomiting, and drowsiness. Less frequently, seizures, cranial nerve abnormalities, and parenchymal dysfunction supervene. Ford (1966) noted that hemianopia, hemiplegia, hemianasthesia, chorea, myoclonus, and ataxia are all rare. Acute cerebellar ataxia in association with mumps infection has been reported, however, with a benign outcome (Cohen et al., 1992). Resolution of the meningoencephalitis often occurs over the course of 3 to 10 days. The case fatality rate for mumps encephalitis is usually below 2% (Center for Disease Control, 1978). Estimates of the frequency of significant neurological sequelae vary and are partially dependent on estimating the incidence of encephalitis. Johnstone et al. (1972), in a review of a 10-year period, found 137 cases of meningitis and 2 cases of encephalitis, one of which was followed by severe psychomotor retardation. Other sequelae include paralysis, vision loss, cranial nerve palsies, seizures, and personality changes (reviewed in Levitt et al., 1970). Deafness as a sequela, although rare, may come as a result of direct and often sudden involvement of the middle ear.

In addition to meningoencephalitis, mumps may affect the nervous system and sensory apparatus in other ways. Loss of hearing may be sudden and may be associated with poor recovery. Myelitis may occur (Nussinovitch et al., 1992), as well as cases resembling mild paralytic poliomyelitis (Lennette et al., 1960). Finally, the potential role of mumps infection of the ependyma as a cause of clinical aqueductal stenosis and hydrocephalus has been considered (Timmons and Johnson, 1970).

In cases in which parotid swelling precedes meningoencephalitis, the diagnosis poses little problem. However, because adenitis, suppurative parotitis, Stensen's duct calculus, various tumors, and sarcoid and other viral infections can produce or simulate salivary gland swelling, confirmatory viral studies should be performed. When neurological involvement occurs before or in the absence of signs of parotitis (Table 5.3), viral diagnostic studies are crucial. Viral isolation attempts and viral identification by PCR can be done on saliva, CSF, and urine (Afzal et al., 1997). Nested PCR on CSF for mumps virus has been shown to be a rapid and sensitive means of diagnosis (Poggio et al., 2000). Ig ELISA for anti-mumps antibody in serum and CSF is rapid, sensitive, and specific (Glikmann et al., 1986; Sharief and Thompson, 1990). Serum amylase, while nonspecific, can be an indicator of salivary gland or pancreatic involvement and peaks within the first week of the disease (Krugman and Ward, 1968). A negative result is of no value.

The CSF in mumps frequently demonstrates a pleocytosis, even in the absence of signs of meningoencephalitis (Bang and Bang, 1943). Furthermore, persistent pleocytosis and oligoclonal IgG can be demonstrated in CSF (Vandvik et al., 1978). Diffusely slow EEG patterns are commonly found in mumps meningoencephalitis (McDonald et al., 1989). Because the pathogenesis of mumps encephalitis may be infectious or parainfectious, an MRI to seek the white matter lesions of ADEM is advised (Sugita et al., 1991).

There is no specific antiviral therapy for mumps. Fortunately, the great majority of cases are benign and self-limited, although rare cases of chronic mumps encephalitis have been reported (Ito et al., 1991). In those cases in which the clinical and MRI patterns suggest a parainfectious immunological process, consideration may be given to steroid therapy. Vaccination with the attenuated Jeryl-Lynn strain is the key to prevention. Substitution of the Urabe strain, now withdrawn in some countries, was associated with vaccine-related meningoencephalitis (McDonald et al., 1989; Colville and Pugh, 1992). Isolation of infectious

cases can be practical, as virus is shed for a week or so following symptoms. However, it should be recognized that virus is also shed for 2 days prior to symptoms.

EBV—IM—GLANDULAR FEVER

The understanding of the diseases caused by Epstein-Barr virus (EBV) has advanced in stages, sometimes logically and sometimes serendipitously (Ross and Cohen, 1997; Nalesnick, 1999; Cohen, 2000; Tselis, in press). Filatov and Pfeiffer are separately credited with describing a syndrome of fever, lymphadenopathy, and hepatosplenomegaly, which Pfeiffer called "glandular fever" in 1895. The term "infectious mononucleosis" (IM) was introduced by Sprunt and Evans in 1920 when abnormal lymphocytes were described. The syndrome was shown by Paul and Bunnell in 1932 to be associated with the presence of heterophile antibodies, the direct descendant of which is the "monospot" assay. The virus itself, however, was first observed in the 1960s by electron microscopy of Burkitt's lymphoma tissue and named after the investigators. The association with IM was recognized soon thereafter when a technician in a virology laboratory developed IM with a serological response to EBV. Study of the replication cycle and the latency phase of EBV has identified several classes of antigen, the antibodies to which serve to identify the stage of the infection. These antibodies have also served to identify numerous tumors, many of which involve chronically infected B cells. EBV replication and EBV-associated tumors and conditions are markedly increased in HIV-infected individuals (Cohen, 2000; also see chapter 12 of this volume).

Manifestations of EBV infection in the nervous system are pleomorphic and have been recognized since the early 1930s (Tselis, in press). The syndromes range from aseptic meningitis to primary CNS lymphoma in AIDS patients (Hochberg et al., 1983) (see chapter 12). They include various combinations of CNS and PNS disorders, as well as some unique presentations such as the "Alice in Wonderland" syndrome, and can have remarkably benign outcomes following the most desperate-appearing clinical states. The pathogenesis of the neurological syndromes is incompletely understood. Some pathological observations and MRI changes in white matter suggest an immune-mediated pathogenesis. However, the capacity to produce nonlytic infection of cells and the finding of the virus in CSF by PCR keep open the possibility of a direct infection of the brain as a pathogenic mechanism. Quantitative CSF PCR studies support that both mechanisms, infectious and postinfectious immune mediated, may be at work in separate cases (Weinberg et al., 2002). Two other potential mechanisms include a "bystander" effect, in which the products of antigen-specific T cells recognizing clinically infected B cells injure neural cells, and the possibility of a vasogenic mechanism, as is observed in the migraine-associated "Alice in Wonderland" phenomena.

Systemic Disease

The distribution of EBV infection is worldwide, and infection occurs in an endemic fashion. In tropical countries infection occurs in the first decade of life and is relatively asymptomatic. In industrially developed nations with a temperate climate, infection is usually delayed until 15 to 25 years of age and is frequently associated with IM. Ultimately, 90% or more of the world's population is infected. Both sexes and all races appear to be equally susceptible.

Transmission of EBV infection in the adolescent and young adult age groups requires intimate oral contact, hence the appellation "the kissing disease." Casual household contact is not sufficient for effective transmission. The mode of infection in younger age groups is not well understood, though transmission by infected saliva seems likely. The incubation period for IM is highly variable. It is shortest in the youngest age groups, but 4 to 7 weeks is common. Similarly, the period of infectiousness is variable, and it may be quite extended. Viral shedding may continue for weeks or months, beginning with the acute illness.

The clinical spectrum of IM is broad, ranging from an insidious onset of lassitude and fatigue to a rapidly evolving syndrome of fever, headache, pharyngitis, cervical adenopathy, petechial hemorrhage, hepatitis, and splenomegaly. Diagnosis has been based on the findings of fever, pharyngitis, and cervical adenopathy in the presence of a positive slide agglutination or solid-phase immunoassay for EBV. If a rapid Paul-Bunnell heterophile test is negative, EBV-specific antibodies should be sought when clinical suspicion merits (Nalesnik, 1999). Resolution of the process is variable, ranging from days to weeks. Fatalities are rare, resulting from splenic rupture, neurological complications, respiratory compromise, and progressive disease in the face of immunodeficiency, including X-linked lymphoproliferative disease.

Atypical lymphocytes (Downey cells) and a relative lymphocytosis are the characteristic hematological abnormalities in IM. Early in the process, infected B lymphocytes stimulate the proliferation of reactive T lymphocytes (reviewed in Cohen, 2000). Infected B cells harbor virus-specific nuclear antigen (EBNA), and viral shedding from the oropharynx can be demonstrated. After resolution of the acute infection, B lymphocytes continue to harbor the EBV genome.

Serological confirmation of IM is achieved with either virus-specific or nonspecific assays. The time-honored heterophile test is nonspecific and may become positive in some cases without EBV infection. It measures antibodies to sheep or horse erythrocytes that are not adsorbed by guinea pig cells but are adsorbed with ox cells. The assay has been adapted for rapid diagnosis with various slide agglutination kits. Depending on the reagents used, it will remain positive from weeks to more than a year after the onset of infection. Several tests of the virus-specific antibody are available and may be used for different purposes. They are particularly valuable for cases in which the heterophile test is negative and for neurological disease occurring in the absence of clinical IM. In general, assays that measure EBV-specific IgM are useful for the diagnosis of acute infection because such antibodies tend to disappear after weeks to months. Virus-specific antibodies of the IgG class tend to persist and are useful indicators of individual immunity and the prevalence of exposure in various populations.

Encephalitis
Pathology
There are very few reports on the pathology of the CNS complications of IM due to EBV infection. Perivascular

mononuclear cells have been described in the brain in occasional reports (Ricker et al., 1947; Sworn and Urich, 1972; Ringelstein et al., 1984; Roulet-Perez et al., 1993). One such case showed serological evidence of recent infection with both EBV and measles, though there was no clinical evidence of measles infection (Melbye et al., 1983). In other cases merely edema and congestion (Dolgopol and Husson, 1949; Bergin, 1960; Carter and Penman, 1969) or pathological features of perivenous encephalitis (Ambler et al., 1971) have been found in the brain. Virus has not been recovered from the brain, but viral antigen was demonstrated by immunofluorescence in the case of a 13-year-old girl with an encephalitic illness associated with acute EBV infection. Measles antigen, paramyxoviruslike nucleocapsids, and herpeslike particles were demonstrated in the same brain (Hochberg et al., 1976), suggesting that the virus had been present in the CNS. In another fatal case in which an autopsy revealed widespread perivascular lymphocytic infiltrates consisting predominantly of B cells, most of these cells were found by in situ hybridization to contain EBV DNA (Schellinger et al., 1999).

Diagnosis and Management
The understanding of the pathogenesis of the CNS involvement in EBV is incomplete, and we do not have a clear idea of the rate of neurological complications in EBV infection. There have, however, been estimates of the incidence of neurological complications in clinical IM. Gautier-Smith (1965) quoted an overall figure of 1% as generally accepted while finding complications in 7.3% of hospitalized patients with EBV. The temporal relationship of neurological complications in IM is highly variable. Walsh et al. (1954) reported an 8-year-old boy with severe encephalitis that appeared on the 13th day of IM. The nervous system complications may also precede or be the major manifestation of clinical IM (Silverstein et al., 1972). In a case described by Schiff et al. (1982), no signs of systemic illness were found at the onset of cerebral dysfunction, which was characterized by disorientation, stupor, multifocal myoclonic jerks, paratonia, and an extensor plantar response. Rapid neurological improvement ensued, and only on the sixth hospital day were enlarged cervical lymph nodes and a spleen tip palpable. The report of Grose et al. (1975) emphasized the appearance of neurological complications of EBV infection in the absence of signs of IM and in the absence of a positive heterophile test. This is particularly apt to occur in children. The message from these observations is that EBV infection must be considered in any undiagnosed encephalitis. Virus-specific antibody studies should be performed, particularly those of the IgM class.

The range of clinical signs and symptoms of neurological dysfunction in EBV infection is diverse (Table 5.4). Headache and fever are frequently observed. The level of consciousness may be only mildly impaired, or coma may ensue. In contrast to HSE, coma in EBV infection does not necessarily portend a poor outcome. In the case described by Walsh et al. (1954), episodes of coma and opisthotonos were followed by complete recovery. As in other types of encephalitis, agitation and disorientation can occur in isolation or in combination with more focal signs. Personality changes and manifestations of a psychological disorder

TABLE 5.4 Neurological complications and associations with EBV[a]

Aseptic meningitis
  Uniphasic
  Mollaret's recurrent meningitis
Encephalitis/encephalopathy
  Focal, multifocal
  Diffuse
  "Alice in Wonderland" syndrome
  Cerebellitis
  Opsoclonus-myoclonus
  Brain stem encephalitis
Parainfectious syndromes
  ADEM
  Myelitis
  Neuropathy
  Guillain-Barré syndrome
  Sensory
  Autonomic
  Cranial, including Bell's palsy
  Encephalomyeloradiculopathy
Lymphoproliferative disorders during immunosuppression
Primary CNS lymphoma in AIDS (chapter 12)

[a] Modified from Tselis (in press).

may simulate HSE. Visual distortions can occur in IM, and seizures are frequently reported (Gautier-Smith, 1965). The EEG may be mildly or markedly abnormal, with generalized or focal abnormalities (Schnell et al., 1966). A complicating feature of seizure therapy in IM is that the clearance of anticonvulsants may be increased during the illness (Leppik et al., 1979). Focal neurological dysfunction is often present. Hemiplegia, hemispheric dysfunction, and acute ataxia of childhood have been reported (Tselis, in press). Deep gray structure dysfunction can be manifest as chorea (Friedland and Yahr, 1977) or other movement disorders. The opsoclonus-myoclonus syndrome (chapter 10) has been described following EBV infection (Verma and Brozman, 2002).

The "Alice in Wonderland" syndrome of metamorphopsia, distortions of body sense and the external environment, were described by Lewis Carroll (Charles Dodgson) in his novel of that name. Lippman (1952) recorded several migraine case histories with such distortions of perception and noted that Dodgson himself suffered from migraine headaches. Cooperman (1977) described three cases of the Alice in Wonderland syndrome as a consequence of IM. Numerous reports since that time have confirmed that association and failed to determine the pathogenesis. The distortions are episodic, lasting on the order of 5 to 20 min, occurring at variable intervals from many each day to 2 or 3 weekly, tapering and clearing without neurological residua after weeks to months (Lahat et al., 1999; Cooperman, 1977). EEGs may be normal or abnormal; the latter clear over time. CSF may reveal a lymphocytic pleocytosis. Neuroimaging, including CT and MRI, has been unremarkable (Lahat et al., 1999). Neurodiagnostic abnormalities have included high-amplitude waveforms on visual evoked potentials (Lahat et al., 1999) and impaired cerebral perfusion to SPECT investigations (Kuo et al., 1998). The differential diagnosis includes migraine headache, epilepsy, use of hallucinogenic drugs, schizophrenia, and delirium

associated with fever (Cooperman, 1977). Signs and symptoms of IM are characteristically present, and serological markers of EBV infection are positive. Often frightening, the condition is benign in outcome, and reassurance and management of anxiety are indicated.

Many of the instances of neurological dysfunction in association with EBV infection appear to have the pattern of postinfectious illness. The evidence includes MRI findings of white matter abnormalities, multilevel distribution, and timing with respect to systemic illness. However, the finding of CSF PCR positivity for EBV DNA indicates that the pathogenesis may be complex. As Tselis (in press) has observed, "... 'infectious' and 'postinfectious' may not be completely distinct from each other." Examples include combinations of CNS and PNS disorders (Morgenlander, 1996) such as encephalomyeloradiculopathy (Tselis et al., 1997; Merelli et al., 1997; Majid et al., 2002) and myeloradiculitis (Majid et al., 2002).

The tempo of the onset of neurological dysfunction is variable. Encephalitic signs may appear de novo or may evolve in the presence of systemic signs of IM. A remarkable feature is the rapidity and completeness with which severe neurological dysfunction can clear. Rapid reversal of neurological signs in an undiagnosed encephalitis should raise the suspicion of an EBV-related syndrome. Cases have also been recorded in which chronic (Caruso et al., 2000) or recurrent (Shoji et al., 1992) illness occurred. However, the prognosis is good. Bernstein and Wolff (1950) quoted a figure of 85% for complete recovery in IM-related neurological complications. Both of these features, rapid reversal and complete recovery, suggest the absence of significant structural damage in IM encephalitis in the majority of cases. However, persistent focal neurological defects and cognitive impairments with MRI abnormalities have been documented in some cases (Caruso et al., 2000).

Etiologic studies in every case of undiagnosed viral encephalitis should include tests of EBV-specific antibodies and CSF PCR. This is particularly the case in immunocompromised individuals (Weinberg et al., 2002). Isolation of EBV is technically difficult but CSF PCR should be attempted. Interpretation of CSF pleocytosis in IM is problematic. Cells may be present in cases of IM apparently uncomplicated by clinical neurological involvement. Conversely, the CSF can be acellular in the face of neurological complications clearly related to IM. However, pleocytosis and protein elevation are usually found. As noted above, the EEG is often abnormal but without specific features to suggest IM. Abnormalities on neuroimaging can be absent (Lahat et al., 1999) or on occasion fleeting and changing (Tolly et al., 1989). When abnormalities are found, MRI is the more sensitive test. It can show abnormalities of white and/or gray matter (Shian and Chi, 1996; Donovan and Zimmerman, 1996; Paskavitz et al., 1995).

Although acyclovir can reduce EBV replication, it has not been demonstrated to be useful in the neurological complications of EBV infection. Steroids have been employed to treat the neurological complications of EBV infection when they appear to be of an immune-mediated pathogenesis. Weinberg et al. (2002) have suggested that severe EBV encephalitis might benefit from treatment with both an antiviral and immunosuppressive therapy directed against T cells.

However, no large prospective randomized trial has been undertaken of the treatment of CNS complications of EBV infection.

Other Neurological Complications

The most frequent neurological complication of IM is aseptic meningitis (Gautier-Smith, 1965). There is also a remarkable capacity to involve peripheral and cranial nerves. EBV is one of the virus infections associated with the Guillain-Barré syndrome, Bell's palsy (Grose et al., 1975), and lumbosacral radiculoplexopathy (Sharma et al., 1993). Moreover, brachial plexitis and mononeuritis (Schnell et al., 1966), painful radiculopathy (Gautier-Smith, 1965), and autonomic neuropathy (Yahr and Frontera, 1975) have been recorded in connection with EBV. Involvement of each of the cranial nerves in IM has been reported (reviewed in DeSimone and Snyder, 1978; Grose, 1989). The potential association of EBV and MS has received attention (e.g., Ascherio et al., 2001).

ADENOVIRUS

Forty-nine adenovirus types grouped into six subgenera are associated with several clinical syndromes. These include acute respiratory tract infections, gastroenteritis, pharyngoconjunctival fever, keratoconjunctivitis, hemorrhagic cystitis, and unlocalized fever (Ruuskanen et al., 1997). Neurological complications of adenovirus infections, however, appear to be infrequent, and the settings in which CNS complications occur have been relatively restricted. The majority of cases of adenovirus encephalitis have occurred in children with respiratory disease, most frequently in association with adenovirus type 7. Other neurological complications have also been described, including transient encephalopathy in infants (R. Straussberg, L. Harel, Y. Levy, and J. Amir, Abstr., *Pediatrics* **107**:1168, 2001) and febrile convulsions in children (Rantala et al., 1990).

Systemic Disease

Several rather distinctive syndrome clusters, often occurring in epidemics, have been associated with a small group of adenovirus types (Ruuskanen et al., 1997). Acute respiratory disease in military recruits is most often associated with types 4 and 7. It is usually a self-limited disease of about 10 days' duration with fever, malaise, sore throat, cough, and coryza. However, occasional deaths have been reported (Dudding et al., 1972). A bivalent vaccine of types 4 and 7 has been available for U.S. military recruits. In 1994 a lapse in immunization resulted in an outbreak of acute respiratory disease due to adenovirus type 4 in military trainees (Barraza et al., 1999). In 1996 manufacture of the vaccine stopped, and supplies were used up. As a consequence, roughly 10 to 12% of U.S. military recruits have become ill with adenovirus infections during basic training, including one death due to encephalitis (Centers for Disease Control and Prevention, 2001). A previously healthy 21-year-old male recruit developed upper respiratory symptoms (day 0), was found unconscious in the barracks on day 4, and expired on day 13. Histopathology revealed encephalitis and acute pulmonary disease. PCR identified adenovirus in the lung and brain, and serological changes were demonstrated against adenovirus types 4 and 7 (Centers for Disease Control and Prevention, 2001).

Epidemic keratoconjunctivitis has been associated with adenovirus types 8, 19, and 37 (Ruuskanen et al., 1997) in group settings such as factories, nursing homes, military bases, camps, and hospitals. It can be spread by eye care using inadequately sterilized instruments. Pharyngoconjunctival fever has been most commonly associated with adenovirus types 3 and 7. Clusters of infections have occurred at group swimming facilities with inadequate chlorination. Fever, conjunctivitis, and pharyngitis follow an incubation period of 6 to 9 days.

In contrast to these distinctive syndromes, adenovirus is a frequent cause of respiratory disease in infants and children that cannot be clinically distinguished from respiratory disease produced by other viruses (Ruuskanen et al., 1997). Adenoviruses are often associated with endemic respiratory disease in infants and children. A range of symptom complexes including pharyngitis, tonsillitis, bronchitis, bronchiolitis, croup, and pneumonia can be produced. Transmission is principally fecal-oral, although respiratory transmission also occurs. The usual incubation period for adenovirus syndromes is 6 to 9 days. The duration of illness varies from roughly a week for pharyngitis to a range of 10 to 20 days for pneumonia. Although usually benign, permanent lung damage sometimes occurs, and deaths have been recorded in adenovirus pneumonia of infants. Adenoviruses are associated with gastroenteritis in children and are the second most frequent cause of diarrhea in infants (Ruuskanen et al., 1997). Other syndromes have included acute hemorrhagic cystitis associated with type 11 and undifferentiated fever. Adenoviruses are significant causes of illness in immunocompromised patients such as bone marrow and liver transplant recipients (Ruuskanen et al., 1997). While infection with adenoviruses can be demonstrated in HIV-infected patients, it appears not to be a significant cause of morbidity in this population.

Encephalitis

The most frequently reported cause of adenovirus-associated encephalitis is type 7 in children with respiratory disease. Lelong et al. (1956) reported CNS findings in five children during an outbreak of respiratory disease in France. Gabrielson et al. (1966) reported a family cluster of acute gastroenteritis associated with adenovirus type 7. One of the children developed encephalitis that progressed to coma, followed by recovery and no disability. Simila et al. (1970) reported an outbreak of adenovirus type 7 in Finland with a high percentage of CNS involvement. Of 32 children hospitalized for adenovirus infection, 8 had CNS complications. These included one patient with meningitis and seven patients with encephalitis, of whom three died. All cases of CNS involvement were associated with respiratory disease. Fever was present in eight, stupor in seven, nuchal rigidity in four, and loss of consciousness and seizures in three. The CSF revealed more than three cells in two of seven patients and protein values over 45 mg/100 ml in two of six patients. EEGs were abnormal in all four patients tested. It was thought that the outlook for survivors was good. Sutton et al. (1976) reported that encephalitis complicated the course of 42 cases of adenovirus type 7 infections in England and Wales between 1971 and 1974. Nonneurological findings and symptoms included sore throat, cervical adenopathy, conjunctivitis, and abdominal pain. The mean age of infected persons was 9 years. Two case reports of CNS involvement were given, both of which were in children. It is of concern that type 7 adenovirus infection has increased markedly in Japan since 1995 (Yamadera et al., 1998). While pharyngoconjunctival fever, influenzalike illness, and gastroenteritis accounted for over half of the cases, aseptic meningitis (2%), encephalitis (1%), and encephaloplathy (0.9%) were observed.

Other adenovirus types have also been identified in neurological disorders. Kelsey (1978) isolated types 6, 7A, and 12 from CSF of children with meningoencephalitis. Type 11 was isolated from a fatal neonatal case of pneumonia and encephalitis (Osamura et al., 1993). A syndrome of transient encephalopathy of infants, associated with fever, depressed consciousness, abnormal EEGs, and normal CSF, was reported by Straussberg et al. (abstr.). They used immunofluorescence on samples from nasopharynx, rectal swab, conjunctiva, and sputum for viral identification. In five of seven patients, serotyping revealed type 3. Rantala et al. (1990) identifed the association of untyped adenovirus in 18 of 144 cases of febrile convulsions, including viral isolations of adenovirus from CSF in three cases.

Uncomplicated adenovirus encephalitis in adults is extremely rare. Adenovirus similar to type 32 was recovered from the brain of a 42-year-old patient with a subacute focal encephalitis who died with lymphosarcoma (Roos et al., 1972; Chou et al., 1973). Large basophilic intranuclear inclusion bodies were seen in cortical neurons (Chou et al., 1973). Adenovirus type 12 was isolated from the CSF of a 36-year-old woman with concomitant lead toxicity (Kelsey and McLean, 1979). Signs included seizures, resistance to neck flexion, fever, confusion, and agitation. The mental status cleared on treatment with calcium disodium versenate. An isolate of type 7 adenovirus was reported from autopsied brain tissue of a 71-year-old patient with chronic schizophrenia without evidence of encephalitis (Lord et al., 1975). Adenovirus type 2 was isolated from the brain biopsy of a patient with encephalitis and concurrent EBV infection (West et al., 1985). Zagardo et al. (1998) described a 53-year-old woman with acute myelogenous leukemia treated with chemotherapy who developed brain stem and cerebellar signs. CSF revealed a mononuclear pleocytosis, and an MRI revealed T2 abnormalities in the brain stem and cerebellum with patchy enhancement. Adenovirus was isolated from the CSF. The patient improved concomitant with Ig infusion. In an unpublished case, adenovirus type 7 was recovered from the throat and stool of a previously healthy 52-year-old woman with encephalitis (M. Landry, personal communication, 1984). The patient developed seizures, lethargy, an abnormal EEG, and a CSF pleocytosis in the setting of a febrile respiratory illness. No underlying illness was known, and the patient recovered uneventfully during a hospitalization of 9 days. The patient refused venipuncture for the convalescent-phase serum sample. Although some types of adenovirus can be recovered from tonsils and adenoids and from stool in the absence of disease, type 7 is not usually among them (Jackson and Muldoon, 1973). Therefore, it is reasonable to assume that adenovirus type 7 was the cause of encephalitis in this case. A second case of uncomplicated adenovirus encephalitis in a previously healthy adult was reported by Landry and Hsiung (1988). A 31-year-old physician developed gastroenteritis followed by meningoencephalitis and atypical pneumonia from which he fully recovered. Adenovirus type 1 was isolated from CSF, and a type-specific rise in neutralizing antibody was shown. Nuchal rigidity and confusion cleared after 2 to 4 days, and full recovery ensued. A third case of uncomplicated adenovirus encephalitis with a fatal outcome in a previously healthy adult (Centers for Disease Control and Prevention, 2001) was noted above in an unvaccinated military recruit.

Laboratory diagnosis of adenovirus encephalitis is complicated by the capacity of the virus to remain latent in throat and stool. CSF isolations can be obtained (Kelsey, 1978); however, they may be negative in patients with isolations from other sites and in the presence of CNS symptoms (Sutton et al., 1976). Ideally, virus isolation or identification should be combined with a diagnostic antibody rise in a patient with CNS symptoms. Virus isolation can be achieved on cell cultures commonly employed in diagnostic virology laboratories (Landry and Hsiung, 1988; West et al., 1985). Alternatively, adenovirus can be identified by PCR (Centers for Disease Control and Prevention, 2001), fluorescent antibody (Straussberg et al., abstr.), or enzyme immunoassay (Rantala et al., 1990).

GASTROENTERITIS—ROTAVIRUSES

In contrast to viral exanthems (Table 5.1) in which numerous viral infections also produce encephalitis, the viruses associated with gastroenteritis are very infrequent causes of encephalitis. Fluid and electrolyte disturbances can result in transient encephalopathy. There are, however, a few case reports of rotavirus encephalitis/encephalopathy in the literature.

Rotaviruses are worldwide ubiquitous pathogens infecting most children by age five (Matson et al., 2000). Gastroenteritis associated with rotaviruses typically occurs between 6 months and 2 years of age. In underdeveloped countries in which childhood nutrition is poor and access to rehydration therapy is unavailable or delayed, death may ensue. An estimated 875,000 deaths worldwide are attributed to rotavirus infections annually.

Rotaviruses contain 11 double-stranded segments of RNA (Matson et al., 2000). The name derives from the wheel-like (rota) appearance of the virion on electron microscopy. Diarrhea results from a virus attack on enterocytes in the small intestine. Experimental evidence in mice supports a role for the enteric nervous system in rotavirus-induced fluid loss (Lundgren et al., 2000). The most common onset of the clinical illness is vomiting in infants and young children, followed by watery diarrhea and fever. The total duration of illness is usually about 4 to 5 days, with a range of seriousness of illness from asymptomatic to dehydration with metabolic acidosis and death (Matson et al., 2000).

In temperate climates, the incidence peaks in the winter. Rotaviruses are a common cause of hospitalization for watery diarrhea in infants and young children.

Starting with the report of Salmi et al. (1978), several authors have noted an effect on the CNS in association with the gastroenteritis. Most case reports are of infants about 2 years of age, but ages range from 9 months to 3 years. Salmi et al. (1978) reported a case of Reye's syndrome and a case of encephalitis. Rotavirus does not appear to be a common cause of Reye's syndrome. The case of encephalitis was in a 3-year-old girl who developed clonic seizures 48 h after the onset of gastroenteritis. The second lumbar puncture (LP) revealed a leukocytosis and protein of 540 mg/liter. The first EEG revealed a very slow basic rhythm. The patient also experienced tetanic cramps, confusion, incoordination, and an inability to talk. Improvement was slow, and some disability of speech and movement was still present at 3 months. Diagnostic workup demonstrated rotavirus particles by EM on anal swab and a serological antibody rise against a cross-reacting rotavirus. Diagnostic methods have evolved. In the following case, diagnosis was made by ELISA on CSF. Ushijima et al. (1986) reported a 9-month-old boy who developed seizures, loss of consciousness, and a bulging anterior fontanelle. Brain CT revealed cerebral edema, and the EEG showed a suppression burst pattern. The patient developed infantile spasms and suffered pronounced developmental delay. EM demonstration of rotavirus particles in CSF was reported in one of two cases of rotavirus encephalopathy reported by Keidan et al. (1992). Both cases manifested an apathetic stuporous state without focal neurological signs. EEGs during the acute phase revealed slowing, the CSFs were acellular, no electrolyte disturbances were found, and a CT scan on one of the patients was normal. Clinically, both patients recovered promptly. More recent case reports of CNS dysfunction associated with rotavirus gastroenteritis have utilized PCR on CSF (Yoshida et al., 1995; Pang et al., 1996).

Seizures are commonly but not universally demonstrated. They have been thought to be febrile (Pang et al., 1996), to mimic afebrile benign convulsions (Hongou et al., 1998), or to reflect direct brain parenchymal involvement (Ushijima et al., 1986). Depression of level of consciousness is common, as is slowing on the EEG. The CSF may be acellular or demonstrate a mild to moderate pleocytosis. Neuroimaging may be normal or reveal cerebral edema. The diagnosis of rotavirus infection should be suspected in an infant or young child developing seizures and a depressed level of consciousness in the context of an acute gastroenteritis. Fluid and electrolyte abnormalities should be sought and corrected. Investigations of the cause of the gastroenteritis can include identification of virus in stool. Many assays are available, but typically ELISA or latex agglutination assays are used. If the evidence suggests a direct effect of virus on the brain, PCR examination of CSF would be the assay of choice, if available. Otherwise, immunoelectron microscopy on concentrated CSF samples or differential antibody responses in CSF compared to serum with controls for transudation could be attempted. Management consists mainly of fluid and electrolyte restoration, with care given to the possible existence of cerebral edema, and seizure management. No specific antiviral therapy is available for rotavirus infection, and a vaccine has been withdrawn in the United States.

HEPATITIS VIRUSES

Neurological dysfunction in the context of severe liver disease is well known. Hepatic encephalopathy or chronic portal systemic encephalopathy and fulminant hepatic failure are each associated with cerebral dysfunction (Lockwood, 1995). Each can be caused by viral infection. However, the CNS dysfunction derives from the metabolic abnormalities of liver function rather than from the direct action of viral infection. Reye's syndrome is an acute disorder of cerebral and liver function (see chapter 8). It is triggered by viral infection, most commonly influenza virus or VZV, often in association with aspirin use. This is also a metabolic disorder. Certain viruses are commonly associated with hepatic dysfunction, such as EBV, CMV, and yellow fever virus. However, attention here is directed to agents specifically identified as hepatitis viruses, which are distinguished as A through E, and more specifically to hepatitis A virus (HAV), hepatitis B virus (HBV), and hepatitis C virus (HCV). Encephalitis in association with these agents is rare, the literature is fragmentary, and the pathogenesis is incompletely understood (Table 5.5).

Acute hepatitis infection is associated with fever, malaise, headache, anorexia, nausea, and vomiting. Dark urine, clay-colored stools, yellowish discoloration of sclera and skin, and an enlarged tender liver are typically found, with laboratory evidence of impaired hepatic function. Neurological abnormalities including encephalitis can be found before or after the appearance of icterus (Friedlander, 1956). The development of viral hepatitis-specific assays has allowed some characterization of syndromes associated with specific hepatitis viruses.

HAV

HAV is a small RNA virus transmitted by the fecal-oral route, with an incubation period of 4 to 6 weeks. Infection is self-limiting, with liver function abnormalities lasting 3 to 4 weeks. A chronic carrier state is not established (Anderson, 2000). Diagnosis is made by identification of serum anti-HAV IgM. A transient alteration of cerebral function as a prodrome to acute hepatitis A was reported by Hammond et al. (1982) in a 34-year-old man who became confused, delirious, and agitated. The syndrome started to reverse within a day. There was no stiff neck or focal neurological findings. The CSF contained 13 neutrophils/mm^3, a head CT was normal, and the EEG showed high amplitude and slow wave activity. Liver function tests were abnormal, and radioimmunoassay was positive for HAV. Mental status and liver function tests normalized over a 2-week period.

Bromberg et al. (1982) described a patient with significantly more severe and persistent encephalitis associated with acute HAV infection. A 56-year-old man who was hospitalized with jaundice and impaired mental acuity developed coma and bilateral Babinski signs and required intubation. LP demonstrated a mononuclear pleocytosis of

TABLE 5.5 Comparison of hepatitis viruses[a]

	HAV	HBV	HCV
Virus family	*Picornavirus*	*Hepadnavirus*	*Flavivirus*
Transmission	Fecal-oral	Parenteral	Parenteral
	Personal contact	IVDA[b]	IVDA
	Food	Unscreened blood products	Blood products[c]
		Perinatal	
		Sexual	
Hepatitis	Acute	Acute and chronic	Chronic
PNS/cranial nerves	Guillain-Barré [d]	Guillain-Barré	Polyneuropathy
	Auditory and vestibular	Mononeuritis multiplex	Guillain-Barré
CNS	Encephalitis	CNS complications of periarteritis nodosa	Vascular occlusions
	Myeloradiculopathy	Seizures	Leukoencephalopathy
			Encephalomyelitis

[a] After Lauer and Walker, 2001; Tabor, 1987; Tembl et al., 1999; and Petty et al., 1996.
[b] IVDA, intravenous drug abuse.
[c] Blood products before screening of blood supply (in 1990 in United States).
[d] Challenged by Xie et al., 1988.

24 cells/mm^3, the head CT was unremarkable, and the EEG demonstrated bilateral symmetric slowing. Although neurological improvement started in the second week, physical and mental incapacities persisted and continued to improve following discharge at 10 weeks.

In the absence of neuropathology, the mechanism of encephalitis is not at all clear. Davis et al. (1993) studied a 7-year-old girl who developed confusion, combativeness, lethargy, and incoherence in the context of an acute hepatitis associated with HAV. CT and MRI were normal, and EEG demonstrated diffuse bilateral slowing. The CSF had 15 white blood cells/mm^3, 97% of which were mononuclear. The CSF contained a low titer (1:2) of IgG antibody against HAV and was negative for the HAV genome. A full clinical recovery was made a month after the start of improvement at 5 days. The authors proposed a postviral pathogenesis. In sum, based on a few clinical reports, the encephalitis of HAV infection can result in marked depression of consciousness but allow full recovery. Neuroimaging has been negative, CSF has shown a mild pleocytosis, and bilateral high-amplitude slow waves are found on EEG. Therapy is supportive. A vaccine is available to those likely to reside or travel in areas of high endemicity.

HBV

Serum hepatitis, caused by HBV, a DNA virus, can produce acute and chronic infection of the liver. Previously undetectable until the discovery of the Australian antigen, it had been a major risk to the blood supply. Presently, blood supplies are screened, a battery of diagnostic tests are used, and a vaccine is available to persons at risk, such as health care workers. HBV can be transmitted perinatally by infected mothers, sexual intercourse, intravenous drug abuse, or accidental exposure in health care settings. The incubation period ranges from 6 weeks to 3 months or longer, and typical symptoms of hepatitis may persist for 2 or 3 weeks or much longer (Bendinelli et al., 2000). Risk for the development of chronic infection is strongly age dependent; it is greatest for infants infected at the time of birth and less for adults. The feared complications of chronic hepatitis are

decompensated cirrhosis and hepatocellular carcinoma. It is to be hoped that interferon therapy combined with antiviral drugs such as lamivudine will reduce these complications and the consequent need for liver transplantation.

Extrahepatic complications include the development of polyarthritis and vasculitis (Sergent et al., 1976; Duffy et al., 1976), including periarteritis nodosa (Michalak, 1978). Injury to the PNS and CNS can result from HBV antigen-induced vasculitis. The Guillain-Barré syndrome has been reported in association with acute HBV infection, and mononeuritis multiplex in the context of periarteritis nodosa has been found in chronic HBV infection (Tabor, 1987).

There are few reports of acute encephalitis associated with acute or chronic HBV infection. Brooks (1977) reported a 21-year-old male who developed anorexia, nausea, and vomiting followed by fatigue, dark urine, and light stools. The patient had a single tonic-clonic seizure 1 week into the illness. There were no focal signs on neurological exam. The second CSF revealed 9 lymphocytes/mm^3. An EEG showed intermittent slowing in the 2 to 4 Hz range. Abnormal liver function studies normalized within 6 weeks, as did the EEG. No further seizures occurred. Abnormal EEGs have also been described in patients with HBV infection but without seizures (Lanzinger-Rossnagel and Kommerell, 1980).

In contrast, Rosenberg et al. (1976) reported a fatal case in a 19-year-old woman who presented to the emergency room in coma with bilateral decerebration. There was a history of arthralgias and urticaria with a positive hepatitis B surface antigen 6 weeks earlier. Evaluation revealed serum chemistries of liver damage, signs of raised intracranial pressure, acellular CSF, and a diffusely slow EEG. The patient's course included seizure on the second day and some neurological improvement on the fourth day, but her course was complicated by airway obstructions, and she died of respiratory failure. The autopsy revealed minimal cerebral edema, no CNS vasculitis, and mild resolving hepatitis. Because cryoprecipitable hepatitis B surface antigen-antibody complexes were found during life, the authors speculated that they played a role in the production of the encephalopathy.

Duffy et al. (1976) described an acute multisystem disorder associated with serological evidence of HBV infection but with a prolonged course. PNS and CNS disorders were found, as were arthritis, renal, heart, and intestinal disease and skin manifestations. Diffuse signs of stupor and confusion were seen in one patient, focal signs including aphasia in another, and seizures with headache, nausea, and vomiting in a third. EEGs were diffusely slowed in all three patients, and CSF protein was elevated in one. The first patient responded to steroid therapy but later died from a stroke, the second improved spontaneously, and the third patient remained unchanged.

Sergent et al. (1976) described nine patients with hepatitis B-associated necrotizing vasculitis. Three patients died of vasculitis, one of whom from widespread CNS vasculitis. A fourth patient died of chronic hepatitis years after vasculitis that had left permanent neurological residua. Two others had residual neurological defects. Although there was a high percentage of CNS disability in this group of patients related to HBV antigenemia, these patients presented as a chronic rheumatological disease with vasculitis, not as encephalitis.

HCV

The story of hepatitis C is remarkable (DiBisceglie and Bacon, 1999). Following the identification of hepatitis B and the screening of the blood supply, a large number of unidentified posttransfusion cases of hepatitis, termed non-A, non-B, were recognized. Hepatitis C was finally identified in 1989, and screening of the blood supply led to a marked drop in new infections in the United States. Currently, the most common causes of HCV transmission are injection drug use and high-risk sexual practices. Prevalence studies have suggested that 3.9 million people in the United States are infected (Alter et al., 1999) and that 170 million people may be chronically infected worldwide (Lauer and Walker, 2001).

An RNA virus in the *Flavivirus* family along with arboviruses such as yellow fever and dengue fever viruses, HCV achieves transmission in blood without a mosquito vector or a replication cycle in mosquitoes. In direct contrast to HAV infection, acute infection with HCV is usually asymptomatic, and chronic infection occurs in an estimated 80% of cases. Decades after acute infection, some patients develop cirrhosis and a smaller number develop hepatocellular carcinoma. Alcohol use and coinfection with HIV accelerate the process. It is not known whether treatment with alpha interferon and ribavirin will reduce the percentage of long-term complications.

Although HCV has been found in CSF (Morsica et al., 1997; Maggi et al., 1999) and in the CNS (Bolay et al., 1996; Radkowski et al., 2002), clinical involvement of the PNS and CNS appears to be primarily immunologically mediated through mechanisms such as cryoglobulinemia (Petty et al., 1996; Origgi et al., 1998; Tembl et al., 1999), anticardiolipin antibody (Malnick et al., 1997), and ischemic events. The most common site of attack appears to be the PNS, as is the case in Guillain-Barré syndrome. Tembl et al. (1999) reported that neuropathic signs including dysesthesiae and paresthesiae were observed in eight of nine studied patients.

Axonal polyneuropathy was the most common electrodiagnostic finding. These patients had a motor as well as a sensory component of their clinical syndrome. Neuropathies as complications of chronic HCV infection were attributed to vasculitis by Heckmann et al. (1999).

CNS findings were described in three of the nine patients reported by Tembl et al. (1999). Acute and subacute diffuse encephalopathic signs were reported, including somnolence, confusion, stupor, dysarthria, dysphagia, and incontinence. One patient demonstrated dementia and gait difficulties. Neuroimaging studies (CT and MRI) in these patients showed scattered small lesions. Acute inflammatory episodes were treated with steroids or cyclophosphamide with symptomatic improvement. Alpha interferon with or without ribavirin was judged to be helpful in some patients. The authors pointed out that a vascular pathogenesis was supported by the concomitant findings of neuropathy, purpura, and cryoglobulinemia.

Similar findings in CNS were previously reported by Origgi et al. (1998) in three patients with chronic HCV and cryoglobulinemia. One patient demonstrated a mild hyperreflexic tetraparesis, hemiparetic gait, bilateral Babinski signs, dysmetria, and nystagmus. MRI revealed multiple lacunar infarctions. The clinical abnormalities resolved. The second patient, whose history included chronic hepatitis due to HCV and breast carcinoma, demonstrated mild right-side facial weakness, left-side hypoesthesia, and nystagmus, among various neurological findings. An MRI showed punctiform ischemic lesions. The third patient, who had had slight hemiparesis and sensory impairment and was evaluated for recurrent episodes of dizziness, was also found on MRI to have many punctiform lesions. These were interpreted as compatible with ischemic lesions.

The original report of cerebral ischemia associated with mixed cryoglobulinemia in HCV-infected patients was published by Petty et al. (1996). Two patients were described, one of whom was found to have multiple intracranial artery narrowings when studied following a cerebral infarction and the other of whom was found on cerebral biopsy to have had an infarction. The latter patient also had membranoglomerulonephritis and hypocomplimentemia. The authors suggested that cerebral ischemia may be the initial manifestation of the mixed cryoglobulinemia associated with HCV. Heckmann et al. (1999) reported a patient with leukoencephalopathy in the context of severe systemic vasculitis.

Yet another mechanism for stroke in association with chronic HCV infection is the production of anticardiolipin antibodies. Malnick et al. (1997) described a 54-year-old man who developed the sudden onset of a left lower quadrant field defect. CT exam revealed a hypodense area in the posterior radiation of the right internal capsule compatible with a lacunar infarction. Laboratory evaluation revealed elevated serum transaminases and serology, RNA positive for HCV, and the presence of anticardiolipin antibodies. Mitral valve prolapse with minimal mitral regurgitation was also found, which the authors felt did not explain the ischemic event. Treatment with alpha interferon was associated with normalization of the liver transaminases, loss of detectable serum HCV RNA, and disappearance of the anticardiolipin antibody. No change in the quadrantanopsia occurred, but no more ischemic events ensued. The authors further noted that they had found anticardiolipin antibodies in almost half of their patients with chronic HCV hepatitis.

Thus, as with HBV, PNS and CNS abnormalities in chronic HCV infection appear to relate to serological immune moieties. In the case of HCV, cryoglobulins and anticardiolipin antibodies have been associated with MRI findings and CNS events compatible with cerebral ischemia. Finally, while apparently very rare, ADEM (Sacconi et al., 2001) and progressive encephalomyelitis with rigidity (Bolay et al., 1996) have been reported in association with HCV infection.

REFERENCES

Afzal, M. A., J. Buchanan, J. A. Dias, M. Cordiero, M. L. Bentley, C. A. Shorrock, and P. D. Minor. 1997. RT-PCR based diagnosis and molecular characterization of mumps viruses derived from clinical specimens collected during the 1996 mumps outbreak in Portugal. *J. Med. Virol.* **52:**349–353.

Agut, H., H. Collandre, J.-T. Aubin, D. Guetard, V. Favier, D. Ingrand, L. Montagnier, and J.-M. Huraux. 1989. In vitro sensitivity of human herpesvirus-6 to antiviral drugs. *Res. Virol.* **140:**219–228.

Ahtiluoto, S., L. Mannonen, A. Paetau, A. Vaheri, M. Koskiniemi, P. Rautiainen, and M. Muttilainen. 2000. In situ hybridization detection of human herpesvirus 6 in brain tissue from fatal encephalitis. *Pediatrics* **105:**431–433.

Albright, A. V., E. Lavi, J. B. Black, S. Goldberg, M. J. O'Connor, and F. Gonzalez-Scarano. 1998. The effect of human herpesvirus-6 (HHV-6) on cultured human neural cells: oligodendrocytes and microglia. *J. Neurovirol.* **4:**486–494.

Alter, M. J., D. Druszon-Moran, O. V. Nainan, G. M. McQuillan, F. Gao, L. A. Moyer, R. A. Kaslow, and H. S. Margolis. 1999. The prevalence of hepatitis C virus infection in the United States, 1988 through 1994. *N. Engl. J. Med.* **341:**556–562.

Ambler, M., J. Stoll, A. Tzamaloukas, and M. M. Albala. 1971. Focal encephalomyelitis in infectious mononucleosis. *Ann. Intern. Med.* **75:**579–583.

Anderson, D. A. 2000. Waterborne hepatitis, p. 295–305. *In* S. Specter, R. L. Hodinka, and S. A. Young (ed.), *Clinical Virology Manual*, 3rd ed. ASM Press, Washington, D.C.

Anderson, M. J., S. F. Jones, S. P. Fisher-Hoch, E. Lewis, S. M. Hall, C. L. R. Bartlett, B. J. Cohen, P. P. Mortimer, and M. S. Pereira. 1983. Human parvovirus, the cause of erethema infectiosum (Fifth Disease). *Lancet* **i:**1378.

Ascherio, A., K. L. Munger, E. T. Lennette, D. Spiegelman, M. A. Hernan, M. J. Olek, S. E. Hankinson, and D. J. Hunter. 2001. Epstein-Barr virus antibodies and risk of multiple sclerosis. A prospective study. *JAMA* **286:**3083–3088.

Azimi, P. H., H. G. Cramblett, and R. E. Haynes. 1969. Mumps meningoencephalitis in children. *JAMA* **207:**509–512.

Bakshi, N., J. Lawson, R. Hanson, C. Ames, and H. V. Vinters. 1996. Fatal mumps meningoencephalitis in a child with severe combined immunodeficiency after bone marrow transplantation. *J. Child Neurol.* **11:**159–162.

Balfour, H. H., Jr., G. M. Schiff, and J. E. Bloom. 1970. Encephalitis associated with erythema infectiosum. *Pediatrics* **77:**133–136.

Bang, H. O., and J. Bang. 1943. Involvement of the central nervous system in mumps. *Acta Med. Scand.* **63:**487–505.

Barah, F., P. J. Vallely, M. L. Chiswick, G. M. Cleator, and J. R. Kerr. 2001. Association of human parvovirus B-19 infection with acute meningoencephalitis. *Lancet* **358:**729–730.

Barraza, E. M., S. L. Ludwig, J. C. Gaydos, and F. Brundage. 1999. Reemergence of adenovirus type 4 acute respiratory disease in military trainees: report of an outbreak during a lapse in vaccination. *J. Infect. Dis.* **179:**1531–1533.

Bech, E., J. Lycke, P. Gadeberg, M. J. Hansen, C. Malmestrom, O. Anderson, T. Christensen, S. Eckholm, S. Haahr, P. Hoolsberg, T. Bergstrom, B. Svennerholm, and J. Jakobsen. 2002. A randomized double blind, placebo-controlled MRI study of anti-herpes virus therapy in MS. *Neurology* **58:**31–36.

Bendinelli, M., M. Pistello, F. Maggi, and M. Vatteroni. 2000. Blood-borne hepatitis viruses: hepatitis B, C, D and G viruses and T.T. virus, p. 306–337. *In* S. Specter, R. L. Hodinka, and S. A. Young (ed.), *Clinical Virology Manual*, 3rd ed. ASM Press, Washington, D.C.

Bergin, J. D. 1960. Fatal encephalopathy in glandular fever. *J. Neurol. Neurosurg. Psychiatr.* **23:**69–73.

Bernstein, T. C., and H. G. Wolff. 1950. Involvement of the nervous system in infectious mononucleosis. *Ann. Intern. Med.* **335:**1120–1138.

Bistrian, B., C. A. Phillips, and I. S. Kaye. 1972. Fatal mumps meningoencephalitis. Isolation of virus pre-mortem and post-mortem. *JAMA* **222:**478–479.

Bolay, H., F. Soylemezoglu, G. Nurlu, S. Tuncer, and K. Varli. 1996. PCR detected hepatitis C virus genome in brain of a case with progressive encephalomyelitis with rigidity. *Clin. Neurol. Neurosurg.* **98:**305–308.

Bosi, A., M. Zazzi, A. Amantini, M. Cellerini, A. M. Vannucchi, A. De Milito, S. Guidi, R. Saccardi, L. Lombardini, D. Laszlo, and P. Rossi Ferrini. 1998. Fatal herpesvirus 6 encephalitis after unrelated bone marrow transplant. *Bone Marrow Transplant* **22:**285–288.

Bossolasco, S., R. Marenzi, H. Dahl, L. Vago, M. R. Terreni, F. Broccolo, A. Lazzarin, A. Linde, and P. Cinque. 1999. Human herpesvirus 6 in cerebrospinal fluid of patients infected with HIV: frequency and clinical significance. *J. Neurol. Neurosurg. Psychiat.* **67:**789–792.

Braun, D. K., G. Dominguez, and P. E. Pellett. 1997. Human herpesvirus 6. *Clin. Microbiol. Rev.* **10:**521–567.

Bromberg, K., D. N. Newhall, and G. Pater. 1982. Hepatitis A and meningoencephalitis. *JAMA* **247:**815.

Brooks, B. R. 1977. Viral hepatitis type B presenting with seizure. *JAMA* **237:**472–473.

Brown, K. E. 2000. Parvoviridae parvovirus B-19, p. 1685–1693. *In* J. E. Bennett and R. Dolin (ed.), *Principles and Practice of Infectious Diseases*, 5th ed. Churchill Livingstone, Philadelphia, Pa.

Campadelli-Fiume, G., P. Mirandola, and l. Menotti. 1999. Human herpesvirus-6: an emerging pathogen. *Emerg. Infect. Dis.* **5:**353–366.

Carrigan, D. R., D. Harrington, and K. K. Knox. 1996. Subacute leukoencephalitis caused by CNS infection with human herpesvirus-6 manifesting as acute multiple sclerosis. *Neurology* **47:**145–148.

Carter, R. L., and H. G. Penman. 1969. *Infectious Mononucleosis.* Blackwell Scientific Publications, Oxford, United Kingdom.

Caruso, J. M., G. A. Tung, G. G. Gascon, J. Rogg, L. Davis, and W. D. Brown. 2000. Persistent preceding focal neurologic deficits in children with chronic Epstein-Barr virus infections. *J. Child. Neurol.* **15:**791–796.

Caserta, M. T., and C. B. Hall. 1997. Human herpesvirus-6, p. 129–138. *In* W. M. Scheld, R. J. Whitley, and D. T. Durack (ed.), *Infections of the Central Nervous System*, 2nd ed. Lippincott, Raven, Philadelphia, Pa.

Caserta, M. T., C. B. Hall, K. Schnabel, K. McIntyre, C. Long, M. Costanzo, S. Dewhurts, R. Insel, and L. G. Epstein. 1994. Neuroinvasion and persistence of human herpesvirus 6 in children. *J. Infect. Dis.* **170:**1586–1589.

Center for Disease Control. 1978. Mumps—United States. *Morb. Mortal. Wkly Rep.* **27:**379–381.

Centers for Disease Control and Prevention. 2001. Two fatal cases of adenovirus-related illness in previously healthy young adults—Illinois, 2000. *Morb. Mortal. Wkly. Rep.* **50:**553–555.

Challoner, P. B., K. T. Smith, J. D. Parker, D. L. MacLeod, S. N. Coulter, T. M. Rose, E. R. Shultz, L. Benneti, R. L. Garber, M. Chang, P. A. Schad, P. A. Steward, R. C. Nowinski, J. P. Brown, and G. C. Burmer. 1995. Plaque-associated expression of human herpesvirus-6 in multiple sclerosis. *Proc. Natl. Acad. Sci. USA* **92:**7440–7444.

Chou, S. M., R. Roos, R. Burrell, L. Gutmann, and J. B. Harley. 1973. Subacute focal adenovirus encephalitis. *J. Neuropath. Exp. Neurol.* **32:**34–50.

Cohen, H. A., A. Ashkenazi, M. Nussinovitch, J. Amia, J. Hart, and M. Frydman. 1992. Mumps-associated acute cerebellar ataxia. *Am. J. Dis. Child.* **146:**930–931.

Cohen, J. I. 2000. Epstein-Barr virus infection. *N. Engl. J. Med.* **343:**481–492.

Cole, P. D., J. Stiles, F. Boulad, T. N. Small, R. J. O'Reilly, D. George, P. Szaboles, T. E. Kiehn, and N. A. Kernan. 1998. Successful treatment of human herpesvirus 6 encephalitis in a bone marrow transplant recipient. *Clin. Infect. Dis.* **27:**653–654.

Colville, A., and S. Pugh. 1992. Mumps meningitis and measles, mumps, and rubella vaccine. *Lancet* **340:**768.

Cooperman, S. M. 1977. "Alice in Wonderland" syndrome as a presenting symptom of infectious mononucleosis in children. *Clin. Pediatr.* **16:**143–146.

Cossart, Y. E., A. M. Field, B. Cant, and D. Widdows. 1975. Parvovirus-like particles in human sera. *Lancet* **i:**72–73.

Daibata, M., N. Hatakeyama, M. Kamioka, Y. Nemoto, M. Hiroi, I. Miyoshi, and H. Taguchi. 2001. Detection of human herpesvirus 6 and JC virus in progressive multifocal leukoencephalopathy. *Am. J. Hematol.* **67:**200–205.

Davis, L. E., L. E. Brown, B. H. Robertson, B. Khanna, and L. B. Polish. 1993. Hepatitis A post-viral encephalitis. *Acta Neurol. Scand.* **87:**67–69.

DeSimone, P. A., and D. Snyder. 1978. Hypoglossal nerve palsy in infectious mononucleosis. *Neurology* **28:**844–847.

DiBisceglie, A. M., and B. R. Bacon. 1999. The unmet challenges of hepatitis C. *Sci. Am.* **October:**80–85.

Dolgopol, V. B., and G. S. Husson. 1949. Infectious mononucleosis with neurologic complications: report of fatal cases. *Arch. Intern. Med.* **83:**179–196.

Donovan, W. D., and R. D. Zimmerman. 1996. MRI findings of severe Epstein-Barr virus encephalomyelitis. *J. Comput. Assist. Tomogr.* **20:**1027–1029.

Drobyski, W. R., K. K. Knox, D. Majewski, and D. R. Carrigan. 1994. Brief report: fatal encephalitis due to variant B human herpes-6 infection in bone marrow transplant recipient. *N. Engl. J. Med.* **330:**1356–1360.

Dudding, B. A., S. C. Wagner, A. Zellerj, J. T. Gmelich, G. R. French, and F. H. Top, Jr. 1972. Fatal pneumonia associated with adenovirus type 7 in three military trainees. *N. Engl. J. Med.* **286:**1289–1292.

Duffy, J., M. D. Lidsky, J. T. Sharp, J. S. Davis, D. A. Person, F. B. Hollinger, and K.-W. Min. 1976. Polyarthritis, polyarteritis, and hepatitis B. *Medicine* **55:**19–37.

Faden, H., G. W. Gary, Jr., and M. Korman. 1990. Numbness and tingling of fingers associated with parvovirus B-19 infection. *J. Infect. Dis.* **161:**354–355.

Feldman, H. A. 1982. Mumps, p. 419–440. *In* A. S. Evans (ed.), *Viral Infections of Humans, Epidemiology and Control*, 2nd ed. Plenum Press, New York, N.Y.

Ford, F. R. 1966. Mumps meningoencephalitis, p. 391–397. *In Diseases of the Nervous System in Infancy, Childhood and Adolescence*, 5th ed. Thomas, Springfield, Ill.

Frieden, I. J., and S. D. Resnick. 1991. Childhood exanthems, old and new. *Pediatr. Clin. N. Am.* **38:**859–887.

Friedland, R., and M. D. Yahr. 1977. Meningoencephalopathy secondary to infectious mononucleosis. Unusual presentation with stupor and chorea. *Arch. Neurol.* **34:**186–188.

Friedlander, W. J. 1956. Neurologic signs and symptoms as prodrome to virus hepatitis. *Neurology* **6:**574–578.

Gabrielson, M. O., C. Joseph, and G. D. Hsiung. 1966. Encephalitis associated with adenovirus type 7 occurring in a family outbreak. *J. Pediatr.* **68:**142–144.

Gautier-Smith, P. C. 1965. Neurological complications of glandular fever (Infectious Mononucleosis). *Brain* **88:**323–334.

Glikmann, G. A., M. Pedersen, and C.-H. Mordhorst. 1986. Detection of specific immunoglobulin M to mumps virus in serum and cerebrospinal fluid samples from patients with acute mumps infection, using an antibody-capture enzyme immunoassay. *Acta Pathol. Microbiol. Immunol. Scand. Sect. C* **94:**145–156.

Gnann, J. W., Jr. 1997. Meningitis and encephalitis caused by mumps virus, p. 169–180. *In* M. W. Scheld, R. J. Whitley, and D. T. Durrack (ed.), *Infections of the Central Nervous System*, 2nd ed. Lippincott-Raven, Philadelphia, Pa.

Grose, C., W. Henle, G. Henle, and P. M. Feorino. 1975. Primary Epstein-Barr virus infections in acute neurological diseases. *N. Engl. J. Med.* **292:**392–395.

Grose, C. 1983. Neurologic complications of infectious mononucleosis, p. 49–68. *In* D. Schlossberg (ed.), *Infectious Mononucleosis*, 2nd ed. Springer-Verlag, New York, N.Y.

Hall, C. B., and F. A. Horner. 1977. Encephalopathy with erythema infectiosum. *Am. J. Dis. Child.* **131:**65–67.

Hall, C. B., C. E. Long, K. C. Schnabel, M. T. Caserta, K. M. McIntyre, M. A. Costanzo, A. Knott, S. Dewhurst, R. A. Insel, and L. G. Epstein. 1994. Human herpesvirus-6 infection in children. A prospective study of complications and reactivation. *N. Engl. J. Med.* **331:**432–438.

Hammond, G. W., B. K. MacDougall, F. Plummer, and L. H. Seka. 1982. Encephalitis during the prodromal stage of acute hepatitis A. *Can. Med. Assoc. J.* **126:**269–270.

Heckmann, J. G., C. Kayser, D. Heuss, B. Manger, H. E. Blum, and B. Nenndorfer. 1999. Neurological manifestations of chronic hepatitis C. *J. Neurol.* **246:**486–491.

Heegard, E. D., and K. E. Brown. 2002. Human parvovirus B19. *Clin. Microbiol. Rev.* **15:**485–505.

Herndon, R. M., R. T. Johnson, L. E. Davis, and L. R. Descalzi. 1974. Ependymitis in mumps virus meningitis. Electron microscopical studies of cerebrospinal fluid. *Arch. Neurol.* **30:**475–479.

Hochberg, F. H., J. R. Lehrich, E. P. Richardson, P. M. Feorino, and K. E. Astrom. 1976. Mononucleosis-associated subacute sclerosing panencephalitis. *Acta Neuropathol.* (Berlin) **34:**33–40.

Hochberg, F. H., G. Miller, R. T. Schooley, M. S. Hirsch, P. Feorino, and W. Henle. 1983. Central-nervous-system lymphoma related to Epstein-Barr virus. *N. Engl. J. Med.* **309:**745–748.

Hongou, K., T. Konishi, S. Yagi, K. Araki, and T. Miyawaki. 1998. Rotavirus encephalitis mimicking afebrile benign convulsions in infants. *Pediatr. Neurol.* **18:**354–357.

Ito, M., T. Go, T. Okundo, and H. Mikawa. 1991. Chronic mumps virus encephalitis. *Pediatr. Neurol.* **7:**467–470.

Ito, M., J. V. Baker, D. J. Mock, A. D. Goodman, B. M. Blumberg, D. A. Shrier, and J. M. Powers. 2000. Human herpesvirus 6-meningoencephalitis in an HIV patient with progressive multifocal leukoencephalopathy. *Acta Neuropathol.* (Berlin) **100:**337–341.

Jackson, G. G., and R. L. Muldoon. 1973. Viruses causing common respiratory infection in man. IV. Reoviruses and Adenoviruses. *J. Infect. Dis.* **128:**811–866.

Johnstone, J. A., C. A. C. Ross, and M. Dunn. 1972. Meningitis and encephalitis associated with mumps infection. A ten year survey. *Arch. Dis. Child.* **47:**647–651.

Kamei, A., S. Ichinohe, R. Onuma, S. Hiraga, and T. Fujiwara. 1997. Acute disseminated demyelination due to primary human herpesvirus-6 infection. *Eur. J. Pediatr.* **156:**709–712.

Katsafanas, G. C., E. C. Schirmer, L. S. Wyatt, and N. Frenkel. 1996. In vitro activation of human herpesviruses 6 and 7 from latency. *Proc. Natl. Acad. Sci. USA* **93:**9788–9792.

Keidan, I., I. Shif, G. Keren, and J. H. Passwell. 1992. Rotavirus encephalopathy: evidence of central nervous system involvement during rotavirus infection. *Pediatr. Infect. Dis. J.* **11:**773–774.

Kelsey, D. S. 1978. Adenovirus meningoencephalitis. *Pediatrics* **61:**291–293.

Kelsey, D. S., and W. T. McLean. 1979. Adenoviral meningoencephalitis in a patient with lead toxicity. *Arch. Neurol.* **36:**384–385.

Knox, K. K., and D. R. Carrigan. 1995. Active human herpesvirus (HHV-6) infection of the central nervous system in patients with AIDS. *J. Acquir. Immune Defic. Syndr. Hum. Retrovirol.* **9:**69–73.

Knox, K. K., D. P. Harrington, and D. R. Carrigan. 1995. Fulminant human herpesvirus six encephalitis in a human immunodeficiency virus-infected infant. *J. Med. Virol.* **45:**288–292.

Knox, K. K., J. H. Brewer, J. M. Henry, D. J. Harrington, and D. R. Carrigan. 2000. Human herpesvirus-6 and multiple sclerosis: systemic active infections in patients with early disease. *Clin. Infect. Dis.* **31:**894–903.

Kondo, K., T. Kondo, T. Okuno, M. Takahashi, and K. Yamanishi. 1991. Latent human herpesvirus 6 infection of human monocytes/macrophages. *J. Gen. Virol.* **72:**1401–1408.

Krugman, S., and R. Ward. 1968. Mumps (epidemic parotitis), p. 184–198. *In Infectious Diseases of Children.* C. V. Mosby Co., St. Louis, Mo.

Kuo, Y. T., N.-O. Chiu, E. Y. Shen, C.-S. Ho, and M. C. Wu. 1998. Cerebral perfusion in children with Alice in Wonderland syndrome. *Pediatr. Neurol.* **19:**105–108.

Lahat, E., M. Berkovitch, J. Barr, G. Paret, and A. Barzilai. 1999. Abnormal visual evoked potentials in children with "Alice in Wonderland" syndrome due to infectious mononucleosis. *Child. Neurol.* **14:**732–735.

Landry, M. L., and G. D. Hsiung. 1988. Adenovirus-associated meningoencephalitis in a healthy adult. *Ann. Neurol.* **23:**627–628.

Lanzinger-Rossnagel, G., and B. Kommerell. 1980. EEG changes in acute viral hepatitis. *Electroenceph. Clin. Neurophysiol.* **50:**96–101.

Lauer, G. M., and B. D. Walker. 2001. Hepatitis C virus infection. *N. Engl. J. Med.* **345:**41–52.

Lelong, M., P. Lepine, F. Alison, P. Le-Tan-Vinh Satge, and C. Chany. 1956. La pneumonie A virus du group A.P.C. chez de nourrison isolement du virus: les lisions anatomohistologiques. *Arch. Fr. Pediatr.* **13:**1092–1096.

Lennette, E. H., G. E. Caplan, and R. L. Magoffin. 1960. Mumps virus infection simulating paralytic poliomyelitis. A report of 11 cases. *Pediatrics* **25:**788–797.

Leppik, I. E., V. Ramani, R. J. Sawchuk, and R. J. Gumnit. 1979. Increased clearance of phenytoin during infectious mononucleosis. *N. Engl. J. Med.* **300:**481–482.

Levitt, L. P., T. A. Rich, S. W. Kinde, A. L. Lewis, E. H. Gates, and J. O. Bond. 1970. Central nervous system mumps. A review of 64 cases. *Neurology* **20:**829–834.

Lippman, C. W. 1952. Certain hallucinations peculiar to migraine. *J. Nerv. Ment. Dis.* **116:**346–351.

Ljungman, P., F. Z. Wang, D. A. Clark, V. C. Emery, M. Remberger, O. Ringden, and A. Linde. 2000. High levels of human herpesvirus 6 DNA in peripheral blood leucocytes are correlated to platelet engraftment and disease in allogeneic stem cell transplant patients. *Br. J. Haematol.* **111:**774–781.

Lockwood, A. H. 1995. Hepatic encephalopathy and other neurological disorders associated with gastrointestinal disease, p. 247–266. *In M. J. Aminoff (ed.), Neurology and General Medicine.* Churchill Livingstone, New York, N.Y.

Lord, A., N. P. Sutton, and J. A. N. Corsellis. 1975. Recovery of adenovirus type 7 from human brain cell cultures. *J. Neurol. Neurosurg. Psychiatr.* **38:**710–712.

Love, S., and C. A. Wiley. 2002. Viral infections, p. 1–106. *In D. I. Graham and P. L. Lantos (ed.), Greenfield's Neuropathology.* Arnold, London, United Kingdom.

Lundgren, O., A. T. Peregrin, K. Persson, S. Kordasti, I. Uhnoo, and L. Svensson. 2000. Role of the enteric nervous system in the fluid and electrolyte secretion of rotavirus diarrhea. *Science* **287:**491–495.

Luppi, M., P. Barozzi, A. Maiorana, R. Marasca, and G. Torelli. 1994. Human herpes 6 infection in normal human brain tissue. *J. Infect. Dis.* **169:**943–944.

Lycke, J., B. Svennerholm, E. Hjeimquist, L. Frisen, G. Badr, M. Andersson, A. Vahlne, and O. L. Andereson. 1966. Acyclovir treatment of relapsing-remitting multiple sclerosis. A randomized placebo-controlled, double-blind study. *J. Neurol.* **243:**214–224.

MacKenzie, I. R. A., D. R. Carrigan, and C. A. Wiley. 1995. Chronic myelopathy associated with human herpesvirus-6. *Neurology* **45:**2015–2017.

Maggi, F., M. Giorgi, C. Fornai, A. Morrica, M. L. Vatteroni, M. Pistello, G. Sieiliano, A. Nuecorini, and M. Bendinelli. 1999. Detection and quasispecies analysis of hepatitis C virus in the cerebrospinal fluid of infected patients. *J. Neurovirol.* **5:**319–323.

Majid, A., S. L. Galetta, C. J. Sweeney, C. Robinson, R. Mahalingam, J. Smith, B. Forgham, and D. H. Gilden. 2002. Epstein-Barr virus myeloradiculitis and encephalomyeloradiculitis. *Brain* **125:**159–165.

Malnick, S. D. H., Y. Abend, E. Evron, and Z. M. Sthoeger. 1997. HCV hepatitis associated with anticardiolipin antibody and a cerebrovascular event. Response to interferon therapy. *J. Clin. Gastroenterol.* **24:**40–42.

Matson, D. O., M. L. O'Ryan, X. Jiang, and D. K. Mitchell. 2000. Rotavirus, enteric adenoviruses, calciviruses, astroviruses, and other viruses causing gastroenteritis, p. 270–275. *In S. Specter, R. L. Hodinka, and S. A. Young (ed.), Clinical Virology Manual,* 3rd ed. ASM Press, Washington, D.C.

McCullers, J. A., F. D. Lakeman, and R. J. Whitley. 1995. Human herpesvirus 6 is associated with focal encephalitis. *Clin. Infect. Dis.* **21:**571–576.

McDonald, J. C., D. L. Moore, and P. Quennec. 1989. Clinical and epidemiologic features of mumps meningoencephalitis and possible vaccine-related disease. *Pediatr. Infect. Dis. J.* **8:**751–755.

Melbye, M., P. Ebbesen, N. Jacobsen, and C. H. Mordhorst. 1983. Simultaneous primary infections with Epstein-Barr virus and measles virus in fatal acute encephalitis. *Br. Med. J.* **286:**521–522.

Merelli, E., R. Bedin, P. Sola, M. Gentilini, P. Pietrosemoli, M. Meacci, and M. Portolani. 1997. Encephalomyeloradiculopathy associated with Epstein-Barr virus: primary infection or reactivation? *Acta Neurol. Scand.* **96:**416–420.

Michalak, T. 1978. Immune complexes of hepatitis B surface antigen in the pathogenesis of periarteritis nodosa. *Am. J. Pathol.* **90:**619–628 and following figures.

Mookerjee, B. P., and G. Vogelsang. 1997. Human herpesvirus-6 encephalitis after bone marrow transplantation: successful treatment with ganciclovir. *Bone Marrow Transplant.* **20:**905–906.

Morgenlander, J. C. 1996. A syndrome of concurrent central and peripheral nervous system involvement due to Epstein-Barr virus infection. *Muscle Nerve* **19:**1037–1039.

Morsica, G., M. T. Bernardi, R. Novati, C. U. Foppa, A. Castagna, and A. Lazzarin. 1997. Detection of hepatitis C virus genomic sequences in the cerebrospinal fluid of HIV infected patients. *J. Med. Virol.* **53:**252–254.

Naides, S. J. 2000. Parvoviruses, p. 487–500. *In* S. Specter, R. L. Hodinka, and S. A. Young (ed.), *Clinical Virology Manual*, 3rd ed. ASM Press, Washington, D.C.

Nalesnik, M. A. 1999. Epstein-Barr virus, p. 385–407. *In* E. H. Lennette and T. F. Smith (ed.), *Laboratory Diagnosis of Viral Infections*, 3rd ed. Marcel Dekker, New York, N.Y.

Novoa, L. J., R. M. Nagra, T. Nakawatase, T. Edwards-Lee, W. W. Tourtellotte, and M. E. Cornford. 1997. Fulminant demyelinating encephalomyelitis associated with productive HHV-6 infection in an immunocompetent adult. *J. Med. Virol.* **52:**301–308.

Nussinovich, M., N. Brand, M. Frydman, and I. Varsano. 1992. Transverse myelitis following mumps in children. *Acta Paediatr.* **81:**183–184.

Origgi, L., M. Vanoli, A. Carbone, M. Grasso, and R. Scorza. 1998. Central nervous system involvement with HCV-related cryoglobulinemia. *Am. J. Med. Sci.* **315:**208–210.

Osamura, T., R. Mizuta, H. Yoshioka, and S. Fushiki. 1993. Isolation of adenovirus type 11 from the brain of a neonate with pneumonia and encephalitis. *Eur. J. Pediatr.* **152:**496–499.

Pang, X.-L., J. Joensuu, and T. Vesikar. 1996. Detection of Rotavirus RNA in cerebrospinal fluid in a case of Rotavirus gastroenteritis with febrile seizures. *Pediatr. Infect. Dis. J.* **15:**543–545.

Paskavitz, J. R., C. A. Anderson, C. H. Filley, B. K. Kleinschmidt-DeMasters, and K. L. Tyler. 1995. Acute arcuate fiber demyelinating encephalopathy following Epstein-Barr virus infection. *Ann. Neurol.* **38:**127–131.

Petty, G. W., J. Duffy, and J. Huston III. 1996. Cerebral ischemia in patients with hepatitis C virus infection and mixed cryoglobulinemia. *Mayo Clin. Proc.* **71:**671–678.

Poggio, G. P., C. Rodriguez, D. Cisterna, M. C. Freire, and J. Cello. 2000. Nested PCR for rapid detection of mumps virus in cerebrospinal fluid from patients with neurological disease. *J. Clin. Microbiol.* **38:**274–278.

Poppe, M., W. Bruck, G. Hahn, B. Weissbrick, G. Heubner, H. H. Goebel, and H. Todt. 2001. A fulminant course in a case of diffuse myelinoclastic encephalitis—a case report. *Neuropediatrics* **32:**41–44.

Radkowski, M., J. Wilkenson, M. Nowicki, D. Adair, H. Vargas, C. Ingui, J. Rakela, and T. Laskus. 2002. Search for hepatitis C virus negative strand RNA sequences and analysis of viral sequences in the central nervous system: evidence of replication. *J. Virol.* **76:**600–608.

Rantala, H., M. Uhari, and H. Tuokko. 1990. Viral infections and recurrences of febrile convulsions. *J. Pediatr.* **116:**195–199.

Rezza, G., M. Dorrucci, M. Andreoni, C. Arpino, A. DeLuca, P. Monini, E. Nicastri, M. B. Alliegro, P. Pezzoti, and B. Ensoli for the Italian HIV-Seroconversion Study. 1999. Does HHV-8 have a protective role on the development of HIV encephalopathy? *Neurology* **53:**2032–2036.

Ricker, W., A. Blumberg, C. H. Peters, and A. Widerman. 1947. The association of the Guillain-Barré syndrome with infectious mononucleosis, with a report of two fatal cases. *Blood* **2:**217–226.

Ringelstein, E. B., H. Sobczak, B. Pfeifer, and W. Hacke. 1984. [Polyradiculomeningo-encephalitis caused by Epstein-Barr virus infection—description of a case with fatal outcome]. *Fortschr. Neurol. Psychiatr.* **52:**73–82.

Roos, R., S. M. Chou, N. G. Rogers, M. Basnight, and D. C. Gaidusek. 1972. Isolation of an adenovirus 32 strain from human brain in a case of subacute encephalitis. *Proc. Soc. Exp. Biol. Med.* **139:**636–640.

Rosenberg, R. N., E. A. Neuwelt, J. Kirkpatrick, and P. Kohler. 1976. Encephalopathy associated with cryoprecipitable Australia antigen. *Ann. Neurol.* **1:**298–300.

Ross, J. P., and J. I. Cohen. 1997. Epstein-Barr virus, p. 117–127. *In* W. M. Scheld, R. J. Whitley, and D. T. Durack (ed.), *Infections of the Central Nervous System*, 2nd ed. Lippincott-Raven, Philadelphia, Pa.

Roulet-Perez, E., P. Maeder, J. Cotting, A. C. Eskenazy-Cottier, and T. Deonna. 1993. Acute fatal parainfectious cerebellar swelling in two children. A rare or an overlooked situation? *Neuropediatrics* **24:**346–351.

Ruuskanen, O., O. Meurman, and G. Akusjarvi. 1997. Adenoviruses, p. 525–547. *In* D. D. Richman, R. J. Whitley, and F. G. Hyden (ed.), *Clinical Virology*. Churchill Livingstone, New York, N.Y.

Sacconi, S., L. Salviati, and E. Merelli. 2001. Acute disseminated encephalomyelitis associated with hepatitis C virus infection. *Arch. Neurol.* **58:**1679–1681.

Salahuddin, S. Z., D. V. Ablashi, P. D. Markham, S. F. Josephs, S. Sturzenegger, M. Kaplan, G. Halligan, P. Biberfeld, F. Wong-Staal, G. Kramarsky, and R. C. Gallo. 1986. Isolation of a new virus, HBLV, in patients with lymphoproliferative disorders. *Science* **234:**596–601.

Salmi, T. T., P. Arstila, and A. Koivikko. 1978. Central nervous system involvement in patients with rotavirus gastroenteritis. *Scand. J. Infect. Dis.* **10:**29–31.

Schellinger, P. D., C. Sommer, F. Leithauser, S. Schwab, B. Storch-Hagenlocher, W. Hacke, and M. Kiessling. 1999. Epstein-Barr virus meningoencephalitis with a lymphoma-like response in an immunocompetent host. *Ann. Neurol.* **45:**659–662.

Schiff, J. A., A. Schaeferj, and E. Robinson. 1982. Epstein-Barr virus in cerebrospinal fluid during infectious mononucleosis encephalitis. *Yale J. Biol. Med.* **55:**59–63.

Schnell, R. G., P. J. Dyck, E. J. W. Bowie, D. W. Klass, and H. F. Taswell. 1966. Infectious mononucleosis: neurologic and EEG findings. *Medicine* **45:**51–63.

Schwarz, G. A., D. C. Yang, and E. L. Noone. 1964. Meningoencephalomyelitis with epidemic parotitis. *Arch. Neurol.* **11**:453–462.

Sergent, J. S., M. D. Lockshin, C. L. Christian, and D. J. Gocke. 1976. Vasculitis with hepatitis B antigenemia. Long-term observations in nine patients. *Medicine* **55**:1–18.

Sharief, M. K., and E. J. Thompson. 1990. A sensitive ELISA system for the rapid detection of virus specific IgM antibodies in the cerebrospinal fluid. *J. Immunol. Methods* **130**:19–24.

Sharma, K. R., S. Sriram, T. Fries, H. J. Bevan, and W. G. Bradley. 1993. Lumbosacral radiculoplexopathy as a manifestation of Epstein-Barr virus infection. *Neurology* **43**:2550–2554.

Shian, W. J., and C. S. Chi. 1996. Epstein-Barr virus encephalitis and encephalomyelitis: MR findings. *Pediatr. Radiol.* **26**:690–693.

Shoji, H., T. Kusuhara, Y. Honda, K. Kojima, T. Abe, and M. Watanabe. 1992. Relapsing acute disseminated encephalomyelitis associated with chronic Epstein-Barr virus infection: MRI findings. *Neuroradiology* **34**:340–342.

Silverstein, A., G. Steinberg, and M. Nathanson. 1972. Nervous system involvement in infectious mononucleosis. The heralding and/or major manifestation. *Arch. Neurol.* **26**:353–358.

Simila, S., R. Jouppila, A. Salmi, and R. Pohionen. 1970. Encephalomeningitis in children associated with an adenovirus Type 7 epidemic. *Acta Pediatr. Scand.* **59**:310–316.

Skaff, P. T., and D. M. Labiner. 2001. Status epilepticus due to human parvovirus B-19 in an immunocompetent adult. *Neurology* **57**:1336–1337.

Staud, R., R. A. Davidson, and L. C. Corman. 1995. Brachial plexitis in a patient with acute parvovirus B-19 infection. *Br. J. Rheumat.* **34**:480–481.

Suga, S., T. Yoshikawa, Y. Asano, T. Kozawa, T. Nakashima, I. Kobayashi, T. Yazaki, M. Yamamoto, Y. Kajita, T. Ozaki, Y. Nishimura, T. Yamanaka, A. Yamada, and J. Imanishi. 1993. Clinical and virological analyses of 21 infants with exanthem subitum (roseola infantum) and central nervous system complications. *Ann. Neurol.* **33**:597–603.

Suga, S., K. Suzuki, M. Ihira, T. Yoshikawa, Y. Kajita, T. Ozaki, K. Iida, Y. Saito, and Y. Asano. 2000. Clinical characteristics of febrile convulsions during primary HHV-6 infection. *Arch. Dis. Child.* **82**:62–66.

Sugita, K., M. Ando, K. Minamitani, H. Miyamoto, and H. Niimi. 1991. Magnetic resonance imaging in a case of mumps post infectious encephalitis with asymptomatic optic neuritis. *Eur. J. Pediatr.* **150**:773–775.

Sutton, R. N. P., H. J. M. Pullen, P. Blackledge, E. H. Brown, L. Sinclair, and P. N. Swift. 1976. Adenovirus Type 7; 1971-4. *Lancet* **ii**:987–991.

Sworn, M. J., and H. Urich. 1972. Acute encephalitis in infectious mononucleosis. *J. Pathol.* **100**:201–205.

Tabak, F., A. Mert, R. Ozturk, V. Koksal, I. Akbas, and Y. Aktuglu. 1999. Prolonged fever caused by parvovirus B-19-induced meningitis: case report and review. *Clin. Infect. Dis.* **29**:446–447.

Tabor, E. 1987. Guillain-Barré syndrome and other neurologic syndromes in hepatitis A, B, and non-A, non-B. *J. Med. Virol.* **21**:207–216.

Taylor, F. B., and W. E. Toreson. 1963. Primary mumps meningoencephalitis. *Arch. Intern. Med.* **112**:216–221.

Tembl, J. I., J. M. Ferrer, M. T. Sevilla, A. Lago, F. Mayordomo, and J. J. Vilchez. 1999. Neurologic complications associated with hepatitis C virus infection. *J. Clin. Gastroenterol.* **24**:40–42.

Tiacci, E., M. Luppi, P. Barozzi, G. Gurdo, A. Tabilio, S. Ballanti, G. Torelli, and F. Aversa. 2000. Fatal herpesvirus-6 encephalitis in a recipient of a T-cell-depleted peripheral blood stem cell transplant from a 3-loci mismatched related donor. *Haematologica* **85**:94–97.

Timmons, G. D., and K. P. Johnson. 1970. Aqueductal stenosis and hydrocephalus after mumps encephalitis. *N. Engl. J. Med.* **283**:1505–1507.

Tolly, T. L., R. G. Wells, and J. R. Sty. 1989. MR features of fleeting CNS lesions associated with Epstein-Barr virus infection. *J. Comput. Assist. Tomogr.* **20**:1027–1029.

Tselis, A. Epstein-Barr virus and the nervous system. *In* A. Nath and J. Berger (ed.), *Clinical Neurovirology.* Marcel Dekker, New York, N.Y., in press.

Tselis, A., R. Duman, G. A. Storch, and R. P. Lisak. 1997. Epstein-Barr virus encephalomyelitis diagnosed by polymerase chain reaction: detection of genome in the CSF. *Neurology* **48**:1351–1355.

Uesugi, H., H. Shimizu, T. Maehara, N. Arai, and H. Nakayama. 2000. Presence of human herpesvirus 6 and herpes simplex virus detected by polymerase chain reaction in surgical tissue from temporal lobe epileptic patients. *Psychiatry Clin. Neurosci.* **54**:589–593.

Ushijima, H., K. Bosu, T. Abe, and T. Shinozaki. 1986. Suspected Rotavirus encephalitis. *Arch. Dis. Child.* **61**:692–694.

Vandvik, B., E. Norrby, J. Steen-Johnsen, and K. Stensvold. 1978. Mumps meningitis: prolonged pleocytosis and occurrence of mumps virus-specific oligoclonal IgG in the cerebrospinal fluid. *Eur. Neurol.* **17**:13–22.

Verma, A., and B. Brozman. 2002. Opsoclonus-myoclonus syndrome following Epstein Barr virus infection. *Neurology* **58**:1131–1132.

Wagner, M., J. Muller-Berghaus, R. Schroeder, S. Sollberg, J. Luka, N. Leyssens, B. Schneider, and G. R. Krueger. 1997. Human herpesvirus-6 (HHV-6)-associated necrotizing encephalitis in Griscelli's syndrome. *J. Med. Virol.* **53**:306–312.

Wainwright, M. S., P. L. Martin, R. P. Morse, M. Lacaze, J. M. Provenzale, R. E. Cdeman, M. A. Morgan, C. Hulette, J. Kurtzberg, C. Bushnell, L. Epstein, and D. V. Lewis. 2001. Human herpes 6 limbic encephalitis after stem cell transplantation. *Ann. Neurol.* **50**:612–619.

Walsh, F. C., C. M. Poser, and S. Carter. 1954. Infectious mononucleosis encephalitis. *Pediatrics* **13**:536–543.

Wang, J., K. Huff, R. McMasters, and M. E. Cornford. 1999. Sudden unexpected death associated with HHV-6 in an adolescent with tuberous sclerosis. *Pediatr. Neurol.* **21**:488–491.

Watanabe, T., M. Satoh, and Y. Oda. 1994. Human parvovirus B-19 encephalopathy. *Arch. Dis. Child.* **70**:71.

Weinberg, A., S. Li, M. Palmer, and K. L. Tyler. 2002. Quantitative PCR in Epstein-Barr virus infections of the central nervous system. *Ann. Neurol.* **52**:543–548.

West, T. E., C. J. Papsian, B. H. Park, and S. W. Parker. 1985. Adenovirus type 2 encephalitis and concurrent Epstein-Barr virus infection in an adult man. *Arch. Neurol.* **42**:815–817.

Wierenga, K. J. J., B. E. Serjeant, and G. R. Serjeant. 2001. Cerebrovascular complications and parvovirus infection in homozygous sickle cell disease. *J. Pediatr.* **139**:438–442.

World Health Organization. 2001. Mumps virus vaccines. WHO position paper. *Wkly. Epidemiol. Rec.* **76**:346–355.

Xie, J., Y. Cai, and L. E. Davis. 1998. Guillain-Barré syndrome and Hepatitis A: lack of association during a major epidemic. *Ann. Neurol.* **24**:697–698.

Yahr, M. D., and A. T. Frontera. 1975. Acute autonomic neuropathy. Its occurrence in infectious mononucleosis. *Arch. Neurol.* **32**:132–133.

Yamadera, S., K. Yamashita, M. Akatsuka, N. Kato, and S. Inouye. 1998. Trend of adenovirus type 7 infection, an emerging disease in Japan. *Jpn. J. Med. Sci. Biol.* **51:**43–51.

Yamanishi, K., T. Okuno, K. Shiraki, M. Takahashi, T. Kondo, Y. Asano, and T. Kurata. 1988. Identification of human herpesvirus-6 as a causal agent for exanthem subitum. *Lancet* **i:**1065–1067.

Yoshida, A., T. Kawamitu, R. Tanaka, M. Okumura, S. Yamakura, Y. Takasaki, H. Hiramatsu, T. Momoi, M. Lizuka, and S. Nakagomi. 1995. Rotavirus encephalitis: detection of the virus genomic RNA in the cerebrospinal fluid of a child. *Pediatr. Infect. Dis. J.* **14:**914–916.

Yoto, Y., T. Kudoh, K. Haseyama, and H. Tsutsumi. 2001. Human parvovirus B-19 and meningoencephalitis. *Lancet* **358:**2168.

Zagardo, M. T., C. B. Shanholtz, G. H. Zoarski, and M. I. Rothman. 1998. Rhombencephalitis caused by adenovirus: MR imaging appearance. *Am J. Neuroradiol.* **19:**1901–1903.

6

Encephalitis Viruses Transmitted from Animals

Many viruses that infect humans have animal reservoirs or have an important cycle in animal hosts. The major diagnostic consideration here is that contact with various types of animals can result in significant viral infection of the central nervous system (CNS). Therefore, careful evaluation of contacts with pets and domestic and wild animals, and exposure to vectors of viruses from animals must be part of the workup of every case of encephalitis. The history should also include type of employment, recreational activities, location and type of residence, and travel history. In addition to the viruses considered in this chapter, Nipah virus (chapter 10) is transmitted to humans from swine.

SPORADIC ARBOVIRUS INFECTION

Epidemic encephalitis caused by the arboviruses is discussed in chapter 11. Important in the present context is the occasional presentation as sporadic, apparently isolated, cases of encephalitis in areas not usually associated with arboviral infections. There appear to be two common mechanisms. First, the patient may be infected in an endemic or epidemic area and become sick after traveling to an area free of the disease. Second, the territory in which the virus is prevalent may enlarge. Experience in Connecticut and Rhode Island illustrates these mechanisms. In a case reported by Bia et al. (1980) a 17-year-old boy became ill in Connecticut with signs and symptoms suggestive of herpes simplex encephalitis. Brain biopsy was negative for herpes simplex virus (HSV); however, the diagnosis of Western equine encephalitis was made by seroconversion. Exposure had occurred while on a camping trip in the western United States. In another case, an infant with encephalitis was transferred to a Connecticut hospital from Rhode Island. Biopsy yielded Eastern equine encephalitis, and viral particles were observed on electron microscopy (Kim et al., 1985). Whereas Eastern equine encephalitis has been previously well known in the neighboring state of Massachusetts, it had not previously been known to infect humans in Rhode Island (Center for Disease Control, 1983). It is axiomatic, therefore, that a careful travel history be obtained in any case of encephalitis. Furthermore, it is necessary to know what viral activity is occurring, not only in one's own area, but also in adjacent regions. We therefore contact the state virology laboratory to learn the present viral activity in our own and adjacent regions during the evaluation of any case of encephalitis.

TABLE 6.1 Arenaviruses that can cause human neurological disease[a]

Virus	Disease
LCMV	Lymphocytic meningitis
Lassa fever	Lassa fever
Junin	Argentine hemorrhagic fever
Machupo	Bolivian hemorrhagic fever
Guanarito	Venezuelan hemorrhagic fever

[a] Buchmeier et al., 2001; Lehmann-Grube, 1989.

TABLE 6.2 Representative neurological and sense organ abnormalities associated with infection by LCMV

Congenital[a]
  Hydrocephalus
  Chorioretinitis
  Psychomotor retardation
  Sensorineural deafness
Acquired
  Aseptic meningitis
  Hydrocephalus
  Meningoencephalitis
  Encephalomyelitis

[a] Barton et al., 1995.

LCMV

Lymphocytic choriomeningitis (LCM) virus (LCMV) is a member of the *Arenavirus* family, so named because of the presence of sandlike internal granules on electron microscopy. The arenaviruses include other viruses associated with diseases in humans (Table 6.1). The principal host for LCMV is the mouse. CNS dysfunction can be observed to varying degrees with these other arenaviruses (Lehmann-Grube, 1989; Buchmeier et al., 2001).

LCMV is an important human pathogen and has also served as an experimental probe in immunobiology (reviewed in Peters, 1994). Ironically, LCMV was first isolated during the 1933 outbreak of St. Louis encephalitis in St. Louis, Mo. Soon thereafter, it was the first virus to be associated with Walgren's syndrome of aseptic meningitis. At about the same time, it was shown by Traub to establish a chronic persistent infection in mice. Subsequently, it was demonstrated that although newborn mice are tolerant of LCMV infection, disease in older mice is immune mediated. The mechanism of disease production in the human CNS, however, has not been fully elucidated.

General Disease Characteristics

Most human infections with LCMV probably arise from inadvertent and unrecognized exposures to mice. There is a low and variable prevalence of antibody to LCMV in human populations—4% in Nova Scotia, 4.7% in inner-city Baltimore, and 2.38% in Santa Fe province in Argentina (reviewed by Marrie and Saron, 1998). These figures suggest that many LCMV infections of humans are clinically inapparent or insignificant. The capacity of the virus to establish chronic infections in animal colonies has resulted in several outbreaks among animal handlers in biomedical facilities. The virus can be introduced into mouse and hamster colonies and persist unnoticed in the absence of active surveillance (Gregg, 1975; Dykewicz et al., 1992). An outbreak in owners of pet hamsters was traced to a single source (Gregg, 1975).

LCMV infection of humans can present with a grippelike syndrome, meningitis, meningoencephalitis, and encephalomyelitis (Table 6.2). There is a fairly wide spectrum of signs and symptoms of systemic illness in the initial phase preceding neurological involvement. The incubation period between exposure and the onset of grippelike symptoms has been estimated to be 6 to 13 days or longer (Lehmann-Grube, 1989). Fever, headache, myalgia, anorexia, and malaise are commonly noted. Estimates of the duration of grippelike symptoms prior to neurological involvement have varied from 1 to 3 weeks (Farmer and Janeway, 1942) to 10 days (Buchmeier et al., 2001). Fever may fluctuate. The onset of neurological involvement may appear in a second phase of illness, or the grippelike phase may not be manifested. Peters (1994) has summarized data indicating that about 16% of patients with confirmed LCMV aseptic meningitis will develop encephalitis.

Pathology

There are reports of occasional fatalities in cases of encephalitis due to LCMV. Autopsy studies are limited to six reported cases. In three cases with death in the acute stage of infection, there were extensive areas of parenchymal necrosis (Howard, 1940). The spinal cord was severely involved in one case, with many neutrophils present in the spinal leptomeninges (Howard, 1940). The cerebral cortex and subcortical white matter were extensively replaced by inflammatory cells in one of the other two acute cases. In the third case, inflammatory changes were most severe in the medulla and pons. Viral antigen was demonstrated in the meninges and neurons by immunofluorescence, and virus was isolated from the brain in this case (Warkel et al., 1973). A fatal case without clinical evidence of CNS involvement showed perivascular lymphocytic infiltration of the meninges and brain (Smadel et al., 1942). A case with a history of 9 years' progressive neurological disease following an acute illness showed at autopsy extensively thickened leptomeninges and changes in the brain from perivenous encephalitis (Baker, 1947).

LCMV infection in mice has been the subject of detailed study. Neurological disease in mice is not due to a direct cytopathic effect of the virus but to an immune response to viral antigens. Mice infected in utero, as occurs under natural conditions, are tolerant of the virus and are asymptomatic carriers of it. But if the virus is inoculated into the brains of previously uninfected adult mice, a symptomatic, sometimes severe, meningoencephalitis results. The infection is cleared primarily through the effects of CD8 lymphocyte cytotoxicity (Buchmeier et al., 1980; Borrow and Oldstone, 1997).

Meningoencephalitis and Encephalomyelitis—Diagnosis and Management

Historically, LCMV was the first specific virus to be associated with the syndrome of aseptic meningitis. In an early survey of the causes of aseptic meningitis, Adair et al. (1953) found that approximately 9% of 854 cases were associated with LCMV infection. Headache, fever, and stiff neck were virtually ubiquitous findings. Prodromal symptoms, most often of a grippelike nature, were recorded in the preceding 10 days in approximately 35% of cases. In the majority of cases the meningeal signs were noted first. Other reports have described a biphasic illness in which systemic symptoms cleared prior to the onset of meningeal signs (Armstrong et al., 1969). The cerebrospinal fluid (CSF) often contained between 650 and 1,500 cells per mm^3—predominantly lymphocytes—and a peak mean protein value of 118 mg per 100 ml (Adair et al., 1953). Of particular interest was the finding of low CSF glucose, less than 50 mg per 100 ml in 19 of 72 samples. The importance of this observation has been borne out in other studies (for example, Biggar et al., 1975). The conclusion of Farmer and Janeway in 1942 remains apt: "A story of mouse contact, a prodromal illness and a spinal fluid lymphocyte count over 600/mm^3 have been found useful criteria of infection due to this specific virus." When present, a low CSF glucose adds to the suspicion of LCMV as the cause of the aseptic meningitis.

There does not appear to be a consistent clinical profile of LCM encephalitis. It may manifest as meningoencephalitis, encephalitis, encephalomyelitis, or myelitis. In the report of Biggar et al. (1975), of 49 patients for whom adequate clinical information was available, 3 had evidence of encephalomyelitis. Dysfunction included delirium and disorientation, ataxia, dysphasia, amnesia for the illness, and an atonic bladder. In two cases described by Hirsch et al. (1974), dysphasia and signs of spatial disorientation were found in one and a spontaneously resolving mild hydrocephalus was found in the other. Metamorphopsia has been described by Lewis and Utz (1961) in a case of LCM encephalitis associated with prostatitis and orchitis. In the fatal case described by Warkel et al. (1973), an acute mental status change was followed by opisthotonos, a right Babinski sign, coma, signs of severe brain dysfunction, and nuchal rigidity. An isotopic brain scan revealed bilateral parietal lobe uptake.

By and large, the encephalitis associated with LCMV infection has been followed by complete recovery. In the study of Meyer et al. (1960), only 1 of 20 patients of LCM encephalitis suffered severe sequelae, and none died. Conversely, in two fatal cases described by Smadel et al. (1942), although LCMV was isolated from autopsied brain tissue of both cases, clinical signs of meningoencephalitis had been absent.

The diagnosis of LCM encephalitis is critically dependent on clinical thoroughness. A history of exposure to mice or hamsters, a grippelike prodromal illness, and a CSF revealing greater than 600 mononuclear cells per mm^3 with a low glucose level are useful clues. The clinical presentation and electroencephalogram (EEG) are not specific. There is a frustrating paucity of neuroimaging data. The diagnosis is made by the demonstration of the virus in the CSF or blood and/or by the demonstration of a specific antibody rise. Isolation in mice, guinea pigs, or cell culture is complicated and not employed in most diagnostic labs. PCR, if standardized and widely applied, would likely expand the number of cases recognized. As noted by Buchmeier et al. (2001), immunofluorescent assay, enzyme-linked immunosorbent assay, and neutralization assays are each used for serological diagnosis.

The great majority of LCMV-infected patients survive without residua. While LCMV is sensitive to ribavirin in cell culture, it has been recommended only in special circumstances such as in presentations resembling hemorrhagic fever or in immunosuppressed cancer patients (Peters, 1994). Steroids and immunosuppressants are not recommended (Peters, 1994). Aggressive supportive medical management is indicated.

Other Neurological Disease

LCMV infection has been associated with hydrocephalus. Hirsch et al. (1974) described a spontaneously resolving hydrocephalus in an adult infected with LCMV. Larsen et al. (1993) described a case of acquired LCMV-associated hydrocephalus treated with a ventricular reservoir. Magnetic resonance imaging (MRI) showed enlargement of the lateral ventricles and increased periventricular signal. Computerized tomography (CT) scans were also useful. Komrower et al. (1955) described the probable transplacental transmission of LCMV infection in a fatal case, and Sheinbergas (1976) reported on 14 children with hydrocephalus in whom prenatal infection with LCMV was said to have been serologically confirmed. More recently, Barton et al. (1995) reported congenital abnormalities associated with LCMV in five infants. These consisted of nonobstructive hydrocephalus with periventricular calcifications, chorioretinitis, and psychomotor retardation in all and sensorineural deafness in one. Cardiac abnormalities were not found.

RABIES

Perhaps the most feared of all the encephalitides, rabies is almost always transmitted to people by the bite of a virus-bearing animal and is almost always fatal in humans. Globally, approximately 50,000 human cases occur annually, most of them in underdeveloped countries (Crepin et al., 1998). The disease in animals was described as early as 500 B.C. by Democritus, and its transmission as hydrophobia in humans was described by Celsus in A.D. 100 (Johnson, H. N., 1965).

Although stringent control of the canine population has eliminated rabies from locations such as Great Britain, it is principally an enzootic disease of wild animals. Territories of rabies viruses, associated with specific terrestrial mammals, occur in geographically defined areas (Krebs et al., 1999). Bats have emerged as the most important reservoir for transmission to humans in North America. More specifically, virus variants associated with the small silver-haired or eastern pipistrelle bats are most commonly found. Despite the dramatic explosion of raccoon-associated rabies on the Eastern Seaboard after its translocation from the southeastern United States, it has not been associated with human disease (Fishbein and Robinson, 1993; Noah et al., 1998).

Pathology

Rabies virus is a single-stranded negative-sense RNA rhabdovirus described as bullet shaped when viewed with the electron microscope. The genome contains five genes. These code for the external membrane glycoprotein (G protein), which is the major antigenic determinant and is essential for pathogenicity. G protein binds to the nicotinic acetylcholine receptor (nAChR) expressed by muscle, thereby allowing the virus to gain entry to muscle, where it is capable of replicating. Apart from muscle and salivary and lachrymal glands, the virus otherwise replicates exclusively in nerve cells. Entry to muscle via the nAChR is blocked by α-bungarotoxin, d-tubocurarine, and monoclonal antibodies to the α-subunit of the acetylcholine receptor (AChR) (Burrage et al., 1985). In experimental studies, a single amino acid substitution in the G protein at position 333 dramatically reduced neurovirulence of the virus (Dietzschold et al., 1983; Seif et al., 1985), and two substitutions rendered the virus unable to penetrate the nervous system (Coulon et al., 1998). A second protein, the matrix (M) protein, lines the inner surface of the virion membrane and shows variation that forms the basis of a subtype classification of the virus. The other three proteins are contained in the nucleocapsid.

Replication of the virus takes place in nerve cell cytoplasm, though some viral RNA enters the nucleus, where it blocks host cell DNA and RNA synthesis to promote viral synthesis. The nucleocapsids and the envelope are synthesized separately and come together to form a whole virus particle as a separate step. Before this happens, there is an opportunity for the bare nucleocapsids to be transported along axons and across synapses to spread infection throughout the nervous system (Gosztonyi, 1994). Paradoxically, for a virus that produces an almost invariably fatal encephalitis, the virus displays little cytopathic effect in tissue culture.

Naked-eye examination of the brain in the majority of human cases of rabies reveals no abnormality other than congestion. Microscopically, typical features of encephalitis are found but tend to be scanty in the majority of cases, including neuronophagia, perivascular cuffs of inflammatory cells, and more diffuse microglial proliferation. Focal collections of microglial cells, termed Babe's nodules, may be seen (Tangchai et al., 1970). These changes are distinctly more common in gray than in white matter and are found in greatest concentration in the brain stem, particularly the pons and medulla. The hypothalamus and cervical spinal cord are also frequently affected, followed by the thalamus, basal ganglia, cerebral cortex, hippocampus, and cerebellum. The perivascular inflammatory cells consist of lymphocytes, macrophages, plasma cells, and, in rare cases, neutrophils. The astrocytic reaction is slight or negligible. The meninges show merely slight lymphocytic cuffing. Thrombi in small vessels and associated small hemorrhagic infarcts or petechial hemorrhages have been described in congested parenchyma in some patients (Tangchai et al., 1970).

The most characteristic feature of the pathology of rabies is the presence of Negri bodies (see Fig. 1.4d and 1.11a in chapter 1)—intracytoplasmic inclusions first described by Negri (1903). The observation of these inclusion bodies is generally considered to make the diagnosis certain, but some doubt has been cast on their specificity (Derakhshan et al., 1978). In their absence, rabies cannot be definitely distinguished from other forms of encephalitis on the basis of the light microscopic features alone. Negri bodies were found in 71% of the series of cases studied by Dupont and Earle (1965)

and in 96% of those studied by Tangchai et al. (1970). They are shown by hematoxylin and eosin staining or by Mann's and Schleifenstein's stains on fixed and embedded material and by Sellar's stain on fresh smears. They are easier to see after Formalin fixation and consist of intracytoplasmic eosinophilic structures, 2 to 10 μm across, usually round, but sometimes irregular in shape. They contain some discernible internal structure, a feature that distinguishes them from similar bodies, Lyssa bodies, which are also characteristic of rabies infection. Single or occasionally multiple Negri bodies are identified most frequently in pyramidal neurons of the hippocampus and in Purkinje cells of the cerebellum, but they may be seen in almost any large neurons. In a few cases of rabies, they occur in the complete absence of any inflammatory change and are easier to find in relatively uninflamed areas. Negri bodies have been shown by immunofluorescence to contain rabies virus antigen (Fig. 1.4d, chapter 1) (Goldwasser and Kissling, 1958; Johnson, R. T., 1965) and by electron microscopy to contain viral particles (Morecki and Zimmerman, 1969; Gonzalez Angulo et al., 1970; Ho Sung et al., 1976).

It is not clear that the presence of Negri bodies is associated with neuronal damage. The older literature frequently commented on the topographical dissociation between the Negri bodies and the inflammatory infiltrate, including the foci of neuronophagia. Neurons containing Negri bodies do not necessarily show any degenerative changes (Aksel, 1958). Dupont and Earle (1965) considered them to be more common in the later stages of the disease. What does seem clear from the immunofluorescence studies is that viral antigen is not confined to cells containing Negri and Lyssa bodies but is widespread throughout the brain. It is almost entirely confined to neurons. Immunofluorescence and immunoperoxidase techniques have now largely replaced the classical techniques that relied on searching for Negri bodies for diagnostic purposes. Immunofluorescence carried out on fresh frozen tissue has greater sensitivity than immunoperoxidase on Formalin-fixed, paraffin-embedded tissue (Palmer et al., 1985; Torres-Anjel et al., 1987; Fekadu et al., 1988).

Virus is not confined to the brain in rabies encephalitis. In experimental infections and humans, it has been shown to spread centrifugally along nerves from the brain to the salivary glands, gut, heart, adrenals, pancreas, and skin in the later stages of infection (Fischman and Schaeffer, 1971; Metze and Feiden, 1991; Warrell et al., 1988; Li et al., 1995). It is of course the salivary infection, combined with the altered psychological state, which includes an increased tendency to bite, that leads to the unique mode of spread of the virus. Infection of the nerves supplying the hair follicles of the back of the neck provides a possible means of making the diagnosis by skin biopsy and immunofluorescence staining in human cases (Warrell et al., 1988). Return of virus to peripheral organs via their nerve supply makes use of organs for transplantation from subjects with undiagnosed fatal encephalitis hazardous. Such cases have led to transmission of rabies in corneal transplants (Houff et al., 1979; Hemachudha, 1989; Fishbein and Robinson, 1993).

In a few cases in which the clinical presentation is of a rapidly ascending paralysis resembling the Guillain-Barré syndrome, the main pathological changes are found in the spinal roots, ganglia, and cord (Hurst and Pawan, 1931, 1932; Love, 1944; Chopra et al., 1980). The ganglia show inflammation, degeneration of axons and ganglion cells, and proliferation of satellite cells (Tangchai and Vejjajjva, 1971). Neuronal damage and proliferation of satellite cells in sensory ganglia have been noted to occur with great regularity in all cases of rabies and may be a useful diagnostic feature in cases lacking Negri bodies (Hertzog, 1945). The diagnosis of rabies depends on the demonstration of viral antigen in the brain, using immunofluorescence or immunoperoxidase techniques and specific antisera, and viral culture in vitro or by animal inoculation. The histological demonstration of Negri bodies is also a useful adjunct in diagnosis. It should be noted that some cases are not clinically recognized—usually when no recognized animal bite has occurred—and the diagnosis may be made only at autopsy. This occurred in 27% of the cases reported by Dupont and Earle (1965).

Pathogenesis

The well-recognized occurrence of neuritic pain referable to the site of the original bite during the incubation period of the disease, or as its presenting symptom, led to the suggestion that the virus may travel to the CNS along peripheral nerves, producing irritation of sensory nerve fibers as it does so. There is no more than such circumstantial evidence of neural spread of the virus in humans, but in experimental animal infection, this mode of spread of the virus is now well established (Johnson, H. N., 1965; Murphy et al., 1973).

Rabies has an exceptionally long incubation period. Most patients develop symptoms within 30 to 60 days of exposure to infection, but occasional cases take as long as a year or more to declare themselves (Hemachudha and Mitrabhakdi, 2000; Smith et al., 1991). This long incubation period has been attributed in part to persistent infection of skeletal muscle at the site of entry of the virus (Baer and Cleary, 1972; Charlton et al., 1997). After initial replication at the site of exposure, the virus may remain undetectable for weeks or months (Baer, 1975).

As indicated above, the AChR receptor at skeletal muscle motor end plates may act as a peripheral receptor for rabies virus (Watson et al., 1981; Lentz et al., 1982). Neural spread is thought to occur along axons and can be prevented experimentally by neurectomy, colchicine, and vinblastine (Murphy, 1977); once the CNS is reached, the virus spreads remarkably rapidly among neuron populations. There have been few attempts to relate the distribution of lesions in the CNS to the site of the bite (Perl, 1975), and opinions on this differ. For example, some early studies concluded that the distribution of lesions was dependent on the location of the bite (Schaffer, 1912), while others concluded that the two were independent (Aksel, 1958). Some cases of rabies are acquired by aerosol exposure in caves inhabited by rabid (sometimes symptom-free) bats (Constantine, 1967), in laboratory accidents, or by handling infected carcasses (Tariq et al., 1991; Kureishi et al., 1992).

The role played by immune mechanisms during the incubation period and later in protection from or enhancement of disease has received considerable attention. In experimental infection of rats, successful and rapid clearance of virus from the CNS requires both cellular and humoral

immunity (Miller et al., 1978; Dietzschold et al., 1992; Hooper et al., 1998). However, patients with active T-cell immunity to rabies and elevated serum levels of interleukin-2 (IL-2) receptor and IL-6 succumb faster and suffer more frequently from "furious" rabies than others (Hemachudha et al., 1988, 1993; Hemachudha, 1994; Sugamata et al., 1992; Weiland et al., 1992; Ceccaldi et al., 1996). An immune response to the virus does not normally develop naturally during the incubation period of the disease, presumably because the small amount of virus at that stage is confined to muscle and nerve. Postexposure immune prophylaxis is designed to make up for this and thus prevent the virus from reaching the CNS (see below). Only about 25% of subjects with clinical rabies develop neutralizing antibody despite the fact that the nucleocapsid of rabies contains a humoral immunity-promoting superantigen with adjuvant properties (Lafon et al., 1992, 1994; Astoul et al., 1996). But if defective humoral immunity is in part responsible for the near 100% mortality in humans, it is disappointing that attempts to boost this response have been ineffective (Hemachudha, 1994). It is noteworthy that in the five worldwide survivors, very high serum antibody titers were generated by prophylaxis (Hemachudha and Mitrabhakdi, 2000).

The extent of the neuronal damage and its cause in rabies encephalitis remain a matter of some debate. Clearly, where neuronophagia is visible, neurons have died. This occurs most regularly in the brain stem but can be quite widespread. Some authors have described nonspecific degenerative changes in neurons, such as chromatolysis and vacuolation of cytoplasm, and degenerative changes in nuclear chromatin in many parts of the brain (Lowenberg, 1928; Riesman et al., 1933). This is said to occur in the absence of inflammation. A cytopathic effect of the virus would seem the most likely explanation for such degeneration, as viral antigen is also known to extend beyond the inflamed areas. However, in tissue culture, the virus exhibits little cytopathic effect (Johnson, 1982). Other authors (Dupont and Earle, 1965) are not convinced that there is widespread neuronal degeneration and believe the virus is relatively noncytopathic, in keeping with its behavior in tissue culture. In this case an explanation needs to be sought for the localized cell death that occurs chiefly in the brain stem. In experimental infection of mice, apoptosis occurred and was most marked in hippocampal pyramidal neurons and scattered neocortical neurons (Jackson and Rossiter, 1997; Threerasurakarn and Ubol, 1998). It was more severe in suckling than in adult mice (Jackson and Park, 1998) and was unrelated to the amount of local viral antigen, so it may be mediated by an indirect mechanism. One possible mediator could be nitric oxide production (Van Dam et al., 1995). In one study, levels of nitric oxide produced by macrophages and microglial cells correlated with symptoms (Hooper et al., 1995). Production of IL-1β and tumor necrosis factor alpha by macrophages and microglia has also been demonstrated in rabies-infected rat brain, but this did not correlate with presence of virus (Marquette et al., 1996).

It is tempting to speculate whether there may be a selective toxic mechanism that operates on certain functional groups of neurons, perhaps related to neurotransmitter content or receptor expression. In this context it is interesting to note that rabies virus is capable of modulating expression of immediate-early genes such as *junB* and c-*fos* and late-response genes encoding enkephalin in some brain regions (Fu et al., 1993; Dietzschold et al., 1996). Other neurotransmitter-related changes associated with rabies infection are impairment of muscarinic AChR confined to hippocampus and brain stem in rabies-infected dogs (Dumrongphol et al., 1996), decreased potassium-evoked 5-HT release in rat cortical synaptosomes (Bouzamondo et al., 1993), and modification to 5-HT 1D receptor affinity in rabies-infected rat brains (Ceccaldi et al., 1993). In connection with the latter two findings, Hemachudha and Mitrabhakdi (2000) point out a clinical similarity between furious rabies and the serotonin syndrome (Bodner et al., 1995).

Of similar possible relevance to disease mechanisms in human rabies is a study of acute and persistent rabies virus infection of mouse neuroblastoma–rat glioma hybrid cells (Koschel and Munzel, 1984). In these cells a loss of affinity of opiate receptors (though their number is unchanged) and reduction of the normal opiate receptor coupling to an inhibitory regulatory protein of adenylate cyclase have been demonstrated (Koschel and Munzel, 1984). This study points to a disruption of regulation of cell functions normally influenced by opiate receptors, and it is noteworthy that the limbic system, whose function is altered in rabies infection, contains a large number of neurons bearing opiate receptors.

It is sometimes necessary to distinguish on a neuropathological basis between rabies encephalitis and the effects of postexposure antirabies immunization. In rabies, as already indicated, the inflammatory changes are most severe in the gray matter, while in allergic forms of encephalitis resulting from antirabies immunization, the inflammation is most severe in the white matter (chapter 7). Neuronophagia does not occur in allergic perivenous encephalitis but does occur in rabies. Perivenous demyelination characterizes the allergic encephalitis but does not occur in rabies. Negri bodies are a feature of rabies but are not seen in the allergic encephalitis that may complicate rabies immunization.

The Disease

In the underdeveloped world, where the vast majority of human rabies cases are of canine origin, a history of a dog bite in an individual experiencing hydrophobia or aerophobia strongly suggests a rabies diagnosis. In the United States, however, control of canine rabies has been extremely effective since the 1940s and 1950s. From 1990, 20 of 22 cases of domestic-acquired rabies, as described in 1999, were associated with bats. In only one case was there history of an animal bite (Krebs et al., 1999). Furthermore, of 32 laboratory-confirmed cases in the United States from 1980 to 1996, hydrophobia, aerophobia, agitation, or confusion was recorded in only 11 cases (Noah et al., 1998). More often than not, the clinician in the industrial developed world must evaluate cases of rabies presenting as encephalitis, encephalomyelitis, or a Guillain-Barré-like syndrome, without the telltale history of a bite or the clinical findings of hydrophobia/aerophobia. Characteristic history and findings may occur, however, in travelers returning from underdeveloped countries.

Disease expression in animals takes various forms. Dog rabies can be "furious," with agitated menacing behavior. It is the most dangerous form because of undirected random biting and snapping. The duration of the disease to death is usually 3 to 5 days (Johnson, H. N., 1965). "Dumb" rabies is less dangerous because the animal is relatively immobile and random biting is less frequent. Hydrophobia does not occur in dogs, but dysphagia and a change in the quality of the bark and howl do occur (Johnson, H. N., 1965). Changes in the usual behavior patterns of wild animals, such as the loss of fear of humans, apparent docility, or daytime activity of nocturnal animals, are cause for concern but are not diagnostic. However, some species do not necessarily appear ill at the time of biting. In particular, bats sustain virus in the saliva for considerable periods in the absence of disease (Shope, 1982).

The disease in humans has a variable incubation period and expression (Hattwick and Gregg, 1975). Several features modify the incidence, such as the site and severity of the bite, virus titer in the saliva, and whether the bite occurred through clothing. Bites about the head and face produce the highest incidence of disease. Severe bites that deliver large quantities of virus occur with the attack of rabid wolves. A reduction of the amount of the inoculated virus and hence a lowered risk of the disease occur when the bite is through clothing. The incubation period of disease is also influenced by several factors. Bites on the head and face are estimated to have the briefest incubation periods and those on the legs the longest. Although incubation periods of 2 weeks or less and 1 year or more have been reported, the usual incubation time is between 20 and 90 days. Unfortunately, a history of a bite may not be obtained at the time of illness and the diagnosis may not be suspected, particularly in the case of bat bites. The puncture wound of a bite from a silver-haired or eastern pipistrelle bat is small and can be missed or dismissed as trivial (Jackson and Fenton, 2001).

On rare occasions, infection can occur by other mechanisms. People entering caves heavily contaminated by infected bats and laboratory workers handling infected material under conditions that produce an aerosol are at risk of infection by the olfactory route. Electron micrographic demonstration of viral particles in the olfactory bulb has been reported in one such case (Conomy et al., 1977). Several cases of transmission by corneal transplant are known (e.g., Houff et al., 1979). In each of these cases, the donor suffered the paralytic form of the disease. Any patient suffering from an undiagnosed neurological disease should be rejected as a tissue or organ donor.

Gowers (1893) gave a succinct descriptive summary of human rabies: "Thus the disturbance in the act of swallowing liquids, which constitutes as it were the first symptom and key note of the disease, spreads, on the one hand, to mental disturbance, and on the other to extensive muscular spasms." However, rabies can present in many neurological guises, and history of an animal bite may not be forthcoming. It is useful to consider signs and symptoms of the prodrome, presentation, and evolution of the disease, recognizing that the appearance and sequence of dysfunction may be inconstant. After a variable period of incubation, usually 20 to 90 days, a prodrome of 2 to 10 days may be recognized. Rarely, very much longer incubation periods may be observed. If the person has been particularly disconcerted by an animal bite, much of the prodrome symptomology may appear to be part of the rabies phobia syndrome. Thus agitation, depression, sleeplessness, headache, nausea, and anxiety are seen in both circumstances. Itching, tingling, and pain at the wound site or neuritic discomfort in the region of the bite are useful signs of rabies and occur in about 30% of patients (Hemachudha and Mitrabhakdi, 2000). Low-grade fever may be present but is an inconstant early manifestation. Great sensitivity to tactile, auditory, and visual stimulation is frequently described. The course of the disease in the unsupported patient usually runs from 7 to 14 days. Hydrophobia and aerophobia have been emphasized as diagnostic signs. Hemachudha and Mitrabhakdi (2000) found them to be present in all cases of furious rabies but in only one-half of patients with the paralytic form, nor were they commonly found in the most recent United States experience (Noah et al., 1998).

The most common form of human rabies is the excited or furious form. It is characterized by attacks of agitation or frenzy lasting 1 to 5 min, alternating with periods of lucidity. Seizures, hallucinations, and muscular contractions occur. As the disease progresses, fever of increasing degree is a more constant feature. Signs of excess activity of the autonomic nervous system include fluctuations in blood pressure and temperature, excess salivation, sweating, abnormal pupils, and lacrimation. Irregularities of cardiac rhythm are observed, and the patient is at risk of expiring during a cardiac arrest. The disease may progress into a paralytic phase prior to death. Progressive apathy, stupor, and coma may precede the demise.

The disease starts as paralytic (or dumb) in less than one-fifth of patients (Warrell, 1983). It may present as an ascending paralysis or as a flaccid myelitis with slight changes in sensation and sphincter impairment progressing to brain stem involvement. Hydrophobia is rare, and the course can be prolonged for a month. This form presents particular diagnostic difficulties in the absence of a history of an animal bite. It is most likely to be confused with the ascending paralysis of Guillain-Barré or with polio. The cases involving

corneal transplants cited above are particularly tragic examples of the paralytic form. An outbreak of vampire bat-transmitted rabies in Trinidad was characterized by the paralytic form of the disease (van Rooyen and Rhodes, 1940).

Increasingly, atypical features characteristic of neither the furious nor the paralytic forms are observed, particularly in cases of insect- or fruit-eating bat-associated rabies virus. Focal weakness or sensory loss, hemiparesis, myoclonus, and brain stem and cranial nerve abnormalities are found (Roine et al., 1988; Hemachudha and Mitrabhakdi, 2000). Thus, bat-associated cases of rabies virus often present very significant diagnostic challenges. While rabies itself has not been found in Australia, a nonrabies lyssavirus associated with fruit bats has caused human deaths. Signs of brain stem and cerebellar involvement were prominent with ataxia, slurred speech, diplopia, dysphagia, bilateral facial weakness, and quadraparesis (Samaratunga et al., 1998). European bat lyssavirus 2 was the cause of death of a person handling bats in Scotland in 2002. This was the first case of a rabies-like infection acquired in the United Kingdom in a century (Eurosurveillance, 2002).

Clinical rabies is almost uniformly fatal in humans. Both the furious and paralytic forms progress to coma, as do the atypical forms. Inspiratory respiratory spasms are found, as are cardiac arrhythmias. Cardiac arrhythmias may be the cause of death in patients who do not appear to experience a brain death. Roine et al. (1988) noted brain stem death in their patient before cortical brain death. While a few cases of survival have been described, fewer than half a dozen are published, so they are regarded as atypical (Hemachudha and Mitrabhakdi, 2000).

Diagnosis and Management

There are two broad circumstances in which the clinician is called upon to make critical decisions for rabies. In the first, care for the patient who has suffered possible rabies exposure requires a decision about postexposure prophylaxis (Table 6.3). In the second, diagnostic evaluation and management decisions are required for the patient who has

TABLE 6.3 Rabies postexposure prophylaxis guide[a,b]

Animal species	Condition of animal at time of attack	Treatment of exposed person[c]
Dog, cat, and ferret	Healthy and available for 10 days of observation	None, unless animal develops rabies
	Rabid or suspected rabid	Vaccination and RIG
	Unknown (escaped)	Consult public health officials
Skunk, bat, raccoon, fox, and most other carnivores	Regard as rabid unless proven negative by laboratory tests; sacrifice animal immediately, without a holding period, for testing	Consider immediate vaccination and RIG
Livestock, rodents, rabbits, hares, woodchucks, beavers, and other mammals	Consider individually. Local and state public health officials should be consulted on questions about the need for rabies prophylaxis. Bites of squirrels, hamsters, guinea pigs, gerbils, chipmunks, rats, mice, other small rodents, rabbits, and hares almost never call for antirabies prophylaxis.	

[a] Modified from Centers for Disease Control and Prevention, 1999.

[b] Take into account the animal species involved, the circumstances of the bite or other exposure, the vaccination status of the animal, and the presence of rabies in the region. Local or state public health officials should be consulted.

[c] All bites and wounds should be thoroughly cleansed immediately with soap and water, debrided if necessary, and treated with an antiviral solution such as 70% ethanol, iodine, or povidone-iodine. If antirabies treatment is indicated, both RIG and rabies vaccine should be given as soon as possible, regardless of the interval from exposure. Discontinue vaccine if tests of the biting animal are negative. During the usual holding period of 10 days, begin treatment at first sign of rabies in the animal that has bitten someone. The symptomatic animal should be killed immediately and tested.

developed a CNS syndrome in which rabies is in the differential diagnosis.

Postexposure Prophylaxis

Pasteur's development of rabies vaccine for animals culminated in the historic postexposure prophylaxis of 9-year-old Joseph Meister in 1885 (van Rooyen and Rhodes [1940]; this book also includes a 1938 photo of the adult Joseph Meister, when he was concierge at the Institut Pasteur in Paris). Early vaccines developed in animal CNS were often complicated by neuroparalytic events due to the presence of neural tissue. Applebaum et al. (1953) found that neuroparalytic events occurred in 1 of 2,025 recipients of the Semple vaccine in New York City. These took the form of encephalitic, myelitic, or neuritic complications. The majority occurred between 8 and 21 days after the first inoculation. Currently used preparations in the United States are safe and efficacious (Centers for Disease Control and Prevention, 1999). The human diploid cell vaccine has been associated with three cases of a Guillain-Barré-like syndrome, which cleared fully, and no other peripheral nervous system or CNS causally related illnesses (Centers for Disease Control and Prevention, 1999).

There are six steps to be followed in every case of an animal bite or other suspected exposure in which postexposure prophylaxis will be undertaken:

1. Treat the wound. Thoroughly wash the wound immediately. Extensive soap and water washing, with encouragement of bleeding to rid the wound of virus, should be prolonged. Foreign matter should be removed, and surgical debridement may be necessary. Many authorities advise against suturing the wound immediately (e.g., Hemachudha and Mitrabhakdi, 2000). Painting the wound with a viricidal solution such as 70% alcohol, iodine, or a povidone-iodine solution is recommended. Antibacterial therapy and antitetanus therapy should be considered as part of the wound therapy to protect against disease from other microbial pathogens.

2. Secure the biting or suspect animal. Disposition of the animal will depend on the recommendations of the local health authorities.

3. Contact the local health authority. Advice will be needed concerning sacrifice of the biting animal and shipment to a virus diagnostic center or observation of the animal, the relative likelihood of the animal being rabid, and supplies of vaccine and antiserum.

4. Treat with antiserum. If postexposure prophylaxis is required based on estimate of risk through consultation with the local health authorities, unimmunized individuals will require antiserum. Human rabies immunoglobulin (RIG) is recommended (20 IU/kg of body weight). If possible, the whole amount should be delivered to the wound site. Any remainder should be given intramuscularly. Pain at the site and low-grade fever may result. For persons with a history of allergy to human serum, the public health authorities must be consulted. Purified equine RIG, used in some developing countries, has a low incidence (0.8 to 6.0%) of adverse reactions, most of which are minor (Centers for Disease Control and Prevention, 1999).

5. Administer vaccine. The U.S. Advisory Committee on Immunization Practices recommends a schedule of intramuscular inoculations into the deltoid area on days 0, 3, 7, 14, and 28 for those not previously vaccinated and on days 0 and 3 for those previously vaccinated (Centers for Disease Control and Prevention, 1999). The vaccine should be inoculated in the deltoid at a site remote from the sites of antiserum inoculation. The gluteal region should not be used. The anterolateral thigh may be used in children, if necessary. Pregnancy is not considered a contraindication. Management of patients with potentially serious allergic responses should be conducted in consultation with the local health authorities. For preexposure regimens for persons at risk of exposure to the virus, recommendations of the U.S. Advisory Committee on Immunization Practices should be consulted (Centers for Disease Control and Prevention, 1999).

6. Collect serum. Prior to the administration of immune serum, the patient should be bled for an acute-phase serum sample. This should be stored frozen for later use should another illness be considered. It is not recommended to routinely test for the development of antirabies antibodies after standard immunization unless the person is immunosuppressed (Centers for Disease Control and Prevention, 1999).

Differential Diagnosis in the Postexposure-Treated Patient

In the period following a bite and postexposure prophylaxis, several syndromes may present themselves. Hysterical rabies can manifest several of the signs of rabies. Agitation, restlessness, depression, and headache are seen in both rabies and hysterical rabies. A brief incubation period (hours to a few days), a prolonged time course, absence of objective findings of neurological dysfunction, and a response to tranquilizing medication are found in hysterical rabies. "Rage de laboratoire," in which infection results from inadequately inactivated vaccine, has been controlled by manfacturing processes but would require management as clinical rabies. Illness from infection with another agent as a result of the original bite, such as tetanus, must be considered. Tetanus is characterized by trismus, muscle rigidity, normal CSF, and a usual incubation period of 15 days or less (Warrell, 1983). If the biting animal was a monkey, B-virus infection can appear after an incubation period of 10 to 20 days, and treatment with acyclovir or ganciclovir should be instituted (see below). In the case of paralytic rabies, both Guillain-Barré and polio must be considered. In agitated or furious rabies, the presence of hydro- or aerophobia, coupled with periods of frenzied activity separated by lucid intervals, is reasonably specific. Atypical rabies may not be distinguishable from encephalitis or myelitis associated with numerous other agents.

With the use of vaccines approved in developed countries, the incidence of serious vaccine-related neurological events is exceedingly rare. Localized pain, redness, and swelling can be found at the injection site in 30 to 74% of cases. Systemic allergic reactions of headache, nausea, muscle aches, and dizziness have been reported in 5 to 40% of cases (Centers for Disease Control and Prevention, 1999). If exposure to rabies has occurred, immunization should not be stopped. However, continued immunization should include measures to control the systemic allergic reaction. If a patient develops a neuroparalytic accident from another type of rabies vaccine (Semple, duck embryo, suckling mouse brain) as a result of treatment in an underdeveloped country, the distinction must be made from rabies itself. The onset of a neuroparalytic accident is usually between 8 and 21 days after the first inoculation, whereas the usual latency period for rabies is between 20 and 90 days from the time of the exposure, with rare incubation periods of much greater duration. Neuroparalytic accidents present as transverse or ascending myelitis, mononeuritis multiplex, meningoencephalitis, or a combination of forms. The timing and the form of the disease will therefore often help to distinguish a vaccine-related neuroparalytic accident. Measurement of serum antibodies may be useful in diagnosis and management. In all such cases, consultation with the U.S. public health authorities is necessary to decide how to proceed.

Diagnostic Studies

General neurodiagnostic studies in human rabies encephalitis are nonspecific. The CSF may be abnormal with elevated protein and a pleocytosis, but these assays are often within normal limits (Johnson, H. N., 1965). The EEG may show nonspecific slowing and/or paroxysmal activity. Neuroimaging may be negative, particularly CT scanning. Abnormalities in the pons and medulla on MRI of a patient who died from rabies virus associated with the Mexican free-tailed bat were reported by Pleasure and Fischbein (2000). Thus, the neurodiagnostic studies, while often supporting the clinical impression of encephalitis, are not etiologically specific and are variable.

Considerable persistence may be required to make an agent-specific diagnosis of rabies because of the inconsistency of the appearance of viral antigen at various sites and because antibody may not appear until well into the clinical stage. Reverse transcriptase PCR (RT-PCR) on saliva and nuchal skin biopsy at the hairline, to contain a minimum of 10 hair follicles, for fluorescent-antibody studies are recommended (Smith and Neill, 1999). A records review of U.S. and French cases demonstrated that corneal smears were insensitive for clinical diagnosis (Crepin et al., 1998). Collection of serum and CSF for antibody determinations is recommended (Smith and Neill, 1999). Based on their review of intravitam assays for rabies diagnosis, Crepin et al. (1998) recommended that skin biopsy (nuchal) be sent for fluorescent-antibody examination for virus, that saliva be sent for RT-PCR assay at the early stage of the clinical illness, and that serum samples be examined for antibodies after 1 week of the illness. Wacharapluesadee and Hemachuda (2001) have described a nucleic acid sequence-based amplification assay to detect rabies RNA in saliva and CSF. The test can be done rapidly and can detect the virus early in the disease course. Serial CSF and saliva samples are recommended.

Acute Management

Once the disease has started, vaccine and antibody administration are of no benefit. Therefore, in the absence of a specific antiviral drug, therapy is directed toward patient comfort and management of complicating factors. Hypoxia increases the likelihood of cerebral edema and has a detrimental effect on cardiac function. Therefore, scrupulous pulmonary toilet, including tracheostomy with frequent suctioning, is important. Irregularities of cardiac rhythm are frequent and myocarditis occurs. Cardiac arrest may be one of the principal causes of death. Therefore, cardiac monitoring in an intensive care unit is required. Seizure control is important, particularly in light of the observation that death may occur during a seizure (Johnson, H. N., 1965). As pointed out by Baltazard (1970), the abject horror experienced by patients during lucid intervals should be ameliorated with appropriate medication. Analgesics are also often necessary. Except for corneal transplants, no human-to-human transmission has been documented (Centers for Disease Control, 1984). However, care should be exercised by medical personnel, particularly against bites from patients during frenzied activity and exposure of mucous membranes and skin lesions to saliva. Isolation procedures are recommended for the management of patients with rabies, with the use of face masks, gloves, and gowns (Bernard and Hattwick, 1985). Rabies prophylaxis is not recommended for the medical staff unless potentially infectious body fluids come in contact with mucous membranes or nonintact skin (Centers for Disease Control and Prevention, 1999).

Rabies Prevention

Immunization of domestic dogs and enforcement of leash laws since the 1940s and 1950s have had a remarkably strong effect on reducing canine transmission of rabies to humans in the United States. Strictly enforced quarantine regulations, such as in England, have protected some island regions from rabies. As a zoonosis, rabies is adapted to several species. Hence, various strategies are required. Remarkable success using an oral vaccine has been achieved against the main host of rabies in Europe, the red fox (World Health Organization, 1995). Controlling rabies in hematophagous, insectivorous, and fruit-eating bats will prove a greater challenge.

HERPES B VIRUS OF MONKEYS— *HERPESVIRUS SIMIAE*—CERCOPITHECINE HERPESVIRUS

In October 1932, "Dr. W. B." was bitten on the fingers of the left hand by a normal *Macacus* rhesus monkey during experimental studies on polio (Sabin and Wright, 1934). He died 17 days later after suffering a febrile ascending myelitis that developed into an encephalitis. In the course of the illness, vesicles appeared at the site of the bite and regional lymphadenopathy developed. Death occurred as a result of respiratory failure. Pathology revealed focal necrosis in the spleen, adrenals, and regional lymph nodes. Acute inflammatory changes were present in the brain and spinal cord, with the most marked changes in the medulla and spinal cord. A virus was isolated that reproduced the disease in rabbits and was designated "B virus" from the victim's last name (Weigler, 1992).

By the early 1990s, almost 40 cases of B-virus infection had been reported, three-quarters of which were encephalomyelitis, and of those, over two-thirds were fatal

(Davenport et al., 1994). Enzootic in macaque monkeys, B virus is an occupational hazard for monkey handlers and those working with monkey cells. Guidelines for prevention and treatment of human B-virus infections have been promulgated (Holmes et al., 1995; Kaplan, 1987; Centers for Disease Control and Prevention, 1998).

Pathology

Herpes B virus is closely related to HSV and causes a latent infection in healthy rhesus monkeys. The virus has been identified in monkey saliva. It appears to spread to the CNS along peripheral nerves from the site of inoculation and initially usually infects the spinal cord. Here, it produces a focal but rapidly spreading myelitis and lower brain stem encephalitis. Inclusion bodies and destructive changes are seen in neurons and oligodendrocytes, with associated inflammation. Frank necrosis rapidly follows (Thomas and Henschel, 1960). White as well as gray matter of the spinal cord shows inflammatory cell cuffing, but neuronophagic nodules are most frequent in the gray matter of the posterior and lateral horns. In one case there was spread of virus to the eye, where it caused a multifocal necrotizing retinitis (Nanda et al., 1990).

Diagnosis and Management

The lesions in monkeys that result from B-virus infection are quite similar to the lesions that occur in the oral pharynx during primary infection with HSV in humans. A chronic infection is established with intermittent asymptomatic shedding of virus (Palmer, 1987). The percentage of seropositive monkeys increases during captivity. Persons handling these animals and tissues taken from them are at risk of being infected. At least one case of likely human-to-human spread has been reported (Holmes et al., 1990).

Although a specific bite or scratch has often been identified, several cases have had minimal or no demonstrable inoculation. One of the cases reported by Davidson and Hummeler (1960) was a chemist whose only contact had been to clean the skull of a rhesus monkey, without gloves, 2 weeks prior to the illness. In another case there was no known contact with monkeys or their tissue in the 6 months preceding the illness (Fierer et al., 1973). However, a history of extensive monkey handling 10 years in the past raised the issue of whether herpes B virus can cause an active infection of the CNS after establishing latency in humans. More recently, a fatal infection followed a splash injury to the eye, possibly from fecal material (Centers for Disease Control and Prevention, 1998).

The several thousand people who have handled monkeys and their tissues without illness suggest that susceptibility to B-virus infection in humans is low and raises the possibility that differing serotypes may have differences in human virulence (Smith et al., 1998). The incubation period is usually 2 to 5 weeks and can be as short as 2 days (Centers for Disease Control and Prevention, 1998). Longer periods are on record, in some instances raising the possibility of activation from latency. Headache, malaise, and nausea are frequently observed. Vesicles, either at the site of the bite or in the oropharynx, and lymphadenopathy are inconstant features. Signs of a febrile ascending myelitis frequently, but not

always, appear first. Regional pain, paraparesis, sensory loss, and urinary retention are frequent. The disease progresses to signs of brain stem and cortical involvement. Difficulty in swallowing, diplopia, facial weakness, and ataxia, as well as impaired consciousness, seizures, and coma are well described (Davidson and Hummeler, 1960). On occasion the CNS presentation has been with cerebral signs. The course ranges from 3 days to 3 weeks with mortality of over two-thirds of patients and with significant sequelae in survivors. Prompt wound treatment and antiviral therapy may reduce the mortality and sequelae (Davenport et al., 1994; Holmes et al., 1995).

Although the febrile patient with an ascending myelitis or encephalitis subsequent to the bite of a monkey is assumed to have a B-virus infection, other causes must be excluded. Tetanus, poliolike manifestations of enteroviruses, and rabies must be considered. Conversely, in the absence of a clear history of a wound, any animal handler, laboratory investigator, or other person in proximity to monkeys or their cells must be considered at risk for herpes B. For example, concern has been expressed over exposure to monkeys kept illegally as pets (Ostrowski et al., 1998). Exposures are theoretically possible at zoos and wildlife parks.

Examination of the CSF shows a lymphocytic pleocytosis, except in the presence of focal tissue necrosis, when neutrophils can predominate, and protein elevation. Glucose can be reduced in the presence of tissue necrosis (Davenport et al., 1994). EEGs may be normal or nonspecifically abnormal. Studies of somatosensory evoked potentials in one patient demonstrated impaired conduction through the brain stem (Davenport et al., 1994). Head CT scans have been less sensitive than MRIs. Serial MRIs have shown the progressive development of lesions principally in the spinal cord and brain stem, but also in the cerebrum, deep gray matter, and cerebellum (Davenport et al., 1994; Centers for Disease Control and Prevention, 1998).

Viral diagnostic studies are complicated by difficulties in virus isolation and in distinguishing the serological response from HSV and by the biosafety needs associated with a CDC/NIH Biosafety Level 4 pathogen. The Centers for Disease Control and Prevention has recommended that diagnostic specimens in the United States be routed to the B Virus Research and Resource Laboratory at Georgia State University in Atlanta (telephone 404-651-0808 [Centers for Disease Control and Prevention, 1998]). Guidelines recommend culturing of the wound site, lesions, conjunctivae, and oropharynx, with acute-phase serum samples taken for serology and convalescent-phase samples taken 2 to 3 weeks later (Holmes et al., 1995).

Thorough prevention, wound treatment, and clinical management guidelines have been developed for persons at risk to be injured in the course of monkey handling (Holmes et al., 1995; Kaplan, 1987; Centers for Disease Control and Prevention, 1998). Prompt scrubbing and irrigation of the wound for at least 15 min or irrigation of mucosal sites for at least 15 min is key. That first step is to be followed by specimen collection and evaluation by a physician experienced in the management of animal-inflicted injuries. The reader is referred to the aforementioned guidelines for details of evaluation and management.

There is insufficient clinical experience on which to base unequivocal antiviral treatment guidelines. Current recommendations include high-dose oral acyclovir as prophylaxis following a wound, depending on risk status (Holmes et al., 1995). If the patient becomes symptomatic, hospitalization with blood and fluid precautions and treatment with intravenous acyclovir or ganciclovir is recommended (Holmes et al, 1995; Jainkittivong and Langlais, 1998). Following resolution of infection, long-term oral viral suppressant therapy may be necessary (Davenport et al., 1994; Holmes et al., 1995). Consultative advice should be sought through the Centers for Disease Control and Prevention in the United States and through national public health services in other countries.

In light of the high mortality and morbidity, albeit in a disease of low incidence, adherence of laboratory animal facilities to the prevention guidelines (Kaplan, 1987) is crucial. Nonoccupational exposures can theoretically occur with illicit pet monkeys and free-ranging monkey populations in various settings. Caution must be exercised because macaque monkey behavior is unpredictable and can become aggressive. Children are at particular risk (Ostrowski et al., 1998).

REFERENCES

Adair, C. V., R. L. Gauld, and J. E. Smadel. 1953. Aseptic meningitis, a disease of diverse etiology: clinical and etiologic studies on 854 cases. *Ann. Intern. Med.* **39:**675–704.

Aksel, I. S. 1958. Pathologische Anatomie der Lyss, p. 418–435. *In* O. Lubarsch, F. Henke, and R. Rossle (ed.), *Handbuch der spez. Path Anatomie und Histologie*, vol. 13, 2A. Springer, Berlin, Germany.

Anderson, L. J. , K. G. Nicholson, R. V. Tauxe, and W. G. Winkler. 1984. Human rabies in the United States, 1960 to 1979: epidemiology, diagnosis, and prevention. *Ann. Intern. Med.* **100:**728–735.

Applebaum, E., M. Greenberg, and J. Nelson. 1953. Neurological complications following antirabies vaccination. *JAMA* **151:**188–191.

Armstrong, D., J. G. Fortner, W. P. Rowe, and J. C. Parker. 1969. Meningitis due to lymphocytic choriomeningitis virus endemic in a hamster colony. *JAMA* **209:**265–267.

Astoul, E., M. Lafage, and M. Lafou. 1996. Rabies superantigen as a VB T-dependent adjuvant. *J. Exp. Med.* **183:**1623–1631.

Baer, G. M. 1975. Pathogenesis to the central nervous system, p. 181–197. *In* G. M. Baer (ed.), *The Natural History of Rabies*, vol. 1. Academic Press, New York, N.Y.

Baer, G. M., and W. F. Cleary. 1972. A model in mice for the pathogenesis and treatment of rabies. *J. Infect. Dis.* **125:**520–527.

Baker, A. B. 1947. Chronic lymphocytic choriomeningitis. *J. Neuropathol. Exp. Neurol.* **6:**253–264.

Baltazard, M. 1970. Rabies, p. 138–154. *In* R. Debre and J. Celers (ed.), *Clinical Virology, the Evaluation and Management of Human Viral Infections*. W. B. Saunders, Philadelphia, Pa.

Barton, L. L., C. J. Peters, and T. G. Ksiazek. 1995. Lymphocytic choriomeningitis virus: an unrecognized teratogenic pathogen. *Emerg. Infect. Dis.* **1:**152–153.

Bernard, K. W., and M. A. W. Hattwick. 1985. Rabies virus, p. 897–909. *In* G. L. Mandell, R. G. Douglas, Jr., and J. E. Bennett (ed.), *Principles and Practice of Infectious Diseases*, 2nd ed. John Wiley & Sons, New York, N.Y.

Bernard, K. W., P. W. Smith, J. F. Kader, and J. Moran. 1982.

Neuroparalytic illness and human diploid cell rabies vaccine. *JAMA* **248:**3136–3138.

Bia, F. J., G. F. Thornton, A. J. Main, C. K. Y. Fong, and G. D. Hsiung. 1980. Western equine encephalitis mimicking Herpes simplex encephalitis. *JAMA* **244:**367–369.

Biggar, R. J., J. P. Woodall, P. D. Walter, and G. E. Haughie. 1975. Lymphocytic choriomeningitis outbreak associated with pet hamsters. Fifty-seven cases from New York State. *JAMA* **232:**494–500.

Bodner, R. A., T. Lynch, L. Lewis, and D. Kahn. 1995. Serotonin syndrome. *Neurology* **45:**219–223.

Borrow, P., and M. B. A. Oldstone. 1997. Lymphocytic choriomeningitis virus, p. 593–619. *In* N. Nathanson (ed.), *Viral Pathogenesis*. Lippincott-Raven, Philadelphia, Pa.

Bouzamondo, E., A. Ladogana, and H. Tsiang. 1993. Alteration of potassium-evoked 5-HT release from virus-infected rat cortical synaptosomes. *Neuroreport* **4:**555–558.

Buchmeier, M. J., R. M. Welsch, F. J. Dutko, and M. B. A. Oldstone. 1980. The virology and immunobiology of lymphocytic choriomeningitis infection. *Adv. Immunol.* **30:**275–331.

Buchmeier, M. J., M. D. Bowen, and C. J. Peters. 2001. Adenaviridae: the viruses and their replication, p. 1635–1668. *In* D. M. Knipe and P. M. Howley (ed.), *Fields Virology*, 4th ed. Lippincott, Williams & Wilkins, Philadelphia, Pa.

Burrage, T. G., G. H. Tignor, and A. L. Smith. 1985. Rabies virus binding at neuromuscular junctions. *Virus Res.* **2:**273–289.

Ceccaldi, P. E., M. P. Fillion, A. Ermine, H. Tsiang, and G. Fillion. 1993. Rabies virus selectively alters 5-HT1 receptor subtypes in rat brain. *Eur. J. Pharmacol.* **245:**129–138.

Ceccaldi, P. E., C. Marquette, P. Weber, P. Gourmelon, and H. Tsiang. 1996. Ionizing radiation modulates the spread of an apathogenic rabies virus in mouse brain. *Int. J. Radiat. Biol.* **70:**69–75.

Center for Disease Control. 1983. Arboviral encephalitis—United States, 1983. *Morb. Mortal. Wkly. Rep.* **32:**557–560.

Centers for Disease Control. 1984. Rabies prevention—United States, 1984. *Morb. Mortal. Wkly. Rep.* **33:**393–408.

Centers for Disease Control and Prevention. 1998. Fatal cercopithecine herpesvirus 1 (B Virus) infection following a mucocutaneous exposure and interim recommendations for worker protection. *Morb. Mortal. Wkly. Rep.***47:**1073–1083.

Centers for Disease Control and Prevention. 1999. Human rabies prevention—United States, 1999. *Morb. Mortal. Wkly. Rep.* **48:**RR-1.

Charlton, K. M., S. Nadin-Davis, G. A. Casey, and A. I. Wandeler. 1997. The long incubation period in rabies: delayed progression of infection in muscle at the site of exposure. *Acta Neuropathol.* **94:**73–77.

Chopra, J. S., A. K. Banerjee, J. M. K. Murthy, and R. Pal. 1980. Paralytic rabies—a clinico-pathological study. *Brain* **103:**789–802.

Conomy, J. P., A. Leibovitz, W. McCombs, and J. Stinson. 1977. Airborne rabies encephalitis: demonstration of rabies virus in the human central nervous system. *Neurology* **27:**67–69.

Constantine, D. G. 1967. Bat rabies in the southwestern United States. *Public Health Rep.* **82:** 867–888.

Coulon, P., J. P. Ternaux, A. Flamand, and C. Tuffereau. 1998. An avirulent mutant of rabies virus is unable to infect motoneurons in vivo and in vitro. *J. Virol.* **72:**273–278.

Crepin, P., L. Audry, Y. Rotivel, A. Gacoin, C. Caroff, and H. Bourhy. 1998. Intravitam diagnosis of human rabies by PCR using saliva and cerebrospinal fluid. *J. Clin. Microbiol.* **36:**1117–1120.

Davenport, D. S., D. R. Johnson, G. P. Holmes, D. A. Jewett, S. C. Ross, and J. K. Hilliard. 1994. Diagnosis and management of human B Virus (Herpesvirus simiae) infection in Michigan. *Clin. Infect. Dis.* **19:**33–41.

Davidson, W. L., and K. Hummeler. 1960. B Virus infection in man. *Ann. N.Y. Acad. Sci.* **85:**970–979.

Derakhshan, I., A. Fayaz, M. Bahmanyar, S. Noorsalehi, M. Mohammad, and P. Ahouraii. 1978. Light microscopical diagnosis of rabies. A reappraisal. *Lancet* **i:**302–303.

Dietzschold, B., W. H. Wunner, T. J. Wiktor, A. D. Lopes, M. Lafon, C. L. Smith, and H. Koprowski. 1983. Characterization of an antigenic determinant of the glycoprotein that correlates with pathogenicity of rabies virus. *Proc. Natl. Acad. Sci. USA* **80:**70–74.

Dietzschold, B., M. Kao, Y. M. Zheng, Z. Y. Chen, G. Maul, Z. F. Fu, C. E. Rupprecht, and H. Koprowski. 1992. Delineation of putative mechanisms involved in antibody-mediated clearance of rabies virus from the central nervous system. *Proc. Natl. Acad. Sci. USA* **89:**7252–7256.

Dietzschold, B., C. E. Rupprecht, and Z. F. Fu. 1996. Rhabdoviruses, p. 1137–1159. *In* B. N. Fields, D. M. Knipe, and P. M. Howley (ed.), *Fields Virology,* 3rd ed. Lippincott-Raven, Philadelphia, Pa.

Dumrongphol, H., A. Srikiatkhachorn, T. Hemachudha, N. Kotchabhakdi, and P. Govitrapong. 1996. Alteration of muscarinic acetylcholine receptors in rabies viral-infected dog brains. *J. Neurol. Sci.* **137:**1–6.

Dupont, J. R., and K. M. Earle. 1965. Human rabies encephalitis. A study of forty-nine cases with a review of the literature. *Neurology* **15:**1023–1034.

Dykewicz, C. A., V. M. Dato, S.-P. Fisher-Hoch, M. V. Howarth, G. I. Perez-Oronoz, S. W. Ostroff, H. Gary, Jr., L. B. Schonberger, and J. B. McCormick. 1992. Lymphocytic choriomeningitis outbreak associated with nude mice in a research institute. *JAMA* **267:**1349–1353.

Eurosurveillance. 2002. Rabies-like infection in Scotland. *Eurosurveill. Wkly.* **6(50):**12.

Farmer, T. W., and C. A. Janeway. 1942. Infections with the virus of lymphocytic choriomeningitis. *Medicine* **21:**1–63.

Fekadu, M., P. W. Greer, F. W. Chandler, and D. W. Sanderlin. 1988. Use of the avidin-biotin peroxidase system to detect rabies antigen in formalin-fixed paraffin-embedded tissues. *J. Virol. Methods* **19:**91–96.

Fierer, J., P. Bazeley, and A. I. Braude. 1973. Herpes B Virus encephalomyelitis presenting as ophthalmic zoster. A possible latent infection reactivated. *Ann. Intern. Med.* **79:**225–228.

Fischman, H. R., and M. Schaeffer. 1971. Pathogenesis of experimental rabies as revealed by immunofluorescence. *Ann. N.Y. Acad. Sci.* **177:**78–97.

Fishbein, D. B., and L. E. Robinson. 1993. Rabies. *N. Engl. J. Med.* **329:**1632–1638.

Fu, Z. F., E. Weihe, Y. M. Zheng, M. K. Schafer, H. Sheng, S. Corisdeo, R. J. Rauscher, III, H. Koprowski, and B. Dietzschold. 1993. Differential effects of rabies and borna disease viruses on immediate-, early-, and late-response gene expression in brain tissues. *J. Virol.* **67:**6674–6681.

Goldwasser, R. A., and R. E. Kissling. 1958. Fluorescent antibody staining of street and fixed rabies virus antigen. *Proc. Soc. Exp. Biol. Med.* **98:**219–223.

Gonzalez Angulo, A., H. Marquez Monter, A. Feria-Velasco, and B. J. Zavala. 1970. The ultrastructure of Negri Bodies in Purkinje neurons in human rabies. *Neurology* **20:**323–328.

Gosztonyi, G. 1994. Reproduction of lyssaviruses: ultrastructural composition of lyssavirus and functional aspects of pathogenesis. *Curr. Top. Microbiol. Immunol.* **187:**43–68.

Gowers, W. R. 1893. Hydrophobia, p. 922–942. *In Diseases of the Nervous System,* vol. 2. *Diseases of the Brain and Cranial Nerves*

and Functional Diseases of the Nervous System, 2nd ed. Blakiston, Son & Co., Philadelphia, Pa.

Gregg, M. B. 1975. Recent outbreaks of lymphocytic choriomeningitis in the United States of America. *Bull. W. H. O.* **52:**549–552.

Hattwick, M. A. W., and M. B. Gregg. 1975. The disease in man, p. 281–304. *In* G. M. Baer (ed.), *The Natural History of Rabies,* vol. 2. Academic Press, New York, N.Y.

Hemachudha, T. 1989. Rabies, p. 383–404. *In* P. J. Vinken, G. W. Bruyn, and H. L. Klawan (ed.), *Handbook of Clinical Neurology,* revised series. Elsevier Science, Amsterdam, The Netherlands.

Hemachudha, T. 1994. Human rabies: clinical aspects, pathogenesis, and potential therapy, p. 121–143. *In* C. E. Rupprecht, B. Dietzschold, and H. Koprowski (ed.), *Lyssaviruses.* Springer-Verlag, New York, N.Y.

Hemachudha, T., and E. Mitrabhakdi. 2000. Rabies, p. 401–444. *In* L. E. Davis and P. G. E. Kennedy (ed.), *Infections of the Nervous System.* Butterworth, Heinemann, Oxford, United Kingdom.

Hemachudha, T., P. Phanuphak, B. Sriwanthana, S. Manutsathit, K. Phanthumchinda, W. Siriprasomsup, C. Ukachoke, S. Rasameechan, and S. Kaoroptham. 1988. Immunologic study of human encephalitic and paralytic rabies. Preliminary report of 16 patients. *Am. J. Med.* **84:**673–677.

Hemachudha, T., T. Panpanich, P. Phanuphak, S. Manatsathit, and H. Wilde. 1993. Immune activation in human rabies. *Trans. R. Soc. Trop. Med. Hyg.* **87:**106–108.

Hertzog, E. 1945. Histologic diagnosis of rabies. *Arch. Pathol.* **39:**279–280.

Hirsch, M. S., R. C. Moellering, Jr., H. G. Pope, and D. C. Poskanzer. 1974. Lymphocytic-Choriomeningitis-Virus infection traced to a pet hamster. *N. Engl. J. Med.* **291:**610–612.

Holmes, G. P., J. K. Hilliard, K. C. Klontz, A. H. Rupert, C. M. Schindler, E. Parrish, G. Griffin, G. S. Ward, N. D. Bernstein, T. W. Bean, M. R. Ball, Sr., J. A. Brady, M. H. Wilder, and J. E. Kaplan. 1990. B virus (Herpesvirus simiae) infection in humans: epidemiologic investigation of a cluster. *Ann. Intern. Med.* **112:**833–839.

Holmes, G. P., L. E. Chapman, J. A. Stewart, S. E. Straus, J. K. Hilliard, D. S. Davenport, and the B Virus Working Group. 1995. Guidelines for the prevention and treatment of B-Virus infections in exposed persons. *Clin. Infect. Dis.* **20:**421–439.

Hooper, D. C., S. T. Ohnishi, R. Kean, Y. Numagami, B. Dietzschold, and H. Koprowski. 1995. Local nitric oxide production in viral and autoimmune diseases of the central nervous system. *Proc. Natl. Acad. Sci. USA* **92:**5312–5316.

Hooper, D. C., K. Morimoto, M. Bette, E. Weihe, H. Koprowski, and B. Dietzschold. 1998. Collaboration of antibody and inflammation in clearance of rabies virus from the central nervous system. *J. Virol.* **72:**3711–3719.

Ho Sung, J., M. Hayano, A. R. Mastri, and T. Okagaki. 1976. A case of human rabies and ultrastructure of the Negri body. *J. Neuropathol. Exp. Neurol.* **35:**541–559.

Houff, S. A., R. C. Burton, R. W. Wilson, T. E. Henson, W. T. London, G. M. Baer, L. J. Anderson, W. G. Winkler, D. L. Madden, and J. L. Sever. 1979. Human-to-human transmission of rabies virus by corneal transplant. *N. Engl. J. Med.* **300:**603–604.

Howard, M. E. 1940. Infection with the virus of choriomeningitis in man. *Yale Biol. Med.* **13:**161–180.

Hurst, M. E., and J. L. Pawan. 1931. Outbreak of rabies in Trinidad without a history of bites and with symptoms of acute ascending myelitis. *Lancet* **ii:**622–628.

Hurst, E. W., and J. L. Pawan. 1932. A further assessment of the

Trinidad outbreak of acute rabic myelitis: histology of the experimental disease. *J. Pathol. Bacteriol.* **35**:301–321.

Jackson, A. C., and M. B. Fenton. 2001. Human rabies and bat bites. *Lancet* **357**:1714.

Jackson, A. C., and H. Park. 1998. Apoptotic cell death in experimental rabies in suckling mice. *Acta Neuropathol.* **95**:159–164.

Jackson, A. C., and J. P. Rossiter. 1997. Apoptosis plays an important role in experimental rabies virus infection. *J. Virol.* **71**:5603–5607.

Jainkittivong, A., and R. Langlais. 1998. Herpes B infection. *Oral Surg. Oral Med. Oral Pathol.* **85**:399–403.

Johnson, H. N. 1965. Rabies virus, p. 814–840. *In* F. L. Horsfall and I. Tamm (ed.), *Viral and Rickettsial Infections of Man*, 4th ed. J. B. Lippincott Co., Philadelphia, Pa.

Johnson, R. T. 1965. Experimental rabies. Studies of cellular vulnerability and pathogenesis using fluorescent antibody staining. *J. Neuropathol. Exp. Neurol.* **24**:662–674.

Johnson, R. T. 1982. Viruses and virus-cell interactions, p. 9–35. *In Viral Infections of the Nervous System.* Raven Press, New York, N.Y.

Kaplan, J. E. 1987. Guidelines for prevention of herpesvirus simiae (B-virus) infection in monkey handlers. *Lab. Anim. Sci.* **37**:709–712.

Kim, J. H., J. Booss, E. E. Manuelidis, and C. C. Duncan. 1985. Human eastern equine encephalitis: electron microscopic study of a brain biopsy. *Am. J. Clin. Pathol.* **84**:223–227.

Komrower, G. M., B. L. Williams, and P. B. Stones. 1955. Lymphocytic choriomeningitis in the newborn. Probable transplacental infection. *Lancet* **i**:697–698.

Koschel, K., and P. Munzel. 1984. Inhibition of opiate receptor-mediated signal transmission by rabies virus in persistently infected NG-108-15 mouse neuroblastoma rat glioma hybrid cells. *Proc. Natl. Acad. Sci. USA* **81**:950–954.

Krebs, J. W., J. S. Smith, C. E. Rupprecht, and J. E. Childs. 1999. Rabies surveillance in the United States during 1998. *JAMA* **215**:1786–1798.

Kureishi, A., L. Z. Xu, H. Wu, and H. G. Stiver. 1992. Rabies in China: recommendations for control. *Bull. W. H. O.* **70**:443–450.

Lafon, M., M. Lafage, A. Martinez-Arends, R. Ramirez, F. Vuillier, D. Charron, V. Lotteau, and D. Scott-Algara. 1992. Evidence for a viral superantigen in humans. *Nature* **358**:507–510.

Lafon, M., D. Scott-Algara, P. N. Marche, P. A. Cazenave, and E. Jouvin-Marche. 1994. Neonatal deletion and selective expansion of mouse T cells by exposure to rabies virus nucleocapsid superantigen. *J. Exp. Med.* **180**:1207–1215.

Larsen, T. D., S. A. Chartrand, K. M. Thomashek, L. G. Hauser, and T. G. Ksiazek. 1993. Hydrocephalus complicating lymphocytic choriomeningitis virus infection. *Pediatr. Infect. Dis. J.* **12**:528–531.

Lehmann-Grube, F. 1989. Diseases of the nervous system caused by lymphocytic choriomeningitis virus and other arenaviruses, p. 355–381. *In* R. R. McKendall, (ed.), *Handbook of Clinical Neurology.* Elsevier Science Publishers, B. V., Amsterdam, The Netherlands.

Lentz, T. L., T. G. Burrage, A. L. Smith, J. Crick, and G. H. Tignor. 1982. Is the acetylcholine receptor a rabies virus receptor? *Science* **215**:182–184.

Lewis, J. M., and J. P. Utz. 1961. Orchitis, parotitis and meningoencephalitis due to lymphocytic choriomeningitis virus. *N. Engl. J. Med.* **265**:776–780.

Li, Z., Z. Feng, and H. Ye. 1995. Rabies viral antigen in human tongues and salivary glands. *J. Trop. Med. Hyg.* **98**:330–332.

Love, S. V. 1944. Paralytic rabies: a review of literature and report of case. *Pediatrics* **24**:312–325.

Lowenberg, K. 1928. Rabies in man. Microscopic observations. *Arch. Neurol. Psychiatr.* **19**:638–646.

Marquette, C., A. M. Van Dam, P. E. Ceccaldi, P. Weber, F. Haour, and H. Tsiang. 1996. Induction of immunoreactive interleukin-1 beta and tumor necrosis factor-alpha in the brains of rabies virus infected rats. *J. Neuroimmunol.* **68**:45–51.

Marrie, T. J., and M.-F. Saron. 1998. Seroprevalence of lymphocytic choriomeningitis virus in Nova Scotia. *Am. J. Trop. Med. Hyg.* **58**:47–49.

Metze, K., and W. Feiden. 1991. Rabies virus ribonucleoprotein in the heart. *N. Engl. J. Med.* **324**:1814–1815.

Meyer, H. M., Jr., R. T. Johnson, I. P. Crawford, H. E. Dascomb, and N. G. Rogers. 1960. Central nervous system syndromes of viral etiology. A study of 713 cases. *Am. J. Med.* **129**:334–347.

Miller, A., H. C. Morse, J. Winkelstein, and N. Nathanson. 1978. The role of antibody in recovery from experimental rabies. 1. Effect of depletion of B and T cells. *J. Immunol.* **121**:321–326.

Morecki, R., and H. M. Zimmerman. 1969. Human rabies encephalitis. Fine structure study of cytoplasmic inclusions. *Arch. Neurol.* **20**:599–604.

Mrak, R. E., and L. Young. 1994. Rabies encephalitis in humans: pathology, pathogenesis and pathophysiology. *J. Neuropathol. Exp. Neurol.* **53**:1–10.

Murphy, F. A. 1977. Rabies pathogenesis. A brief review. *Arch. Virol.* **54**:279–297.

Murphy, F. A., A. K. Harrison, W. G. Winn, and S. P. Bauer. 1973. Comparative pathogenesis of rabies and rabies-like viruses. Infection of the nervous system and centrifugal spread of virus to peripheral tissues. *Lab. Invest.* **29**:1–16.

Nanda, M., V. T. Curtin, J. K. Hilliard, N. D. Bernstein, and R. D. Dix. 1990. Ocular histopathologic findings in a case of human herpes B virus infection. *Arch. Ophthalmol.* **108**:713–716.

Negri, A. 1903. Beitrag zum Studium der Aetiologie der Tollwuth. *Z. Hyg-Infekt.* **43**:507–528.

Noah, D. L., C. L. Drenzek, J. S. Smith, J. W. Krebs, L. Orciari, J. Shaddock, D. Sanderlin, S. Whitfield, M. Fekadu, J. G. Olson, C. E. Rupprecht, and J. E. Childs. 1998. Epidemiology of human rabies in the United States, 1980 to 1996. *Ann. Intern. Med.* **128**:922–930.

Ostrowski, S. R., M. J. Leslie, T. Parrott, S. Abelt, and P. E. Percy. 1998. B-virus from pet macaque monkeys: an emerging threat in the United States? *Emerging Infect. Dis.* **4**:117–121.

Palmer, A. E. 1987. B virus *Herpesvirus simiae*: historical perspective. *J. Med. Primatol.* **16**:99–130.

Palmer, D. G., P. Ossent, M. M. Suter, and E. Ferrari. 1985. Demonstration of rabies viral antigen in paraffin tissue sections: comparison of the immunofluorescence technique with the unlabelled antibody enzyme method. *Am. J. Vet. Res.* **46**:283–286.

Perl, D. P. 1975. The pathology of rabies in the central nervous system, p. 235–272. *In* G. M. Baer (ed.), *The Natural History of Rabies,* vol. 1. Academic Press, New York, N.Y.

Peters, C. J. 1994. Arenavirus infections, p. 621–637. *In* R. R. McKendall and W. G. Stroop (ed.), *Handbook of Neurovirology.* Marcel Dekker, Inc., New York, N.Y.

Pleasure, S. J., and J. Fischbein. 2000. Correlation of clinical and neuroimaging findings in a case of rabies encephalitis. *Arch. Neurol.* **57**:1765–1769.

Prabhakar, B. S., and N. Nathanson. 1981. Acute rabies death mediated by antibody. *Nature* **290**:590–591.

Reisman, D., B. J. Alpers, and D. A. Cooper. 1933. Hydrophobia. Report of two fatal cases with pathologic studies in one. *Arch. Intern. Med.* **51**:643–655.

Roine, R. O., M. Hillbom, M. Valle, M. Haltia, L. Ketonen, E. Neuvonen, J. Lumio, and J. Lahdevirta. 1988. Fatal encephalitis caused by a bat-borne rabies-related virus. Clinical findings. *Brain* **111**:1505–1516.

Sabin, A. B., and A. M. Wright. 1934. Acute ascending myelitis following a monkey bite, with isolation of a virus capable of reproducing the disease. *J. Exp. Med.* **59**:115–136 and 15 plates.

Samaratunga, H., J. W. Searle, and N. Hudson. 1998. Non-rabies lyssavirus human encephalitis from fruit bats: Australian bat Lyssavirus (pteroid Lyssavirus) infection. *Neuropathol. Appl. Neurobiol.* **24**:331–335.

Schaffer, K. 1912. p. 980–991. *In* M. von Lewandowsky (ed.), *Handbuch der Neurologie*, vol. 3. Springer, Berlin, Germany.

Seif, I., P. Coulon, P. E. Rollin, and A. Flamand. 1985. Rabies virulence: effect on pathogenicity and sequence characterization of rabies virus mutations affecting antigenic site III of the glycoprotein. *J. Virol.* **53**:926–934.

Sheinbergas, M. M. 1976. Hydrocephalus due to prenatal infection with the lymphocytic choriomeningitis virus. *Infection* **4**:185–191. [NB: *This report has been incorrectly indexed.*]

Shope, R. E. 1982. Rabies, p. 455–470. *In* A. S. Evans (ed.), *Viral Infections of Humans. Epidemiology and Control*, 2nd ed. Plenum Press, New York, N.Y.

Sikes, R. K., W. F. Cleary, H. Koprowski, T. J. Wiktor, and M. M. Kaplan. 1971. Effective protection of monkeys against death from street virus by post-exposure administration of tissue culture rabies vaccine. *Bull. W.H.O.* **45**:1–11.

Smadel, J. E., R. H. Green, R. M. Paultaub, and T. A. Gonzales. 1942. Lymphocytic choriomeningitis: two human fatalities following an unusual febrile illness. *Proc. Soc. Exp. Biol. Med.* **49**:683–686.

Smith, A. L., D. H. Black, and R. Eberle. 1998. The existence of differing monkey B Virus genotypes with possible implications for degree of virulence in humans. *Lab. Anim. Sci.* **49**:10–11.

Smith, J. S., and S. U. Neill. 1999. Rabies virus, p. 745–760. *In* E. H. Lennette and T. F. Smith (ed.), *Laboratory Diagnosis of Viral Infections*. Marcel Dekker, New York, N.Y.

Smith, J. S., D. B. Fishbein, C. E. Rupprecht, and K. Clark. 1991. Unexplained rabies in three immigrants in the United States. A virologic investigation. *N. Engl. J. Med.* **324**:205–211.

Sugamata, M., M. Miyazawa, S. Mori, C. J. Spangrude, L. C. Ewalt, and D. L. Lodmell. 1992. Paralysis of street rabies virus-infected mice is dependent on T lymphocytes. *J. Virol.* **66**:1252–1260.

Tangchai, P., and A. Vejjajjva. 1971. Pathology of the peripheral nervous system in human rabies. A study of 9 autopsy cases. *Brain* **94**:299–306.

Tangchai, P., D. Yenbutr, and A. Vejjajjva. 1970. Central nervous system lesions in human rabies. A study of twenty-four cases. *J. Med. Assoc. Thailand* **53**:471–486.

Tariq, W. U., M. S. Shafi, S. Jamal, and M. Ahmad. 1991. Rabies in man handling infected calf. *Lancet* **337**:1224.

Theerasurakarn, S., and S. Ubol. 1998. Apoptosis induction in brain during the fixed strain of rabies virus infection correlates with onset and severity of illness. *J. Neurovirol.* **4**:407–414.

Thomas, E., and E. Henschel. 1960. Uber die Herpes B Myelitis und Encephalitis beim Menschen. *D. Z. Nervenheilk.* **181**:494–516.

Torres-Anjel, M. J., D. C. Blenden, J. W. Frost, M. Raisbeck, J. K. Oakman, and D. Volz. 1987. Retrospective evaluation of the immunoreactivity of viral antigens after several years of "formalin" fixation at ambient temperature: a rabies virus-immunoperoxidase model. *Rev. Latinoam. Microbiol.* **29**:337–344.

Van Dam, A. M., J. Bauer, A. H. W. K. Man, C. Marquette, F. J. Tilders, and F. Berkenbosch. 1995. Appearance of inducible nitric oxide synthase in the rat central nervous system after rabies virus infection and during experimental allergic encephalomyelitis but not after peripheral administration of endotoxin. *J. Neurosci. Res.* **40**:251–160.

van Rooyen, C. E., and A. J. Rhodes. 1940. Trinidad rabies, p. 651–655. *In Virus Diseases of Man*. Oxford University Press, London, United Kingdom.

Wacharapluesadee, S., and T. Hemachuda. 2001. Nucleic acid sequence based amplification in the rapid diagnosis of rabies. *Lancet* **359**:892–893.

Warkel, R. L., C. F. Rinaldi, W. H. Bancroft, R. D. Cardiff, G. E. Holmes, and R. E. Wilsnack. 1973. Fatal acute meningoencephalitis due to lymphocytic choriomeningitis virus. *Neurology* **23**:198–203.

Warrell, D. A. 1983. Rhabdoviruses: rabies and rabies-related viruses, p. 5, 93–99. *In* D. J. Weatherall, J. G. G. Ledingham, and D. A. Warrell (ed.), *Oxford Textbook of Medicine*. Oxford University Press, Oxford, United Kingdom.

Warrell, M. J., S. Looareesuwan, S. Manatsathit, N. J. White, P. Phuapradit, A. Vejjajiva, C. H. Hoke, D. S. Burke, and D. A. Warrell. 1988. Rapid diagnosis of rabies and post-vaccinal encephalitides. *Clin. Exp. Immunol.* **71**:229–234.

Watson, H. D., G. H. Tignor, and A. L. Smith. 1981. Entry of rabies virus into the peripheral nerves of mice. *J. Gen. Virol.* **56**:372–382.

Weigler, B. J. 1992. Biology of B Virus in Macaque and human hosts: a review. *Clin. Infect. Dis.* **14**:555–567.

Weiland, F., J. H. Cox, S. Meyer, E. Dahme, and M. J. Reddeshase. 1992. Rabies virus neuritic paralysis: immunopathogenesis of nonfatal paralytic rabies. *J. Virol.* **66**:5096–5099.

World Health Organization. 1995. Veterinary public health. Oral immunization of foxes in Europe in 1994. *Wkly. Epidemiol. Rec.* **70**:89–91.

ACUTE PARAINFECTIOUS IMMUNE-MEDIATED ENCEPHALOMYELITIS

Pathology of Allergic Forms of Encephalomyelitis

The concept of allergic damage to the nervous system arose with Pasteur's vaccine against rabies, first used in 1884. This vaccine was prepared from the dried and fixed spinal cord of an experimentally infected rabbit. People at risk of developing rabies were given repeated injections of this material, and although they were protected from developing rabies, they sometimes developed other serious neurological complications. These "neuroparalytic accidents" prompted investigation of their cause. A natural supposition that they were due to modified rabies virus was found to be mistaken. Experiments on the effects of injecting uninfected brain tissue into animals showed that this procedure alone was capable of producing similar changes. Rivers and Schwentker (1935) showed in monkeys that this resulted in inflammation accompanied by demyelination—the first demonstration of an experimentally induced autoimmune disease. Following recognition that an inflammatory demyelinating process may occur in the human brain after antirabies immunization, descriptions started to appear of essentially the same condition occurring occasionally after smallpox vaccination (Glanzmann, 1927; van Bogaert, 1932; de Vries, 1960) and various exanthematous diseases. The same pathological state has also been described after nonspecific upper respiratory tract infections and in the absence of overt preceding infection. We shall refer to this pathological condition as perivenous encephalitis (PVE) and to its clinical counterpart as acute disseminated encephalomyelitis (ADEM). Hurst (1941) described a particularly fulminating clinical variant of this disease in which there were hemorrhagic as well as inflammatory demyelinating lesions in the brain. This form of the disease will be referred to as acute hemorrhagic leukoencephalitis (AHLE).

Whereas in the case of encephalitis following antirabies immunization immune-mediated damage could be understood as a consequence of the inclusion of central nervous system (CNS) antigens in the inoculum, cases of PVE arising after smallpox vaccination or other infections were not so readily explained. The mechanism whereby a variety of virus infections may trigger an immune reaction against CNS antigens is not understood (see below). Regardless of the setting in which allergic encephalitis occurs, the pathology is quite similar. Detailed recent reviews of the pathology and pathogenesis of PVE and AHLE have been published by Prineas et al. (2002) and Johnson (1998).

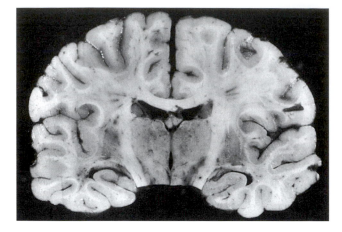

FIGURE 7.1 Macroscopic appearance of coronal slice from a case of PVE. Vascular markings are prominent, and lateral and third ventricles are reduced in size.

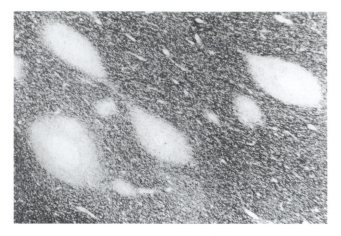

FIGURE 7.2 Low-power view of cerebral white matter from a case of PVE. Myelin stain shows loss of myelin around veins.

PATHOLOGY OF HUMAN PVE (ADEM)

PVE is an acute monophasic disease; in most fatal cases, death occurs within the first 3 weeks of the onset of neurological disease. The naked-eye appearance of the brain is nonspecific. It appears swollen, sometimes with uncal and tonsillar herniation. The leptomeninges are usually congested and minimally cloudy. In slices of the fixed brain the ventricles appear narrow and the cerebral white matter edematous (Fig. 7.1). Venous congestion and occasional small petechial hemorrhages may be noted. The hindbrain shows no abnormality apart from possible swelling.

Microscopic Appearance

In contrast to the absence of specific features on naked-eye examination, the microscopic appearances are diagnostic. There are two essential features, inflammation and demyelination, both of which are mainly confined to perivenous and perivenular tissues. White matter is particularly severely affected, but similar, though less severe, changes are frequently present in gray matter. The white matter of the centrum ovale is almost invariably severely involved, and in most cases the changes extend into the brain stem and spinal cord. Cases presenting clinically as acute transverse myelitis may show more severe pathology in the spinal cord than in the brain.

The demyelination takes the form of a narrow sleeve around inflamed perivenous and perivenular spaces (Fig. 7.2). In the presence of edema the myelin in general stains poorly, but the pallor is most obvious around small veins. In the demyelinated perivascular regions, bare axons can be seen completely stripped of myelin or with a few fragments of irregular, apparently bubbly, myelin sheaths remaining. Some axons may be destroyed or damaged, but they are much better preserved than the myelin. Many inflammatory cells are usually seen in the demyelinated zone, spilling over into the parenchyma from deep cuffs of cells within the adjacent perivenous spaces. Occasionally, these cells are scarce, but there are invariably increased numbers of macrophagelike cells in the region.

In hematoxylin-and-eosin-stained sections, the myelin loss may be difficult to detect, but attention is immediately attracted to the perivenous regions where inflammatory cells form compact cuffs around veins and venules and extend into immediately adjacent parenchyma (Fig. 7.3 and 7.4). The inflammatory cells consist predominantly of mononuclear cells, most of them lymphocytes and macrophages, but there may be a few neutrophil polymorphs as well. Some of the macrophages contain fragments of phagocytosed myelin that stain with the usual myelin stains. They contain little or no neutral fat unless the length of the illness has exceeded a week. The lymphocytes are small with scanty cytoplasm and consist predominantly of cytotoxic-suppressor T cells (Weiner and Hauser, 1982; Esiri, unpublished observations). Plasma cells are rarely seen. Mitotic figures are not difficult to find in these perivascular cuffs. The veins and venules lying at their center are usually patent and the walls are usually intact, although the endothelial cells are often swollen and there may be exudation of plasma proteins, indicating breakdown of the blood-brain barrier. Capillaries and arterioles, as well as veins and venules, are congested, and some

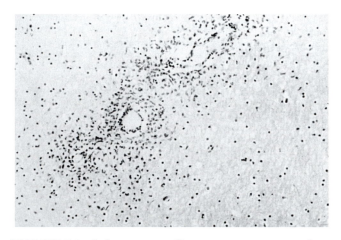

FIGURE 7.3 Inflammatory cells in perivenous space and immediately surrounding white matter from a case of PVE. Hematoxylin and eosin stain.

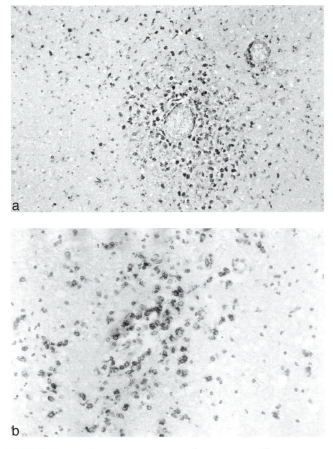

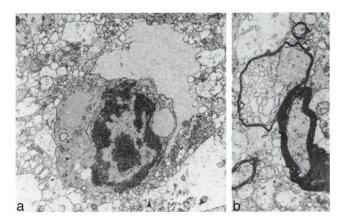

FIGURE 7.5 Electron micrograph of cerebrum (a) and spinal cord (b) from two autopsy cases of PVE. Complete (a) or incomplete (b) vesicular dissolution of myelin with axons remaining intact. Lead citrate and uranyl acetate stain. Magnification, ×19,800.

FIGURE 7.4 Immunostaining inflammatory cells in perivenous space and adjacent white matter from a case of PVE showing (a) macrophages stained for CD68 and (b) leukocytes (mainly lymphocytes) stained for leukocyte common antigen. Both counterstained with hematoxylin.

1939; Berard-Badier et al., 1961; Toro et al., 1977). Widened perivascular spaces are seen in cerebral white matter, marking the sites of previous inflammatory cuffing. The parenchyma around them is attenuated, and there is confluent deficiency of myelin and, to a lesser extent, of axons, accompanied by intense fibrillary gliosis.

Electron Microscopy

Electron microscopic appearances in PVE have not been reported in the literature. In two personally examined cases, at autopsy the most striking finding was of vesicular dissolution of myelin sheaths, sometimes in the absence of infiltrating inflammatory cells (Fig. 7.5). Capillaries and venules show endothelial cell swelling, gaps between endothelial cells, and occasional deposits of fibrin in and around the walls.

In summary, pathological studies reveal a generally intense but frequently short-lived inflammatory process associated with localized demyelination followed by glial scarring. The demyelination occurs early, within the first few days of onset, when the majority of the inflammatory cells that have accumulated are T lymphocytes and macrophages.

PATHOLOGY OF AHLE

General

Naked-eye appearances in this variant of allergic encephalomyelitis are more dramatic than in the nonhemorrhagic type described above (Fig. 7.6). The brain is congested and swollen, usually symmetrically so, but sometimes with sufficient asymmetry to produce midline shift. Bilateral uncal and tonsillar herniation often occur, and the leptomeninges are usually clear. Cut slices of the fixed brain show narrowed lateral ventricles and numerous petechial hemorrhages speckling the cerebral white matter. The white matter itself is soft and edematous or yellowish and necrotic. These abnormalities are most marked in the centrum ovale but extend variably into the corpus callosum and internal capsule. The cerebral cortex, basal ganglia, and thalamus

extravasation of red blood cells may be apparent around capillaries, but this is not extensive.

Moving away from the regions of perivenous demyelination and inflammation, the parenchyma may appear edematous but is otherwise relatively normal. There is some reactive astrocytosis around the demyelinated zones from the end of the first week. Neuron cell bodies are almost invariably well preserved even in the most severely affected areas unless there has been a complicating factor such as hypoxia secondary to respiratory depression, epilepsy, or hypostatic pneumonia. The leptomeninges frequently contain a moderate mononuclear inflammatory infiltrate.

Occasionally, a patient survives the acute phase of the disease only to die later of some complication such as bronchopneumonia. In patients dying a few weeks after the onset of the disease, perivenous inflammation is still present but is less intense than in patients dying earlier. Inflammation is now largely confined to the perivascular spaces and consists of a mixed population of mononuclear cells. Demyelination is still present as relatively narrow sleeves around inflamed veins and venules and is accompanied by slight axonal loss and considerable reactive gliosis. In patients dying years later, the inflammation has largely subsided (Malamud,

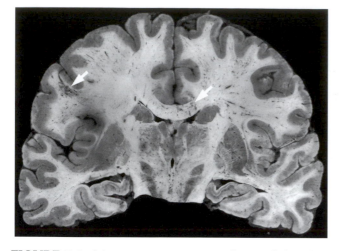

FIGURE 7.6 Macroscopic appearance of coronal slice from a case of AHLE. Vascular markings and swelling are even more marked than in Fig. 7.1, and there are foci of petechial hemorrhage (white arrows).

appear relatively well preserved. The brain stem may be involved, in which case it is swollen and blotchily discolored, and petechial hemorrhages may be present. The cerebellar white matter and the spinal cord are sometimes affected; the thoracic region usually shows the most severe abnormalities, including hemorrhagic necrosis.

Microscopic Appearance

Microscopic lesions are present in the areas that appear abnormal macroscopically and beyond; the white matter is predominantly affected. The histology varies somewhat according to the length of time the patient has been ill. Most patients have died within 5 days of the onset. If death has occurred in the first 3 days, the most striking change consists of necrosis of small venules, capillaries, and arterioles, with surrounding narrow zones of necrotic parenchyma and ring or ball hemorrhages around veins and venules. In the necrotic area myelin staining is lost, axons are fragmented, and glial nuclei appear pyknotic. Fibrin is often demonstrable in necrotic vessel walls, together with marked exudation of plasma proteins into surrounding parenchyma. Inflammatory cells at this stage consist chiefly of neutrophil polymorphs found in and around necrotic vessels and infiltrating the zone of necrotic parenchyma (Fig. 7.7). Fibrin thrombi are not usually found in these necrotic vessels. Later, from about the fourth day, the character of the lesions changes slightly. Although foci of vascular necrosis, hemorrhage, and neutrophil infiltration are still seen in areas, the more characteristic lesions at this stage resemble those of PVE described above. In these, the small vessels are congested and endothelial cells are swollen, but there is no necrosis. There is a variable but frequently intense inflammatory infiltrate surrounding these vessels, which may include some neutrophils and now many macrophages and lymphocytes. The surrounding parenchyma is not necrotic but shows selective demyelination and edema and clear evidence of damage to axons in the form of swollen axons that immunostain for β-amyloid precursor protein (Fig. 7.8),

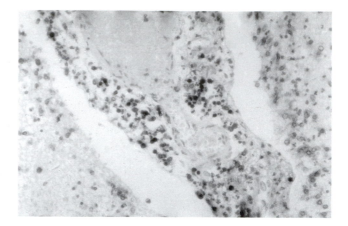

FIGURE 7.7 Perivascular cells from a case of AHLE. Note that many are polymorphonuclear leukocytes. Hematoxylin counterstain on preparation immunostained for leukocyte common antigen.

perhaps with early reactive astrocytosis. The leptomeninges are congested and show some exudation of both neutrophils and mononuclear cells. The cerebral cortex and other areas of gray matter show changes that are less pronounced but otherwise similar to those seen in the white matter.

Electron microscopy of biopsy specimens has shown edema and diapedesis of erythrocytes, lymphocytes, and macrophages in white matter. The macrophages in perivascular parenchyma contained phagocytosed myelin remnants (Cox and Luse, 1963).

Although the pathologies of PVE and AHLE have been described as distinct variants of allergic CNS disease, it is apparent from the description of the microscopy that there is considerable overlap between them. Furthermore, it is not unusual to find the typical appearances of both variants in different regions of the same brain (Russell, 1955).

ACUTE PARAINFECTIOUS ENCEPHALOPATHY

In addition to being associated with the inflammatory conditions described above, many of the same infections have also

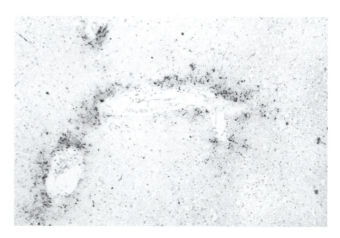

FIGURE 7.8 Immunostain for β-amyloid precursor protein to mark damaged axons in a case of AHLE. Perivenous axons are selectively damaged. Counterstained with hematoxylin.

been associated with an acute encephalopathy that differs from Reye's syndrome in lacking evidence of hepatic pathology or hypoglycemia (Lyon et al., 1961). In these cases the brain at autopsy is edematous but shows none of the inflammatory or hemorrhagic changes described above. The etiology of this condition is unknown, but most authors are unconvinced of its immune basis, though some favor the idea of a common immune-based vascular insult both in this condition and as a prerequisite for the inflammatory conditions (Poser, 1969, 1978; Reik, 1980). The possibility that direct virus-inflicted vascular damage may have a part to play must also be considered.

PATHOGENESIS OF ALLERGIC ENCEPHALITIS

There are few reports of immunological investigation in patients with allergic encephalitis, partly on account of their rarity but also because of the difficulty in reaching a diagnosis during life. The illnesses are of short duration, and there are no confirmatory laboratory tests. Magnetic resonance imaging examination is often consistent with but not diagnostic of the condition. Most clinicians and pathologists are impressed by the very close similarities in time course and histopathology between these inflammatory diseases and experimental allergic encephalomyelitis (EAE). This condition therefore warrants brief consideration here. Further details can be found in several recent reviews, for example, those of Bradl and Linington (1996) and Gold et al. (2000).

As already indicated, it was shown in the 1930s that an inflammatory demyelinating disease of the CNS could be produced in monkeys subjected to repeated injections of CNS antigens (Rivers and Schwentker, 1935). Development of this disease was facilitated by combining the CNS antigen with Freund's adjuvant (Kabat et al., 1947). Subsequent work with several different laboratory animals demonstrated that the main relevant sensitizing antigen is myelin basic protein (Kies and Alvord, 1959) and that its encephalitogenic activity resides in a defined, relatively short sequence of amino acids (Hashim, 1978). Other myelin components or their immunodominant domains have been recognized as encephalitogenic as well: myelin proteolipid protein and myelin oligodendroglial glycoprotein (Miller and Karpus, 1994; Tuohy et al., 1994).

The pathology consists initially of perivenular inflammatory cell infiltration with lymphocytes, plasma cells, and macrophages within the CNS, particularly in the white matter (Waksman and Adams, 1962). Their appearance is rapidly followed by the development of demyelination in the vicinity of these cells (Wisniewski et al., 1969; Lampert, 1969, 1978). Confirmation that these lesions are the result of an immune reaction came with the demonstration that the disease can be transferred passively to normal syngeneic animals by the passage of lymph node cells (Paterson, 1960; Stone, 1961; Astrom and Waksman, 1962), more specifically with T lymphocytes (Bernard et al., 1976; Ben-Nun and Lindo, 1983; Swanborg, 1983).

Further analysis of this animal model has shown that the species, strain, and age of the animal to be immunized and the composition of the inoculum, particularly the amount and proportions of antigen to adjuvant and the nature of the

adjuvant, all decisively influence the outcome in terms of the disease produced. For example, a form of acute disease resembling AHLE can be produced by substituting pertussis vaccine for Freund's adjuvant in the inoculum (Levine and Wenk, 1964, 1965). It is now possible to produce a spectrum of clinical and pathological changes in animals that ranges from acutely fatal disease through more subacute forms of allergic encephalitis to chronic relapsing disease (Lassmann and Wisniewski, 1979; Miller and Karpus, 1994; Tuohy et al., 1994).

There is general agreement that the conventional form of acute EAE is an experimental counterpart to human PVE. The time course of the two diseases is similar, and the histopathological lesions strikingly so. In this experimental model one of the major immunological reactions is that of delayed cell-mediated hypersensitivity, and it seems likely that the same may be true for human PVE. Certainly, the latent period of 10 to 14 days that most characteristically elapses between vaccination and the onset of symptoms of postvaccinal PVE would be consistent with this suggestion. There are also a few reports of lymphocyte sensitivity to myelin basic protein in patients with postinfectious encephalitis (Behan et al., 1968; Lisak et al., 1974; Lisak and Zweiman, 1977; Johnson et al., 1984) and neurological complications of postexposure rabies immunization (Johnson et al., 1984). This would imply that the damage to myelin in PVE is mediated in part by T lymphocytes, as it is in EAE. The inflammatory reaction in EAE is thought to commence with the passage of activated antigen-specific T helper 1 (Th1) and/or Th2 cells across the blood-brain barrier, where they encounter recognized antigen presented by perivascular, major histocompatibility complex (MHC) class II-expressing macrophages (Table 7.1). (Th1 lymphocytes produce cytokines that facilitate cell-mediated immune responses such as alpha interferon, interleukin-2, interleukin-12, and tumor necrosis factor alpha, whereas Th2 lymphocytes produce cytokines that predominantly influence humoral responses such as interleukins-4, -5, -6, and -10 [Biernacki et al., 2001].) This stimulates release of cytokines and chemokines from T cells, macrophages, and astrocytes (Ransohoff et al., 1993; Godiska et al., 1995; Glabinski et al., 1995), which, in turn, activate endothelial cells to interact with circulating leukocytes and prompts an invasion of nonspecific inflammatory cells into the CNS.

In passively transferred EAE, radiolabeling of antigen-specific T cells showed that radiolabeled cells constituted less than 4% of the perivascular inflammatory cells and did not penetrate into the CNS parenchyma (Cross et al., 1990, 1993). Onset of symptoms of EAE coincided with the influx of many more nonspecific inflammatory cells into the CNS parenchyma. Many of these cells were macrophages. There is evidence that macrophages play an important role in damaging myelin in EAE. For example, administering the selective macrophage toxin silica quartz by intraperitoneal injection on days 8 and 11 after sensitization resulted in protection of 80% of Lewis rats at risk of developing allergic encephalitis, and a single injection given just after the onset of clinical signs produced a very significant slowing in the clinical expression of the disease (Brosnan et al., 1979). Likewise, use of myelin oligodendroglial glycoprotein or S100β as

TABLE 7.1 Steps envisaged as occurring in development of PVE, based on experimental studies of EAE, and interventions that are effective in preventing or reducing clinical expression of the disease

Step	Counteracted by:
Stimulation of T lymphocytes specifically responding to myelin antigens ↓ Passage of activated myelin-specific T lymphocytes into CNS perivascular spaces ↓	← Antibodies to leukointegrin such as VLA-4
Further stimulation of myelin-specific T lymphocytes by encounter with antigens presented by MHC class II-expressing macrophages ↓ Production of proinflammatory cytokines, chemokines, and matrix metalloproteinases by macrophages, microglia, T lymphocytes, and astrocytes ↓	← Matrix metalloproteinase inhibitors and chemokine antibodies
Lowering of blood-brain barrier and entry of many more antigen-nonspecific lymphocytes and macrophages into perivascular spaces and CNS parenchyma; entry of immune-related proteins such as complement and immunoglobulins into CNS parenchyma from blood ↓	← Macrophage toxins
Myelin destruction mediated by a combination of mechanisms involving macrophages, lymphocytes, and antibody	

immunogen was associated with much reduced production of the macrophage chemokines macrophage chemotactic protein-1 (MCP-1) and macrophage inflammatory protein (MIP)-1α, greatly reduced macrophage infiltration of the CNS, and only mild clinical symptoms of EAE (Kojima et al., 1994; Linington et al., 1993; Bradl and Linington, 1996). Humoral antibodies may also play a part. Serum from animals with EAE was capable of producing demyelination in organotypic cultures of CNS tissues (Bornstein and Appel, 1961; Bornstein, 1978). This appears to be a complement-dependent antibody effect (Grundke-Iqbal et al., 1980). Demyelinating antibody appears to be directed against galactocerebroside, a glycolipid myelin antigen, or against myelin oligodendroglial glycoprotein, rather than against myelin basic protein (Dubois-Dalcq et al., 1970; Fry et al., 1974; Lassmann et al., 1988). Yet another mechanism of demyelination is suggested by in vivo studies using the rabbit eye, in which interaction of mononuclear cells with specific immune serum was required to induce demyelination (Brosnan et al., 1977).

In the hemorrhagic forms of human and animal allergic encephalitis, the appearance of the lesions strongly suggests the occurrence of an Arthus reaction. In this reaction vascular damage occurs at the site of contact within the vascular compartment of antigen with excess circulating specific antibody in the blood. Continual turnover of myelin basic protein with passage of small amounts into the blood is presumed to provide the opportunity for this antigen to combine with antibody to form intravascular immune complexes once antibody appears in the blood. These complexes are deposited locally and damage the vascular wall through activation of the complement pathway, allowing influx of inflammatory cells and plasma proteins into the parenchyma. Further myelin breakdown results, thus amplifying the reaction. Although such a sequence of events may well occur during the development of AHLE, there is disappointingly

little evidence for the presence of circulating immune complexes to myelin basic protein, but attempts to find them have been few. For example, in the case investigated by Behan and Lamarche (1969), immunological studies were in favor of a delayed hypersensitivity reaction because transfer of lymphoid cells, but not serum, resulted in allergic encephalitis in a monkey. However, even in animals with hemorrhagic allergic encephalitis, the condition is transferable only with lymphoid cells, and the recipients must have been treated with pertussis vaccine, suggesting that some modification of cellular reactivity is required to produce this variant of allergic disease (Levine and Wenk, 1967).

The EAE models, with their resemblance to human allergic encephalitis, offer the chance of demonstrating the possible immunoregulatory factors involved. For example, strains of certain animal species differ in their susceptibility to EAE, and differences in behavior of lymphoid cells in response to induction of EAE in these different strains can uncover factors of importance in pathogenesis. Furthermore, rats that have recovered from EAE induced by an injection of myelin basic protein and complete Freund's adjuvant are then resistant to reinduction of the disease; this model can be used to explore suppressor mechanisms responsible for this resistance. Injections of myelin basic protein, particularly when incorporated into liposomes, are also capable of inducing suppression of EAE (Strejan et al., 1984).

These and similar lines of investigation offer important opportunities to dissect immune and nonspecific inflammatory responses that are responsible for inducing the types of processes that may well be responsible for human PVE and AHLE and may suggest methods for their control. For example, injection of antibody to the macrophage chemokine MIP-1α (but not MCP-1) prevents development of passive transfer EAE (Karpus et al., 1995) (Table 7.1); inhibitors of matrix metalloproteinases reduce injury to the blood-brain barrier in EAE (Gijbels et al., 1994); and antibodies to leukointegrins such as VLA-4 prevent passage of antigen-specific T cells through the blood-brain barrier (Cannella et al., 1993; Yednock et al., 1992).

From the pathogenetic viewpoint no discussion of the different forms of human allergic encephalitis would be complete without a mention of multiple sclerosis (MS). Some cases of MS are clinically indistinguishable from ADEM at first presentation, and in a recent series of 40 patients initially diagnosed with ADEM, no fewer than 35% developed clinically definite MS over a mean follow-up period of 38 months (Schwarz et al., 2001). In MS there is selective demyelination in the form of multiple plaques, many of which are centered on veins or venules. These plaques differ from the sleeves of demyelination seen in PVE principally in being confined to shorter lengths of the vessels, extending more widely into the parenchyma, showing less (though still appreciable) inflammation, and in the evidence of chronicity in some of the lesions. However, in the more acute forms of MS, many small perivenous lesions are present, and there is an intense mononuclear inflammatory infiltrate in perivenous spaces and within plaque parenchyma. The pathological resemblance to PVE can therefore be quite striking. Further indications that there may be a close pathogenetic relationship between the two come from occasional reports of lesions of both PVE and MS occurring together (Carpenter and Lampert, 1972; Oppenheimer, 1976). Among cases of post-rabies vaccine encephalitis were some in which large plaquelike demyelinated lesions as well as more typical perivenous sleeves of demyelination were seen (Uchimura and Shiraki, 1957; Toro et al., 1977). Finally, the demonstration that chronic relapsing varieties of EAE, which form part of the same spectrum as acute disease, show convincing parallels to MS clinically, pathologically, and immunologically strengthens the view that MS similarly belongs in the spectrum of human immune-mediated CNS diseases (Hartung and Grossman, 2001).

The question of how a preceding viral infection initiates the series of immune reactions that result in allergic encephalitis remains unanswered. It is quite possible to envisage viral induction of an immune response to neural antigens if viral epitopes share amino acid sequences with myelin, if infection of CNS cells alters host cell membrane antigens, or if such antigens are incorporated in the outer envelope of those viruses that possess one. However, it is not known whether viral invasion of the CNS is necessary for human PVE or AHLE to develop. Recovery of vaccinia virus from the brain or CSF has been reported in some patients with postvaccinal encephalitis (Turnbull and McIntosh, 1926; von Siegert, 1957; Tyler, 1957; Angulo et al., 1964; Gurvich and Vilesova, 1983), and measles virus has been rarely recovered in patients with postmeasles encephalitis (Purdham and Batty, 1974). In most cases, however, attempts to recover viruses have been unsuccessful. This does not, however, exclude the possibility that virus may have been present in the CNS before the onset of symptoms of PVE. The case reports that describe PVE in conjunction with another form of encephalitis in which presumptive or certain virus-inflicted CNS damage also occurs suggest that the presence of virus in the CNS can indeed trigger such an immune reaction.

There are a number of examples of naturally occurring and experimental CNS viral infections in animals in which demyelination and inflammation occur (reviewed by Dal Canto and Rabinowitz, 1982; Johnson, 1998). In some of these infections, demyelination is thought to involve immunopathological mechanisms and not simply to result from lytic infection of oligodendroglia. For example, in the case of infection with certain temperature-sensitive mutants of coronavirus JHM in rats, there is a subacute demyelinating encephalomyelitis that resembles chronic EAE (Wege et al., 1984). Lymph node cells from animals with this disease have been shown to be specifically stimulated to proliferate when cultured in the presence of myelin basic protein, and these cells are then capable of adoptively transferring mild clinical and histological abnormalities characteristic of EAE to normal recipients. These observations support the suggestion that virus infections of the CNS can trigger autoimmune responses to myelin if the virus strain and the age and strain of the host are appropriate.

On the other hand, a careful study of postmeasles encephalomyelitis failed to detect intrathecal synthesis of antimeasles antibody or measles virus antigen in brain tissues, observations that were interpreted as suggesting that measles virus replication in the CNS is not a prerequisite for the development of this disease (Johnson et al., 1984; Gendelman et al., 1984). An alternative explanation for the triggering of autoimmune neurological disease by a variety of infections is entertained by Johnson et al. and Gendelman et al., who note that many of the infectious agents implicated are capable of replicating in host leukocytes and may therefore produce alterations in immune regulation independent of nervous system invasion. Such a mechanism might explain why a wide variety of viruses can trigger a similar pathological process, but the reason why CNS antigens, in particular myelin antigens, are the target for attack in such reactions remains obscure. One possible explanation might lie in the vulnerability of myelin to "bystander damage" or to provoking autoimmunity in association with an ongoing immune response to another antigen, perhaps viral. A recent study using the sensitive in situ PCR technique to search for virus-specific nucleic acid sequences in AHLE reports finding evidence of a variety of viruses in the brain (An et al., 2002).

REFERENCES

An, S. F., M. Groves, L. Martinian, and F. Scaravilli. 2002. Detection of infectious agents in brain of patients with acute hemorrhagic leucoencephalitis. *J. Neurovirol.* **8:**439–446.

Angulo, J. J., E. Pimenta de Campos, and L. F. de Salles-Gomes. 1964. Post-vaccinal meningo-encephalitis. Isolation of the virus from the brain. *JAMA* **187:**151–153.

Astrom, K. E., and B. H. Waksman. 1962. The passive transfer of experimental allergic encephalomyelitis and neuritis with living lymphoid cells. *J. Pathol. Bacteriol.* **83:**89–106.

Behan, P. O., and J. B. Lamarche. 1969. Passive transfer of allergic encephalitis from man to primates. *Neurology* **19:**321–322.

Behan, P. O., N. Geschwind, J. B. Lamarche, R. P. Lisak, and M. W. Kies. 1968. Delayed hypersensitivity to encephalitogenic protein in disseminated encephalomyelitis. *Lancet* **ii:**1009–1012.

Ben-Nun, A., and Z. Lindo. 1983. Detection of autoimmune cells proliferating to myelin basic protein and selection of T cell lines that mediate EAE. *J. Immunol.* **130:**1205–1209.

Berard-Badier, M., H. Gastaut, and H. Payan. 1961. Comparative clinico-pathological study of one early and two late cases of measles encephalitis (with an electroencephalographic study of one case), p. 106–123. *In* L. van Bogaert, J. Radermecker, J. Hozay, and A. Lowenthal (ed.), *Encephalitides*. Elsevier, Amsterdam, The Netherlands.

Bernard, C. C. A., J. Leydon, and I. R. MacKay. 1976. T cell necessity in the pathogenesis of experimental autoimmune encephalomyelitis in mice. *Eur. J. Immunol.* **6:**655–660.

Biernacki, K., A. Prat, M. Blain, and J. P. Antel. 2001. Regulation of Th1 and Th2 lymphocyte migration by human adult brain endothelial cells. *J. Neuropathol. Exp. Neurol.* **60:**1127–1136.

Bornstein, M. B. 1978. Immunobiology of demyelination, p. 313–336. *In* S. G. Waksman (ed.), *Physiology and Pathology of Axons*. Raven Press, New York, N.Y.

Bornstein, M. B., and S. H. Appel. 1961. The application of tissue culture to the study of experimental allergic encephalomyelitis. Patterns of demyelination. *J. Neuropathol. Exp. Neurol.* **20:**141–147.

Bradl, M., and C. Linington. 1996. Animal models of demyelination. *Brain Pathol.* **6:**303–311.

Brosnan, C. F., G. L. Stoner, B. R. Bloom, and H. M. Wisniewski. 1977. Studies on demyelination by activated lymphocytes in the rabbit eye. 2. Antibody-dependent cell-mediated demyelination. *J. Immunol.* **118:**2103–2110.

Brosnan, C. F., M. B. Bornstein, and B. R. Bloom. 1979. The effects of macrophage depletion on the expression of EAE in the Lewis rat. *J. Neuropathol. Exp. Neurol.* **38:**305.

Cannella, B., A. H. Cross, and C. S. Raine. 1993. Anti-adhesion molecule therapy in experimental autoimmune encephalomyelitis. *J. Neuroimmunol.* **46:**43–55.

Carpenter, S., and P. W. Lampert. 1972. Post infectious perivenous encephalitis and acute hemorrhagic leukoencephalitis, p. 2260–2269. *In* J. Minckler (ed.), *Pathology of the Nervous System*. McGraw-Hill, New York, N.Y.

Cox, W. S., and S. A. Luse. 1963. Acute haemorrhagic leukoencephalitis. A clinical and electron microscopic report of 2 patients treated with surgical decompression. *J. Neurosurg.* **20:**584–596.

Cross, A. H., B. Cannella, C. F. Brosnan, and C. S. Raine. 1990. Homing to central nervous system vasculature by antigen-specific lymphocytes. I. Localization of 14C-labeled cells during acute, chronic, and relapsing experimental allergic encephalomyelitis. *Lab. Investig.* **63:**162–170.

Cross, A. H., T. O'Mara, and C. S. Raine. 1993. Chronologic localization of myelin-reactive cells in the lesions of relapsing EAE: implications for the study of multiple sclerosis. *Neurology* **43:**1028–1033.

Dal Canto, M. C., and S. G. Rabinowitz. 1982. Experimental models of virus induced demyelination of the central nervous system. *Ann. Neurol.* **11:**109–127.

de Vries, E. 1960. *Postvaccinal Perivenous Encephalitis*. Elsevier, Amsterdam, The Netherlands.

Dubois-Dalcq, M., B. Niedieck, and M. Buyse. 1970. Action of anti-cerebroside sera on myelinated nervous tissue cultures. *Pathol. Eur.* **5:**331–347.

Fry, J. M., S. Weissbarth, G. M. Lehrer, and M. B. Bornstein. 1974. Cerebroside antibodies inhibit sulphatide synthesis and myelination and demyelinate cord tissue cultures. *Science* **183:**540–542.

Gendelman, H. E., J. S. Wolinsky, R. T. Johnson, N. J. Pressman, G. H. Pezeshkpour, and G. F. Boisset. 1984. Measles

encephalomyelitis: lack of evidence of viral invasion of the central nervous system and quantitative study of the nature of demyelination. *Ann. Neurol.* **15:**353–360.

Gijbels, K., R. E. Galardy, and L. Steinman. 1994. Reversal of experimental autoimmune encephalomyelitis with a hydroxamate inhibitor of matrix metalloproteases. *J. Clin. Investig.* **94:**2177–2182.

Glabinski, A. R., M. Tani, V. K. Tuohy, R. J. Tuthill, and R. M. Ransohoff. 1995. Central nervous system chemokine mRNA accumulation follows initial leukocyte entry at the onset of acute murine experimental autoimmune encephalomyelitis. *Brain Behav. Immunol.* **9:**315–330.

Glanzmann, E. 1927. Die nervosen Komplikationen der Varicellen variola und Vakzine. *Schweiz. Med. Wochenschr.* **57:**145–154.

Godiska, R., D. Chantry, G. N. Dietsch, and P. W. Gray. 1995. Chemokine expression in murine experimental allergic encephalomyelitis. *J. Neuroimmunol.* **58:**167–176.

Gold, R., H. P. Hartung, and K. V. Toyka. 2000. Animal models for autoimmune demyelinating disorders of the nervous system. *Mol. Med. Today* **6:**88–91.

Grundke-Iqbal, I., H. Lassmann, and H. M. Wisniewski. 1980. Immunohistochemical studies in chronic relapsing experimental allergic encephalomyelitis. *Arch. Neurol.* **37:**651–656.

Gurvich, E. B., and I. S. Vilesova. 1983. Vaccinia virus in postvaccinial encephalitis. *Acta Virol.* **27:**154–159.

Hartung, H. P., and R. I. Grossman. 2001. ADEM: distinct disease or part of the MS spectrum? *Neurology* **56:**1257–1260.

Hashim, G. A. 1978. Myelin basic protein: structure, function and antigenic determinants. *Immunol. Rev.* **39:**60–107.

Hurst, E. W. 1941. Acute haemorrhagic leucoencephalitis: a previously undefined entity. *Med. J. Austr.* **28:**1–6.

Johnson, R. T. 1998. *Viral Infections of the Nervous System*, 2nd ed. Lippincott-Raven, Philadelphia, Pa.

Johnson, R. T., D. E. Griffin, R. L. Hirsch, J. S. Wolinsky, S. Roedenbeck, I. Lindo de Soriano, and A. Vaisberg. 1984. Measles encephalomyelitis—clinical and immunologic studies. *N. Engl. J. Med.* **310:**137–141.

Kabat, E. A., A. Wolf, and A. E. Bezer. 1947. The rapid production of acute disseminated encephalomyelitis in rhesus monkeys by injection of heterologous and homologous brain tissue with adjuvants. *J. Exp. Med.* **85:**117–130.

Karpus, W. J., N. W. Lukacs, B. L. McRae, R. M. Strieter, S. L. Kunkel, and S. D. Miller. 1995. An important role for the chemokine macrophage inflammatory protein-1 alpha in the pathogenesis of the T cell-mediated autoimmune disease, experimental autoimmune encephalomyelitis. *J. Immunol.* **155:**5003–5010.

Kies, M. W., and E. C. Alvord. 1959. Encephalolitogenic activity in guinea pigs of water soluble protein fractions of nervous tissue, p. 239–299. *In* M. W. Kies and E. C. Alvord (ed.), *Allergic Encephalomyelitis*. Thomas, Springfield, Ill.

Kojima, K., T. Berger, H. Lassmann, D. Hinze-Selch, Y. Zhang, J. Gehrmann, K. Reske, H. Wekerle, and C. Linington. 1994. Experimental autoimmune panencephalitis and uveoretinitis transferred to the Lewis rat by T lymphocytes specific for the S100 beta molecule, a calcium binding protein of astroglia. *J. Exp. Med.* **180:**817–829.

Lampert, P. W. 1969. Mechanism of demyelination in experimental allergic neuritis. Electron microscopic studies. *Lab. Investig.* **20:**127–138.

Lampert, P. W. 1978. Autoimmune and virus-induced demyelinating diseases. A review. *Am. J. Pathol.* **91:**175–208.

Lassmann, H., and H. M. Wisniewski. 1979. Chronic relapsing experimental allergic encephalomyelitis: morphological sequence of myelin degradation. *Brain Res.* **169:**357–368.

Lassmann, H., C. Brunner, M. Bradl, and C. Linington. 1988. Experimental allergic encephalomyelitis: the balance between encephalitogenic T lymphocytes and demyelinating antibodies determines size and structure of demyelinated lesions. *Acta Neuropathol.* (Berlin) **75:**566–576.

Levine, S., and E. J. Wenk. 1964. Allergic encephalomyelitis: a hyperacute form. *Science* **146:**1681–1682.

Levine, S., and E. J. Wenk. 1965. A hyperacute form of allergic encephalomyelitis. *Am. J. Pathol.* **47:**61–88.

Levine, S., and E. J. Wenk. 1967. Hyperacute allergic encephalomyelitis: lymphatic system as site of adjuvant effect of pertussis vaccine. *Am. J. Pathol.* **50:**465–483.

Linington, C., T. Berger, L. Perry, S. Weerth, D. Hinze-Selch, Y. Zhang, H. C. Lu, H. Lassmann, and H. Wekerle. 1993. T cells specific for the myelin oligodendrocyte glycoprotein mediate an unusual autoimmune inflammatory response in the central nervous system. *Eur. J. Immunol.* **23:**1364–1372.

Lisak, R. P., and B. Zweiman. 1977. In vitro cell-mediated immunity of cerebrospinal fluid lymphocytes to myelin basic protein in primary demyelinating diseases. *N. Engl. J. Med.* **297:**850–853.

Lisak, R. P., P. O. Behan, B. Zweiman, and T. Shetty. 1974. Cell-mediated immunity of myelin basic protein in acute disseminated encephalomyelitis. *Neurology* **24:**560–564.

Lyon, G., P. R. Dodge, and R. D Adams. 1961. The acute encephalopathies of obscure origin in infants and children. *Brain* **84:**680–708.

Malamud, N. 1939. Sequelae of postmeasles encephalomyelitis; a clinicopathological study. *Arch. Neurol. Psychiatr.* **41:**943–954.

Miller, S. D., and W. J. Karpus. 1994. The immunopathogenesis and regulation of T-cell-mediated demyelinating diseases. *Immunol. Today* **15:**356–361.

Oppenheimer, D. R. 1976. Demyelinating diseases, p. 470–499. *In* W. Blackwood and J. A. N. Corsellis (ed.), *Greenfield's Neuropathology*, 3rd ed. Edward Arnold Publ. Ltd., London, United Kingdom.

Paterson, P. Y. 1960. Transfer of allergic encephalomyelitis in rats by means of lymph node cells. *J. Exp. Med.* **111:**119–136.

Poser, C. M. 1969. Disseminated vasculomyelinopathy: a review of the clinical and pathologic reactions of the nervous system to hyperergic diseases. *Acta Neurol. Scand. Suppl.* **37:**1–44.

Poser, C. M. 1978. Diseases of the myelin sheath, p. 80–104. *In* A. B. Baker and L. H. Baker (ed.), *Clinical Neurology*, vol. 2. Harper and Row, New York, N.Y.

Prineas, J. W., W. I. McDonald, and R. J. Franklin. 2002. Demyelinating diseases, p. 471–550. *In* D. I. Graham and P. L. Tantos (ed.), *Greenfield's Neuropathology*, 7th ed., vol. II. Arnold, London, United Kingdom.

Purdham, D. R., and P. F. Batty. 1974. A case of acute measles meningoencephalitis with virus isolation. *J. Clin. Pathol.* **27:**994–996.

Ransohoff, R. M., T. A. Hamilton, M. Tani, M. H. Stoler, H. E. Shick, J. A. Major, M. L. Estes, D. M. Thomas, and V. K. Tuohy. 1993. Astrocyte expression of mRNA encoding cytokines IP-10 and JE/MCP-1 in experimental autoimmune encephalomyelitis. *FASEB J.* **7:**592–600.

Reik, L. J. 1980. Disseminated vasculomyelinopathy: an immune complex disease. *Ann. Neurol.* **7:**291–296.

Rivers, T. M., and F. F. Schwentker. 1935. Encephalomyelitis accompanied by myelin destruction experimentally produced in monkeys. *J. Exp. Med.* **61:**689–702.

Russell, D. S. 1955. The nosological unity of acute haemorrhagic leucoencephalitis and acute disseminated encephalomyelitis. *Brain* **78:**369–376.

Schwarz, S., M. Knauth, A. Mohr, B. Wildemann, C. Sommer, B. Storch-Hagenlocher. 2001. Acute disseminated encephalomyelitis (ADEM). *Nervenarzt* **72:**241–254.

Stone, S. H. 1961. Transfer of allergic encephalomyelitis by lymph node cells in inbred guinea pigs. *Science* **134:**619–620.

Strejan, G. H., D. H. Percy, and J. St. Louis. 1984. Suppression of experimental allergic encephalomyelitis in Lewis rats treated with myelin basic protein-liposome complexes: clinical, histopathological and cell-mediated immune complexes. *Cell. Immunol.* **84:**171–184.

Swanborg, R. H. 1983. Autoimmune effector cells. 5. A monoclonal antibody specific for rat helper T lymphocytes inhibits adoptive transfer of autoimmune encephalomyelitis. *J. Immunol.* **130:**1503–1505.

Toro, G., L. Vergara, and G. Roman. 1977. Neuroparalytic accidents of antirabies vaccinations with suckling mouse brain vaccine. *Arch. Neurol.* **34:**694–700.

Tuohy, V. K., R. B. Fritz, and A. Ben-Nun. 1994. Self-determinants in autoimmune demyelinating disease: changes in T-cell response specificity. *Curr. Opin. Immunol.* **6:**887–891.

Turnbull, H. M., and J. McIntosh. 1926. Encephalomyelitis following vaccination. *Br. J. Exp. Pathol.* **7:**181–222.

Tyler, H. R. 1957. Neurological complications of rubella (measles). *Medicine* **36:**147–167.

Uchimura, I., and H. Shiraki. 1957. A contribution to the classification and the pathogenesis of demyelinating encephalitis. *J. Neuropathol. Exp. Neurol.* **16:**139–208.

van Bogaert, L. 1932. Essai d'interpretation des manifestations nerveuses au cours de la vaccination de la maladie serique et des maladies eruptives. *Rev. Neurol.* **58:**1–26.

von Siegert, R. 1957. Das Verhalten des Vakzinevirus im organismus bei zentralnervosen Impfschaden. *Deutsch. Med. Wochenschr.* **82:**2021–2024.

Waksman, B. H., and R. D. Adams. 1962. A histologic study of the early lesion in experimental allergic encephalomyelitis in the guinea pig and rabbit. *Am. J. Pathol.* **41:**135–162.

Wege, H., R. Watanabe, and V. ter Meulen. 1984. Coronavirus JHM infection of rats as a model for virus induced demyelinating encephalomyelitis, p. 13–21. *In* E. C. Alvord, M. W. Kies, and A. J. Suckling (ed.), *Experimental Allergic Encephalomyelitis: A Useful Model for Multiple Sclerosis*. Alan R. Liss Inc., New York, N.Y.

Weiner, H. L., and S. L. Hauser. 1982. Neuroimmunology. 1. Immunoregulation in neurological disease. *Ann. Neurol.* **11:**437–439.

Wisniewski, H. M., J. Prineas, and C. S. Raine. 1969. An ultrastructural study of experimental demyelination and remyelination in the peripheral and central nervous system. 1. Acute experimental allergic encephalomyelitis. *Lab. Investig.* **21:**105–118.

Yednock, T. A., C. Cannon, L. C. Fritz, F. Sanchez-Madrid, L. Steinman, and N. Karin. 1992. Prevention of experimental autoimmune encephalomyelitis by antibodies against alpha 4 beta 1 integrin. *Nature* **356:**63–66.

Clinical Syndromes Including Smallpox and Measles

This chapter focuses on the central nervous system (CNS) syndromes that can follow in the wake of viral infections but may also present after immunization or without a recognized preceding event. The CNS dysfunction does not appear to result from viral replication in the brain but rather from a host immune response in the brain in the wake of a systemic infection. With the cessation of smallpox vaccination and the decline of recognizable childhood illnesses because of the implementation of measles-mumps-rubella and varicella-zoster virus (VZV) vaccination in the industrialized nations, many of the identifiable precedents to this class of encephalitis have been eliminated. As a consequence, many of these syndromes are found after nonspecific febrile illnesses associated with gastrointestinal, respiratory, or poorly defined systemic complaints. The immunological mechanisms thought to underlie this cluster of syndromes, and their pathologies, are discussed in the preceding chapter.

Smallpox has reared its head as a potential weapon of bioterrorism. Measles remains an enormous problem worldwide in developing nations. Hence, smallpox, its vaccination, and measles are specifically covered in the present chapter.

ADEM

Acute disseminated encephalomyelitis (ADEM) can follow a heterogeneous group of precipitating factors (Tselis and Lisak, 1998). When preceded by viral or bacterial infection, ADEMs are termed parainfectious or postinfectious encephalomyelitis (Miller et al., 1956). However, the same types of clinical manifestations and histopathological changes can be induced by other types of infection, immunizations (Fenichel, 1982), various therapies, and some medications. Viral causes of ADEM that are dealt with in other chapters include infectious mononucleosis and mumps (chapter 5) and influenza (chapter 10). Clearly, the discussion of certain causes of virus encephalitis as parainfectious or as ongoing infection is problematic. There appears to be evidence for each mechanism for a number of viruses. Hence, it is often difficult to determine clinically if a case is encephalitis with viral replication or if it is immune-mediated ADEM. The finding of multiple lesions on magnetic resonance imaging (MRI), usually in the white matter, is of great diagnostic benefit (Murthy et al., 1999).

Many viruses can induce ADEM. Many clinical forms can be induced by any of several viruses. In histopathologically termed perivenous encephalitis (chapter 7), there may be diffuse or multifocal lesions, many of which may not have been manifest clinically. The CNS illness can present as a diffuse encephalitis, brain stem dysfunction, cerebellar disease, and myelitis. Coupled with CNS disease can be evidence of radicular, peripheral nerve, or cranial nerve disease. Various combinations of loci of dysfunction can occur simultaneously or in succession. When the illness presents in a multifocal distribution over a prolonged period, differentiation from multiple sclerosis (MS) may be difficult, particularly if systemic signs of infection are absent (McAlpine, 1931).

An accurate history of preceding events is crucial to distinguishing parainfectious encephalomyelitis from encephalitis resulting from ongoing viral replication. The preceding illness may be poorly remembered, so questions concerning absence from school or work in the previous 3 to 4 weeks are useful. The health of family members, work or school contacts, and social contacts should be questioned to help determine if the patient suffered from a shared systemic infection. Not infrequently, the illness may have been relatively nondescript. In a study by Kennard and Swash (1981), 15 of 19 patients had malaise, fever, and myalgia, and some had nasal congestion. A history of immunizations, various therapies, and drugs must also be sought. The symptoms just named tend to occur in the first to third week prior to CNS signs. Specific viral infection, upper respiratory infection, and Semple antirabies vaccination occurred 3 days to 3 weeks prior to onset in the study of Murthy et al. (1999). Sixty-eight percent occurred within 11 days in the study of Kennard and Swash (1981). When the preceding illness is more than 4 weeks prior to CNS dysfunction, it becomes more difficult to suggest an etiologic link. Conversely, the initial illness may appear to merge with the CNS illness. This point often requires considerable effort to clarify because there are cases of encephalitis due to ongoing viral replication that start off with a systemic prodrome or minimal signs of meningeal irritation or cerebral dysfunction prior to eruption of clearly encephalitic signs. The clinical diagnosis of parainfectious ADEM is greatly facilitated by defining a period of good health following systemic illness and prior to CNS signs; such a period should be carefully sought. Multifocal findings on MRI help substantiate the clinical suspicion (Singh et al., 1999).

The patterns of onset and evolution of CNS dysfunction are pleomorphic. Headache, fever, stiff neck, and vomiting may be present. Depression of the level of consciousness, coma, seizures, and hemiparesis may occur. Optic neuritis may be found in ADEM (Apak et al., 1999) and is not a feature of encephalitis due to ongoing viral replication. Other cranial nerve dysfunction and ataxia are often present when the brain stem and cerebellum are affected. Paraparesis, quadraparesis, incontinence, and sensory loss are manifestations of a myelitic component. Although the course is usually monophasic, there are many case reports that describe more than one separate event. Miller and Evans (1953) reported the case of a woman who developed a fatal encephalopathic component 10 days after the onset of myelitic

signs. The course of the illness is also highly variable, perhaps reflecting a variety of pathogenic mechanisms. Rapid reversal in a few days or, rarely, a chronic progressive course can occur.

Representative modern figures for survival are difficult to assess. Death certainly occurs, for example, in the fulminant forms such as the acute leukoencephalopathy of Hurst (Case Records, 1999). Of 25 cases of ADEM, Murthy et al. (1999) reported no fatalities and 17 full recoveries. In the series of Kennard and Swash (1981), 1 of 19 (5%) died, 10 recovered fully and, of the 8 with residual disability, 4 could lead independent lives.

The issues of relapse and recurrence are important in differentiating ADEM from MS. This is difficult to do, particularly considering the white matter lesions seen on MRI in both conditions. However, various clinicians have made a case for relapsing ADEM as distinct from MS (Miller and Evans, 1953; Durston and Milnes, 1970). More recently, Dale et al. (2000) have differentiated ADEM and multiphasic disseminated encephalomyelitis from MS on the basis of clinical and diagnostic exams.

MRI has greatly facilitated the diagnosis of ADEM (Fig. 8.1). This is particularly so in countries in which childhood immunization is extensively implemented. The stigmata of diseases such as measles, mumps, chicken pox, and German measles as the triggering event are not present but are often replaced by nonspecific symptoms of upper respiratory or gastrointestinal illness. The appearance of multiple white and gray matter lesions on T2-weighted images with or without contrast enhancement clarifies the clinical diagnosis. While the distinction from multiple white matter lesions of MS must be made (Kesselring et al., 1990), the clinical setting following a viral illness and the absence of other episodes point toward ADEM. Although white matter lesions have been emphasized, gray matter involvement is often found, particularly in deep structures such as thalami and basal ganglia (Baum et al., 1994). This feature may be useful too in the differentiation from MS. It is important to emphasize that a negative MRI does not eliminate the diagnosis of ADEM and that serial MRIs may be required to demonstrate late-developing abnormalities (Murray et al., 2000). Conversely, while lesion resolution occurs, some may persist well after clinical recovery, as long as 18 months in the study of Kesselring et al. (1990).

Of the diagnostic methods, MRI has proven to be the most useful. Computerized tomography (CT) scanning is not as sensitive to changes in ADEM as MRI. This is unfortunate in light of the much wider availability of CT. Early reports of CT were optimistic because of the findings of white matter changes in cases of ADEM (e.g., Lukes and Norman, 1983). However, lesion definition by CT scanning in ADEM does not approach that on MRI. The cerebrospinal fluid (CSF) typically demonstrates a moderate pleocytosis and a moderate protein elevation, although a benign CSF does not mitigate against the diagnosis. The electroencephalogram (EEG) typically demonstrates bilateral slow wave activity, although unilateral predominance, sharp activity, or normality may also be found. The EEG may be useful in following the course, particularly in prolonged cases. Viral diagnostic studies are usually unrewarding. Virus isolation

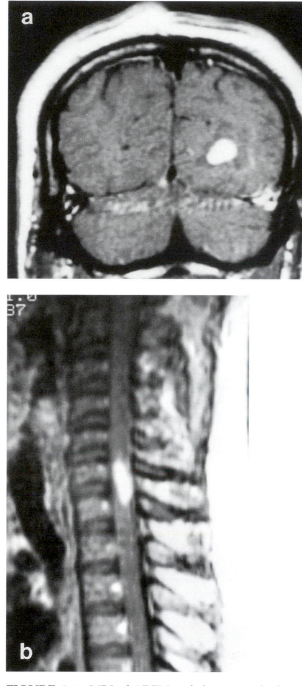

FIGURE 8.1 MRI of ADEM with lesions in the brain and spinal cord. (a) T1-weighted MRI of brain with contrast, demonstrating enhancing lesion surrounded by an area of hypointensity consistent with nonenhancing portion of lesion and edema. (b) T1-weighted MRI with contrast of cervical spinal cord, demonstrating enhancing lesion. Courtesy of Gordon Sze, Yale University School of Medicine.

attempts are almost uniformly negative, and only occasional serologic evidence for specific infection has been reported. In a research setting, CSF PCR may help to determine if minute amounts of virus serve to trigger an ADEM.

In cases in which there are clinical signs of active inflammation and in which the disease is principally of the cerebral hemispheres, differentiation from encephalitis with ongoing viral infection of the brain is crucial. The most useful diagnostic points for ADEM are a period of good health between the preceding illness and CNS dysfunction and evidence for disease at multiple sites in the nervous system. In general, the MRI will show multifocal white matter disease in ADEM, whereas contiguous areas of gray matter involvement are seen in active viral encephalitis. In cases in which clinical signs of inflammation are absent and clinical expression is clearly multifocal, differentiation from a first attack of MS may be difficult. Abrupt onset, seizures, and clouded consciousness favor ADEM. Schwarz et al. (2001) studied 40 adult patients with a discharge diagnosis of ADEM for evidence of MS on follow-up. A history of preceding infection or immunization was not required for a diagnosis of ADEM, and 35% developed clinically definite MS on follow-up at 38 months. No useful criteria to distinguish a first attack of MS from ADEM were found. A study of children by Hynson et al. (2001) concluded that a viral prodrome, ataxia, MRI demonstration of many lesions, including in deep gray matter, and the absence of oligoclonal bands favored a diagnosis of ADEM. Hartung and Grossman (H.-P. Hartung and R. I. Grossman, Editorial, *Neurology* **56:**1257–1260, 2001) noted the inability of MRI to distinguish ADEM, MS, and other white matter diseases and emphasized that reliance on MRI criteria alone would result in misdiagnosis and inappropriate therapy for MS. Hence, in cases in which the clinical and MRI distinction of ADEM and MS is ambiguous, serial follow-up will be required. Even so, recurrent episodes of ADEM need to be distinguished from MS (McDonald et al., 2001).

There has been a general tendency to treat cases of ADEM with corticosteroids. Use of these agents was originally predicated on the analogy of ADEM with experimental allergic encephalomyelitis, an immune-mediated process (chapter 7) that can be prevented by pretreatment with steroids. Early studies in the ADEM following measles were encouraging (Applebaum and Abler, 1956; Allen, 1957), but subsequent studies failed to demonstrate any benefit (Karelitz and Eisenberg, 1961; Ziegra, 1961). In the series of Ziegra (1961), the majority of patients were allocated to treatment or control groups in a sequential alternating pattern. Thus, some degree of controlled study was achieved, and no benefit was found. In studies with cases following diverse infections, the effects of steroid therapy are even less likely to be clear. However, Pasternak et al. (1980) described a group of seven children with slowly progressive disease that was interrupted by treatment with steroid therapy. In addition, there are many reports containing anecdotal experience of apparently dramatic disease reversal. Potential dangers of steroid therapy include the amplification of virus replication, the increased possibility of bacterial complications, chemical diabetes, and aggravation of stress ulcers.

More recently, other immune-based interventions have gained attention in case reports. In light of its use in acute relapses in MS, high-dose pulse therapy with intravenous (i.v.) methylprednisolone is a logical intervention. Straub et al. (1997) reported the prompt reversal of symptoms in a 27-year-old man treated with 1 g of i.v. methylprednisolone daily for 3 days. Treatment was started on the second day of neurological symptoms. No relapse followed the pulse therapy. In cases in which high-dose pulse steroid has failed or in which relapse occurred, i.v. immunoglobulin (Ig) or plasmapheresis has been reported to be successful. Pradhan et al. (1999) reported the reversal of symptoms on treatment with i.v. Ig of four children initially treated with 10 or 15 mg of i.v. methylprednisolone per kg of body weight for 3 or 5 days. The children received 5-day courses of 0.4 g/kg/day i.v. Ig and demonstrated improvement within 2 to 4 days of treatment. Sahlas et al. (2000) described two adult patients in whom high-dose pulse steroids apparently failed but who experienced symptom reversal with i.v. Ig therapy. The doses were 30 g/day for 5 days and 50 g/day for 2 days, respectively. Reasoning that steroid therapy could complicate a viral encephalitis, Nishikawa et al. (1999) successfully used i.v. Ig primary therapy in three children with ADEM. A dose of 400 mg/kg was given daily for 5 days. Consciousness was recovered from 14 h to 4 days. The authors emphasized the usefulness of i.v. Ig in cases in which a viral encephalitis cannot be distinguished.

Plasmapheresis has also been applied to the treatment of ADEM that failed i.v. steroid therapy. Kanter et al. (1995) reported two adult cases with extensive manifestations of ADEM in which i.v. steroid therapy was followed by plasma exchange. The first patient had five daily one-volume exchanges, whereas the second patient required seven daily one-volume exchanges followed by three more a week later after a clinical plateau was observed. Shah et al. (2000) reported a case of ADEM in a woman in the third trimester of pregnancy who failed to respond following high-dose i.v. corticosteroids. Following an induced delivery, symptoms improved with plasmapheresis. Relapses responded to repeat courses of plasmapheresis.

The mechanisms whereby i.v. Ig or plasmapheresis might interrupt an immune-mediated process in the CNS are multiple. Blockage of Fc receptors on macrophages, functional alteration of natural killer cells, increased function of suppressor T cells, alteration of cytokine pathways, neutralization of the complement pathway, immunoregulation by antiidiotype antibodies, blockage of antigenic sites on nerves, and promotion of remyelination have each been suggested as the mode of action for i.v. Ig (Pradhan et al., 1999; Nishikawa et al., 1999). Reciprocally, plasmapheresis may alter immune effector or regulatory mechanisms or remove toxic substances. Pradhan et al. (1999) noted that plasmapheresis in children may cause hemodynamic complications. However, i.v. Ig is also not without neurological complications. In a case report and a review of the literature, Gille et al. (1998) found reports of aseptic meningitis, cerebral infarction, and acute encephalopathy associated with i.v. Ig therapy. A large controlled clinical trial comparing high-dose pulse i.v. steroid, i.v. Ig, and plasmapheresis, including a second-stage intervention as indicated, is badly needed. Until such time, we favor the use of high-dose pulse steroid as the initial intervention in properly selected and monitored patients. On failure to respond, the selection of a repeat course of pulse steroids, i.v. Ig, or plasmapheresis will depend on particular clinical characteristics, availability, and the clinical experience of the treating center.

ACUTE CEREBELLAR ATAXIA AND RELATED SYNDROMES

General

The parainfectious syndrome resulting in acute ataxia is sufficiently dramatic in presentation that it is identified as a distinct syndrome. Usually occurring in children, it has been variously termed acute ataxia of childhood, acute cerebellar ataxia, acute cerebellar encephalitis, or pontocerebellitis. Clinical and MRI evidence demonstrates a preponderance of cerebellar and/or pontine involvement. However, clinical or imaging evidence may also demonstrate other sites of involvement in the CNS (Griffith, 1921; Maggi et al., 1997; Klockgether et al., 1993). Griffith (1921) found that preceding infection had been recorded in about three-fourths of patients, and that over half the cases occurred between 6 and 12 years of age. More recently, Connolly et al. (1994) found that 60% of the children were 2 to 4 years old. In particular, chicken pox appears as a frequent precedent, as does Epstein-Barr virus (EBV). When exanthemata are specifically excluded, approximately half of the cases are preceded by a nonspecific undiagnosed illness; the majority of these are found in infants between 1 and 2 years of age (Weiss and Carter, 1959). The interval between the preceding illness and the ataxia is usually from 1 day to 3 weeks. The ataxia is dramatic in onset and is most severe in the legs, impairing gait. Associated abnormalities include tremor and nystagmus. Depending on the expression of the particular case, alteration of consciousness, seizures, speech disturbances, and motor and cranial nerve abnormalities may be found. Fever and/or stiff neck may be found in some cases.

Spontaneous regression of the ataxia is found in the majority of patients. Weiss and Carter (1959) found that a third of the patients were asymptomatic in 3 weeks and half were asymptomatic in 3 months. However, a third were found to be symptomatic in follow-up periods ranging from 9 months to 6.5 years. The long-term defects included ataxia, eye movement disorders, speech impairment, mental retardation, and behavioral abnormalities. Griffith (1921) reported that approximately a quarter of the studied patients had some form of mental defect at the time of the last observation. Connolly et al. (1994) found that 5 of 60 patients followed up for more than 4 months had sustained learning disabilities. However, mortality is not a feature of the syndrome.

Many laboratory studies are unrevealing. In the study of Weiss and Carter (1959), tests on blood and urine were normal, and only 2 of 10 patients had elevations of the erythrocyte sedimentation rate. Lumbar punctures and EEGs were each found to be normal in two-thirds of the patients (Weiss and Carter, 1959). Lesions in the cerebellum (Pasternak et al., 1980) and in the pons (Ruutu et al., 1983) have been described on CT scan. Findings on MRI are frequently normal (Murthy et al., 1999; Connolly et al., 1994) but can demonstrate focal lesions (Maggi et al., 1997) or swelling (Bakshi et al., 1998). Neuroimaging is clearly important to exclude a posterior fossa mass.

Opsoclonus-Myoclonus Syndrome

A related but clinically distinct syndrome involving ocular oscillations and trunkal myoclonus was reported by Baringer and his colleagues (1968); it has been termed opsoclonus-myoclonus, or dancing eyes-dancing feet (Imtiaz and Vora, 1999). The syndrome is characterized by rapid intermittent oscillations of the eyes, which are increased by visual fixations; coarse jerking of the head, neck, and trunk on attempting to sit or stand; and trunkal ataxia with widespread myoclonus. Reported in eight patients who ranged in age from 5 to 38 years, it was preceded by signs suggestive of an infectious illness 4 days to 3 weeks earlier (Baringer et al., 1968). Rapid improvement occurred in the first week, most patients were asymptomatic at 6 weeks, and no recurrences were noted. Moderate CSF pleocytosis and protein elevation were found, and EEGs were normal. While the infectious agent is rarely identified, EBV has been identified in a few cases (Verma and Brozman, 2002). Symptomatic treatment such as clonazepam has been employed, as has immune-based therapy such as i.v. Ig or steroids (Imtiaz and Vora, 1999). The most important differential diagnostic consideration is systemic cancer such as neuroblastoma in children, often thoracic.

BRAIN STEM ADEM, INCLUDING BICKERSTAFF'S BRAIN STEM ENCEPHALITIS

Brain stem findings commonly occur in cases with widespread lesions of ADEM. At times, the brain stem features predominate. Lukes and Norman (1983) included a case report of a 26-year-old man who developed neurologic illness 2 weeks after a febrile illness. Findings included gaze paresis, dysarthria, emotional lability, ataxia, weakness of the face, jaw, and tongue, and weakness of three extremities. CT scan revealed swelling of the midbrain. Full recovery followed steroid treatment.

In 1951, Bickerstaff and Cloake reported three patients with a dramatic clinical picture. Ptosis, external ophthalmoplegia, facial weakness, and bulbar weakness gave a moribund appearance. However, though drowsy, the patients could be roused to a full conscious response, and no limb weakness was present. Commenting on one of the patients who had reduced hearing, the authors noted that "It was an unforgettable sight to see an apparently moribund patient, her wireless set at full volume, occasionally turning on the motor of her sucker to clear her own nasopharynx" (Bickerstaff and Cloake, 1951). Each of the patients recovered fully, although two experienced fresh symptomatology during the recovery period. Further observations underscored the generally favorable outcome. Bickerstaff identified this aspect in the subtitle of his second report (1957), "Further observations on a grave syndrome with benign prognosis." Thus, what has come to be known as Bickerstaff's encephalitis has a subacute onset with prominent signs of brain stem dysfunction in the relative absence of hemispheral dysfunction, and significant recovery often occurs. Variations in the clinical configuration occur (Al-Din et al., 1982), yet the clinical presentation is sufficiently distinct to allow recognition by others (Sandyk and Brennan, 1983; Yaqub et al., 1990; Yuki et al., 1993; M. M. Siccoli, C. W.

Hess, and C. L. Bassetti, Abstr., *Neurology* **56**(Suppl. 3): A97, 2001).

A prodromal period of 1 to 3 weeks is characterized by muscle aches, fever, malaise, and lethargy. Most series note a preceding viral or febrile illness. All six of the patients of Yaqub et al. (1990) had a febrile illness, and 6 of 10 reported by Siccoli et al. (abstr., 2001) had a "flu-like prodrome." The stage of progressive CNS dysfunction ranges from 1 to 8 weeks in duration, with an average of 2 weeks. Drowsiness, from which the patient may be aroused, reasserts itself on cessation of stimuli. Ptosis and complete or virtually complete external ophthalmoplegia evolve, sparing only downward gaze. Impairment of pupillary responses occurs. Weakness of the jaw and facial muscles with intact facial sensation is a frequent component. Paralysis of the palate, pharynx, tongue, and sternocleidomastoid muscles is observed with somewhat less frequency than facial weakness. Ataxia is a frequent finding. The deep tendon reflexes are most frequently reduced but may be increased and may be seen in combination with upgoing plantar responses. Reduced hearing has occurred, but loss of somatic sensory function is relatively unusual. In contrast to bulbar polio, dysfunction of medullary respiratory centers is not a feature of the illness.

The stage of maximal disability varies from 5 days to 4 weeks. The importance of vigorous nursing, prevention of infection, and adequate nutrition at this stage has been emphasized to prevent complications in an illness that often has a good outcome (Bickerstaff, 1978). Much improvement occurs during the first 3 weeks of recovery, although continuing restoration may go on for up to 18 months. During the recovery period, transient parkinsonism and transient psychotic states have been observed. In separate reports, one of eight (Bickerstaff, 1957) and 2 of 18 (Al-Din et al., 1982) patients expired. Significant sequelae in survivors have not been reported in this syndrome.

Laboratory studies offer no specifically diagnostic tests. The CSF may demonstrate a moderate pleocytosis and/or a moderate protein elevation. However, the CSF was normal in 8 of 17 patients studied in one series (Al-Din et al., 1982). The EEG was abnormal in 10 of 13 patients, with bilateral slow activity the principal abnormality. CT scans were performed on nine patients; results were normal for six, but demonstrated low-density lesions in the midbrain in two and in the medulla in one (Al-Din et al., 1982). MRI changes, when found, included hyperintense lesions in the brain stem (Yaqub et al., 1990; Siccoli et al., abstr., 2001). Yaqub et al. (1990) found brain stem auditory evoked potential abnormalities compatible with an upper brain stem localization. Viral studies have not revealed a consistent etiology. Most reports suggest an immune process. Yuki et al. (1993) found antiganglioside antibodies similar to those they have found in the Miller Fisher syndrome. Absent consistent virological evidence, a postinfectious immune-mediated pathogenesis appears most likely.

In light of the generally benign outlook, therapy must be vigorously supportive. Clinicians may consider the use of immune intervention such as pulse steroid, i.v. Ig, or plasmapheresis. However, there is no body of experience to evaluate such intervention. Although respiratory centers are not involved in this syndrome, the presence of medullary signs requires careful observation for the need for assisted respiration. Prevention of superinfection, venous thrombosis, and nutritional compromise is paramount. Management of symptomatology appearing in the recovery period, such as parkinsonism or behavioral change, should be symptomatic.

MILLER FISHER SYNDROME

It appears that Bickerstaff's encephalitis overlaps clinically with other syndromes. In particular, the relationship to the Miller Fisher syndrome has provoked controversy over the years. The triad of ophthalmoplegia, ataxia, and reflexia has come to be known as Miller Fisher syndrome (Fisher, 1956). Whether peripheral or central lesions, or both, underlie the symptomatology has been a matter of discussion and contention since the syndrome's first description. Fisher came down in favor of peripheral mechanisms and argued that it was a variant of idiopathic polyneuritis, the Guillain-Barré syndrome. Others have contended that the syndrome can result from a brain stem encephalitis (Al-Din et al., 1982).

Each of the three originally reported cases had symptoms of respiratory infection prior to the onset of neurological symptomatology. Similar precedent symptoms have been reported in subsequent series (Elizan et al., 1971). Once started, the evolution of neurological dysfunction tends to be swift, with maximum disability usually occurring within the first few days. External ophthalmoplegia may be associated with ptosis and varying degrees of pupillary paralysis. Ataxia may be midline or principally of the extremities, and reduced or absent deep tendon reflexes are usually found. However, variations of the clinical picture with signs of additional neurological dysfunction can be found. Elizan et al. (1971) reported 11 cases, four of which had other cranial nerve involvement. Weakness in the distribution of the facial nerve was most common, but impairment of cranial nerves V, IX, X, and XII was also found. Two patients with quadraparesis and six with impairment of vibratory sensation were included. The first patient described by Fisher (1956) had weakness in chewing, hoarseness, sensory loss, and facial weakness in addition to the three highlighted findings. Fisher (1956) noted the tendency for complete recovery, which often started within a few days of the height of disability. Nine of the patients reported on by Elizan et al. (1971) were evaluated at 1 year and were found to be normal or have only minor defects. Thus the outlook for complete or virtually complete recovery in those patients whose disease closely approximates the clinical triad is excellent. The period of recovery ranges from weeks to months (Elizan et al., 1971). The benign outlook was confirmed in a recent series of 50 patients, including 28 who received no immunotherapy (Mori et al., 2001).

Laboratory studies are useful to delineate the extent of the syndrome and to assist differential diagnosis. Only 2 of 10 patients reported on by Elizan et al. (1971) had a CSF pleocytosis, whereas 9 of 11 had an elevated CSF protein. The EEG was normal in all seven patients in whom it was performed. The EEG can be abnormal in patients with clear-cut evidence of CNS involvement. Ten of 13 patients were found to have abnormal EEGs in cases of brain stem encephalitis

(Al-Din et al., 1982). CT, MRI, and brain stem auditory evoked potential studies may be useful to define lesions.

The majority of cases appear to follow prodromes of infectious diseases. If the mechanism is parainfectious, there is the temptation to treat a presumed immunologic pathogenesis with i.v. Ig, plasmapheresis, or immunoadsorption. However, in light of the usually benign outcome, the risks of intervention must be balanced against the potential benefits (Cida et al., 1998; Mathy et al., 1998; Turner and Wills, 2000).

ATM

When myelitis appears in concert with signs of encephalitis closely following a well-defined viral illness, one is reasonably secure in the diagnosis of parainfectious ADEM. Confirmation should be sought by MRI. However, the rapid onset of transverse myelitis in the absence of signs of disseminated lesions in the nervous system is a different situation. Neuroimaging should be performed promptly to rule out a compressive mass lesion requiring intervention.

Acute transverse myelitis (ATM) is a rare illness; 1.34 cases per million inhabitants per year were found by Berman et al. (1981) and 4.6 cases per million per year were found by Jeffrey et al. (1993). Males and females were equally affected, and the ages ranged from 1.5 to 80 years. The incidence of a recognized preceding infection varies from 30 to 60%, depending on the series. In general, it appears that children have a higher incidence of a recognized preceding infection. The preceding event is often an upper respiratory illness thought to be viral in nature, but it may also be a bacterial infection, immunization, or simply a period of nonspecific malaise. Other factors such as minor trauma and obstetric delivery have been reported. The infection may precede neurological symptoms by less than 1 week to about 3 weeks. Diagnostic criteria and a diagnostic algorithm have been proposed that distinguish ADEM, MS, idiopathic or disease-associated ATM, or Devic's disease (Transverse Myelitis Consortium Working Group, 2002).

The onset of ATM may be rapid, sometimes catastrophically rapid. The fully developed syndrome of functional transection of spinal cord function may sometimes occur in under an hour. In a review of 52 patients, Ropper and Poskanzer (1978) found that 36 had a relatively smooth development of neurological dysfunction that took a maximum of 2 weeks. A subacute staccato progression, with stabilization over 10 days to 4 weeks, was found in five. Eleven had the catastrophic onset with the fully developed syndrome apparent within 12 h, but it was often complete in less than an hour. Paresthesias, back pain that is often intrascapular in location, leg weakness, and urinary retention may be found initially. At the height of the illness, most patients have sensory loss below the lesion, motor weakness, and sphincter dysfunction. From the onset to stabilization, there may be an ascending course. Lesion expansion or tissue responses to the original lesion extend both up and down the cord. However, downward extension of the lesion is clinically silent due to the damage above, hence the pattern of ascending myelitis. Fever and stiff neck are reported in a minority of patients.

The prognosis has been shown to be related to the rapidity of onset and severity of damage to the cord. Wilmshurst et al. (1998) found that rapid-onset paralysis in under 6 h, the extent of hyperintensity on MRI imaging, and electrophysiological evidence of anterior horn cell involvement portended an adverse prognosis. The potential etiologic role of fibrocartilaginous emboli in this subgroup was raised. Misra and Mandal (1998) found that severity of weakness and electrophysiological changes, including denervation, unrecordable central motor conduction time, and tibial somatosensory evoked potentials were associated with a poor outcome. Mortality is usually due to predictable causes. Urinary tract infection is common and may result in life-threatening urosepsis. Venous thrombosis occurs because of immobilization and can lead to a fatal pulmonary embolus. Respiratory insufficiency of life-threatening proportions occurs with involvement of cervical segments supplying the diaphragm and also with extension to the respiratory centers in the medulla. Aspiration or stasis pneumonia may complicate management. If these hurdles are cleared, recovery may begin between 1 and 3 months after the onset. Berman and colleagues (1981) found that no recovery could be expected unless it had started by 3 months after onset. In a compilation of the results in several reports, the outcome has been characterized as good in 42%, fair in 38%, and poor in 20% (Ropper and Poskanzer, 1978). A poor outcome was characterized as being chair- or bed-bound with urinary incontinence.

The crucial diagnostic study is neuroimaging to rule out a treatable mass lesion. Findings on MRI range from normal to high-intensity lesions over several segments with cord swelling. Al Deeb et al. (1997) found abnormal MRI exams in 10 of 20 patients studied. Diffuse high-signal-intensity T2 intramedullary lesions were found with swelling on T1-weighted images and patchy enhancement after contrast administration. Abnormalities may range from one to several spinal cord segments. Findings in the CSF are variable; however, Al Deeb et al. (1997) found pleocytosis or elevated protein or both in 94% of cases. Ropper and Poskanzer (1978) found the peripheral white blood cell count to be over 11,000 in 16 of 42 patients and the erythrocyte sedimentation rate to be less than 25 mm/h in most patients. In the absence of a well-defined viral infection preceding the ATM, viral diagnostic studies have not been systematically applied. However, attempts at CSF virus isolation or PCR identification should be made to exclude myelitis secondary to viral replication, such as VZV, herpes simplex virus (HSV), cytomegalovirus (CMV), or, rarely, human herpesvirus 6, requiring antiviral therapy.

When myelitis occurs in the presence of a defined infection for which antiviral therapy is available, antiviral compounds should be used to protect against viral destruction of the cord. The use of steroids in ATM has not been evaluated in a systematically controlled fashion, yet they are frequently used. There would appear to be two major reasons to consider their use. First, some cases of ATM are likely caused by an immune-mediated response. Second, the limiting constraints of the meninges may aggravate tissue destruction by compression as the cord swells. Autopsied specimens may show liquefaction of the spinal cord (Hughes, 1978). Therefore, the arguments for the use of steroids include interruption of an immune-mediated process and reduction of edema

and swelling in a confined space. The dangers of aggravating a superimposed bacterial infection or of extending a primary viral infection must be considered. Lahat et al. (1998) treated 10 children promptly after the establishment of the diagnosis with high-dose pulse i.v. methylprednisolone for 5 days. Recovery was rapid, with ambulation reacquired after a median period of 5.5 days. The need for a controlled trial was emphasized.

The possibility of ATM being the first manifestation of MS is important because of the potential role of immunotherapy in modulating the disease course of MS (Jacobs et al., 2000). Ropper and Poskanzer (1978) found that only 7 of 52 patients went on to a diagnosis of MS, as did only 1 of the 62 patients reviewed by Berman et al. (1981). In a retrospective analysis of transverse myelitis, Jeffrey et al. (1993) found that 21% had developed MS. MS-associated cases were clinically less severe in onset than the parainfectious cases, did not have cord swelling on MRI, and could have oligoclonal bands in the CSF. Overall, one gains the impression that patients with incomplete myelitis with selective and less severe dysfunction are at greater risk of later developing MS than severe onset cases with complete ablation of function. The occurrence of optic neuritis with myelitis in neuromyelitis optica (Devic's syndrome) may cause clinical uncertainty on occasion because viral illness or immunization can be found as an antecedent event in some cases (Wingerchuck et al., 1999).

The syndrome of sacral myeloradiculitis with urinary retention should be mentioned in the present context. Vanneste et al. (1980) described three female patients with acute onset of urinary retention who were found to have a CSF pleocytosis. The urinary dysfunction spontaneously resolved in all. Sacral hypalgesia may also be found. Pradhan et al. (1998) described similar symptoms in a syndrome they termed "parainfectious conus myelitis" and emphasized the diagnostic importance of axial views on MRI of the conus-epiconus region. The syndrome has also been recognized in men and women with anal-genital HSV infection (chapter 4). CMV radiculomyelitis, described in chapter 13 on immunocompromise, must be vigorously sought because antiviral therapy may interrupt progression of the illness. The differential diagnosis also includes other illnesses that involve the cauda equina, sacral roots, conus, or discrete descending tracts to the bladder.

ACUTE HEMORRHAGIC LEUKOENCEPHALOPATHY (HURST)

Acute hemorrhagic leukoencephalopathy (Hurst) is a rare but fulminant disorder of white matter felt to be a hyperacute form of parainfectious encephalomyelitis. Usually brief in duration and often fatal in outcome, the diagnosis has been difficult to make. However, the clinical configuration and neuroimaging findings can be sufficiently distinct to strongly suggest the diagnosis. Findings on cerebral biopsy or from specimens taken during surgical decompression can confirm the diagnosis and exclude other processes requiring different forms of therapy.

A preceding event, often a viral respiratory infection, has been identified in 80% of cases. Behan and Currie (1978) found that a viral or presumed viral illness preceded the onset in 28 of 49 patients. Bacterial infections were noted in eight, pertussis immunization in one, and drug reactions in two. No preceding event was noted in 10. The disease has also been found in association with ulcerative colitis, thrombotic thrombocytopenic purpura, acute rheumatism, asthma, and the generalized Schwartzman reaction. Roughly a quarter of the patients will have a symptom-free interval prior to the onset of neurological symptoms. The range of this interval varies widely but has an average of 4 days (Kulick, 1960). The neurological illness afflicts men more frequently than women and has its highest incidence in the third and fourth decades of life (Geerts et al., 1991).

The onset of neurologic dysfunction is often heralded by headache, malaise, and generalized weakness. The evolution is usually rapid, with the appearance of fever, depression of consciousness, vomiting, and stiff neck. Manifestations of a unilateral space-occupying lesion are frequently found. Hemiparesis or unilateral motor weakness is found in up to 50% of cases. Seizures are present in a third of the cases. Less commonly, the brunt of the illness can be on the cerebellum, the brain stem, or rarely, in the spinal cord. In the great majority of cases the illness progresses to coma with signs of increased intracranial pressure (ICP). The risk of death from lateral or central herniation is great (Gosztonyi, 1978). In fatal cases the duration of the neurological phase averages 5 days, of which only 2 days are in the precomatose state (Kulick, 1960). Although there is significant variation in the duration of the illness, there is little time for clinical indecision because the mortality rate is about 70% (Behan and Currie, 1978).

Laboratory studies offer considerable help. The peripheral white blood cell count is usually elevated, with an excess of neutrophils. The erythrocyte sedimentation rate may be elevated and albumin may be found in the urine. The CSF is usually under increased pressure and contains a pleocytosis with polymorphonuclear cells often predominating and with an elevated protein level. However, normal values for lumbar puncture have been reported in some cases. Viral isolation studies have been negative. The EEG most frequently demonstrates bilateral slowing, often with a lateralized emphasis in cases presenting as an expanding unilateral mass. Neuroimaging is crucial in the evaluation of suspected cases (Watson et al., 1984). In three histopathologically confirmed cases, Valentine et al. (1982) found the CT to be characterized by a regional hypodense swelling. Only a small area of contrast enhancement was found in one of the studies. One of the patients was a 29-year-old woman in whom the diagnosis was made by biopsy and who survived with no clinical residual found on examination at 1 year. Rothstein and Shaw (1983) reported a histopathologically verified fatal case in that the CT demonstrated a unilateral hypodense lesion that produced a mass effect. Contrast resulted in a generalized enhancement of the gray matter. Findings of diffuse edema on CT scanning, with white matter hypodensity, multifocal gray matter hypodensities, and obscuration of the gray-white matter border, were presented in a more recent case discussion (Case Records, 1999).

The clinician should have a high index of suspicion when an infection is followed by swiftly evolving hemispheral

dysfunction in the presence of fever, peripheral leukocytosis, and a CSF pleocytosis of polymorphonuclear cells. The differential diagnosis will include cerebral abscess, meningitis, subdural empyema, dural sinus thrombosis, epidural abscess, cerebral tumor, and other space-occupying lesions. The CT findings should raise the issue of acute hemorrhagic leukoencephalopathy and viral encephalitis. Consideration of biopsy is justified, despite the considerable hazards, under these grave circumstances because substantially different therapies could be indicated. Characteristic histopathological findings include vessel necrosis with fibrin impregnation and ring and ball hemorrhages. Perivascular and parenchymal infiltrates, often polymorphonuclear in type, can be found along with edema and demyelination. Characteristically, the white matter U fibers are not significantly involved. Therapy is directed towards aggressive reduction of cerebral swelling, which may be monitored by ICP measurement, combined with immunosuppressive treatment such as high-dose i.v. corticosteroids, together with plasmapheresis and cyclophosphamide (Seales and Greer, 1991; Markus et al., 1997).

ACUTE ENCEPHALOPATHY, INCLUDING REYE'S SYNDROME

General

A heterogeneous collection of cases of encephalopathy may be found in infants, children, and adults after specific viral infections, immunizations, and unidentified causes of febrile illness. Reviews of the CNS complications of specific viral infections such as influenza and rubella include descriptions of cases in which there is an absence of inflammation. Reporting a group of cases of encephalopathy of obscure origin in children, Lyon et al. (1961) found no significant evidence of inflammation in the CNS.

It is difficult to characterize a composite clinical course of encephalopathy in adults and children following nonspecific febrile illnesses. The courses range in severity from a relatively brief period of clouding of consciousness or delirium to coma with massive cerebral swelling and death. Lyon et al. (1961) pointed out the likely relationship of acute toxic encephalopathy to febrile delirium. The clinician must seek signs of a specifically treatable process. First, a broad spectrum of other disorders that can present in a similar fashion must be considered (Table 8.1). Second, the complications of the primary process and aggravating conditions must be addressed. Typical cases usually develop in the course of or soon after a febrile illness. The onset is often relatively swift, with confusion, headache, and obscuration of consciousness. Signs of diffuse cerebral dysfunction predominate, but focal and multifocal signs may be superimposed. Hyperactive deep tendon reflexes and upgoing plantar responses reflect diffusely elevated ICP. Seizures may presage the rest of the clinical picture or may appear during the course. They are frequently difficult to control during the acute stage of the illness. The lumbar puncture, often normal except for elevated pressure, may reveal slightly elevated protein. The EEG usually reveals bilateral dysfunction. The peripheral white cell count may be elevated.

TABLE 8.1 Types of disorders to be considered in the evaluation of acute toxic encephalopathy[a]

Oxygen deprivation, including anoxia and ischemia
Disordered glucose metabolism
Fluid and electrolyte imbalance
Endocrine imbalance
Toxin ingestion
Disordered temperature regulation
Drug reaction or overdose
Other organ infections
Organ failure, including hepatic encephalopathy
Hypertensive encephalopathy
Inborn errors of metabolism
Encephalitis with an acellular CSF
ADEM without CSF pleocytosis
Reye's syndrome
Idiopathic seizures, recurrent or continuous in the absence of a
    focus of infection

[a] Modified from DeVivo, 1982, and Parke, 1999.

Management principles include strict control of fluid and electrolytes to prevent exacerbation of cerebral edema. Maintenance of oxygenation and prevention of elevated partial CO_2 pressure, which will aggravate cerebral swelling, may require assisted respiration. As ICP rises, it is crucial to maintain cerebral perfusion pressure (see chapter 3). This may be attempted by corticosteroid therapy and by small pulses of mannitol to reduce cerebral edema. CT studies and careful clinical monitoring for signs of rostro-caudal compression of the brain stem are required. The use of ICP monitoring does not appear to have been applied in the systematic way in which it has been in Reye's syndrome.

The outcome is equally unpredictable. Rapid reversal may occur from the most desperate-appearing circumstances, death may supervene, or a gradual recovery with or without sequelae may evolve. The clinical description is apt to remain poorly delineated until a unifying mechanism is identified or until discrete subgroups based on pathogenesis can be defined.

Reye's Syndrome

Reye's syndrome is a life-threatening encephalopathy of childhood associated with hepatic dysfunction that usually follows influenza A or B, VZV, or other viral infection. At its peak incidence, the Center for Disease Control estimated that 600 to 1,200 cases occurred annually in the United States, with a fatality rate of 20 to 30% (Center for Disease Control, 1982). First described in 1963 by Reye et al. in Australia and Johnson et al. in the United States, its association with the use of salicylates in children for virus-induced fevers was reported by Starko et al. (1980). Confirmation was followed by the U.S. Surgeon General's advising against the use of salicylates and salicylate-containing medications in children with influenza or chicken pox (Center for Disease Control, 1982) and the addition of warnings to medication labels in 1986 (A. S. Monto, Editorial, *N. Engl. J. Med.* **340**:1423–1424, 1999). Studies in the United Kingdom (Hardie et al., 1996) and in the United States (Belay et al., 1999) have documented a remarkable decline in Reye's syndrome cases since the association with aspirin was

recognized. From 1994 to 1997, only two or fewer cases that met the case definition were reported annually through the voluntary National Reye's Syndrome Surveillance System in the United States (Belay et al., 1999).

The onset of Reye's syndrome is heralded by recurrent vomiting in a child who is recovering from a viral illness. This may be followed within a few hours or a day or two by lethargy, confusion, or irritability. Early hospitalization with glucose and electrolyte replacement may arrest progression of the illness. At the outset, fever is not present and clinical jaundice is not apparent. However, serum studies will demonstrate elevated transaminases, ammonia, and prothrombin time in the face of normal bilirubin values. Liver enlargement may be present on physical examination. Diagnostic criteria include an acute encephalopathy with the absence of evidence for infection in the CSF, liver dysfunction as manifested by fatty metamorphosis on histological examination, or a threefold elevation of hepatic transaminases or ammonia. If a child presents for medical care in the more frankly encephalopathic stages, encephalitis will be considered. However, the configuration of encephalopathy, elevated hepatic enzymes, and benign CSF in the absence of disseminated viral disease points clearly at Reye's syndrome. In cases in which the diagnosis is not clear, liver biopsy is indicated after correction of coagulation defects. On light microscopy a panlobular accumulation of lipid droplets is seen in the absence of necrosis, inflammation, and cholestasis. Low serum glucose may be seen, particularly in infants. An elevated white cell count with excess granulocytes may be found.

Rapid worsening of the encephalopathy is common and must be dealt with on an emergency basis. Clinical staging based on responses to stimuli is important to direct therapy (National Institute of Neurological and Communicative Disorders and Stroke, 1982). The critical therapeutic goal is the maintenance of cerebral perfusion by controlling raised ICP. Cerebral pathology in fatal cases has revealed cerebral swelling in the absence of inflammation with evidence of multifocal ischemia, which is often laminar in pattern (Manz and Colon, 1982). Therefore, the mean arterial pressure must remain at least 60 mm Hg above the ICP. Hence, ICP monitoring is often indicated.

Two messages are clear: avoidance of the use of aspirin for virus-induced fever in children and prompt hospitalization when the diagnosis of Reye's syndrome is suspected. However, it is unsettling to reflect that we do not understand the pathogenesis of the syndrome. Recent clusters of influenza-associated encephalopathy in Japan in children presenting with convulsions and slight to moderate liver dysfunction (Fujimoto et al., 1998) suggest that Reye's syndrome may be a special case in a spectrum of virus-associated encephalopathy in children. Further, related syndromes may exist in adults (Davis and Kornfeld, 1980).

POSTVIRAL STROKE

Stroke can occur in several types of viral infection (Table 8.2). Acute viral infection in childhood is one of the many causes of acute hemiplegia of childhood (Gold and Carter, 1976). The abrupt or subacute onset of hemiparesis

TABLE 8.2 Representative viral infections and mechanisms of stroke

Virus	Mechanisms	Reference
VZV	Necrotizing arteritis,	Mackenzie et al., 1981
	Granulomatous arteritis	Berger et al., 2000
	Giant cell arteritis	
Measles	Infarction in territory of major arterial channels	Tyler, 1957
	Infection of the vascular endothelium	Esolen et al., 1995
Nipah	Vasculitis	Chua et al., 2000
HIV	Aneurysmal dilation, thrombosis, and emboli	Kure et al., 1989
	Vasculitis	Gillams et al., 1997
HBV	Immune complex disease	Duffy et al., 1976
HCV	Mixed cryoglobulinemia	Petty et al., 1996
	Anticardiolipin antibody	Malnick et al., 1997
Rubella	Thrombosis	Connolly et al., 1975
CMV	Vasculitis	Koeppen et al., 1981
Parvo	Aplastic crisis in homozygous sickle cell disease	Wierenga et al., 2001

can be associated with seizures and fever. Tyler (1957) distinguished infarction in the distribution of major arterial channels from encephalitis in association with measles infection of children. He noted that the timing was variable with respect to the rash, ranging from before the appearance of the rash to well after it. Other childhood infections such as rubella virus have also been associated with major cerebral artery thrombosis (Connolly et al., 1975). In the adult age group, acute West Nile virus encephalitis has been found to have a neurovascular-mediated pathogenesis. Histopathological studies from the New York City outbreak in 1999 demonstrated acute microinfarctions in the medulla of the elderly patients who expired (Sampson et al., 2000). Vessel occlusion was associated with viral antigen in the neurovasculature endothelium. The newly emergent Nipah virus encephalitis appears to result from a virus-triggered vasculitis (Chua et al., 2000).

Cerebral infarction can also occur in the context of chronic viral infection. For example, Petty et al. (1996) reported two patients with hepatitis C virus (HCV) infection confirmed by PCR analysis in whom cerebral infarction occurred in association with mixed cryoglobulinemia. Malnick et al. (1997) reported finding anticardiolipin antibodies in a patient with chronic HCV infection who had suffered an infarction with quadranopsia.

While the attribution of neurological defects to comorbid factors is always a diagnostic issue, the observation of stroke and transient ischemic attack in human immunodeficiency virus (HIV)-infected individuals occurs with sufficient regularity to be a clinical issue (Shah et al., 1996; Gilliams et al., 1997). Findings include fusiform aneurysmal dilatation, potentially serving as a site for thromboembolism, and vasculitis. Kure et al. (1989) demonstrated viral antigen in the walls of cerebral vessels, suggesting a direct role for HIV infection in the vascular pathology.

Arteritis associated with hemiparesis weeks to months following contralateral herpes zoster ophthalmicus is a clear example of postviral stroke. Whereas the delay of appearance of ADEM following systemic viral infection is thought to result from the development of the immune response, the delay in the post-herpes zoster ophthalmicus contralateral stroke syndrome is thought to result from the spread of the virus from the trigeminal ganglion or along the branches of the ophthalmic division of the trigeminal nerve to the cerebral arteries (MacKenzie et al., 1981). A syndrome associating cervical VZV infection followed by delayed pontine infarction has also been recognized (Schmutzhard, 1991; Patrick et al., 1995). Migration of VZV from the C2 dorsal root ganglion via neural pathways to the vertebrobasilar circulation was proposed (Patrick et al., 1995). Berger et al. (2000) demonstrated VZV antigen in giant cell arteritis of a 4-year-old girl who succumbed from a progressive stroke syndrome 13 months after primary varicella infection. A significant statistical link between idiopathic arterial ischemic strokes and VZV infection has been demonstrated in a case-controlled study in children by Sebire et al. (1999). The age range of the children was 8 months to 8 years, and the interval after the rash ranged from 1 week to 9 months. In addition to the long delay between the manifestations of varicella or zoster and stroke, cases of stroke without VZV rash have been documented in adults (reviewed by Moriuchi and Rodriguez, 2000). Widely variable stroke syndromes have been attributed to VZV based on viral detection in cerebral vessels by modern methods (Gilden et al., 2000).

Absent isolation of VZV from spinal fluid or a positive PCR therein, intrathecal production of anti-VZV antibodies should be sought (Hausler et al., 1998). Treatment of CNS vasculitis associated with VZV has not been subjected to controlled trial. Four types of intervention are to be considered: antiviral drugs, anticoagulants, antiplatelet aggregation, and steroids (Moriuchi and Rodriguez, 2000). Little risk would appear to be attached to the use of anti-VZV medication and perhaps small risk with concomitant use of steroids. The use of anticoagulants carries some risk in the setting of weakened arterial cells at the sites of VZV vasculopathy. Inhibition of platelet aggregation by aspirin might be a suitable alternative.

SMALLPOX AND ITS VACCINATION

General

In a stunning achievement of organization, international cooperation, and thoroughness, the World Health Organization succeeded in eliminating smallpox in its 1966–1977

TABLE 8.3 Clinical types of smallpox and adverse responses to vaccination

Smallpox—pox characteristics and mortality[a]
   Ordinary—discrete pox <10%
   Ordinary—semiconfluent pox 25–50%
   Ordinary—confluent pox 50–75%
   Flat (malignant)—flat (velvety) pox >90%
   Hemorrhagic—hemorrhagic pox ~100%

Adverse responses to vaccination[b]
   Progressive vaccinia, aka:
      Vaccina necrosum
      Vaccina gangrenosum
   Eczema vaccinatum
   Postvaccinal encephalitis, encephalopathy
   Generalized vaccinia

[a]Modified from Koplan and Foster (1979).
[b]Modified from Goldstein et al. (1975) and Booss and Davis (2003).

campaign (Benenson, 1982). Worldwide in distribution, it had had a cumulative mortality of about 30% in the unimmunized. With its disappearance went the requirement for mass vaccination programs. As a consequence, much of the world's population has no protection against smallpox. Hence, smallpox is one of the most likely agents to be employed in a bioterrorist attack (Table 8.3) (Breman and Henderson, 1998), along with anthrax, tularemia, botulism, pneumonic plague, and viral hemorrhagic fevers (Varkey et al., 2002).

Smallpox (variola) is an enveloped double-stranded DNA virus, brick shaped and approximately 200 by 250 nm in size. Variola major and minor viruses cannot be distinguished by electron microscopic examination but do have different growth characteristics on chorioallantoic membranes in vitro. Other relevant members of the orthopox family of viruses include vaccinia, cowpox, and monkey pox viruses. Variola had no animal reservoir; therefore, eradication in humans allowed its complete elimination. Monkey pox can infect humans but spreads inefficiently in human populations (Jezek et al., 1983; Hutin et al., 2001). Vaccinia vaccination protects against monkey pox. Cowpox can infect humans and protect against smallpox, as Jenner demonstrated by immunizing James Phipps in 1790 (Benenson, 1982). However, vaccinia virus is a different virus, and its origin is unclear (Downie, 1970).

The spread of smallpox depended primarily on person-to-person contact by respiratory droplets and vesicle fluid, but contaminated bedclothes or clothing also contributed. The incubation period ranged from 7 to 17 days, during which time it was thought that the virus replicated in cells of the reticuloendothelial system. Overt illness developed in the toxemic stage, which lasted about 4 days. Onset was abrupt with symptoms that included fever, headache, backache, and malaise. Lysis of cells in which virus had been replicating and the consequent viremia underlay these symptoms. Virus was seeded to the skin and mucous membranes, where the first lesions were in the capillary endothelium. After 2 days, the rash appeared as a consequence of injury to the cells over the involved blood vessels. At first macular in character, the rash evolved through papular, vesicular, pustular, and scabbing

stages in about 2 weeks. It was found first on the face and upper extremities, then proceeded to the lower extremities and trunk. Massive accumulation of subcutaneous fluid could lead to the loss of cutaneous anatomy, depletion of intravascular volume, and renal failure (Kaplan and Foster, 1979). Virus could be isolated from oral mucosal lesions, skin lesions, urine, and occasionally from the eye. However, involvement of internal organs was not typically found. In the unvaccinated, mortality averaged about 30%, whereas in the vaccinated it averaged approximately 3%. Residual scarring in survivors resulted from destruction of sebaceous glands.

Various clinical forms of smallpox were seen (Table 8.3). Asymptomatic infection was demonstrated by virus isolation from the pharynx and serological conversion after clinical contact in apparently well individuals (reviewed by Benenson, 1982). Alastrim, or variola minor, was like variola major except that it was less severe and had a significantly lower mortality, around 1%, than variola major. Moreover, it spread through communities more slowly and was less easily identified; therefore, outbreaks were more prolonged. The hemorrhagic form of variola major had a mortality of over 90%. In the vaccinated, it struck the age groups in which immunity from primary vaccination had waned. Necrosis of small vessels was associated with a prolonged viremia, and death sometimes occurred before a clear-cut clinical diagnosis could be made. Pregnancy was associated with more severe and lethal disease, often hemorrhagic in type. In the flat or malignant form, which was also associated with a high mortality, the skin lesions failed to progress through the usual sequence. They were described as flat and velvety to the touch. The host inflammatory response failed to develop despite the presence of virus at the deeper levels of the skin. Finally, various modified forms of disease were seen in persons exposed to the virus who had some degree of immunity. Often there were reduced or absent skin lesions and a shortened course.

Diagnosis of smallpox depended on observation of the characteristic rash and on laboratory studies. Differentiation from chicken pox included the more superficial lesions, preferential location on the trunk, and successive crops of lesions in the same area by chicken pox (World Health Organization, 2001a). The smallpox rash was usually present on palms and soles, which is not so with chicken pox. A useful World Health Organization PowerPoint slide set to differentiate the rash of smallpox from that of chicken pox can be downloaded at http://www.WHO.int/csr/disease/smallpox/en. Also, The Centers for Disease Control and Prevention has a diagnostic algorithm for smallpox, with photographs, at http://www.bt.cdc.gov/agent/smallpox/diagnosis/evalposter.asp. Laboratory studies should include electron micrographic examination of vesicle scrapings, light microscopic observation of intracytoplasmic Guarnieri bodies in skin lesions, virus isolation in cell cultures, PCR, and antibody studies. Because of the hazard to lab personnel, these studies require Centers for Disease Control and Prevention/National Institutes of Health Biosafety Level 4 facilities. Espy et al. (2002) demonstrated that standard autoclaving eliminates infectivity of vaccinia virus, VZV, and HSV while retaining the capacity to detect viral DNA by PCR. The Centers for Disease Control and Prevention smallpox website (http://www.bt.cdc.gov/agent/smallpox/index.asp) provides information for the general public; http://www.bt.cdc.gov/agent/smallpox/index.asp also provides information for clinicians for evaluating potential smallpox cases.

Therapy can be applied after contact with a known case. Smallpox could be prevented or modified by vaccination up to 4 days after exposure (World Health Organization, 2001a). Previously, treatment with vaccinia-specific globulin or an antiviral compound, thiosemicarbazone, was found to abort the disease (Fenner, 1997; Bauer et al., 1963). The usefulness of each of these steps declined as the time from exposure lengthened. The thiosemicarbazones appear to be no longer available. The antiviral cidofovir has activity against variola, and other compounds are under investigation (LeDuc and Jahrling, 2001).

Smallpox itself was associated with neurological complications that were parainfectious in presentation (Booss and Davis, 2003). Marsden and Hurst (1932) reported 11 cases following modified smallpox, of which they regarded 7 as typical. The interval between the onset of the rash and the neurological symptomatology was 5 to 13 days, with an average of 8 days. The onset included headache, fever, back pain, and stiff neck. Cerebral signs included drowsiness, irritability, trismus, speech disturbances, facial weakness, strabismus, and paralysis. Duration of altered consciousness was between 7 and 14 days. In forms that were principally myelitic, paralysis, sensory loss, and sphincter dysfunction predominated. During recovery, some patients manifested transient emotional lability. Some fluctuations in the clinical course were seen. Of the seven typical patients, three died, and three of the survivors had some degree of spasticity. Pleocytosis, elevated protein, and normal globulins were noted in CSF. Albuminuria in the absence of urinary tract infection was also found. Of the four other cases, three appeared similar to the seven typical cases except that they were less severe in presentation. The fourth case resembled neuromyelitis optica. Future cases, should they occur, should be investigated for the presence of virus by virus isolation and CSF PCR if facilities and assays are available. Hence, while such cases appear to be parainfectious or immune mediated, evidence of the virus would lead to a reconsideration of pathogenesis and treatment with antiviral compounds such as cidofovir.

With the progressive elimination of smallpox, complications following vaccination became relatively more significant (Centers for Disease Control and Prevention, 2003a). As a live vaccine, it could replicate and spread, and in immunosuppressed individuals, fatal vaccinia necrosum could result. If the vaccinated individual or contact suffered from eczema, eczema vaccinatum could ensue. The severity of each of these conditions could be reduced by treatment with vaccinia virus Ig and thiosemicarbazone. Less severe complications included generalized vaccinia and accidental infection. Postvaccinial encephalomyelitis could not be specifically treated and was associated with a significant mortality. Of 15 cases of postvaccinial encephalomyelitis in the United States in 1968, 4 patients died (Lane et al., 1969). Concern about the use of smallpox in bioterrorism has resulted in reevaluation of the population at risk of side

effects of vaccination and in strategies to ameliorate these risks (Engler et al., 2002). Cardiac adverse events emerged during 2003 with the resumption of smallpox vaccination of targeted groups (Centers for Disease Control and Prevention, 2003b).

Postvaccinial Encephalomyelitis

Figures from the United States (Lane et al., 1969) demonstrated 2.9 neurological complications per million individuals receiving primary vaccination. Variations in the frequency with age (Scott, 1967) and type of manifestation seem most compatible with variation of the host response. An encephalopathy was seen in children less than 2 years of age, and the encephalitic response was not found before 2 years of age. In addition, the variation in incidence has been as high as 15-fold (Scott, 1967). These observations suggest that variations in the vaccine itself may have played a role in the genesis of ADEM. Stored live vaccine stocks consist of freeze-dried scraped pulp from animal skin infected with vaccinia, with phenol added (World Health Organization, 2001a). New live virus vaccine will be produced in cell cultures (LeDuc and Jahrling, 2001).

Vaccination produced a spectrum of illness in the nervous system. Thus, of 39 patients with neurological complications among 800,000 persons vaccinated in South Wales in 1962, Spillane and Wells (1964) described several central and peripheral nervous system complications (Table 8.4). Three clinical points should be made. First, although ADEM predominated, cases compatible with an encephalopathy were also seen. Second, when myelitic and encephalitic manifestations occurred simultaneously, the clinical differential was between ADEM and MS. Third, the presence of peripheral nervous system dysfunction in addition to encephalitic signs helped to secure the diagnosis of ADEM.

The incubation period from immunization to the appearance of ADEM was usually between 5 days and 3 weeks. It occurred after primary or booster vaccination (Spillane and Wells, 1964), and there did not appear to be a difference in the incubation period following primary or booster vaccination. The interval preceding the encephalopathic syndrome was more variable and could be seen within 2 days of

TABLE 8.4 Cases of neurological dysfunction following smallpox vaccination[a]

Dysfunction	No. of cases
Onset following vaccination	
Encephalomyelitis	11
Encephalopathy	3
Vasculitic component	1
Meningism	7
Epilepsy	2
Focal CNS dysfunction	3
Polyneuritis	5
Brachial neuritis	2
Exacerbation following vaccination	
Focal CNS disease	3
Epilepsy	1
Myasthenia gravis	2

[a] After Spillane and Wells, 1964.

immunization (Scott, 1967). Spillane and Wells (1964) found local vaccination responses present in all cases of ADEM, and most had axillary adenopathy. The onset in encephalitic cases was associated with confusion and an altered level of consciousness; most had fever and a stiff neck. Although depressed level of consciousness was most common, ataxia, speech disturbances, tremor, and chorea were also found. Cases of encephalopathy often presented with seizures. Others have commented on the abrupt presentation of the encephalopathic type of complication (Scott, 1967). In two of Spillane and Wells's (1964) patients with ADEM, myelitis was the principal presentation.

There was also a wide variation in the severity and type of evolution of the illness. Cases have been reported of meningism in the absence of CNS signs and CSF pleocytosis (Spillane and Wells, 1964). Also reported were cases of focal CNS dysfunction, not always monophasic, but in which other evidence for MS did not present itself. Mortality associated with postvaccinial ADEM was between 25 and 30% (Miller, 1953; Lane et al., 1969). In the cases reviewed by Miller (1953), all the deaths occurred in patients with significant encephalitic signs. Duration of CNS illness prior to death ranged from less than a day to 8 days. Miller (1953) found that the patients with transverse myelitis made a fair recovery but that some residual dysfunction occurred. Of 12 patients recovered from encephalitis, 9 had some degree of psychiatric disturbance.

Laboratory studies produced variable results. CSF pleocytosis with elevated protein was often found in the ADEM following vaccination. In contrast, CSF pleocytosis was not found in cases of encephalopathy (Spillane and Wells, 1964). The peripheral white blood cell count was normal or elevated. The EEG often demonstrated bilateral slowing, but focal features, as well as normal records, could be found. Although virus has been isolated from the brain in a few fatal cases (Angulo et al., 1964; Gurvich and Vilesova, 1983) and viral antigen has been identified in the absence of virus isolation (Kurata et al., 1977), failure to isolate virus from the brain in postvaccinial ADEM has been more common. Future cases should be investigated by CSF PCR for vaccinia virus. In the face of negative laboratory data, the diagnosis of postvaccinial ADEM depended on the clinical configuration and the temporal sequence following vaccination. White matter changes on MRI should be sought in future cases.

Because the roles of virus replication and the immune response in postvaccinial encephalomyelitis are not determined, the therapeutic strategy is unclear and should be subject to investigation (Booss and Davis, in press). Goldstein et al. (1975) reviewed the management of various complications of vaccination. For postvaccinial encephalitis, it was pointed out that vaccinia virus Ig was not effective once the syndrome was established. The use of steroids was mentioned only as a possible treatment for cerebral edema, and no mention was made concerning antiviral therapy. Should virus be isolated from the spinal fluid in postvaccinial encephalomyelitis (Gurvich and Vilesova, 1983) or CSF PCR be positive for vaccinia virus, treatment with an antiviral compound such as cidofovir should be undertaken. Methisazone had been used systemically in other complications of vaccinia virus (Jaroszynska-Weinberger, 1970; McLean,

1977) but is apparently no longer avaliable. Consequently, cidofovir would be the antiviral currently available for use (LeDuc and Jahrling, 2001). It must be emphasized, however, that neither steroid therapy nor antiviral therapy of postvaccinial encephalomyelitis has been subjected to controlled study. Careful management in an intensive care unit may be required.

MEASLES

Measles produces three CNS complications: a parainfectious encephalomyelitis, which is covered here; subacute inclusion body encephalitis (SIME) in immunocompromised children, which is discussed in chapter 13; and subacute sclerosing paraencephalitis (SSPE), which is discussed in chapter 14. Use of the live attenuated measles vaccine has markedly reduced the incidence of measles and the associated ADEM. Fortunately, the vaccine itself is 1,000-fold less likely to induce the encephalitis than natural measles. In the United States, use of the vaccine reduced the incidence of measles from an average of 315 cases per 100,000 population from 1950 to 1962 to 0.6 cases per 100,000 population in 1983 (Centers for Disease Control, 1984). In 1964, 300 cases of measles-associated ADEM were reported to the Center for Disease Control with 46 deaths, whereas in 1978, 13 cases with three deaths were recorded (Center for Disease Control, 1981). This is a particularly fortunate result because the ADEM of measles is the most fatal of those associated with childhood viral infections, and it produces the most significant percentage of sequelae in survivors.

In the year 2000, it was estimated that 30 to 40 million cases of measles occurred worldwide with 777,000 deaths (World Health Organization, 2002). It is the leading cause of vaccine-preventable deaths in children. Moreover, even in countries with widespread implementation of measles immunization programs, vigilance to maintain immunization is required. In the United States between 1989 and 1992, for example, a resurgence of measles resulted in 50,000 cases (Rota et al., 1996). Failure to sustain vaccination, particularly in urban areas, has been cited as a reason. Sequence analysis of the hemagglutinin (H) and nucleoprotein (N) genes, particularly the 450 nucleotides in the N gene coding for the COOH terminus, facilitates determination of the geographic origin of chains of infection (World Health Organization, 2001b). As of 2000, 20 genotypes were recognized among eight clades of viruses. Molecular epidemiologic analysis allowed the demonstration that of the 86 reported confirmed cases of measles in the United States in 2000, 62% could be related to importation (Centers for Disease Control and Prevention, 2002). Large-scale surveillance is facilitated by the assay of salivary IgM specific for measles to avoid the many logistical and human hurdles of serum antibody surveys (Oliveira et al., 1998). A global initiative to reduce measles, involving international, national, and nongovernmental organizations using a fourfold strategy, is under way (World Health Organization, 2002). Vitamin A supplementation with measles vaccination at age 9 months has been demonstrated to boost long-term antibody levels in children in less developed countries (Benn et al., 2002).

Measles is a pleomorphic paramyxovirus with a size range of 120 to 170 nm. It is lipid coated and contains a single-stranded RNA genome and six polypeptides. Because infection induces lifelong immunity, spread of measles requires a population of susceptibles to maintain a chain of infection. Although chronic infection can be established in the brain in SSPE, there is no evidence that the chain of infection can be sustained by other than the acute infection. A labile virus, measles is dependent on direct transmission by respiratory droplets.

Infection occurs on respiratory, nasal, and possibly conjunctival tissues (Christie, 1974). During the incubation of 12 to 14 days, widespread replication, particularly in reticuloendothelial cells, occurs throughout the body. The prodrome occurs 2 to 3 days before the appearance of the rash and is associated with a slight temperature elevation, conjunctival injection, rhinitis, swollen eyelids, and a fretful disposition. Pathognomic at this time are the appearance of Koplik spots on the buccal mucosa. These are small irregular red spots with white centers. A dry, hacking cough and somewhat enlarged cervical nodes are found. The illness is usually recognized with the development of the rash, which starts behind the ears and at the hairline and proceeds down the limbs and trunk in 2 to 3 days. It is maculopapular in type, may become confluent, and fades after 2 to 3 days in the order in which it appeared. The temperature reaches a peak of 103 to 105°F in the absence of superimposed bacterial infection but falls within 2 days. Vigor returns soon thereafter, though the rash may take days to fully fade.

Measles is associated with a significant viremia during the incubation stage, and measurable circulating antibody occurs with the appearance of the rash. Virus has been isolated from blood, urine, tears, nasal secretions, and throat (Black, 1997). The risk of transmission is greatest from a few days before to 2 days after the appearance of the rash. Therefore, patient isolation on recognition of the rash has been relatively ineffective in terminating spread of the infection. Diagnosis is usually based on the clinical recognition of Koplik spots in association with the prodromal symptoms followed by the characteristic rash. Serum IgG and IgM antibodies rise together, but the IgM component disappears within 60 days (Black, 1997). Salivary IgM is useful for disease surveillance (Oliveira et al., 1998). Complications include pneumonia, otitis media, and hemorrhagic measles as well as the neurological complications. Superimposed bacterial pneumonia must be distinguished from viral giant cell pneumonia and the bronchitis commonly associated with measles. Malnourishment has been associated with an increased incidence of superimposed bacterial infections.

Involvement of the CNS in apparently uncomplicated measles may provide clues to the pathogenesis in patients who do develop CNS illness. Thus, Hanninen et al. (1980) confirmed earlier findings that about 30% of patients with measles will have a CSF pleocytosis shortly after the appearance of the rash and 50% will have slowing on the EEG. Almost 20% of autopsied brains of measles patients have been found to have measles virus mRNA in the absence of recoverable virus (Katayama et al., 1998). The role of such findings in the later development of SIME or SSPE is of interest.

In fatal acute measles, Esolen et al. (1995) found evidence of measles in cerebral endothelial cells by in situ hybridization and reverse transcriptase PCR in situ hybridization, evidence for breakdown of the blood-brain barrier, and a reactive microgliosis. Disruption of the blood-brain barrier by infection of the cerebral vascular endothelium could arguably have a role in parainfectious measles encephalomyelitis, as well as in SIME and SSPE.

The percentage of cases of measles that go on to neurological complications varies. A generally accepted figure is 0.1 to 1 per 1,000 cases. The spectrum of neurological complications is broad, but the great majority of cases demonstrate an ADEM. Table 8.5 lists the forms observed. Similar clinical configurations were reviewed by Miller et al. (1956) in their massive compilation of the literature. They found that over 95% of cases were ADEM, less than 3% were predominantly myelitic, and fewer than 2% were principally polyradiculitis. There are no markers to predict the population at risk for any of the complications. They affect children predominantly, reflecting the age of measles incidence. Males and females have been equally affected, and there is no dependence on a preexisting state of immune dysfunction or hyperactivity. Finally, there has been no correlation between the severity of systemic measles and the risk of acute neurological complications.

The interval between the appearance of ADEM and the onset of the rash may vary up to 20 days but averages about 5 days (Johnson et al., 1984; Tyler, 1957; Miller et al., 1956). Neurological dysfunction often occurs after the start of recovery from systemic measles. It may be ushered in abruptly with a resurgence of fever, the appearance of seizures, and the rapid development of coma. Other cases are more gradual, with recrudescence of fever, headache, and meningeal irritation. Still others may be manifest with recurrent fever, agitation, and delirium. Impaired consciousness is seen in virtually all cases with cerebral symptoms. Coma may be seen in up to 45% of cases, and seizures may be seen in almost half of individually described cases (Miller et al., 1956). Hemiplegia was found in 12%, paraplegia in 8%, and ataxia in 10% of the individual cases reviewed by Miller et al. (1956). However, an upgoing plantar response was found in about 70%. Movement disorders were described in slightly over 19%, but sensory loss was rare.

TABLE 8.5 Types of CNS involvement associated with measles infection[a]

Meningitis
ADEM
   Generalized pattern
   Specific features
      Myelitis
      Retrobulbar neuritis
      Cerebellar ataxia
      Seizures
Acute hemorrhagic leukoencephalitis
Acute infantile hemiplegia
Toxic encephalopathy
Isolated retrobulbar neuritis
Toxic delirium

[a] After Tyler, 1957; Ford, 1966; and Pearl et al., 1990.

The evolution of the illness can be rapid. Miller et al. (1956) found that over 90% of the mortality occurred within the first week of neurological illness. In the postantibiotic era, a composite mortality of approximately 15% has been found (Miller et al., 1956). Prognostic features for a poor outcome include prolonged coma and extensive seizures. There has been a wide variability in the reported incidence of sequelae. Miller et al. (1956) found that 50% of survivors were described as fully recovered on discharge. However, this does not appear to have been borne out by more recent follow-up studies. Aarli (1974) found some abnormality on follow-up neurological examination of all 10 patients previously hospitalized for measles ADEM, including four who reported no symptoms. Similarly, only 1 of 10 patients followed up by Johnson et al. (1984) was found to be free of neurological sequelae. Intellectual retardation and psychiatric impairment are particularly serious problems. Seizures and impaired motor function are the other commonly described residuals.

Other neurological complications following measles are also described (Table 8.5). Although signs of spinal cord dysfunction in the presence of encephalitic signs were not uncommon, Tyler (1957) found only one case of pure myelitis among the 67 cases he reported. Similarly, Miller et al. (1956) found that less than 3% of cases were myelitis. Of 24 cases of myelitis, 75% were transverse and 25% were ascending. The onset was usually acute, with back pain, urinary retention, and progressive paraparesis. Sensory loss occurred in slightly over half the cases. Of the five deaths in cases of myelitis, four were associated with bulbar involvement. No cases of polyradiculitis were found in Tyler's series (1957), and less than 2% of cases were found in the review of Miller et al. (1956). The onset was with painful paresthesias in the limbs, which evolved to motor weakness of the limbs. Nine of 10 were reported to have had signs of bulbar dysfunction, but no deaths in cases of polyradiculitis were reported. Although signs of cerebellar ataxia were frequent, the syndrome of acute cerebellar ataxia in the absence of other signs of ADEM was rare. Hemiplegia occurred in the setting of other signs of ADEM. However, hemiplegia also came on abruptly, heralded by a seizure and associated with a poor return of function, suggesting a vascular occlusion. Tyler (1957) reported three cases of fatal toxic encephalopathy. Each was associated with increased ICP but had no focal signs, CSF pleocytosis, or CNS inflammation at autopsy. Acute hemorrhagic leukoencephalitis was reported in a 19-year-old with acute lymphocytic leukemia and measles pneumonia (Pearl et al., 1990). Finally, two relatively benign complications have been recognized. Febrile seizures can be seen, particularly about the time of the appearance of the rash (Christie, 1974), and a transient delirium common to childhood fevers may also be seen (Tyler, 1957).

As noted above, MRI is the diagnostic study of choice, with a high percentage of cases detected (Hung et al., 2000). CT scans are abnormal less frequently. Levy and Roseman (1954) found symmetric slowing on EEG in all 10 cases studied during the acute phase of encephalitis following measles. These changes cleared rapidly except in patients with seizures. Follow-up EEGs 3 to 4 years later revealed dysrhythmias, including spikes. The CSF often contains a moderate number of mononuclear cells, usually 250 or fewer per ml, which declines in the second week (Tyler, 1957). The protein is often moderately elevated, usually less than 100 mg/100 ml (Miller et al., 1956). However, the CSF may also be normal. Johnson et al. (1984) found a normal protein and cell count in 4 of 18 CSFs from patients with ADEM following measles. As noted above, a mild pleocytosis as well as slowing on the EEG can be found in uncomplicated systemic measles (Ojala, 1947; Gibbs et al., 1959; Hanninen et al., 1980).

The diagnosis is dependent on the sequence of an ADEM following clinical measles, with supportive findings on MRI. Virus isolation from the CSF or CNS has been achieved fewer than half a dozen times. These isolates have been challenged by Gendelman et al. (1984) in a study in which they could not identify measles antigens in the CNS. Because antimeasles IgM disappears from the serum within 2 months of infection (Black, 1997), it has been used to confirm the clinical impression of systemic measles infection (Fleischer and Kreth, 1983). Evidence for intrathecal production of antimeasles antibody was found in only 1 of 12 patients by Johnson et al. (1984) but was found in three of four patients by Kennedy and Webster (C. R. Kennedy and A. D. B. Webster, Letter, *N. Engl. J. Med.* **311**:330, 1984). In the study of Johnson et al. (1984), elevation of myelin basic protein was found in 6 of 10 CSF samples.

Sufficiently controlled data do not exist to make a definitive comment on the efficacy of anti-inflammatory or anti-immune therapy such as steroids. Whether treatment with an antiviral such as ribavirin directed against infection of the cerebral vascular endothelium would prove beneficial is speculative at this time. Given the marked reduction of measles-associated ADEM concurrent with use of the attenuated measles vaccine, the best hope would appear to be eradication of human measles through concerted immunization. However, clinicians must be alert to the occasional case of ADEM following immunization and also in association with apparent failure of measles vaccine (Nagai and Mori, 1999).

REFERENCES

Aarli, J. A. 1974. Nervous complications of measles. Clinical manifestations and prognosis. *Eur. Neurol.* **12**:79–93.

Al Deeb, S. M., B. A. Yaqub, G. W. Bruyn, and N. M. Biary. 1997. Acute transverse myelitis. A localized form of postinfectious encephalomyelitis. *Brain* **120**:1115–1122.

Al-Din, A. N., M. Anderson, E. R. Bickerstaff, and I. Harvey. 1982. Brainstem encephalitis and the syndrome of Miller Fisher. A clinical study. *Brain* **105**:481–495.

Allen, J. E. 1957. Treatment of measles encephalitis with adrenal steroids. *Pediatrics* **20**:87–91.

Angulo, J. J., E. Pimenta de Campos, and L. F. de Salles-Gomes. 1964. Postvaccinial meningo-encephalitis. Isolation of the virus from the brain. *JAMA* **187**:151–153.

Apak, R. A., G. Kose, B. Anlar, G. Turanh, H. Topaloglu, and E. Ozdirim. 1999. Acute disseminated encephalomyelitis in childhood: report of 10 cases. *J. Child. Neurol.* **14**:198–201.

Applebaum, E., and C. Abler. 1956. Treatment of measles encephalitis with corticotropin. *Am. J. Dis. Child.* **92**:147–151.

Bakshi, R., V. E. Baes, P. R. Kinkel, L. L. Mechtler, and W. R. Kinkel. 1998. Magnetic resonance imaging findings in acute cerebellitis. *Clin. Imaging* **22**:79–85.

Baringer, J. R., V. P. Sweeney, and G. F. Winkler. 1968. An acute syndrome of ocular oscillations and truncal myoclonus. *Brain* **91**:473–480.

Bauer, D. J., L. St. Vincent, C. H. Kempe, and A. W. Donnie. 1963. Prophylactic treatment of smallpox contacts with N-methylistatin β-thiosemi-carbazone. *Lancet* **ii**:494–496.

Baum, P. A., A. J. Barkovich, T. K. Koch, and B. O. Berg. 1994. Deep gray matter involvement in children with acute disseminated encephalomyelitis. *Am. J. Neuroradiol.* **15**:1275–1283.

Behan, P. O., and S. Currie. 1978. Acute haemorrhagic leucoencephalitis, p. 34–48. *In Clinical Neuroimmunology.* W. B. Saunders Co., London, United Kingdom.

Belay, E. D., J. S. Bresee, R. C. Holman, A. S. Khan, A. Shahriari, and L. B. Schonberger. 1999. Reye's syndrome in the United States from 1981 through 1997. *N. Engl. J. Med.* **340**:1377–1382.

Benenson, A. S. 1982. Smallpox, p. 541–568. *In* A. S. Evans (ed.), *Viral Infections of Humans, Epidemiology and Control,* 2nd ed. Plenum Press, New York, N.Y.

Benn, C. S., A. Balde, E. George, M. Kidd, H. Whittle, I. M. Lisse, and P. Aaby. 2002. Effect of vitamin A supplementation on measles-specific antibody levels in Guinea-Bissau. *Lancet* **359**:1313–1314.

Berger, T. M., J. G. Cadiff, and J.-A. Gebbers. 2000. Fatal varicella zoster virus antigen-positive giant cell arteritis of the central nervous system. *Pediatr. Infect. Dis. J.* **19**:653–656.

Berman, M., S. Feldman, M. Alter, N. Zilber, and E. Kahana. 1981. Acute transverse myelitis: incidence and etiologic considerations. *Neurology* **31**:966–971.

Bickerstaff, E. R. 1957. Brain-stem encephalitis. Further observations on a grave syndrome with benign prognosis. *Br. Med. J.* **1**:1384–1387.

Bickerstaff, E. R. 1978. Brain stem encephalitis (Bickerstaff's encephalitis), p. 605–609. *In* P. J. Vinken and G. W. Bruyn, in collaboration with H. L. Klawans (ed.), *Handbook of Clinical Neurology,* Part II, *Infections of the Nervous System,* vol. 34. North-Holland Publishing Co., Amsterdam, The Netherlands.

Bickerstaff, E. R., and P. C. P. Cloake. 1951. Mesencephalitis and rhombencephalitis. *Br. Med. J.* **2**:77–81.

Black, F. L. 1997. Measles, p. 507–529. *In* A. S. Evans and R. A. Kaslow (ed.), *Viral Infections of Humans. Epidemiology and Control,* 4th ed. Plenum Medical Book Company, New York, N.Y.

Booss, J., and L. B. Davis. 2003. Smallpox and smallpox vaccination: neurological implications. *Neurology* **60**: in press.

Breman, J. G., and D. A. Henderson. 1998. Poxvirus dilemmas—monkeypox, smallpox, and biologic terrorism. *N. Engl. J. Med.* **339**:556–559.

Case Records of the Massachusetts General Hospital. 1999. Case 1–1999. A 53-year-old man with fever and rapid neurologic deterioration. *N. Engl. J. Med.* **340**:127–135.

Center for Disease Control. 1981. Encephalitis surveillance—annual summary 1978.

Center for Disease Control. 1982. Surgeon general's advisory on the use of salicylates and Reye syndrome. *Morb. Mortal. Wkly. Rep.* **31**:289–290.

Centers for Disease Control. 1984. Measles—United States, 1983. *Morb. Mortal. Wkly. Rep.* **33**:105–108.

Centers for Disease Control and Prevention. 2002. Measles—United States, 2000. *Morb. Mortal. Wkly. Rep.* **51**:120–123.

Centers for Disease Control and Prevention. 2003a. Smallpox vaccination and adverse reactions. Guidance for clinicians. *Morb. Mortal. Wkly. Rep.* **52**-(RR-4):1–29.

Centers for Disease Control and Prevention. 2003b. Cardiac adverse events following smallpox vaccination—United States, 2003. *Morb. Mortal. Wkly. Rep.* **52**:248–250.

Christie, A. B. 1980. Measles (Morbilli), p. 357–386. *In Infectious Diseases: Epidemiology and Clinical Practice,* 3rd ed. Churchill Livingstone, Edinburgh, Scotland.

Chua, K. B., W. J. Bellini, P. A. Rota, B. H. Harcourt, A. Tamin, S. K. Lam, T. G. Ksiazek, P. E. Rollin, S. R. Zaki, W.-J. Shieh, C. S. Goldsmith, D. J. Gubler, J. T. Roehrig, B. Easton, A. R. Gould, J. Olson, H. Field, P. Daniels, A. E. Ling, C. J. Peters, L. J. Andereson, and B. W. J. Mahy. 2000. Nipah virus: a recently emergent deadly paramyxovirus. *Science* **288**:1432–1435.

Cida, K., S. Takase, and Y. Itoyama. 1998. Development of facial palsy during immunoadsorption plasmapheresis in Miller Fisher Syndrome: a clinical report of two cases. *J. Neurol. Neurosurg. Psychiatr.* **64**:399–401.

Connolly, J. H., W. M. Hutchinson, I. V. Allen, J. A. Lyttle, M. W. Swallow, E. Dermott, and D. Thomas. 1975. Carotid artery thrombosis, encephalitis, myelitis, and optic neuritis associated with rubella virus infections. *Brain* **98**:583–594.

Connolly, A. M., W. E. Dodson, A. L. Prensky, and R. S. Rust. 1994. Course and outcome of acute cerebellar ataxia. *Ann. Neurol.* **35**:673–679.

Dale, R. C., C. deSousa, W. K. Chong, C. S. Cox, B. Harding, and B. G. R. Neville. 2000. Acute disseminated encephalomyelitis, multiphasic disseminated encephalomyelitis, and multiple sclerosis in children. *Brain* **123**:2407–2422.

Davis, L. E., and M. Kornfeld. 1980. Influenza A virus and Reye's syndrome in adults. *J. Neurol. Neurosurg. Psychiatr.* **43**:516–521.

DeVivo, D. C. 1982. Acute encephalopathies of childhood, p. 1605–1613. *In* A. M. Rudolph, J. I. E. Hoffman, and S. Axelrod (ed.), *Pediatrics,* 17th ed. Appleton Century-Crofts, Norwalk, Conn.

Downie, A. W. 1970. Smallpox, p. 487–518. *In* S. Mudd (ed.), *Infectious Agents and Host Reactions.* W. B. Saunders Co., Philadelphia, Pa.

Duffy, J., M. D. Lidsky, J. T. Sharp, J. S. Davis, D. A. Person, B. Hollinger, and K.-W. Min. 1976. Polyarthritis, polyarteritis, and hepatitis B. *Medicine* **55**:19–37.

Durston, J. H. J., and J. N. Milnes. 1970. Relapsing encephalomyelitis. *Brain* **93**:715–730.

Elizan, T. S., J. P. Spire, R. M. Andiman, F. A. Baughman, Jr., and D. L. Lloyd-Smith. 1971. Syndrome of acute idiopathic ophthalmoplegia with ataxia and areflexia. *Neurology* **21**:281–292.

Engler, R. J. M., J. Kenner, and D. Y. M. Leung. 2002. Smallpox vaccination: risk considerations for patients with atopic dermatitis. *J. Allergy Clin. Immunol.* **110**:357–365.

Esolen, L. M., K. Takahashi, R. T. Johnson, A. Vaisberg, T. R. Moench, S. L. Wesselingh, and D. E. Griffin. 1995. Brain endothelial cell infection in children with acute fatal measles. *J. Clin. Investig.* **96**:2478–2481.

Espy, M. J., J. R. Uhl, L. M. Sloan, J. E. Rosenblatt, F. R. Cockerill, III, and T. F. Smith. 2002. Detection of vaccinia virus, herpes simplex virus, varicella-zoster virus, and bacillus anthracis DNA by LightCycler polymerase chain reaction after autoclaving: implications for biosafety of bioterrorism agents. *Mayo Clin. Proc.* **77**:624–628.

Fenichel, G. M. 1982. Neurological complications of immunization. *Ann. Neurol.* **12**:119–128.

Fenner, F. 1997. Poxviruses, p. 357–373. *In* D. D. Richman, F. J. Whitley, and F. G. Hayden (ed.), *Clinical Virology.* Churchill Livingstone, New York, N.Y.

Fisher, M. 1956. An unusual variant of acute idiopathic polyneuritis (syndrome of ophthalmoplegia, ataxia, and areflexia). *N. Engl. J. Med.* **255:**57–65.

Fleischer, B., and H. W. Kreth. 1983. Clonal expansion and functional analysis of virus-specific T lymphocytes from cerebrospinal fluid in measles encephalitis. *Hum. Immunol.* **7:**239–248.

Ford, F. R. 1966. Intoxications due to infections. Disseminated encephalomyelitis or myelinoclasis following measles, p. 555–569. *In Diseases of the Nervous System in Infancy, Childhood and Adolescence,* 5th ed. Thomas, Springfield, Ill.

Fujimoto, S., M. Kobayashi, O. Uemura, M. Iwasa, T. Ando, T. Katoh, C. Nakamura, N. Maki, H. Togari, and Y. Wada. 1998. PCR on spinal fluid to show influenza-associated acute encephalopathy or encephalitis. *Lancet* **352:**873–875.

Geerts, Y., I. Deheane, and M. Lammens. 1991. Acute hemorrhagic leucoencephalitis. *Acta Neurol. Belg.* **91:**201–211.

Gendelman, H. E., J. S. Wolinsky, R. T. Johnson, N. J. Pressman, G. H. Pezeshkpour, and G. F. Boisset. 1984. Measles encephalomyelitis: lack of evidence of viral invasion of the central nervous system and quantitative study of the nature of demyelination. *Ann. Neurol.* **15:**353–360.

Gibbs, F. A., E. L. Gibbs, P. R. Carpenter, and H. W. Spies. 1959. Electroencephalographic abnormality in 'uncomplicated' childhood diseases. *JAMA* **171:**1050–1055.

Gilden, D. H., B. K. Kleinschmidt-DeMasters, J. J. LaGuardia, R. Mahaling, and R. J. Cohrs. 2000. Neurologic complications of the reactivation of Varicella-Zoster Virus. *N. Engl. J. Med.* **342:**635–645.

Gillams, A. R., E. Allen, K. Hrieb, N. Venna, D. Craven, and A. P. Carter. 1997. Cerebral infarction in patients with AIDS. *Am. J. Neuroradiol.* **18:**1581–1585.

Gille, M. I., M. Van Raemdonck, F. Delbecq, and J. Depre. 1998. Neurological complications of intravenous immunoglobulin (I.V. Ig) therapy: an illustrative case of acute encephalopathy following I.V. Ig therapy and a review of the literature. *Acta Neurol. Belg.* **98:**347–351.

Gold, A. P., and S. Carter. 1976. Acute hemiplegia of infancy and childhood. *Pediatr. Clin. North Am.* **23:**413–433.

Goldstein, J. A., J. M. Neff, J. M. Lane, and J. P. Koplan. 1975. Smallpox vaccination reactions, prophylaxis, and therapy of complications. *Pediatrics* **55:**342–347.

Gosztonyi, G. 1978. Acute haemorrhagic leucoencephalitis (Hurst's disease), p. 587–604. *In* P. J. Vinken and G. W. Bruyn (ed.), in collaboration with H. L. Klawans, *Handbook of Clinical Neurology, Part II, Infections of the Nervous System,* vol. 34. North-Holland Publishing Co., Amsterdam, The Netherlands.

Griffith, J. P. C. 1921. Acute cerebellar encephalitis (acute cerebellar ataxia). *Am. J. Med. Sci.* **162:**781–789.

Gurvich, E. B., and L. S. Vilesova. 1983. Vaccinia virus in postvaccinal encephalitis. *Acta Virol.* **27:**154–159.

Hanninen, P., P. Arstila, H. Lang, A. Salmi, and M. Panelius. 1980. Involvement of the central nervous system in acute, uncomplicated measles virus infection. *J. Clin. Microbiol.* **36:**299–301.

Hardie, R. M., L. H. Newton, J. C. Bruce, J. F. T. Glasgow, A. P. Mowat, J. B. P. Stephenson, and S. M. Hall. 1996. The changing clinical pattern of Reye's Syndrome. 1982–1990. *Arch. Dis. Child.* **74:**400–405.

Hausler, M. G., V. T. Ramaekers, J. Reul, R. Meilicke, and G. Heimann. 1998. Early and late onset of cerebral vasculitis related to varicella zoster. *Neuropediatrics* **29:**202–207.

Hughes, J. T. 1978. Acute necrotic myelopathy, p. 209–217. *In Pathology of the Spinal Cord,* 2nd ed. Lloyd-Luke Ltd., London, United Kingdom.

Hung, K.-L., H.-T. Liao, and M.-L. Tsai. 2000. Postinfectious encephalomyelitis: etiologic and diagnostic trends. *J. Child. Neurol.* **15:**666–670. (Erratum, **15:**802.)

Hutin, Y. J. F., R. J. Williams, P. Malfait, R. Pebody, V. N. Loparev, S. L. Ropp, M. Rodriguea, J. C. Knight, F. K. Tshioko, A. S. Khan, M. V. Szczeniowski, and J. J. Esposito. 2001. Outbreak of human monkeypox, Democratic Republic of Congo, 1996–1997. *Emerg. Infect. Dis.* **7:**434–438.

Hynson, J. L., A. J. Kornberg, L. T. Coleman, L. Shield, A. S. Harvey, and M. J. Kean. 2001. Clinical and neuroradiologic features of acute disseminated encephalomyelitis in children. *Neurology* **56:**1308–1312.

Imtiaz, K. E., and J. P. Vora. 1999. Dancing eyes-dancing feet. *Lancet* **354:**390.

Jacobs, L. D., R. W. Beck, J. H. Simon, R. P. Kinkel, C. M. Brownscheidle, T. J. Murray, N. A. Simonian, P. J. Slasor, and A. W. Sandrock. 2000. Intramuscular interferon Beta-1α therapy initiated during a first demyelinating event in Multiple Sclerosis. *N. Engl. J. Med.* **343:**898–904.

Jaroszynska-Weinberger, B. 1970. Treatment with methisazone of complications following smallpox vaccination. *Arch. Dis. Child.* **45:**573–580.

Jeffrey, D. R., R. N. Mandler, and L. E. Davis. 1993. Transverse myelitis. Retrospective analysis of 33 cases, with differentiation of cases associated with Multiple Sclerosis and parainfectious events. *Arch. Neurol.* **50:**532–535.

Jezek, Z., A. I. Gromyko, and M. V. Szczeniowsk. 1983. Human monkeypox. *J. Hyg. Epidemiol. Microbiol. Immunol.* **27:**13–28.

Johnson, G. M., T. D. Scurletis, and N. B. Carroll. 1963. A study of 16 fatal cases of encephalitis-like disease in North Carolina children. *N. Carolina Med. J.* **24:**464–473.

Johnson, R. T., D. E. Griffin, R. L. Hirsch, J. S. Wolinsky, S. Roedenbeck, I. L. de Soriano, and A. Vaisberg. 1984. Measles encephalomyelitis-clinical and immunological studies. *N. Engl. J. Med.* **310:**137–141.

Kanter, D. S., D. Horenshy, R. A. Sperling, J. D. Kaplan, M. E. Malachowski, and W. H. Churchill, Jr. 1995. Plasmapheresis in fulminant acute disseminated encephalomyelitis. *Neurology* **45:**824–827.

Karelitz, S., and M. Eisenberg. 1961. Measles encephalitis. Evaluation of treatment with adrenocorticotropin and adrenal corticosteroids. *Pediatrics* **27:**811–818.

Katayama, Y., K. Kohso, A. Nishimura, Y. Tatsuno, M. Homma, and H. Hotta. 1998. Detection of measles virus mRNA from autopsied human tissues. *J. Clin. Microbiol.* **36:**299–301.

Kennard, C., and M. Swash. 1981. Acute viral encephalitis. Its diagnosis and outcome. *Brain* **104:**129–148.

Kesselring, J., D. H. Miller, J. A. Robb, B. E. Kendall, I. F. Moseley, D. Kinsley, E. P. G. H. duBoulay, and W. I. McDonald. 1990. Acute disseminated encephalomyelitis. MRI findings and the distinction from multiple sclerosis. *Brain* **113:**291–302.

Klockgether, T., G. Doller, U. Wullner, D. Petersen, and J. Dichgans. 1993. Cerebellar encephalitis in adults. *J. Neurol.* **240:**17–20.

Koeppen, A. H., L. S. Lansing, J.-K. Peng, and R. S. Smith. 1981. Central nervous system vasculitis in cytomegalovirus infection. *J. Neurol. Sci.* **51:**395–410.

Kono, R., N. Uchida, A. Sasagawa, Y. Akao, H. Kodama, J. Mukoyama, and T. Jujwara. 1973. Neurovirulence of acute haemorrhagic conjunctivitis virus in monkeys. *Lancet* **i:**61–63.

Koplan, J. F., and S. O. Foster. 1979. Smallpox: clinical types, causes of death, and treatment. *J. Infect. Dis.* **140:**440–441.

Kulick, S. A. 1960. Acute hemorrhagic leukoencephalitis: report of a case and review of the literature. *Boston Med. Q.* **11:**120–130.

Kurata, T., Y. Aoyama, and T. Kitamura. 1977. Demonstration of vaccinia virus antigen in brains of postvaccinal encephalitis cases. *Jpn. J. Med. Sci. Biol.* **30:**137–147.

Kure, K., Y. D. Park, T.-S. Kim, W. D. Lyman, G. Lantos, S. Lee, S. Cho, A. L. Belman, K. M. Weidenheim, and D. W. Dickson. 1989. Immunohistochemical localization of an HIV epitope in cerebral aneurysmal arteriopathy in pediatric acquired immunodeficiency syndrome (AIDS). *Pediatr. Pathol.* **9:**655–667.

Lahat, E., G. Pillar, S. Ravid, A. Barzilai, A. Etzioni, and E. Shahar. 1998. Rapid recovery from transverse myelopathy in children treated with methylprednisolone. *Pediatr. Neurol.* **19:**279–282.

Lane, J. M., F. L. Ruben, J. M. Neff, and J. D. Millar. 1969. Complications of smallpox vaccination, 1968. National surveillance in the United States. *N. Engl. J. Med.* **281:**1201–1208.

LeDuc, J. L., and P. B. Jahrling. 2001. Strengthening national preparedness for smallpox: an update. *Emerg. Infect. Dis.* **7:**155–157.

Levy, L. L., and E. Roseman. 1954. Electroencephalographic studies of the encephalopathies. III. Serial studies in measles encephalitis. *Am. J. Dis. Child.* **88:**5–14.

Lukes, S. A., and D. Norman. 1983. Computed tomography in acute disseminated encephalomyelitis. *Ann. Neurol.* **13:**567–572.

Lyon, G., P. R. Dodge, and R. D. Adams. 1961. The acute encephalopathies of obscure origin in infants and children. *Brain* **84:**680–708.

Mackenzie, R. A., G. S. Forbes, and W. E. Karnes. 1981. Angiographic findings in herpes zoster arteritis. *Ann. Neurol.* **10:**458–464.

Maggi, G., A. Varone, and F. Alberti. 1997. Acute cerebellar ataxia in children. *Childs Nerv. Syst.* **13:**542–545.

Malnick, S. D. H., Y. Abend, E. Evron, and Z. M. Sthoeger. 1997. HCV hepatitis associated with anticardiolipin antibody and a cerebrovascular accident. *J. Clin. Gastroenterol.* **24:**401–442.

Manz, H. J., and A. R. Colon. 1982. Neuropathology, pathogenesis, and neuropsychiatric sequelae of Reye syndrome. *J. Neurol. Sci.* **53:**377–395.

Markus, R., B. J. Brew, J. Turner, and M. Pell. 1997. Successful outcome with aggressive treatment of acute hemorrhagic leukoencephalitis. *J. Neurol. Neurosurg. Psychiatr.* **63:**551.

Marsden, J. P., and E. W. Hurst. 1932. Acute perivascular myelinoclasis (acute disseminated encephalomyelitis) in smallpox. *Brain* **55:**181–225.

Mathy, I., M. Gille, F. Van Raemdonck, J. Delbecq, and A. Depre. 1998. Neurological complications of intravenous immunoglobulin (IV Ig) therapy: an illustrative case of acute encephalopathy following IV Ig therapy and a review of the literature. *Acta Neurol. Belg.* **98:**347–351.

McAlpine, D. 1931. Acute disseminated encephalomyelitis: its sequelae and its relationship to disseminated sclerosis. *Lancet* **i:**846–852.

McDonald, W. I., A. Compston, G. Edan, D. Goodkin, H.-P. Hartung, F. D. Lublin, H. F. McFarland, D. W. Paty, C. H. Polman, S. C. Rheingold, M. Sandbert-Wollheim, W. Sibley, A. Thompson, S. van den Noort, B. Y. Weinshenker, and J. S. Wolinsky. 2001. Recommended diagnostic criteria for MS: Guidelines from the International Panel on the Diagnosis of MS. *Ann. Neurol.* **50:**121–127.

McLean, D. M. 1977. Methisazone therapy in pediatric vaccinia complications. *Ann. N.Y. Acad. Sci.* **284:**118–121.

Miller, H. G. 1953. Prognosis of neurologic illness following vaccination against smallpox. *Arch. Neurol. Psychiatr.* **69:**695–706.

Miller, H. G., and M. J. Evans. 1953. Prognosis in acute disseminated encephalomyelitis: with a note on neuromyelitis optica. *Q. J. Med.* **22:**347–379.

Miller, H. G., J. B. Stanton, and J. L. Gibbons. 1956. Parainfectious encephalomyelitis and related syndromes. *Q. J. Med.* **25:**427–505.

Misra, K. J., and S. K. Mandal. 1998. Prognostic predictors of acute transverse myelitis. *Acta Neurol. Scand.* **98:**60–63.

Mori, M., S. Kuwabara, T. Fukutake, Y. Nobuhiro, and T. Hattori. 2001. Clinical features and prognosis of Miller Fisher syndrome. *Neurology* **56:**1104–1106.

Moriuchi, H., and W. Rodriguez. 2000. Role of varicella-zoster virus in stroke syndromes. *Pediatr. Infect. Dis. J.* **19:**648–653.

Murray, B. J., D. Apetauerova, and T. E. Scammell. 2000. Severe acute disseminated encephalomyelitis with normal MRI at presentation. *Neurology* **55:**1237–1238.

Murthy, J. M. K., R. Yangala, A. K. Meena, and J. J. Reddy. 1999. Acute disseminated encephalomyelitis: clinical and MRI study from South India. *J. Neurol. Sci.* **165:**133–138.

Nagai, K., and T. Mori. 1999. Acute disseminated encephalomyelitis with probable measles vaccine failure. *Pediatr. Neurol.* **20:**399–402.

National Institute of Neurological and Communicative Disorders and Stroke. 1982. The diagnosis and treatment of Reye's syndrome (consensus development summary). *Conn. Med.* **46:**138–142.

Nishikawa, M., T. Ichiyama, T. Hayashi, K. Ouchi, and S. Furukawa. 1999. Intravenous immunoglobulin therapy in acute disseminated encephalomyelitis. *Pediatr. Neurol.* **21:**583–586.

Ojala, A. 1947. On changes in the cerebrospinal fluid during measles. *Ann. Med. Intern. Fenn.* **36:**321–331.

Oliveira, S. A., M. M. Siqueira, D. W. G. Brown, L. A. B. Comacho, T. Faillace, and B. J. Cohen. 1998. Salivary diagnosis of measles for surveillance: a clinic-based study in Niterói state of Rio de Janeiro, Brazil. *Trans. R. Soc. Trop. Med. Hyg.* **92:**936–938.

Parke, J. T. 1999. Acute encephalopathies, p. 1917–1923. *In* J. A. McMillan, C. D. Deangelis, R. D. Feigin, and J. B. Warshaw (ed.), *Oski's Pediatrics. Principles and Practice.* Lippincott-Williams & Wilkins, Philadelphia, Pa.

Pasternak, J. F., D. C. DeVivo, and A. L. Prensky. 1980. Steroid-responsive encephalomyelitis in childhood. *Neurology* **30:**481–486.

Patrick, J. T., E. Russell, J. Meyer, J. Biller, and J. L. Saver. 1995. Cervical (C2) herpes-zoster infection followed by pontine infarction. *J. Neuroimag.* **5:**192–193.

Pearl, P. L., H. Abu-Farsakh, J. R. Starke, Z. Dreyer, P. T. Louis, and J. B. Kirkpatrick. 1990. Neuropathology of two fatal cases of measles in the 1988–1989 Houston epidemic. *Pediatr. Neurol.* **6:**126–130.

Peatfield, R. C. 1987. Basal ganglia damage and subcortical dementia after possible insidious Coxsackie Virus Encephalitis. *Acta Neurol. Scand.* **76:**340–345.

Petty, G. W., J. Duffy, and J. Huston, III. 1996. Cerebral ischemia in patients with hepatitis C virus infection and mixed cryoglobulinemia. *Mayo Clin. Proc.* **71:**671–678.

Pradhan, S., R. K. Gupta, R. Kapoor, S. Shashank, and M. K. Kathuria. 1998. Parainfectious conus myelitis. *J. Neurol. Sci.* **161:**156–162.

Pradhan, S., R. P. Gupta, S. Shashank, and N. Pandry. 1999. Intravenous immunoglobulin therapy in acute disseminated encephalomyelitis. *J. Neurol. Sci.* **165:**56–61.

Reye, R. D. K., G. Morgan, and J. Baral. 1963. Encephalopathy and fatty degeneration of the viscera. A disease entity in childhood. *Lancet* ii:749–752.

Ropper, A. H., and D. C. Poskanzer. 1978. The prognosis of acute and subacute transverse myelopathy based on early signs and symptoms. *Ann. Neurol.* 4:51–59.

Rota, J. S., J. L. Heath, P. A. Rota, G. E. King, M. L. Celma, J. Carabana, R. Fernandez-Munoz, D. Brown, L. Jin, and W. J. Bellini. 1996. Molecular epidemiology of measles virus: identification of pathways of transmission and implications for measles virus transmission. *J. Infect. Dis.* 173:32–37.

Rothstein, T. L., and C.-M. Shaw. 1983. Computed tomography as a diagnostic aid in acute haemorrhagic leukoencephalitis. *Ann. Neurol.* 13:331–333.

Ruutu, P., M. Partinen, M. Livanainen, K. Aho, and P. Jaatinen. 1983. Pontocerebellitis—a rare manifestation of mononucleosis. *J. Neurol. Neurosurg. Psychiatr.* 46:81–82.

Sahlas, D. J., S. P. Miller, M. Guerin, M. Veilleux, and G. Francis. 2000. Treatment of acute disseminated encephalomyelitis with intravenous immunoglobulin. *Neurology* 54:1370–1372.

Sampson, B. A., C. Ambrosi, A. Charlot, K. Reiber, J. F. Veress, and V. Armbrustmacher. 2000. The pathology of human West Nile Virus infection. *Hum. Pathol.* 31:527–531.

Sandyk, R., and M. J. W. Brennan. 1983. Bickerstaff's brain stem encephalitis in Johannesburg. A case report. *S. Afr. Med. J.* 64:179–180.

Schmutzhard, W. J. 1991. Cervical herpes-zoster and delayed brain stem infarction. *Clin. Neurol. Neurosurg.* 93:245–247.

Schwarz, S., A. Mohr, M. Knauth, B. Wildemann, and B. Storch-Hagenlocher. 2001. Acute disseminated encephalomyelitis. A follow-up study of 40 adult patients. *Neurology* 56:1313–1318.

Scott, T. F. M. 1967. Postinfectious and vaccinal encephalitis. *Med. Clin. North Am.* 51:701–717.

Seales, D., and M. Greer. 1991. Acute hemorrhagic leukoencephalitis. A successful recovery. *Arch. Neurol.* 48:1086–1088.

Scbire, G., L. Meyer, and S. Chabrier. 1999. Varicella as a risk factor for cerebral infarction in childhood: a case-controlled study. *Ann. Neurol.* 45:679–680.

Shah, S. S., R. A. Zimmerman, L. B. Rorke, and L. G. Vezina. 1996. Cerebrovascular complications of HIV in children. *AJNR (Am. J. Neuroradiol.)* 17:1913–1917.

Shah, A. K., A. Tselis, and B. Mason. 2000. Acute disseminated encephalomyelitis in a pregnant woman successfully treated with plasmapheresis. *J. Neurol. Sci.* 174:147–151.

Singh, S., M. Alexander, and I. P. Korah. 1999. Acute disseminated encephalomyelitis: MR imaging features. *AJR Am. J. Roentgenol.* 173:1101–1107.

Spillane, J. D., and C. E. C. Wells. 1964. The neurology of Jennerian vaccination. *Brain* 87:1–44 *and four plates.*

Starko, K. M., C. G. Ray, L. B. Dominguez, W. L. Stromberg, and D. F. Woodall. 1980. Reye's syndrome and salicylate use. *Pediatrics* 66:859–864.

Straub, J., M. Chofflon, and J. Delavelle. 1997. Early high dose intravenous methylprednisolone in acute disseminated encephalomyelitis: a successful recovery. *Neurology* 49:1145–1147.

Transverse Myelitis Consortium Working Group. 2002. Proposed diagnostic criteria and nosology of acute transverse myelitis. *Neurology* 59:499–505.

Tselis, A. C., and R. P. O. Lisak. 1998. Acute disseminated encephalomyelitis, p. 116–147. *In* J. Antel (ed.), *Clinical Neuroimmunology.* Blackwell Science, Oxford, United Kingdom.

Turner, B., and A. J. Wills. 2000. Cerebral infarction complicating intravenous immunoglobulin therapy in a patient with Miller Fisher syndrome. *J. Neurol. Neurosurg. Psychiatr.* 68:790–791.

Tyler, H. R. 1957. Neurological complications of rubeola (measles). *Medicine* 36:147–167.

Valentine, A. R., B. E. Kendall, and B. N. Harding. 1982. Computed tomography in acute haemorrhagic leukoencephalitis. *Neuroradiology* 22:215–219.

Vanneste, J. A. L., P. P. M. Karthaus, and G. Davies. 1980. Acute urinary retention due to sacral myeloradiculitis. *J. Neurol. Neurosurg. Psychiatr.* 43:954–956.

Varkey, P., G. A. Poland, F. R. Cockerill, III, T. F. Smith, and P. T. Hagen. 2002. Confronting bioterrorism: physicians on the front line. *Mayo Clin. Proc.* 77:661–672.

Verma, A., and B. Brozman. 2002. Opsoclonus-myoclonus syndrome following Epstein-Barr virus infection. *Neurology* 58:1131–1132.

Watson, R. T., W. E. Ballinger, Jr., and R. G. Quisling. 1984. Acute hemorrhagic leukoencephalitis: diagnosis by computed tomography. *Ann. Neurol.* 15:611–612.

Weiss, S., and S. Carter. 1959. Course and prognosis of acute cerebellar ataxia in children. *Neurology* 9:711–721.

Wierenga, K. J. J., B. E. Serjeant, and G. R. Serjeant. 2001. Cerebrovascular complications and parvovirus infection in homozygous sickle cell disease. *Pediatrics* 139:438–442.

Wilmshurst, J. M., M. C. Walker, and K. R. E. Pohl. 1998. Rapid onset transverse myelitis in adolescence: implications for pathogenesis and prognosis. *Arch. Dis. Child.* 80:137–143.

Wingerchuck, D. M., W. F. Hogancamp, E. C. O'Brien, and B. G. Weinshenker. 1999. The clinical course of neuromyelitis optica (Devic's syndrome). *Neurology* 53:1107–1114.

World Health Organization. 2001a. Smallpox. Forms of the disease. *Wkly. Epidemiol. Rec.* 76:337–344.

World Health Organization. 2001b. Nomenclature for describing the genetic characteristics of wild-type measles viruses. (Update.) *Wkly. Epidemiol. Rec.* 76:242–247.

World Health Organization. 2002. Global measles mortality reduction and regional elimination, 2000–2001. *Wkly. Epidemiol. Rec.* 77:50–55.

Yaqub, B. A., S. M. Al-Deeb, A. K. Daif, H. S. Sharif, A. R. Shamena, M. Al-Jaber, T. Obeid, and C. C. Panayiotopoulos. 1990. Bickerstaff brain stem encephalitis. A grave nondemyelinating disease with a benign prognosis. *J. Neurol. Sci.* 96:29–40.

Yuki, N., S. Sato, S. Tsuji, I. Hozumi, and T. Miyatake. 1993. An immunologic abnormality common to Bickerstaff's brain stem encephalitis and Fisher's syndrome. *J. Neurol. Sci.* 118:83–87.

Ziegra, S. R. 1961. Corticosteroid treatment for measles encephalitis. *J. Pediatr.* 59:322–323.

9

Varicella-Zoster Virus: The Paradox of Immune Mediation and Immunocompromise

Certainly no virus damages the human nervous system in more diverse ways than does varicella-zoster virus (VZV). Shingles attacks the peripheral nerves and dorsal root ganglia. Cranial nerves are involved in both the Ramsay Hunt syndrome and herpes zoster ophthalmicus (HZO). The former syndrome is associated with motor weakness of the facial nerve. The latter infection may occasionally be followed by cerebral infarction secondary to a vasculitis in the delayed hemiplegia syndrome. Cerebellitis may follow chicken pox on a parainfectious basis, and a vasculopathic encephalitis can occur in the setting of disseminated zoster. The virus attacks the peripheral nervous system as well as the central nervous system (CNS), and disease is mediated through viral lytic, parainfectious, and vascular mechanisms. Both immunologically intact and immunologically compromised hosts, including those with AIDS, can be attacked by VZV.

Neurological complications following the primary infection as chicken pox and following the reactivation infection as zoster will be considered here. The reader is also referrred to chapters 7 and 8, which consider the parainfectious syndromes that can follow several acute viral infections.

VZV causes both chicken pox and zoster (shingles) (Arvin, 1996; Gershon and Silverstein, 1997). It is a double-stranded DNA virus with a lipid coat belonging to the herpesvirus family. It has some gene sequence similarities to those of herpes simplex virus, and its ultrastructural appearance is identical, but its properties are less well understood, in part because it is difficult to grow in culture. Though reasonably labile, it is highly infectious. Following resolution of clinical chicken pox, the virus establishes a state of latency from which it may emerge decades later as shingles. Recent studies indicate that VZV is latent in neurons (Dueland, 1996; Kennedy et al., 1999; LaGuardia et al., 1999). Virus shed at the time of zoster can initiate chicken pox in susceptible children. Accurate figures on the annual incidence of chicken pox are difficult to obtain due to underreporting. However, prior to vaccine use, an annual figure of four million cases in the United States was cited, with a peak occurrence about March (Weller, 1983). Most of the cases in temperate climates occur in children under 10 years of age. A live attenuated virus vaccine was approved for use in the United States in 1995 (Centers for Disease Control and Prevention, 1996, 1999).

CHICKEN POX

Systemic Illness

The incubation period ranges from 11 to 20 days, with an average of 14 to 15 days. Prodromal symptoms consisting of fever and malaise may occur in adults. In children the first sign of illness is the rash. It starts as macular in character and then develops a fine "dewdrop" vesicle. The vesicle evolves to a pustule and finally becomes crusted. Virus may be isolated from the vesicle during the first 3 days, and cells at the base of the vesicle can be demonstrated to have intranuclear inclusions and multinucleate forms. The rash may start on the scalp and face or on the trunk. However, different generations of lesions may appear at any one site. New crops occur over a 2- to 4-day period and are associated with pruritis for 2 or 3 days. Shallow vesicles occur in the mouth and throat. Malaise and mild fever accompany the rash. Mild conjunctivitis and a slight sore throat are often present. The duration of the rash is about 7 to 10 days until separation of scabs.

Chicken Pox Encephalitis and Chicken Pox-Associated Cerebellar Ataxia

Chicken pox is usually considered a benign febrile disease. However, several studies have documented serious complications in previously well children, with an increased frequency of serious complications of chicken pox in adults. A nationwide system of Sentinelle general practitioners in France determined that 95% of cases occurred in children under 14 years of age and that complications occurred in about 2% of cases (Deguen et al., 1998). Respiratory tract and skin infections were the most common; however, neurological injury occurred in 21 of 318 cases. These included encephalitis, cerebellar ataxia, and a case of Guillain-Barré. No case of Reye's syndrome was found in the period studied, 1991 to 1995. In a population-based study in Olmstead County, Minnesota, from 1962 to 1981, Guess et al. (1986) found that acute cerebellar ataxia was the most common neurological complication in children, occurring at a rate of 1 per 4,000 cases of varicella in children under 15 years of age. Reye's syndrome in those years was found to occur at a frequency of 1 case per 10,000 to 15,000 cases of chicken pox in children under 15 years.

Hospital-based surveys confirm the spectrum of complications of chicken pox in previously healthy children. A 1-year survey of pediatric hospitals in 1997 in Germany found that pyogenic bacterial infections of various sites were common but that neurological complications were the most frequent (Ziebold et al., 2001). These included cerebellitis, encephalitis, meningitis, and central facial palsy. No cases of Reye's syndrome were reported in this period. Children who are immunocompromised tend to have more prolonged courses and more complications than do previously healthy children. Studying VZV in 45 human immunodeficiency virus (HIV)-infected children in Romania, Leibovitz et al. (1993) found that in 57% of cases the duration of illness was over 10 days. Complications consisting of skin superinfection, pneumonia, or thrombocytopenia were found in 40%. No cases of encephalitis were reported.

In his review of 119 cases of neurological complications of varicella in the literature, Underwood (1935) found seven cases that he classified as prodromal—that is, each had a seizure prior to the appearance of the rash. All cleared completely. Sixteen cases with meningeal signs predominating were also described. In cases of encephalomyelitis, Applebaum et al. (1953) found the interval between the onset of the rash and CNS symptoms to range from 1 to 21 days, with most occurring between 4 and 8 days after onset of the rash. When the mode of onset was known, it was dramatic in 60%, with headache, vomiting, fever, and an altered sensorium. The 40% with a more gradual onset demonstrated irrational behavior, drowsiness, and/or ataxia. The temperature was usually moderately elevated for a few days. Stiff neck was found in the majority, but seizures were found in only approximately one-fifth of the patients. Miller et al. (1956) found impaired consciousness in about half of studied cases, although coma occurred in about 20%. Ataxia has been found in about one-third of the patients (Miller et al, 1956; Applebaum et al., 1953).

When the cerebellar syndrome is considered separately, several differences emerge. In comparison to the cerebral type, Johnson and Milbourne (1970) found the cerebellar type to be slightly more frequent (29 versus 23 cases) and more benign. Coma and semicoma were not found, and no deaths occurred in the cerebellar type. However, both Underwood (1935) and Miller et al. (1956) found the fatality rate to be around 11%. Sequelae were varied and included ataxia, paralysis, speech disturbances, and intellectual impairment. In the series of Applebaum et al. (1953), 9 of 59 patients (15%) had sequelae at discharge. Of these, two resolved completely and two improved somewhat. Distressingly, however, three of the patients discharged as healthy developed sequelae from 3 months to 3 years later.

Other manifestations are seen. Underwood (1935) included categories of acute cerebral tremor and chorioathetotic forms. Four cases of myelitis were described by Miller et al. (1956) in a review of 134 cases. Paraparesis, upgoing plantar responses, and urinary bladder problems were described. In one patient the brain stem and cerebral hemispheres were also involved. Recovery occurred in all, beginning between 7 and 18 days after onset and taking up to 6 weeks to complete. Polyradiculitis was found in nine cases in the review by Miller et al. (1956). Facial paralysis occurred 7 to 20 days following the rash. Bulbar signs were seen in five patients, and one had spinal cord involvement. However, all had complete recovery between 8 and 16 weeks.

The lumbar puncture characteristically reveals a moderate mononuclear pleocytosis and a normal or moderately elevated protein. Completely normal spinal fluid is occasionally found (Miller et al., 1956). Because Reye's syndrome was not described until 1963 (Reye et al., 1963), the possibility must be entertained that some cases of postvaricella encephalopathy with an acellular cerebrospinal fluid (CSF) in the earlier literature were Reye's syndrome-associated with fatty degeneration of the liver. Takashima and Becker (1979) found that 12 of 32 cases of fatal varicella examined neuropathologically had evidence of fatty metamorphosis of the liver.

Johnson and Milbourne (1970) found diffusely slow electroencephalograms (EEGs) in 10 of 12 cases of cerebral involvement but normal EEGs in 17 of 21 cases involving the cerebellum. Neuroimaging in the cerebellar form is usually normal, although focal lesions and swelling are occasionally found, including in the preeruptive phase (Dangond et al., 1993) (see chapter 8). Neuroimaging of the cerebral forms reported by Darling et al. (1995) included bilateral basal ganglia or diffuse cerebral lesions. Hausler et al. (2002) reported two cases in which multifocal lesions evolved, including involvement of basal ganglia or thalamus, cortical, and subcortical lesions. Magnetic resonance imaging (MRI) has proven useful in the diagnosis and management of myelitis following chicken pox (Rosenfeld et al., 1993).

Virus isolation attempts from CSF in association with CNS complications of chicken pox are usually negative (Johnson and Milbourne, 1970). While the characteristic rash and syndrome usually leave little room for doubt, the virological diagnosis can be confirmed with CSF PCR (Puchhammer-Stockl et al., 1991; Cinque et al., 1997) or antibody indices in which the ratio of antibody specific for VZV in CSF is determined (Hausler et al., 2002). These assays are particularly useful when the CNS syndrome occurs in the preeruptive phase of chicken pox (Dangond et al., 1993) or in the rare case of apparent absence of vesicles (Hausler et al., 2002).

Intervention will be dependent on type of syndrome. Acute VZV cerebellitis is usually a benign illness requiring only supportive care. However, more extensive disease, including cerebral involvement, may require a combination therapy with acyclovir and steroid (Hausler et al., 2002). Clinical and MRI improvement have been associated with steroid and acyclovir therapy of varicella-associated myelitis (Rosenfeld et al., 1993). The appropriate treatment for cerebral vasculitis associated with evidence of varicella zoster infection (Hausler et al., 1998) is not standardized, and therapy must be individualized to particular patients. Steroid and other immunosuppressive therapy, acyclovir, and anticoagulation and antiplatelet therapy can each be considered. Ultimately, therapy will depend on determining the primary and secondary pathogenic mechanisms. Antiviral therapy is indicated if residual viral replication is suspected to be present in vessels. Steroid and/or other immunosuppressive therapy may be indicated to suppress the immune response to the viral antigens. The issue of anticoagulation and/or antiplatelet therapy will need to be judged individually, balancing the risk of thrombosis against hemorrhage from viral infection-weakened vessels.

Congenital and neonatal varicella have been described. Infection in utero in the first trimester of pregnancy can result in a congenital varicella syndrome of limb hypoplasia, eye damage, and gastrointestinal or genitourinary abnormalities (Alkalay et al., 1987; Berrebi et al., 1998; Paryani and Arvin, 1986). Damage to the peripheral nervous system gives rise to denervation, limb hypoplasia, and scarring. Involvement of the CNS also occurs with destructive lesions in all levels of the brain and cord, sometimes accompanied by inflammation but no viral inclusions (Harding and Baumer, 1988; Magliocco et al., 1992; Kustermann et al., 1996). Varicella acquired around the time of birth can result in widely disseminated lesions and a mortality of up to 30% (Mustonen et al., 1998).

ZOSTER

Cutaneous Illness

Hope-Simpson (1965) proposed that following chicken pox, VZV became latent in sensory ganglia, from which it was later activated. Gilden and his colleagues (1983) found evidence in support of this hypothesis. Using a DNA probe, they demonstrated viral DNA in sensory ganglia in the absence of clinical zoster. The incidence of shingles is about 3 to 4 per 1,000 per year (Hope-Simpson, 1965). It increases with age, particularly after 50 years. There is an increased incidence in patients with HIV/AIDS, various types of malignancy, irradiation, immunosuppressive treatment, and chemotherapy. However, a search for malignancy in persons not known to harbor such a process at the time of shingles is generally unproductive. The most common site of shingles is thoracic. Cervical, facial, and lumbar lesions occur less frequently and with approximately equal frequency, roughly 15% each. Sacral lesions occur but are least frequent. Although usually restricted to one dermatome and its adjacent area, the disease may generalize. In the roughly 10% in whom generalization occurs, 65% have serious underlying disease. In contrast, only 16% of the patients in whom the process remains localized have serious underlying disease (Christie, 1980). A small number of scattered vesicles may be found in many cases of localized zoster. Second and extremely rare third attacks may occur.

The rash occurs in a dermatomal distribution, although it may not be clearly bandlike in its initial presentation. It is often preceded by 1 or 2 days of pain in a radicular distribution, followed by the appearance of an erythematous maculopapular rash. New lesions may develop for up to a week, although most are apparent within 2 to 4 days. The lesions usually dry up and crust within 7 to 10 days. Lymphadenopathy can be found in association with the localized lesions. If dissemination is to occur, it often does so in the second week after the appearance of the lesions. Visceral involvement may occur with disseminated lesions. "Zoster sine herpete" refers to a syndrome of radicular pain in the absence of cutaneous lesions (Lewis, 1958).

Virus may be isolated from fresh vesicle fluid and from cells at the base of the vesicle. Humoral antibody rises quickly after appearance of the rash in an amnestic fashion (Miller and Brunell, 1970). During active disease, skin, nerve, and sensory ganglia have been demonstrated to contain viral antigen or viral particles (Esiri and Tomlinson, 1972). CSF pleocytosis has been found in 8 of 21 cases of zoster in the absence of CNS complications, and virus was isolated from the CSF of two of these patients (Gold, 1966). More recently, Haanpaa et al. (1998) evaluated CSF and MRIs in 50 immunocompetent patients with zoster of 18 days or less. None had encephalitis, myelitis, or meningeal signs. Six had motor signs and three had ocular signs, but the majority had only pain and rash. The CSF was abnormal in 28 of 46 patients, with pleocytosis in 21, protein elevation in 12, VZV DNA detected in 10, and anti-VZV immunoglobulin G (IgG) antibody detected in 10. Nine of 16 MRIs had lesions compatible with VZV in the brain stem or cervical cord. Similar findings of a spinal cord abnormality in 13 of 24 patients (asymptomatic in 12) with acute spinal zoster were reported by Steiner et al. (2001). These observations must be borne in mind when evaluating patients with CNS complications of peripheral nervous system zoster.

Postherpetic neuralgia is the most common neurological complication of zoster. It is usually defined as pain persisting for more than 4 to 6 weeks after the onset of zoster. Shingles is more common in those over 50 and may present a difficult pain management challenge. Motor paresis can be observed (Thomas and Howard, 1972; Gardner-Thorpe et al., 1976). The reader is referred to recent discussions of pathogenesis and therapeutic options (Tenser, 2001; Watson, 2000).

Nervous System Complications of Zoster

Pathology and Pathogenesis

The neurological complications of zoster are pleomorphic, ranging, for example, from diaphragmatic paralysis associated with preceding cervical zoster (Stowasser et al., 1990) to fatal leukoencephalitis, cerebral hemorrhage, and cerebral vasculopathy in a patient with AIDS who 10 months previous had suffered a disseminated VZV rash (Case Records, 1996). Emergence from latency is associated with diverse pathogenic mechanisms in the CNS and peripheral nervous system. While infrequent, there is evidence for VZV replication as the basis for certain syndromes, particularly in the immunocompromised patient (McCormick et al., 1969). Immune-mediated mechanisms have long been thought to be involved in light of the "parainfectious" timing of many of the syndromes in relation to the cutaneous manifestations of VZV. A component of cerebral vasculopathy has been recognized for some time, particularly in the syndrome of contralateral hemiplegia following HZO (Booss et al., 1985). More recently, particularly in AIDS patients, the importance of the cerebral vasculopathy has been emphasized (Morgello et al., 1988; Gray et al., 1994; Amlie-Lefond et al., 1995). Kleinschmidt-Demasters et al. (1996) emphasized the separate patterns associated with large and small vessel involvement, and Gilden (D. H. Gilden, Editorial, *J. Neurol. Sci.* **195:**99–101, 2002) offered the view that vasculopathy is the primary lesion in VZV disorders of the nervous system. Finally, it seems reasonable to suspect that an interplay of both low-level viral replication and the host defense response, wherever it is played out—in blood vessels and/or in neuroectodermal cells—has a role in the pathogenesis of zoster complications in the nervous system. This pathogenetic alternative is important because clinicians may elect to intervene therapeutically with both antiviral and immunomodulatory treatment.

Diagnosis and Management

In the abstract, the wide array of neurological syndromes associated with reactivation of VZV is daunting. However, in practice, there are a set of syndromes in which VZV should be suspected and a set of clinical circumstances in which VZV reactivation syndromes may appear (Table 9.1).

While reactivation of zoster is most common among the elderly (Hope-Simpson, 1965), it can occur at any stage of life. For example, Chiappini et al. (2002) described a 2-year-old immunocompetent boy who developed VZV

TABLE 9.1 Neurological complications of zoster: syndromes and circumstances

Syndromes[a]
  Stroke
    HZO with delayed contralateral hemiplegia
    Cervical zoster with posterior circulation infarcts
    Granulomatous angiitis of the basilar artery
    Diffuse small/medium vessel disease
  Aseptic meningitis
  Cranial neuropathy/brain stem encephalitis
    Optic and oculomotor neuropathies/retinitis
    Trigeminal neuronitis, including HZO
    Ramsay Hunt syndrome
    Mononeuritis cranialis of other cranial nerves
    Polyneuritis cranialis
  Cerebellitis—acute cerebellar ataxia
  Encephalitis/encephalopathy
    Encephalomyelitis
    Ventriculoencephalitis
      Multifocal VZV leukoencephalopathy
      Hemorrhagic leukoencephalopathy
      Encephalopathy
      Reye's syndrome
  Myelitis
Circumstances
  AIDS
  Elderly
  Leukemia and lymphoma
  Tumors, chemotherapy, radiation therapy
  Allogeneic bone marrow transplantation
  Organ transplantation
  Chronic immunosuppressive therapy

[a] Syndromes may occur separately or in combination.

encephalitis 20 months after chicken pox at 4 months of age. Second, as already noted, there is CSF and MRI evidence of diffuse spread of VZV to CNS in patients with zoster who are otherwise asymptomatic (Haanpaa et al., 1998; Steiner et al., 2001). Evidence for spread via neural, CSF, and vascular pathways can each be deduced, explaining the presence in certain cases of multiple loci of neurological involvement following zoster. For example, Carroll and Mastaglia (1979) described a 55-year-old man, without known chronic illness or immunosuppressive therapy, who developed polyneuritis cranialis involving facial, auditory, optic, and oculomotor cranial nerve functions, cerebellar ataxia, and possible involvement of the medial longitudinal fasciculus, attributed to VZV.

A crucial factor to consider in the clinical syndromes associated with VZV reactivation is that cutaneous or mucosal vesicles may not occur. For example, each of the cases noted above from Chiappini et al. (2002) and Carroll and Mastaglia (1979) had no described cutaneous vesicles. In supervising the State of Connecticut Virology Laboratory, Mayo noted serological evidence for VZV infection in cases of neurological dysfunction in which no chicken pox or zosteriform lesions were reported (Mayo and Booss, 1989). On investigation, a wide range of neurological disorders without skin lesions was found, including aseptic meningitis, acute polyneuropathy with pleocytosis, cranial polyneuropathy, myelitis, and encephalitis. These cases were equivalent to zoster sine herpete (Lewis, 1958), a term established in the literature of zoster to denote symptoms of zoster without the skin lesions. In 1982 Moller et al. reported two cases of zoster-encephalitis without exanthem. Using serological assays, Echevarria et al. (1987) were able to identify cases of aseptic meningitis due to VZV in the absence of cutaneous vesicles. Recent experience in AIDS demonstrates that neurological syndromes in the absence of or with a temporally distant history of cutaneous lesions attributable to VZV by antibody indices and/or CSF PCR are regularly observed (Gilden et al., 1998; De La Blanchardiere et al., 2000).

VZV-Related Stroke Syndromes

Stroke syndromes in association with VZV infection were first recognized as a rare complication in immunocompetent elderly people with zoster ophthalmicus. A vasculopathy in association with VZV infection is much more common in those who are immunosuppressed, particularly AIDS sufferers. Epidemiologic evidence also associates strokes in children with chicken pox (Askalan et al., 2001; Sébire et al., 1999; Ganesan and Kirkham, 1997; Ichiyama et al., 1990). In immunocompetent elderly people and children, major arteries tend to be affected, whereas in the immunosuppressed a small vessel vasculopathy is more frequent. In fatal cases of contralateral stroke complicating zoster ophthalmicus, a granulomatous inflammatory process has been found in the wall of the thrombosed vessel. In some cases multinucleated giant cells and typical intranuclear viral inclusion bodies as well as viral particles or VZV DNA are detected in association with the adventitia or with the smooth muscle cells of the vessel wall (Doyle et al., 1983; Linneman and Alvira, 1980; Jemsek et al., 1983; Gilden et al., 1996; Eidelberg et al., 1986; Melanson et al., 1996). It is suggested that the virus travels along nerve fibers to reach the vessel wall. In some patients, particularly those who are immunosuppressed and in whom the vessel or vessels affected are widely distributed or unrelated to the site of a skin rash, virus may reach the vessel(s) via the blood. Viral particles have been described rarely in endothelial cells, supporting this rate of spread (Ruppenthal, 1980). In cases of encephalitis in which parenchymal elements of the CNS are infected as well (see below), small vessels may harbor virus, but in this case, it is difficult to say whether the virus spread from brain to vessel or from vessel to brain. Affected vessels may show segments of fibrinoid necrosis as well as thrombosis and inflammation, and the territory of brain supplied by the affected vessel shows ischemic, sometimes hemorrhagic, infarction. In cases of AIDS with zoster vasculopathy, the inflammation may be minimal or absent. Vasculopathy affecting leptomeningeal vessels can be seen associated with brain or spinal cord infarcts (Gray et al., 1994; Chretien et al., 1997; Amlie-Lefond et al., 1995). The extent to which immunopathological mechanisms are involved in mediating VZV-related vasculopathy or vasculitis is not clear.

The best known zoster-associated stroke syndrome is delayed contralateral hemiplegia following HZO. In an early review by Kuroiwa and Furukawa (1981), HZO was found to have preceded the onset of hemiparesis by 8 days to 6 months, with an average interval of 8 weeks. The age of the patients averaged 55 years, but there was a range of 7 to 96 years. When the dominant hemisphere was involved, many patients demonstrated an expressive aphasia. The course of the illness usually has the temporal profile of a stroke with gradual improvement of varying degree. A patient reported on by Doyle et al. (1983) had an apparently uniphasic onset, was treated with and tapered from steroids, but suffered a fatal thrombotic event. At autopsy, necrotizing arteritis was found and herpes-like virions were observed on electron microscopy (Fig. 9.1).

The CSF usually shows a pleocytosis and protein elevation. The EEG often demonstrates lateralized abnormalities. Angiography can demonstrate segmental constriction in the clinically relevant portion of the arterial system (MacKenzie et al., 1981). A necrotizing arteritis may cause the stroke syndrome, which may partially reverse (Fryer et al., 1984). Magnetic resonance angiography can also be used without risk of causing infarction and can show single or multiple areas of interruption of flow (Melanson et al., 1996). Single or multiple ischemic or hemorrhagic areas of ischemia can be seen on MRI or computerized tomography (CT). Serological evidence for systemic vasculitic disease is not found (Booss et al., 1985).

Presumably, because of the timing of the illness in relation to the HZO, virus cannot be isolated from CSF, nor will acute- and convalescent-phase sera and CSF show diagnostic rises in antibody. A case has been reported in which CSF PCR was positive and in which viral DNA was found in cerebral arteries (Melanson et al., 1996). Nonetheless, the clinical diagnosis rests on the observation of a preceding HZO followed by an ipsilateral stroke syndrome, often weeks later.

There is sufficient evidence of the presence of VZV in the walls of the cerebral arteries in this syndrome to merit a course of intravenous (i.v.) acyclovir. Ten to 15 mg/kg of body weight i.v., three times a day for 10 days to 2 weeks, with careful monitoring of renal function, are appropriate parameters in light of the chronic nature of the infection. Because of the inflammatory nature of the vascular lesion, steroid therapy can also be supported despite concerns for its effect on host control of the virus. Unfortunately, there are few data on which to craft this therapy. A recent review has recommended 60 to 80 mg of prednisone for 3 to 5 days (Gilden et al., 2000). In light of the vasculitis, antiplatelet and/or anticoagulation therapy might be considered. Arguing against such therapy is the weakened state of the vessel wall and the propensity for hemorrhagic infarction.

Ross et al. (1991) reported a case of bilateral pontine infarction following zoster in a C2 distribution and reviewed other VZV-associated cases of the posterior circulation. Among these, other vascular syndromes can be observed clinically in association with zoster. Fukumoto et al. (1986) reported subarachnoid hemorrhage from a fusiform aneurysm of the basilar artery in a man with C2 zoster. At autopsy the wall of the aneurysm was found to have granulomatous angiitis, and evidence for VZV was found in histiocytes in the vessel wall. Less clear is the frequency of association of VZV and diffuse granulomatous angiitis of the nervous system. Herpeslike virions have been visualized by

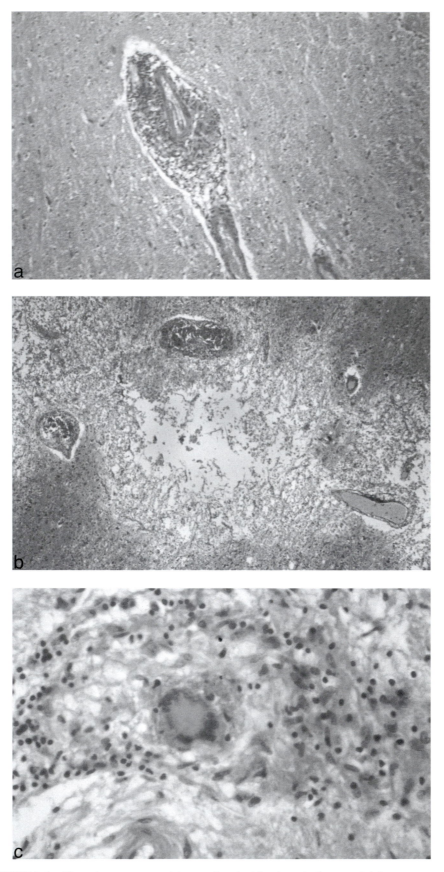

FIGURE 9.1 Granulomatous arteritis associated with trigeminal zoster. (a) Low-power view of perivascular inflammation. (b) Low-power view of small microinfarct in basal ganglia associated with small vessel angiitis at periphery. (c) Higher-power view of inflammation, including a multinucleate giant cell.

electron microscopy in granulomatous angiitis (Reyes et al., 1976; Linneman and Alvira, 1980). This syndrome has a more extensive vascular distribution and progressive clinical course than does HZO with delayed contralateral hemiplegia. Furthermore, it often occurs in the setting of an immunologically compromised host. Unfortunately, it is not always clear at the outset if one is dealing with the uniphasic or the progressive illness.

VZV Cranial Neuropathy and Brain Stem Encephalitis

It is not uncommon for herpes zoster involving spinal ganglia to be accompanied by focal weakness, usually affecting muscles supplied by the same spinal cord segment and on the same side of the body as the rash (Thomas and Howard, 1972). In view of the favorable prognosis, this is likely to be due in most cases to extension of the inflammation from the posterior to the anterior nerve root. However, in some instances a focal myelitis may develop in the spinal cord or brain stem. Even in cases in which motor disturbance is absent or unrecognized, pathological or MRI examination can demonstrate evidence of a myelitis affecting the cord on the same side and at the same level as the ganglionitis (Haanpaa et al., 1998; Steiner et al., 2001). A similar phenomenon also occurs when herpes zoster affects a cranial sensory ganglion, particularly the sensory ganglion of the seventh cranial nerve. Occasionally, the upper cervical segments of the spinal cord may be involved, with an associated brain stem encephalitis (Fig. 9.2). In geniculate herpes, vesicles develop in skin of the external auditory meatus and on the ear drum, and there may be an associated seventh nerve palsy (Ramsay Hunt syndrome). Other lower cranial nerve signs ipsilateral to the affected ganglion may also occur. Involvement of the seventh nerve alone may be due to compression of fibers of the nerve as they pass through the inflamed geniculate ganglion, but a ganglionitis has not always been pathologically

demonstrable in such cases and the involvement of other cranial nerves suggests extension of the inflammatory process to the brain stem. This has been confirmed in only a few autopsy studies in which a focal, predominantly unilateral brain stem encephalitis with intranuclear viral inclusion bodies in neurons and glial cells has been confirmed (Rosenblum, 1989; Schmidbauer et al., 1992; Moulignier et al., 1995).

In a case we studied, the Ramsay Hunt syndrome developed in a 36-year-old woman with chronic renal failure treated by hemodialysis. The illness started with left-sided facial pain, followed after 5 days by left facial palsy and left-sided neural deafness. After a further 6 days, vesicles developed on the left eardrum and the patient had a hoarse voice. Four days later, there were palsies of the left seventh, eighth, ninth, and tenth nerves. These persisted until death from cardiac arrest on the 27th day of the illness. The serum antibody titer to VZV had risen from 1:128 on day 11 to 1:1,024 on day 23 of the illness. Neuropathological examination showed edema, capillary endothelial swelling, lymphocytic perivascular infiltration, and microglial proliferation on the left side of the brain stem, chiefly in the vestibular nuclei and tractus solitarius and its nucleus. No neuronophagia was seen, but a few neurons, including some in the left seventh nerve motor nucleus, were chromatolytic. In addition, there was a neuritis of the seventh nerve proximal and distal to the geniculate ganglion, with demyelination, inflammation, and axonal fragmentation. No viral antigen was detected by immunofluorescence in the ganglion, nerve, or brain stem, and viral culture using material from these sites was unsuccessful.

"Ramsay Hunt Plus." It has been proposed that the term "Ramsay Hunt syndrome" be restricted to those cases in which facial paralysis is associated with herpes zoster oticus (see, for example, Aleksic et al., 1973). However, facial

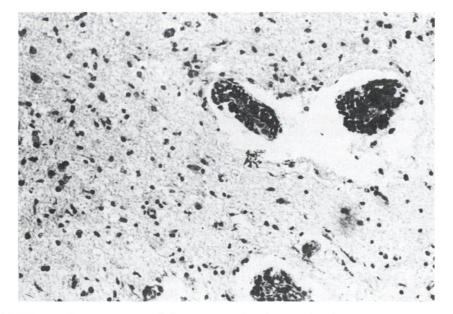

FIGURE 9.2 Brain stem encephalitis associated with geniculate herpes zoster. Perivascular lymphocytic cuffing of the ipsilateral medulla. Hematoxylin and eosin stain. ×350.

paralysis may be seen in association with zoster in several locations about the head. In a review of 36 patients, Heathfield and Mee (1978) found facial paralysis in association with VZV in any of the three territories of the trigeminal nerve on the face, on the hard and soft palate, and on the neck, in addition to about the ear. Cephalic zoster is not infrequently associated with involvement of cranial nerves, in addition to that involved in the skin lesions. In a review of the literature of the Ramsay Hunt syndrome, Aviel and Marshak (1982) found that 74% of cases were associated with evidence of dysfunction of the eighth cranial nerve. Cranial nerves V, VI, IX, and X were also found to have been involved in 10 to 40% of reported cases. Multiple cranial nerves may be involved in any one case, as described above. Morgan-Capner et al. (P. Morgan-Capner, M. A. J. Crofts, and J. C. Sharp, Letter, *Lancet* i:668, 1979) reported a patient with chronic lymphocytic leukemia undergoing chemotherapy who developed disseminated zoster and dysfunction of multiple cranial nerves. Facial weakness, absence of taste, deafness, soft palate weakness, sternocleidomastoid muscle weakness, and tongue deviation were all found. Residual weakness of the face, tongue, and soft palate were present 10 months later. Such cases can be termed "Ramsay Hunt plus."

Special comment should be made about the involvement of zoster and the visual system. VZV is one of the causes of viral retinitis in which the diagnosis can be made by PCR on vitreous specimens (Knox et al., 1998). Rousseau et al. (1993) described two HIV-infected patients in whom HZO was followed by necrotizing retinitis and cerebral vasculitis. Optic neuropathy and oculomotor and cerebellar abnormalities in a patient without reported underlying disease were reported by Carroll and Mastaglia (1979).

Additionally, zoster may be associated with facial nerve weakness and with a cranial polyneuropathy in the absence of demonstrable vesicles (Djupesland et al., 1977). Of 16 patients with facial palsy, only 2 were found to have zoster oticus, but 8 were found to have seriological incidence of recent zoster infection. Six of these had evidence of recent VZV activity. Only 2 patients of the 16 had disease limited to the facial nerve. Dysfunction of the cochlear or vestibular division of the eighth nerve and dysfunction of the fifth nerve were found in the majority. Involvement of the 9th and 10th cranial nerves and the second cervical root was also found. Extensive brain stem involvement and involvement of cranial nerves VI through XI were reported in an HIV-infected man without cutaneous vesicles by Moulignier et al. (1995). Thus, not only is zoster frequently associated with facial weakness, it may also be cryptic, and it is often associated with multiple cranial nerve involvement.

In the diagnosis of cases of cranial neuropathy, particularly those involving the facial nerve, a search for zoster vesicles for viral culture should be made. An acute-phase sample of serum should be taken immediately on presentation, as well as 2 weeks later, because of the rapid amnestic rise of the anti-VZV antibody associated with zoster. CSF should be obtained for PCR for VZV (Puchhammer-Stockl et al., 1991; Quereda et al., 2000) and locally produced anti-VZV antibody (Gilden et al., 1998). Specificity of local CSF production can be gauged by using an antibody index in which the ratio of anti-VZV IgG antibody in CSF compared to serum is itself compared to the ratio of CSF and serum total IgG (Hausler et al., 1998). A significantly greater ratio for anti-VZV IgG antibody than total IgG supports an immune response against VZV in the CNS.

As in the treatment of VZV-associated encephalomyelitis, we believe that treatment with i.v. acyclovir is indicated, 10 to 15 mg/kg three times a day for 10 to 14 days. The use of steroids must be evaluated on a case-by-case basis. Murakami et al. (1997) studied the combined use of i.v. or oral acyclovir and i.v. or oral prednisone. Patients given the combined therapy within 3 days of facial weakness had a significantly higher rate (75%) of complete recovery in comparison to therapy that was started more than 7 days after facial weakness (30%). High-dose-use (oral) acyclovir was found to be as effective as i.v. therapy. Corticosteroid was also used to good benefit in a case of jugular foramen syndrome (cranial nerves IX, X, and XI) associated with VZV and a hypoplastic jugular foramen (Hayashi et al., 2000). In each of these situations, neural edema in the facial canal or in the jugular foramen may have been alleviated by steroid therapy. In other clinical situations not involving edema in confined spaces, however, steroid treatment may be contraindicated, particularly in immunocompromised patients.

Encephalomyelitis

Pathology. There have been few pathological studies of cases clinically diagnosed as disseminated VZV encephalitis (McCormick et al., 1969; Takashima and Becker, 1979; Carmack et al., 1993; Herrold and Hahn, 1994; Horten et al., 1981). Most cases occur in the setting of immunosuppression, particularly AIDS. In some of these cases there was extensive necrosis of deep gray and white matter with viral intranuclear inclusion bodies or viral antigen in neurons and glia (ependymal cells, astrocytes, oligodendrocytes in varying proportion) as well as in the walls of small blood vessels. As already mentioned, one view is that this type of pathology represents a primary cerebral vasculopathy in which the necrosis represents infarction and the virus spreads secondarily from small blood vessels to parenchymal cells (Gilden et al., 2000; Gilden, editorial, 2002). However, where oligodendrocytes are infected and the lesions are at least partly demyelinating, the cerebral damage would seem to be attributable to the parenchymal cell infection as in other forms of viral encephalitis (Scaravilli and Gray, 1993; Gray et al., 1994). Likewise, in VZV myelitis, there is viral infection of the cord parenchyma and a necrotizing process with variable inflammation in the cord (Hogan and Krigman, 1973).

Clinical Manifestations. Prior to the HIV/AIDS epidemic, which resulted in the study of large numbers of patients with opportunistic infections, and prior to the widespread use of CSF PCR and MRI, which each facilitated the laboratory diagnosis of VZV-associated encephalitis, much of the clinical literature related the encephalitis to the appearance of a zosteriform rash. While in most cases neurological dysfunction followed the appearance of the rash, in some cases the sequence was reversed. Applebaum et al. (1962) found the onset of CNS dysfunction to range from 3 weeks before to 11 days after the eruption. Norris et al. (1970) found the range to be 1 week before to 3 weeks after the eruption. In the series of Jemsek et al. (1983), the average interval was about 9 days following the eruption. It was observed that if CNS dysfunction was to follow dissemination of skin lesions, it was likely to do so within 2 days. The mode of onset may be gradual or acute, but Applebaum et al. (1962) found the majority to be acute. Fever, headache, vomiting, stiff neck, altered personality, and altered sensorium were found at the onset.

In the pre-HIV/AIDS era, most cases evolved to resolution over 1 to 3 weeks (Applebaum et al., 1962), although some cases went on in a progressive or fluctuating manner for months (Norris et al., 1970; Jemsek et al., 1983). Fever, particularly at the start, is common although not invariable. The presence of headache, nuchal rigidity, and vomiting varies from one-third to over three-quarters of patients. Personality changes, ranging from irritability through confusion and delirium to psychosis, are described. Similarly, impairment of the level of consciousness is common. Seizures, while reported (for example, Norris et al., 1970), are not common. Ataxia and motor weakness are described. Weakness, sensory loss, and bladder dysfunction are frequently found as part of a myelopathic process. Myelitis can occur on its own in association with zoster or in the context of multiple sites of CNS involvement. Myelitic involvement can be uniphasic or can demonstrate a progressive ascending course over several weeks (Hogan and Krigman, 1973; Corston et al., 1981). The process following zoster may also appear to be essentially a nonfocal encephalopathy. In an elderly febrile patient with an acellular spinal fluid, the clinician may be hard pressed to distinguish a zoster-related encephalitis from a toxic-metabolic encephalopathy. The evolution of focal signs, the persistence of neurological disability, the absence of metabolic imbalance, and the eventual appearance of a CSF pleocytosis would each point toward an encephalitis. The distinction is not trivial because antiviral therapy may be considered.

Mortality in non-HIV zoster-associated encephalomyelitis is sometimes difficult to assess in the presence of an associated malignant disease. In the Applebaum et al. (1962) series of 14 patients, most recovered within 1 to 3 weeks, two had a delayed recovery of months, and one died in the fourth month. Similarly, in a series of eight patients, Norris et al. (1970) reported one death of a patient in whom the CNS symptoms were improving at the time of death from lymphoma. Protracted courses in a minority of cases are reported in many series. Norris et al. (1970) recorded a patient with cerebral involvement who recovered, but 6 months later experienced acute ataxia, hemiparesis, and confusion. Jemsek et al. (1983) described a patient with zoster-associated encephalitis, followed later by a myelitis in the face of improving cerebral function. In survivors, complete or virtually complete recovery may occur. In the Applebaum et al. (1962) series of 14 cases, 3 with sequelae attributable to the encephalitis were found. The disabilities included hemiparesis and psychosis. A case with persistent motor weakness was recorded by Jemsek et al. (1983).

The advent of the HIV/AIDS epidemic resulted in sufficient numbers of cases of VZV infection of the CNS to sort out various patterns of clinical-pathological involvement. Gray et al. (1994) discerned five patterns: multifocal, predominantly white matter encephalitis; ventriculitis with vasculitis; acute hemorrhagic meningomyeloradiculitis with necrotizing vasculitis; focal necrotizing myelitis; and a vasculopathy of the leptomeningeal arteries with cerebral infarcts. Kleinschmidt-Demasters et al. (1996) classified the pathology of VZV encephalitis into three patterns: large and medium cerebral vasculopathy resulting in ischemic or hemorrhagic infarcts, mixed demyelinative ischemic lesions due to small vessel vasculopathy, and ventriculitis/periventriculitis.

Clinically, De La Blanchardiere et al. (2000) reported the results of a multicenter, multiyear study from France in the era prior to highly active antiretroviral therapy. The diagnosis required a positive CSF PCR and that no other pathogen was present in CNS. Of 34 HIV-infected patients, VZV-associated syndromes broke down as follows: encephalitis–37%, myelitis–24%, radiculitis–21%, and isolated meningitis–18%. The cases of encephalitis were further broken down to isolated encephalitis, encephaloradiculomyelomeningitis, encephaloradiculitis, encephalomyelitis, encephalomeningoradiculitis, and thrombotic cerebral vasculitis. Signs and symptoms included confusion, drowsiness, ataxia, focal abnormalities, and seizures. While abnormalities of CSF nucleated cells and/or protein were found in all cases, 12 of the 34 cases had fewer than three white cells per mm^3. MRIs were more useful than CTs in demonstrating brain and spinal cord disease. MRI was abnormal in six of nine studied cases of encephalitis and in three of seven cases of myelitis. All but one of the patients were treated with antivirals. Full recovery occurred in slightly over half, sequelae were found in about 30%, and death occurred in 18%.

Virological diagnosis is dependent on the demonstration of VZV DNA in CSF by PCR (Puchhammer-Stockl et al., 1991; Quereda et al., 2000; Hausler et al., 1998). Preferential antibody production in CSF is demonstrated by comparing the ratio of VZV antibodies in CSF and serum to that of CSF and serum total IgG or to the ratio for antibodies to an unrelated antigen. Local CNS anti-VZV antibody production will be demonstrated if the VZV ratio is clearly greater than that for total IgG or for an unrelated antigen. Treatment consists of i.v. acyclovir at 10 to 15 mg per kg three times a day for 10 to 15 days. Use of steroid may be problematic in light of immunosuppression.

Multifocal VZV Leukoencephalitis

The rare disease multifocal VZV leukoencephalitis was first described by Horten et al. in 1981 in association with Hodgkin's disease and with an ovarian tumor. It has been recognized in the AIDS epidemic neuropathologically (Morgello et al., 1988) and clinically with the use of MRI (Aygun et al., 1998; Weaver et al., 1999) (Fig. 9.3). MRI has also facilitated its recognition in cases of immunosuppression due to other causes (Lentz et al., 1993; Weaver et al., 1999). Clinical presentations have included headache, seizures, hemiparesis, and myelopathy (Weaver et al., 1999). Otero et al. (1998) found 12 cases reported since 1969. The literature review revealed that of the 14 reported cases, including their own, 7 were without cutaneous lesions.

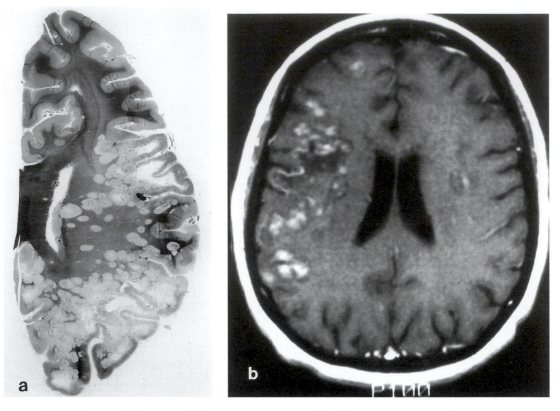

FIGURE 9.3 Multifocal VZV leukoencephalitis. (a) Whole mount stained for myelin demonstrating multiple separate and confluent areas of demyelination. The patient was a woman with underlying Hodgkin's disease. (Courtesy of Marc K. Rosenblum, Memorial Sloan-Kettering Cancer Center, New York, N.Y.). (b) Enhanced T1-weighted MRI image demonstrating multiple foci of demyelination in frontal and parietal lobes, right side (left side of figure) greater than left. Minimal mass effect is seen. The patient was a man with HIV. (Courtesy of Lisa M. DeAngelis, Memorial Sloan-Kettering Cancer Center.)

VZV was identified in these cases by autopsy or biopsy. Prompt recognition is of course facilitated by the MRI findings in combination with the cutaneous lesions. Absent the cutaneous lesions, in the presence of subcortical spherical demyelinating lesions, which can coalesce and show edema and hemorrhage (Weaver et al., 1999; Lentz et al., 1993; Aygun et al., 1998), CSF PCR and antibody indices for VZV should be promptly obtained for early antiviral therapy. The patients of Otero et al. (1998) were the first two treated clinically who recovered and in whom the MRI demyelination resolved. Both patients were treated with i.v. acyclovir, 12.4 mg/kg every 8 h. Weaver et al. (1999) emphasized the distinct nature of the lesions on MRI, facilitating rapid implementation of antiviral therapy.

Myelitis

Myelitis can occur in the immunocompetent or immunosuppressed as part of a complex of signs and symptoms of brain, meninges, spinal roots, and/or cranial nerves, or on its own, with or without cutaneous vesicles. As a consequence, any case of myelitis of undetermined etiology should be examined by spinal cord MRI and CSF PCR for VZV DNA and local antibody production to VZV. Antiviral therapy can result in improvement (DeSilva et al., 1996).

Cerebellitis

While Epstein-Barr virus may be a principal cause of cerebellar encephalitis in adults, in contrast to chicken pox in children, reactivated VZV must also be considered in adults (Klockgether et al., 1993). Although younger and middle-aged patients usually recover well, persistent ataxia may occur in those over 60 years of age. Hence, antiviral therapy and/or steroids should be considered in this age group. A fuller consideration of cerebellitis, otherwise known as acute cerebellar ataxia, is considered among the parainfectious syndromes in chapters 7 and 8.

Circumstances

Certain clinical circumstances that cause compromised immune function are regularly associated with reactivation of VZV (Table 9.1). Compromise of cell-mediated immunity makes the host susceptible to VZV reactivation, such as is found in HIV/AIDS. Myeloablative therapy for bone marrow allografts commonly results in VZV reactivation that can involve the nervous system (Tauro et al., 2000). Chronic therapeutic immunosuppression for other reasons is associated with VZV reactivation (Jemsek et al., 1983). Leukemia and lymphoproliferative disorders have long been recognized as underlying conditions during which VZV reactivates (Jemsek et al., 1983). Children with T-cell acute lymphoblastic leukemia who developed multifocal VZV leukoencephalitis have been reported to be successfully treated with acyclovir (Carmack et al., 1993; Herrold and Hahn, 1994). Hughes et al. (1993) reviewed the neurological complications of VZV associated with systemic cancer at the Mayo Clinic and found that the most common underlying malignancies were chronic lymphocytic leukemia and lymphoma. Except for postherpetic neuralgia, meningoencephalitis was the most common complication of VZV. The response to acyclovir treatment was characterized as generally favorable.

REFERENCES

Aleksic, S. N., G. N. Budzilovich, and A. N. Lieberman. 1973. Herpes zoster oticus and facial paralysis (Ramsay Hunt Syndrome). Clinico-pathologic study and review of literature. *J. Neurol. Sci.* **20:**149–159.

Alkalay, A. L., J. J. Pomerance, and L. Rimoin. 1987. Fetal varicella syndrome. *J. Pediatr.* **111:**320–323.

Amlie-Lefond, C., B. K. Kleinschmidt-DeMasters, R. Mahalingam, L. E. Davis, and D. H. Gilden. 1995. The vasculopathy of varicella-zoster virus encephalitis. *Ann. Neurol.* **37:**784–790.

Applebaum, E., M. H. Rachelson, and V. A. Dolgopol. 1953. Varicella encephalitis. *Am. J. Med.* **15:**223–230.

Applebaum, E., S. I. Kreps, and A. Sunshine. 1962. Herpes zoster encephalitis. *Am. J. Med.* **32:**25–31.

Arvin, A. M. 1996. Varicella-zoster virus. *Clin. Microbiol. Rev.* **9:**361–381.

Askalan, R., S. Laughlin, S. Mayank, A. Chan, D. MacGregor, M. Andrew, R. Curtis, B. Meaney, and G. deVeber. 2001. Chickenpox and stroke in childhood: a study of frequency and causation. *Stroke* **32:**1257–1262.

Aviel, A., and G. Marshak. 1982. Ramsay Hunt Syndrome: a cranial polyneuropathy. *Am. J. Otolaryngol.* **3:**61–66.

Aygun, N., D. A. Finelli, M. S. Rodgers, and R. H. Rhodes. 1998. Multifocal varicella-zoster virus leukoencephalitis in a patient with AIDS: MR findings. *Am. J. Neuroradiol.* **19:**1897–1899.

Berrebi, A., C. Assouline, J. M. Ayoubi, O. Parant, and J. Icart. 1998. Chickenpox in pregnancy. *Arch. Pediatr.* **5:**79–83.

Booss, J., B. B. Haak, and R. F. Leroy. 1985. Delayed contralateral hemiplegia following Herpes zoster ophthalmicus: should antiviral therapy be used? *Eur. Neurol.* **24:**225–228.

Carmack, M. A., J. Twiss, D. R. Enzmann, M. D. Amylon, and A. M. Arvin. 1993. Multifocal leukoencephalitis caused by varicella-zoster virus in a child with leukemia: successful treatment with acyclovir. *Pediatr. Infect. Dis. J.* **12:**402–406.

Carroll, W. M., and F. L. Mastaglia. 1979. Optic neuropathy and ophthalmoplegia in herpes zoster oticus. *Neurology* **29:**726–729.

Case Records of the Massachusetts General Hospital. 1996. Case 36–1996. A 37-year-old man with AIDS, neurologic deterioration, and multiple hemorrhagic cerebral lesions. *N. Engl. J. Med.* **335:**1587–1595.

Centers for Disease Control and Prevention. 1996. Prevention of varicella: recommendations of the Advisory Committee on Immunization Practices (ACIP). *Morb. Mortal. Wkly. Rep.* **45**(RR-11):1–36.

Centers for Disease Control and Prevention. 1999. Prevention of varicella: updated recommendations of the Advisory Committee on Immunization Practices (ACIP). *Morb. Mortal. Wkly. Rep.* **48**(RR-6):1–5.

Chiappini, E., G. Calabri, L. Galli, G. Salvi, and M. de Martino. 2002. Varicella-zoster virus acquired at four months of age reactivates at 24 months and causes encephalitis. *J. Pediatr.* **140:**250–251.

Chretien, F., L. Belec, M. C. Lescs, F. J. Authier, P. De Truchis, F. Scaravilli, and F. Gray. 1997. Central nervous system infection due to varicella and zoster virus in AIDS. *Arch. Anat. Cytol. Pathol.* **45:**142–152.

Christie, A. B. 1980. Herpes zoster, p. 278–287. *In Infectious Diseases: Epidemiology and Clinical Practice*, 3rd ed. Churchill Livingstone, Edinburgh, Scotland.

Cinque, P., S. Bossolasco, L. Vago, C. Fornara, S. Lipari, S. Racca, A. Lazzarin, and K. A. Linde. 1997. Varicella zoster virus (VZV) DNA in cerebrospinal fluid of patients infected with human immunodeficiency virus: VZV disease of the central nervous system or subclinical reactivation of VZV infection? *Clin. Infect. Dis.* **25:**634–639.

Corston, R. N., S. Logsdail, and R. B. Godwin-Austin. 1981. Herpes zoster myelitis treated successfully with vidarabine. *Br. Med. J.* **283:**698–699.

Dangond, F., E. Engle, L. Yessayan, and M. H. Sawyer. 1993. Pre-eruptive varicella cerebellitis confirmed by PCR. *Pediatr. Neurol.* **9:**491–493.

Darling, C. F., M. B. Larsen, S. E. Byrd, M. A. Radkowski, P. S. Palka, and E. D. Allen. 1995. MR and CT imaging patterns in post Varicella encephalitis. *Pediatr. Radiol.* **25:**241–244.

Deguen, S., N. P. Chru, and A. Flahault. 1998. Epidemiology of chickenpox in France (1991–1995). *J. Epidemiol. Community Health* **52**(Suppl. 1):46S–49S.

De La Blanchardiere, A., F. Rozenberg, E. Caumes, O. Picard, F. Lionnet, L. Livartowski, J. Coste, D. Sicard, P. Lebon, and D. Salmon-Ceron. 2000. Neurological complications of varicella zoster virus infection in adults with human immunodeficiency virus infection. *Scand. J. Infect. Dis.* **32:**263–269.

DeSilva, S. M., A. S. Mark, D. H. Gilden, R. Mahalingam, M. Balish, F. Sandbrink, and S. Houff. 1996. Zoster myelitis: improvement with antiviral therapy in two cases. *Neurology* **47:**929–931.

Djupesland, G., M. Degre, R. Stein, and S. Skrede. 1977. Acute peripheral facial palsy. Part of a cranial polyneuropathy? *Arch. Otolaryngol.* **103:**641–644.

Doyle, P. W., G. Gibson, and C. L. Dolman. 1983. Herpes zoster ophthalmicus with contralateral hemiplegia: identification of cause. *Ann. Neurol.* **14:**84–85.

Dueland, A. N. 1996. Latency and reactivation of varicella zoster virus infections. *Scand. J. Infect. Dis. Suppl.* **100:**46–50.

Echevarria, J. M., P. Martinez-Martin, A. Téllez, F. de Ory, J. L. Rapun, A. Bernal, E. Estévez, and R. Nájera. 1987. Aseptic meningitis due to varicella-zoster virus: serum antibody levels and local synthesis of specific IgG, IgM, and IgA. *J. Infect. Dis.* **155:**959–967.

Eidelberg, D., A. Sotrel, D. S. Horoupian, P. E. Neumann, T. Pumarola-Sune, and R. W. Price. 1986. Thrombotic cerebral vasculopathy associated with herpes zoster. *Ann. Neurol.* **19:**7–14.

Esiri, M. M., and A. H. Tomlinson. 1972. Herpes zoster. Demonstration of virus in trigeminal nerve and ganglion by immunofluorescence and electron microscopy. *J. Neurol. Sci.* **15:**35–48.

Fryer, D. G., R. Crane, and M. T. Margolis. 1984. Angiographic changes in intracranial arteries of ophthalmic herpes zoster. *Ann. Neurol.* **15:**311–312.

Fukumoto, S., M. Kinjo, K. Hokamura, and K. Tanaka. 1986. Subarachnoid hemorrhage and granulomatous angiitis of the basilar artery: demonstration of varicella-zoster virus in the basilar artery lesions. *Stroke* **17:**1024–1028.

Ganesan, V., and F. J. Kirkham. 1997. Mechanisms of ischaemic stroke after chicken pox. *Arch. Dis. Child.* **76:**522–525.

Gardner-Thorpe, C., J. B. Foster, and D. D. Barwick. 1976. Unusual manifestations of herpes zoster. A clinical and electrophysiologic study. *J. Neurol. Sci.* **28:**427–447.

Gershon, A. A., and S. J. Silverstein. 1997. Varicella-zoster virus, p. 421–444. *In* D. D. Richman, R. J. Whitley, and F. G. Hayden (ed.), *Clinical Virology.* Churchill Livingstone, New York, N.Y.

Gilden, D. H., A. Vafai, Y. Shtram, Y. Becker, M. Devlin, M. Wellish. 1983. Varicella-zoster virus DNA in human sensory ganglia. *Nature* **306:**478–480.

Gilden, D. H., B. K. Kleinschmidt-DeMasters, M. Wellish, E. T. Hedley-Whyte, B. Rentier, and R. Mahalingam. 1996. Varicella zoster virus, a cause of waxing and waning vasculitis: the *New England Journal of Medicine* case 5-1995 revisited. *Neurology* **47:**1441–1446.

Gilden, D. H., J. L. Bennett, B. K. Kleinschmidt-DeMasters, D. D. Song, A. S. Yee, and I. Steiner. 1998. The value of cerebrospinal fluid antiviral antibody in the diagnosis of neurological disease produced by varicella zoster virus. *J. Neurol. Sci.* **159:**140–144.

Gilden, D. H., J. J. LaGuardia, R. Mahalingam, T. M. White, and R. J. Cohrs. 2000a. Neurological complications of varicella-zoster virus, p. 291–319. *In* L. E. Davis and P. G. Kennedy (ed.), *Infectious Diseases of the Nervous System.* Butterworth Heinemann, Oxford, United Kingdom.

Gilden, D. H., B. K. Kleinschmidt-Demasters, J. J. LaGuardia, R. Mahalingam, and R. J. Cohrs. 2000b. Neurologic complications of the reactivation of varicella-zoster virus. *N. Engl. J. Med.* **342:**635–645.

Gold, E. 1966. Serologic and virus-isolation studies of patients with varicella or Herpes-zoster infection. *N. Engl. J. Med.* **274:**181–185.

Gray, F., L. Bélec, M. C. Lescs, F. Chrétien, A. Ciardi, D. Hassine, M. Flament-Saillour, P. de Truchis, B. Clair, and F. Scaravilli. 1994. Varicella-zoster virus infection of the central nervous system in the acquired immune deficiency syndrome. *Brain* **117:**987–999.

Guess, H. A., D. D. Broughton, L. J. Melton III, and L. T. Kurland. 1986. Population-based studies of varicella complications. *Pediatrics* **78**(Suppl.):723–727.

Haanpaa, M., P. Dastidar, A. Weinberg, M. Levin, A. Miettinen, A. Lapinlampi, P. Laippala, and T. Nurmikko. 1998. CSF and MRI findings in patients with acute herpes zoster. *Neurology* **51:**1405–1411.

Harding, B., and J. A. Baumer. 1988. Congenital varicella-zoster. A serologically proven case with necrotising encephalitis and malformation. *Acta Neuropathol.* **76:**311–315.

Hausler, M. G., V. T. Ramaekers, J. Reul, R. Melicke, and G. Heimann. 1998. Early and late onset manifestations of cerebellar vasculitis related to varicella zoster. *Neuropediatrics* **29:**202–207.

Hausler, M., L. Schaade, S. Kemeny, K. Schweizer, C. Schoenmachers, and V. T. Ramaekers. 2002. Encephalitis related to primary varicella-zoster virus infection in immunocompetent children. *J. Neurol. Sci.* **195:**111–116.

Hayashi, T., S. Murayama, M. Sakurai, and I. Kanazawa. 2000. Jugular foramen syndrome caused by varicella zoster virus in a patient with ipsilateral hypoplasia of the jugular foramen. *J. Neurol. Sci.* **172:**70–72.

Heathfield, K. W. G., and A. S. Mee. 1978. Prognosis of the Ramsay Hunt syndrome. *Br. Med. J.* **1:**343–344.

Herrold, J. M., and J. S. Hahn. 1994. Disseminated multifocal herpes zoster leukoencephalitis and subcortical hemorrhage in an immunosuppressed child. *J. Child. Neurol.* **9:**56–58.

Hogan, E. L., and M. R. Krigman. 1973. Herpes zoster myelitis. Evidence for viral invasion of spinal cord. *Arch. Neurol.* **29:**309–313.

Hope-Simpson, R. E. 1965. The nature of herpes zoster: a long-term study and a new hypothesis. *Proc. R. Soc. Med.* **58:**9–20.

Horten, B., R. W. Price, and D. Jimenez. 1981. Multifocal varicella-zoster virus leukoencephalitis temporally remote from herpes zoster. *Ann. Neurol.* **9:**251–266.

Hughes, B. A., D. W. Kimmel, and A. J. Aksamit. 1993. Herpes zoster-associated meningoencephalitis in patients with systemic cancer. *Mayo Clin. Proc.* **68:**652–655.

Ichiyama, T., S. Houdou, T. Kisa, K. Ohno, and K. Takeshita. 1990. Varicella with delayed hemiplegia. *Pediatr. Neurol.* **6:**279–281.

Jemsek, J., S. B. Greenberg, L. Taber, D. Harvey, A. Gershon, and R. B. Couch. 1983. Herpes zoster associated encephalitis: clinicopathological report of 12 cases and review of the literature. *Medicine* **62:**81–97.

Johnson, R., and P. E. Milbourne. 1970. Central nervous system manifestations of chickenpox. *Can. Med. Assoc. J.* **102:**831–834.

Kennedy, P. G., E. Grinfeld, and J. W. Gow. 1999. Latent varicella-zoster virus in human dorsal root ganglia. *Virology* **258:**451–454.

Kleinschmidt-DeMasters, B. K., C. Amlie-Lefond, and D. H. Gilden. 1996. The patterns of varicella-zoster virus encephalitis. *Hum. Pathol.* **27:**927–938.

Klockgether, T., G. Doller, U. Wullner, D. Petersen, and J. Dichgans. 1993. Cerebellar encephalitis in adults. *J. Neurol.* **240:**17–20.

Knox, C. M., D. Chandler, G. A. Short, and T. P. Margolis. 1998. Polymerase chain reaction-based assays of vitreous samples for the diagnosis of viral retinitis. Use in diagnostic dilemmas. *Ophthalmologia* **105:**37–45.

Kuroiwa, Y., and T. Furukawa. 1981. Hemispheric infarction after herpes zoster ophthalmicus: computed tomography and angiography. *Neurology* **31:**1030–1032.

Kustermann, A., C. Zoppini, B. Tassis, M. Della Morte, G. Colucci, and U. Nicolini. 1996. Prenatal diagnosis of congenital varicella infection. *Prenat. Diagn.* **16:**71–74.

LaGuardia, J. J., R. J. Cohrs, and D. H. Gilden. 1999. Prevalence of varicella-zoster virus DNA in dissociated human trigeminal ganglion neurons and nonneuronal cells. *J. Virol.* **73:**8571–8577.

Leibovitz, E., D. Cooper, D. Giurgiutiu, G. Coman, J. Straus, S. J. Orlow, and R. Lawrence. 1993. Varicella-zoster virus infection in Romanian children infected with the human immunodeficiency virus. *Pediatrics* **92:**838–842.

Lentz, D., J. E. Jordan, G. B. Pike, and D. R. Enzmann. 1993. MRI in varicella-zoster virus leukoencephalitis in the immunocompromised host. *J. Comp. Assist. Tomog.* **17:**313–316.

Lewis, G. W. 1958. Zoster sine herpete. *Br. Med. J.* **2:**418–421.

Linneman, C. C., Jr., and M. M. Alvira. 1980. Pathogenesis of varicella-zoster angiitis in the CNS. *Arch. Neurol.* **37:**239–240.

MacKenzie, R. A., G. S. Forbes, and W. E. Karnes. 1981. Angiographic findings in Herpes zoster arteritis. *Ann. Neurol.* **10:**458–464.

Magliocco, A. M., D. J. Demetrick, H. B. Sarnat, and W. S. Hwang. 1992. Varicella embryopathy. *Arch. Pathol. Lab. Med.* **116:**181–186.

Mayo, D. R., and J. Booss. 1989. Varicella zoster-associated neurologic disease without skin lesions. *Arch. Neurol.* **46:**313–315.

McCormick, W. F., R. L. Rodnitzky, S. S. Schocher, Jr., and A. P. McKee. 1969. Varicella-zoster encephalomyelitis. A morphologic and virologic study. *Arch. Neurol.* **21:**559–570.

Melanson, M., C. Chalk, L. Georgevich, K. Fett, Y. Lapierre, H. Guong, J. Richardson, C. Marineau, and G. A. Rouleau. 1996. Varicella-zoster virus DNA in CSF and arteries in delayed contralateral hemiplegia: evidence for viral invasion of cerebral arteries. *Neurology* **47:**569–570.

Miller, H. G., J. B. Stanton, and J. L. Gibbons. 1956. Para-infectious encephalomyelitis and related syndromes. *Q. J. Med.* **25:**427–505.

Miller, L. H., and P. A. Brunell. 1970. Zoster, reinfection or activation of latent virus? Observations on the antibody response. *Am. J. Med.* **49:**480–483.

Moller, A., R. Ackermann, K. Felgenhauer, and H. Ulm. 1982. Zoster-enzephalitis ohne exanthem. Bericht über zwei Fälle. *Dtsch. Med. Wochenschr.* **107:**822–825.

Morgello, S., G. A. Block, R. W. Price, and C. K. Petito. 1988. Varicella-zoster virus leukoencephalitis and cerebral vasculopathy. *Arch. Pathol. Lab. Med.* **112:**173–177.

Moulignier, A., G. Pialoux, H. Dega, B. Dupont, M. Huerre, and M. Baudrimont. 1995. Brainstem encephalitis due to varicella-zoster virus in a patient with AIDS. *Clin. Infect. Dis.* **20:**1378–1380.

Murakami, S., N. Hato, J. Horiuchi, N. Honda, K. Gyo, and N. Yanagihara. 1997. Treatment of Ramsay-Hunt syndrome with acyclovir-prednisone: significance of early diagnosis and treatment. *Ann. Neurol.* **41:**353–357.

Mustonen, K., P. Mustakangas, M. Smeds, L. Mannonen, L. Uotila, A. Vaheri, and M. Koskiniemi. 1998. Antibodies to varicella zoster virus in the cerebrospinal fluid of neonates with seizures. *Arch. Dis. Child Fetal Neonatal Ed.* **78:**F57-61.

Norris, F. H., Jr., R. Leonards, P. R. Calanchini, and C. D. Calder. 1970. Herpes-zoster meningoencephalitis. *J. Infect. Dis.* **122:**335–338.

Otero, J., E. Ribera, J. Gavalda, A. Rovira, I. Ocaña, and A. Pahissa. 1998. Response to acyclovir in two cases of herpes zoster leukoencephalitis and review of the literature. *Eur. J. Clin. Microbiol. Infect. Dis.* **17:**286–289.

Paryani, S. G., and A. M. Arvin. 1986. Intrauterine infection with varicella-zoster virus after maternal varicella. *N. Engl. J. Med.* **314:**1542–1546.

Puchhammer-Stockl, E., T. Popow-Kraupp, F. X. Heinz, C. W. Mandl, and C. Kunz. 1991. Detection of varicella-zoster virus DNA by polymerase chain reaction in the cerebrospinal fluid of patients suffering from neurological complications associated with chickenpox or herpes zoster. *J. Clin. Microbiol.* **29:**1513–1516.

Quereda, C., I. Corral, F. Laguna, M. E. Valencia, A. Tenorio, J. E. Echeverria, E. Navas, P. Martin-Davila, A. Moreno, V. Morreno, J. M. Gonzalez-Lahoz, J. R. Arribas, and A. Guerrero. 2000. Diagnostic utility of a multiplex herpesvirus PCR assay performed with cerebrospinal fluid from human immunodeficiency virus-infected patients with neurological disorders. *J. Clin. Microbiol.* **38:**3061–3067.

Reye, R. D. K., G. Morgan, and J. Baral. 1963. Encephalopathy and fatty infiltration of the viscera: a disease entity in childhood. *Lancet* **ii:**749–752.

Reyes, M. G., R. Fresco, S. Chokroverty, and E. Q. Salud. 1976. Viruslike particles in granulomatous angiitis of the central nervous system. *Neurology* **26:**797–799.

Rosenblum, M. K. 1989. Bulbar encephalitis complicating trigeminal zoster in the acquired immune deficiency syndrome. *Hum. Pathol.* **20:**292–295.

Rosenfeld, J., C. L. Taylor, and S. W. Atlas. 1993. Myelitis following chickenpox: a case report. *Neurology* **43:**1834–1836.

Ross, M. H., W. K. Abend, R. B. Schwartz, and M. A. Samuels. 1991. A case of C2 herpes zoster with delayed bilateral pontine infarction. *Neurology* **41:**1685–1686.

Rousseau, F., C. Perronne, G. Raguin, D. Thouvenot, A. Vidal, C. Leport, and J. L. Vildé. 1993. Necrotizing retinitis and cerebral vasculitis due to varicella-zoster virus in patients infected with the human immunodeficiency virus. *Clin. Infect. Dis.* **17:**943–944.

Ruppenthal, M. 1980. Changes of the central nervous system in herpes zoster. *Acta Neuropathol.* **52:**59–68.

Scaravilli, F., and F. Gray. 1993. Opportunistic infections. *In* F. Gray (ed.), *Atlas of the Neuropathology of HIV Infection.* Oxford University Press, Oxford, United Kingdom.

Schmidbauer, M., H. Budka, P. Pilz, T. Kurata, and R. Hondo. 1992. Presence, distribution and spread of productive varicella zoster virus infection in nervous tissues. *Brain* **115:**383–398.

Sébire, G., L. Meyer, and S. Chabrier. 1999. Varicella as a risk factor for cerebral infarction in childhood: a case-control study. *Ann. Neurol.* **45:**679–680.

Steiner, I., B. Steiner-Birmanns, N. Levin, K. Hershko, I. Korn-Lubetzki, and I. Biran. 2001. Spinal cord involvement in uncomplicated herpes zoster. *Clin. Diagn. Lab. Immunol.* **8:**850–851.

Stowasser, M., J. Gameron, and W. A. Oliver. 1990. Diaphragmatic paralysis following cervical herpes zoster. *Med. J. Aust.* **153:**555–556.

Takashima, S., and L. E. Becker. 1979. Neuropathology of fatal varicella. *Arch. Pathol. Lab. Med.* **103:**209–213.

Tauro, S., V. Toh, H. Osman, and P. Mahendra. 2000. Varicella zoster meningoencephalitis following treatment for dermatomal zoster in an Allo BMT patient. *Bone Marrow Transplant.* **26:**795–796.

Tenser, R. B. 2001. Herpes zoster infection and postherpetic neuralgia. *Curr. Neurol. Neurosci. Rep.* **1:**526–532.

Thomas, J. E., and F. M. Howard, Jr. 1972. Segmental zoster paresis—a disease profile. *Neurology* **22:**459–466.

Transverse Myelitis Consortium Working Group. 2002. Proposed diagnostic criteria and nosology of acute transverse myelitis. *Neurology* **59:**499–505.

Underwood, E. A. 1935. The neurological complications of varicella: a clinical epidemiological study. *Br. J. Child Dis.* **32:**83–107, 177–196, 241–263.

Watson, C. P. N. 2000. A new treatment for postherpetic neuralgia. *N. Engl. J. Med.* **343:**1563–1565.

Weaver, S., M. K. Rosenblum, and L. M. DeAngelis. 1999. Herpes varicella zoster encephalitis in immunocompromised patients. *Neurology* **52:**193–195.

Weller, T. H. 1983. Varicella and herpes zoster. Changing concepts of the natural history, control and importance of a not-so-benign virus. *N. Engl. J. Med.* **309:**1362–1368, 1434–1440.

Ziebold, C., R. von Kries, R. Lang, J. Weiel, and H. J. Schmitt. 2001. Severe complications of varicella in previously healthy children. *Pediatrics* **108**(e79)**:**1194–1195.

ACUTE EPIDEMIC ENCEPHALITIS

10

Influenza Virus, Enteroviruses, and Other Epidemic Viruses

Epidemic encephalitis was first recognized in the form of von Economo's encephalitis lethargica (EL) in the same decade as World War I and the great pandemic of influenza. In the two following decades, several arboviral encephalitis epidemics were described and the viruses were isolated. These included eastern, western, and Venezuelan equine encephalitis, which demonstrated that human epidemics could be associated with epizootics. It subsequently became clear that epidemics of other viral diseases, such as measles and influenza, which primarily attacked other organ systems, occasionally brought central nervous system (CNS) disease in their wake (Table 10.1). It was also recognized that several enteroviruses, including poliovirus, that cause recurrent epidemics of CNS disease can occasionally produce encephalitis. More recently, enterovirus 71 (EV-71) has caused outbreaks of hand-foot-and-mouth (HFM) disease in association with a rapidly lethal brain stem encephalitis. Remarkably, paramyxoviruses have caused a series of lethal epizootics involving the brains of aquatic and terrestrial mammals in the past two decades. These include Nipah virus, which is highly lethal to workers on pig farms in Malaysia and to abbatoir workers in Singapore. Most significantly, however, a new human lentivirus, one of a family of viruses associated with impairment of reticuloendothelial system function and "slow viral" infection of the CNS, emerged clinically in the last two decades of the 20th century. Human immunodeficiency virus (HIV) has been estimated to have infected over 50 million people, to have killed over 20 million people, and to have disrupted the social fabric of whole continents, most notably Africa. Included among the horrors of this illness is a progressive dementing process due to the direct effect of the virus itself, the AIDS dementia complex. HIV/AIDS will be discussed in chapter 12. The arboviral encephalitides are discussed in chapter 11.

Epidemic encephalitis requires the clinician to investigate circumstances in the community for evidence of contact with disease. Aggregation of children in schools provides the ideal incubator for epidemics of influenza. Movements of people into new environments may spark epidemics, for example, the spread of tick-borne encephalitis when the virgin timberland, the taiga, was developed in Russia. In the north temperate zone, the season will determine which diseases are likely to be epidemic. Thus, influenza occurs during winter months, whereas arboviral and enteroviral infections occur in the summer and early fall. Certain questions are particularly useful when dealing with suspected epidemic disease. Travel, exposure to disease at home, at work, and among social contacts, and animal exposure are

TABLE 10.1 Mechanisms of transmission of epidemic viral and putative viral diseases

Human-to-human transmission
  HIV
  Influenza virus
    Encephalopathy
    Postviral encephalomyelitis
  RSV
  Enteroviruses
    Polioviruses
    Coxsackieviruses
    Echoviruses
    EV-71
    AHC (EV-70)
Animal-to-human transmission
  Hendra virus
  Nipah virus
Arthropod-borne transmission–chapter 11
Unknown means of transmission
  von Economo's encephalitis lethargica
  Epidemic myalgic encephalomyelitis

potential sources of disease. Paul (1966) emphasized the usefulness of a domicillary chart, which is a plot of illness and significant exposures in the family and contacts, as well as in the patient, in a chronological order. The patient may have developed a CNS complication of a systemic illness experienced by other members of the household or contacts. The local health department can tell the clinician which viral diseases are presently active in the community.

HUMAN-TO-HUMAN TRANSMISSION

Influenza Virus

The most important cause of modern acute viral epidemics must certainly be influenza. Significant epidemics occur with influenza A virus every few years, with worldwide pandemics occurring at variable periods up to several decades apart. A small number of cases of encephalopathy and encephalomyelitis occur in these epidemics. More than one pathogenetic mechanism operates, and the exact frequency of CNS complications of influenza is difficult to document. However, a review of case reports from the 1998/1999 influenza season in Japan, using a clinical case definition and laboratory confirmation, uncovered 217 cases of encephalitis or encephalopathy from about 860,000 cases of influenzalike illnesses (Kasai et al., 2000). Over 80% were in children under 5 years of age.

The major difficulty in establishing the etiologic link between influenza and encephalitis has been the infrequency of viral isolation from the brain or cerebrospinal fluid (CSF). For example, in a study of 33 fatal cases of influenza, which included 4 with encephalopathic symptomatology, the two attempts to recover virus from the brain in the encephalopathic cases were unsuccessful (Oseasohn et al., 1959). Swelling was found in the brain but significant signs of inflammation were not. It was concluded that a diagnosis of encephalitis had not been supported and that encephalopathy was a preferable designation. Influenza A virus was isolated from the brain as well as the lung and the liver from a child dying with pneumonia and encephalitis in the British Isles in 1970 (Anonymous, 1970). Recovery of influenza A virus from the CSF has been reported for three Jamaican patients, two of whom had encephalitic signs (Rose and Prabhakar, 1982). Further, Frankova et al. (1977) were able to isolate influenza A virus from the brain in 9 of 77 fatal cases studied at Prague between 1971 and 1975. No clinical neurological details were given, and in all except one case, the cerebral pathology was limited to hyperemia and edema. These investigators isolated virus from brain tissue that lacked evidence of inflammation. More recently, PCR has been used to demonstrate the association of influenza A (Fujimoto et al., 1998) and B (McCullers et al., 1999) with encephalitis/encephalopathy. However, positive findings with PCR were also found to be infrequent (Ito et al., 1999).

Another problem has been the tendency to ascribe encephalitis to influenza based on insufficient evidence. Wells (1971) studied 19 cases of neurological dysfunction following a prodromal illness during an influenza epidemic. Serological evidence compatible with influenza was found in eight cases, but evidence for other specific viruses was found in six cases. Serological confirmation may be difficult to achieve if neurological complications follow the respiratory illness by a sufficient period. Patients may have achieved maximal levels of antibody on first evaluation, as when parainfectious encephalomyelitis follows influenza.

Respiratory Illness

Three influenza strains are recognized. Type A and type B are associated with major epidemics and type C is an infrequent cause of disease. The capacity of type A to cause recurrent major epidemics results from changes in the antigenic configuration of its two major surface glycoproteins, hemagglutinin (H) and neuraminidase (N). Strains of the A viruses thus have an HN designation. Minor changes of antigenicity, which are termed "antigenic drift," result from point mutations in the genes coding for N and/or H and are associated with the more frequent but less intense epidemics seen every 3 to 4 years. Pandemics occurring every 10 to 15 years are associated with major changes resulting from new gene segments coding for H and N, termed "antigenic shift" (Hayden and Palese, 1997). Phenotypic changes are facilitated by reassortment of eight single-stranded RNA segments, with new gene segments derived from birds, and mixing of human and avian segments occurring in pigs. Pandemics may result in infection of over 50% of the exposed populations. Pandemics of the 20th century appeared to have arisen in China (Hayden and Palese, 1997). Reassortment of RNA segments from animals does not appear to occur with type B influenza, and subtypes are not found.

Infection occurs by direct contact and by droplet transmission of nasopharyngeal secretions. The incubation period averages 2 days but ranges from 1 to 4 days. Approximately half of those infected demonstrate clear signs of illness (Davenport, 1982; Cox and Subbarao, 1999). Manifestations of the illness include the abrupt onset of chills and fever, headache, malaise and prostration, muscle pains, and a nonproductive cough. Gastrointestinal (GI) symptomatology can occur in children. Fever often declines by day 3, but it may be diphasic. Full daily activity is usually resumed within a week or 10 days, although a hacking nonproductive cough may continue for weeks. Complications are most likely to occur in the elderly and in those with chronic debilitating disease. The most frequent acute complication is the development of pneumonia. In some cases it results from the virus itself, or it can result from superinfection with bacteria.

The diagnosis of influenza infection (Cox and Subbarao, 1999) had formerly relied on virus isolation from nasopharyngeal and throat swabs or fourfold rises between acute- and convalescent-phase serum samples. However, with the increased range of antiviral therapy, rapid point-of-care diagnostic kits have become available. The comparative sensitivity of these tests continues to be evaluated. Reverse transcription PCR is very sensitive and has proven useful in the evaluation of the acute encephalopathy of influenza.

Antiviral prophylaxis of exposed persons and early treatment of symptomatic individuals are available (Couch, 2000). Amantadine and rimantadine are effective against influenza A in an early stage of viral replication. Zanamivir and oseltamivir are neuroaminidase inhibitors that are effective against both influenza A and B. It is unclear whether treatment of the acute respiratory illness in influenza alters the incidence of neurological complications.

Neuropathology

Reports of single cases or small series of cases have described several diferent types of cerebral pathology associated with influenza infections. First, there is a lymphocytic encephalitis including perivascular mononuclear inflammatory cell cuffs accompanied by some petechial hemorrhages, particularly in the gray matter (Furtado, 1958; Harada, 1966). This seems to be the rarest type of pathology found in influenza-associated neurological disease. The second pathological finding is that of acute hemorrhagic leukoencephalitis, which has been described in association with influenza infection on a few occasions (Hoult and Flewett, 1960; Delorme and Middleton, 1979; Sulkava et al., 1981). Third, perivenous encephalitis has also been described but is exceptionally rare after influenza (Hoult and Flewett, 1960). A fourth type of pathology seen is that of Reye's syndrome and an encephalopathy resembling that seen in Reye's syndrome (Davis and Kornfeld, 1980). Epidemics of influenza B had been associated with marked increases in the numbers of patients presenting with this condition (Linneman et al., 1975). Finally, encephalopathy of a nonspecific nature may be found.

Clinical Manifestations in the CNS

Although the frequency of CNS complications of influenza is low, there are many types of clinical syndromes (Table 10.2). The mechanisms of attack on the nervous system also appear to be varied (Hoult and Flewett, 1960). Syndromes and their pathogeneses resulting from parainfectious immune attack are covered in chapters 7 and 8.

Encephalopathy/Encephalitis. Acute cerebral disease at the height of an attack by influenza, associated with swelling and congestion with or without signs of inflammation in the brain, has been reported by several investigators (Flewett

TABLE 10.2 Neurological syndromes associated with influenza

CNS
Acute encephalitis/encephalopathy
Acute psychosis
Parainfectious processes (chapters 7 and 8)
Encephalomyelitis
Acute necrotizing encephalopathy of childhood
Acute hemorrhagic leukoencephalopathy of Hurst
Transverse myelitis
Acute ataxia of childhood
Reye's syndrome (particularly after influenza B)
Peripheral neuromuscular system
Guillain-Barré syndrome (infection; 1976/1977 swine flu immunization)
Myositis (particularly influenza B)

and Hoult, 1958; Delorme and Middleton, 1979; Kasai et al., 2000). It is found predominantly in children under 5 years of age. Evidence of virus in CSF has been reported in some cases (Fujimoto et al., 1998; Ito et al., 1999), and the role of proinflammatory cytokines such as interleukin-6 (IL-6) has been investigated (Ito et al., 1999; Aiba et al., 2001). While virus has been isolated from brain in fatal cases (Anonymous, 1970; Frankova et al., 1977), whether permissive or nonpermissive replication occurs in the brain is unclear. In animal model studies of influenza B in mice, Davis et al. (1990) found a nonpermissive viral infection of cerebral endothelial cells associated with diffuse cerebral edema.

The onset in children during acute influenzal symptoms usually includes seizures and depression of level of consciousness (Flewett and Hoult, 1958; Kasai et al., 2000; Aiba et al., 2001). Less severe manifestations include a variety of symptoms such as behavioral abnormalities (Delorme and Middleton, 1979). Severe cases evolve rapidly to demonstrate brain stem dysfunction. Aiba et al. (2001) found that elevation of cytokines, particularly serum IL-6, was a useful predictor of severity. The cases reported from Japan also included hepatic and renal abnormalities, as well as disseminated intravascular coagulation and shock (Aiba et al., 2001). Although the CSF may contain a pleocytosis and a protein increase in some cases, the CSF is often normal (Flewett and Hoult, 1958; Delorme and Middleton, 1979). Cranial computerized tomography (CT) scans have revealed cerebral edema (Fujimoto et al., 1998; Fujii et al., 1992). Several reports of acute multifocal abnormalities on imaging studies have been published (Fujii et al., 1992; Nagai et al., 1993; Mizuguchi et al., 1995). Mizuguchi et al. (1995) described acute necrotizing encephalopathy of childhood and reviewed a total of 41 cases in which multiple symmetrically distributed necrotic lesions were found. Seven cases had laboratory evidence of influenza virus infection. The relationship of these cases to diffuse influenzal encephalitis on the one hand and the acute hemorrhagic leukoencephalitis following influenza remains to be determined.

Therapy of acute severe influenzal encephalopathy/encephalitis requires intensive care unit (ICU) management for possible mechanical respiratory support, reduction of intracranial pressure, and seizure management. The role of antiviral therapy has not been systematically reported. However, the occurrence of the encephalopathy/encephalitis at the height of the attack of influenza and the reports of positive CSF PCR in some cases suggest that antiviral compounds should be employed. High-dose dexamethasone therapy would be indicated in severe cases to help manage cerebral swelling and to block a putative neurocytotoxic effect of cytokines (Aiba et al., 2001). The encephalopathy/encephalitis can be highly destructive. Kasai et al. (2000) found that 58 of 217 patients with the diagnosis died and 56 others of the 217 had neurological sequelae. In a series of six cases in which no patients died, Delorme and Middleton (1979) reported that three had sequelae.

Parainfectious Encephalitis. For cases of encephalitis occurring 1 to 3 weeks after the onset of clinical influenza, a parainfectious immune-mediated process is most likely. The role of replicating virus must be excluded in light of the report of virus isolation from the CSF of three patients, two of whom had symptoms of encephalitis (Rose and Prabhakar, 1982). In four cases of postinfectious encephalitis reported by Sulkava et al. (1981), three demonstrated diagnostic serological rises to influenza A virus. Neurological signs developed a week after respiratory symptoms and included depression of level of consciousness, disorientation, confusion, and seizures. Although coma evolved in two, all patients recovered within less than 4 weeks. Lumbar punctures revealed pleocytosis and elevated protein. Electroencephalograms (EEGs) were characterized by generalized slowing, but no abnormalities were found on CT scanning. Kimura et al. (1995) reported two cases of postinfectious focal encephalitis in children manifested by focal motor seizures that became generalized. EEGs revealed delta waves, and the CSF contained a pleocytosis of over 300 cells in both cases. Magnetic resonance imaging (MRIs) revealed T2 high-intensity lesions, predominantly in the cortex. The authors commented that the term acute disseminated encephalomyelitis (ADEM) would not be used because white matter was not primarily involved, hence the term "postinfectious focal encephalitis." Prednisolone therapy was used in one case. An angiopathy was considered based on MRI enhancing lesions and elevated thrombin-antithrombin III complexes. Although steroid therapy in postinfluenzal encephalitis was described as early as 1958 (Flewett and Hoult, 1958), multi-institution controlled trials remain to be done.

Prevention

Current inactivated influenza vaccines include two influenza A subtypes and influenza B. The type A subtypes are based on projections of the likely prevalence in the coming influenza season. Efficacy is 70 to 100% in healthy adults (Couch, 2000). Vaccination is particularly recommended for those at risk of severe disease and complications, such as the elderly, those with chronic debilitating disease, health care workers and others in a position to transmit the virus to high-risk individuals, children on chronic aspirin therapy who might be at risk for Reye's syndrome, and women who will be in the second or third trimester of pregnancy during the influenza season (Centers for Disease Control and Prevention, 2002a). Depending on vaccine availability, vaccination of healthy adults from 50 to 64 years of age is also advisable (Ahmed et al., 2001; Centers for Disease Control

and Prevention, 2002a). Side effects include soreness at the site of injection for 1 to 2 days (Couch, 2000). Persons with egg protein allergy should not be immunized. The vaccine program in 1976 to 1977 (swine strain) was associated with an increased incidence of the Guillain-Barré syndrome (Langmuir et al., 1984), but an increased incidence has not been found in subsequent years (Couch, 2000).

RSV

One of, if not the most, important causes of acute respiratory diseases in infants and children, respiratory syncytial virus (RSV) is an enveloped RNA virus in the *Paramyxovirus* family (Simoes, 1999; Hall, 2001; Mace, 2002). Peak RSV activity is during the winter seasons in temperate climates and in the rainy season in the tropics. Transmitted by aerosol to nose and eyes, it has an incubation period of 2 to 8 days. Disease starts in the upper respiratory tract and quickly moves to the lower respiratory tract, where it is the principal cause of bronchiolitis of infants. Upper respiratory illness, pneumonia, and otitis media are other common manifestations. Severe illness and risk of death are particularly apt to occur in infants with underlying conditions such as prematurity, young age, preexisting pulmonary or cardiac disease, and immunodeficiency. The acute illness runs its course over about 9 to 11 days. The roles of aerosolized ribavirin, steroids, and immunoglobulin in the therapy of infected infants have remained unclear. Infections in adults are less well defined, but it is apparent that RSV is a significant cause of respiratory infection, particularly in the elderly. This odd situation—widespread infection in infants, with virtually 100% seropositive by age three, and common infection in adults—comes about because infection does not produce lifelong immunity and reinfection is common.

The association of encephalopathy with RSV infection of infants has been reported by Ng et al. (2001). In a retrospective study of 487 infants hospitalized for RSV-induced bronchiolitis, 9 were reported to have developed an encephalopathy in the form of seizures. Focal neurological abnormalities were not reported. CSFs revealed no abnormalities, and neuroimaging was within normal limits. Abnormalities were found in the EEGs of five of the nine patients. These consisted of epileptiform discharges, sharp waves, slowing, and spikes. Two of the patients developed status epilepticus. The investigators made the point that the seizures were not febrile convulsions (Hall, 2001). Although hypotonia and transient loss of developmental milestones were noted in two other patients not in the reported series, posthospitalization outcomes were not reported (Ng et al., 2001).

Hirayama et al. (1999) reported on a 3-year-old girl who presented with fever, somnolence, conjugate eye deviation, intention tremor, and truncal ataxia. The CSF contained over 600 white cells per mm^3 and a CSF protein of 157 mg/dl. Serial MRIs revealed multiple lesions in the cerebellum, followed a year later by atrophy. SPECT and PET studies also revealed abnormalities in the cerebellum. An EEG revealed diffuse high-voltage slow waves. While RSV was isolated from a nasal discharge and throat swab and a diagnostic rise in anti-RSV antibodies was documented in serum, no significant respiratory disease was described. In the acute phase of the illness, urinary catheterization was required. Two months after the onset the patient was discharged with mild trunkal ataxia. Although the cerebellum, cerebrum, and spinal cord appeared to be involved, the authors felt that ADEM was less likely than an acute cerebellitis.

The diagnosis of RSV infection is made by isolation of virus, immunofluorescence, or enzyme-linked immunosorbent assay (ELISA) on nasal pharyngeal aspirates or washes. Viral diagnosis is more difficult in the elderly because of a brief period of virus shedding (Simoes, 1999). There appears to be no report of a systematic search for RSV in CSF by PCR, but the literature does contain a report of anti-RSV complement fixing antibodies in a case of meningitis and in three cases of myelitis (Cappel et al., 1975).

Treatment for neurological complications of RSV infection will depend on the nature of the syndrome—anticonvulsants for seizures and steroids if there is evidence of a multifocal ADEM, for example. Vaccines remain under study. A Formalin-inactivated vaccine studied in the 1960s resulted in more severe illness on exposure to natural infection than in controls (Hall, 2001). High-risk infants without cyanotic heart disease are recommended to receive prophylactic RSV hyperimmune globulin or palivizumah, a monoclonal antibody against a viral fusion protein, during the season of RSV prevalence (Hall, 2001).

Enteroviruses

Overview

Aseptic meningitis is the most frequent manifestation, and epidemics of paralytic polio have been the most important manifestation, of enterovirus infection. However, enteroviruses also cause encephalitis, such as a lethal brain stem encephalitis found in association with some outbreaks of HFM disease caused by EV-71.

The enteroviruses are picornaviruses, small RNA viruses. The other major category of picornaviruses of importance to humans is the rhinovirus genus, which is a frequent cause of respiratory illness. Another picornavirus group, the cardioviruses, have been isolated from rodents and on very rare occasions appear to have been associated with CNS disease in humans (Dick et al., 1948). Enteroviruses are subdivided into polioviruses, coxsackie A viruses, coxsackie B viruses, and numbered enteroviruses 68 to 71 (Table 10.3). EV-72—hepatitis A—has been reclassified (Zeichhardt and Grunert, 2000).

Polio was originally an endemic disease of infancy and early childhood. However, improved sanitation practices delayed exposure to the virus until older ages in western countries. As a consequence, epidemics of paralytic disease due to poliovirus developed in the 19th and 20th centuries.

Polio has been a significant stimulus to the development of virology, including the recognition of the other enteroviruses. Originally separated by pathogenesis into coxsackieviruses and echoviruses, so much overlap became apparent that subsequently characterized members were simply identified as numbered enteroviruses. Coxsackieviruses, named for a village in New York State, were distinguished from poliovirus by pathogenicity for newborn mice. Group A is associated with widespread muscle disease, whereas group B is associated with other types of pathological

TABLE 10.3 Enterovirus syndromes

Poliovirus
  Asymptomatic
  "Minor" systemic illness
  "Major" illness
    Aseptic meningitis
    Paralytic illness
  Post-polio syndrome
Coxsackie and echoviruses
  Herpangina—coxsackie A viruses
  Pleurodynia, myocarditis, pericarditis—coxsackie B viruses
  Aseptic meningitis—coxsackie A and B, echo, and numbered
    enteroviruses
  Encephalitis—coxsackie A and B, echo, and numbered
    enteroviruses
    Diffuse
    Focal
  Chronic enteroviral meningoencephalitis in hypo- or
    agammaglobulinemia patients—primarily echovirus
Enteroviruses 68–71
  Acute hemorrhagic conjunctivitis with delayed
    radiculomyelitis—EV-70
  Hand-foot-and-mouth disease with brain stem
    encephalitis—EV-71

lesions. Of clinical significance, however, was the recognition that each group tended to produce certain syndromes. Group A was associated with herpangina, and group B was associated with pleurodynia, pericarditis, and myocarditis (Dalldorf and Melnick, 1965). Both groups occasionally produced paralytic disease, which was usually mild and often transient. Most importantly, both groups caused aseptic meningitis and occasionally produced encephalitis.

Application of tissue culture techniques to the study of poliovirus uncovered the echoviruses. Found as transient residents of the GI tract, originally unassociated with disease, they were termed "enteric cytopathogenic human orphan" viruses, hence the acronym "echo." Although subsequently associated with a variety of clinical syndromes, most notably aseptic meningitis, they highlight an important diagnostic problem. Because enteroviruses are frequently isolated from the GI tract of healthy individuals, particularly during epidemic periods, it is difficult to diagnose an illness based only on virus isolation from the stool. Later, it became apparent that the characteristics to separate group A and B coxsackieviruses and echoviruses were not absolute. Molecular techniques have clarified the relationships of the 66 enteroviruses now recognized (Muir et al., 1998; Oberste et al., 1999).

EV-70 and EV-71 have significant effects on the nervous system. Infection with EV-70 can result in the rapid appearance of an acute hemorrhagic conjunctivitis (AHC). Fortunately, the conjunctivitis is self-limited and leaves no residue. However, in a very small number of cases it has been followed in 1 to 5 weeks by a syndrome of radiculomyelitis. This consists of an often asymmetric flaccid paralysis accompanied at the outset by radicular pains (Hung et al., 1976). Flaccid paralysis and atrophy were often permanent. Monkeys inoculated in the spinal cord and thalamus with EV-70 demonstrated a pathological picture strongly reminiscent of polio infection (Kono et al., 1973). The brain stem encephalitis associated with EV-71 is described separately below.

The distribution of enteroviruses is worldwide. In countries in the temperate zone such as the United States and the United Kingdom, the peak number of epidemic cases occurs in the summer and early fall. However, sporadic cases appear year-round. In the United States, the Centers for Disease Control and Prevention track the incidence and prevalence of enteroviruses through the voluntary National Enterovirus Surveillance System. The report for the period from 1997 to 1999 estimates that enteroviruses caused 10 to 15 million symptomatic infections annually in the United States (Centers for Disease Control and Prevention, 2000a). Of submitted samples with clinical information, 37.6% were for aseptic meningitis, 4.1% were for encephalitis, and 0.2% were for paralytic disease. While there is a bias in favor of sampling more serious illness rather than benign febrile or respiratory illnesses, the data do suggest the relative frequency of processes involving the nervous system. Although there are 66 serotypes of enterovirus, 9 showed up most frequently in surveys from 1970 to 1983 (Strikas et al., 1986), 1993 to 1996 (Centers for Disease Control and Prevention, 1997), and 1997 to 1999 (Centers for Disease Control and Prevention, 2000a). Among the nonpolio enteroviruses, echoviruses 30, 11, 7, and 9, EV-70 and EV-71, and coxsackievirus B5 are the most common neurotropic and neurovirulent agents (Rotbart, 1995). Recently, increased echovirus 13 activity has been found as a cause of aseptic meningitis in Europe, the United Kingdom, and the United States (Centers for Disease Control and Prevention, 2001a). Echoviruses 18 and 13 emerged as the most commonly reported enterovirus serotypes in the United States in 2001 (Centers for Disease Control and Prevention, 2002b).

Transmission of infection is usually by the fecal-oral route, but the apparent incubation period is highly variable. Thus AHC may present less than 24 h after exposure, yet other infections may take 2 to 3 weeks to manifest. In general the incubation time averages 5 to 10 days. In biphasic illnesses the interval preceding neurological involvement varies with the virus. In polio infections the interval between the minor illness and CNS involvement is often 3 to 4 days, but the neurological complications following AHC may appear 5 weeks later. Asymptomatic infection of the GI tract with enteroviruses is a common finding. Hence the ratio of inapparent to apparent infection is usually high, with 90 to 95% of poliovirus infections and a lower proportion for coxsackie and echovirus infections being asymptomatic (Zeichhardt and Grunert, 2000).

Encephalitis

CNS involvement by enteroviruses is accompanied by fever, headache, nausea and vomiting, and stiff neck (Horstmann and Yamada, 1968; Haynes et al., 1969). In an outbreak of echovirus 9 meningoencephalitis in 196 children, Haynes et al. (1969) found that one-third developed lethargy or delirium, six patients had seizures, and one was semicomatose on admission. Males outnumbered females 2.7:1. One patient died and was found at autopsy to have marked cerebral edema. All other patients recovered within 3 weeks. In general, enterovirus encephalitis produces diffuse

involvement of the brain (Modlin et al., 1991). Depression of level of consciousness, confusion, and irritability are found, and coma and seizures may emerge (Rotbart, 1997). However, focal encephalitis may suggest herpes simplex encephalitis (HSE). Modlin et al. (1991) reported on four pediatric patients who presented with focal seizures. On review of the literature, three other cases were considered. Of the seven, four had the acute onset of unilateral weakness and five had focal seizures. Focality was identified by EEG, isotope brain scan, or CT scan in five. The responsible agent was a coxsackie A virus in five of the seven patients. Because the clinical picture of meningoencephalitis is nonspecific, the presence of other signs and symptoms of enteroviral infection is useful to suggest an etiologic diagnosis. Rash, pleurodynia, herpangina, and myocarditis are particularly useful. Enteroviruses can also cause acute ataxia of childhood and acute childhood hemiplegia (Grist et al., 1978).

The outcome of enterovirus encephalitis is usually benign, although a mortality rate of 2.5% has been recorded (Center for Disease Control, 1981). Modlin et al. (1991) commented on the prompt recovery in contrast to HSE. Human pathological studies are limited to an occasional report of perivenous encephalitis associated with isolation of enterovirus from the GI tract (Heathfield et al., 1967). In the immediate convalescent period, irritability, fatigue, and impaired concentration are common complaints. Lepow et al. (1962) emphasized that muscle weakness and tightness may persist for several months following aseptic meningitis. The effect of enteroviral meningoencephalitis during infancy on subsequent development has been controversial. In reviewing the literature, Rotbart (1995) favored the conclusion that no differences between controls and patients could be demonstrated in neurodevelopmental characteristics.

In contrast to enterovirus encephalitis in immunocompetent patients, untreated chronic enteroviral infections of the CNS in patients with congenital antibody deficiency syndromes have a high morbidity and mortality (chapter 13).

Nonviral laboratory studies are supportive of CNS infection but are not specific. Thus the peripheral white cell count may be normal or elevated with an increase in polymorphonuclear cells. The lumbar puncture usually demonstrates a pleocytosis. Polymorphonuclear cells may predominate, particularly in the early stages. CSF protein may be normal or elevated, particularly later in the course of the illness. In an EEG study of acute aseptic meningitis, Gibbs et al. (1962) found slight slowing in 12 to 18% of enteroviral cases and very slow records in 0 to 18%. Focality has occasionally been demonstrated by EEG, CT, or isotopic brain scan (Modlin et al., 1991).

Viral diagnosis had traditionally relied on virus isolation and antibody changes to the isolated virus. Because there are no group-specific antigens and individual virus testing is very time-consuming, routine serological screening of most enteroviral infections is usually not practicable. Therefore, reliance is placed on viral isolation and, more recently, on CSF PCR (Rotbart, 1995). Throat, stool, blood, and CSF specimens are required. Because enteroviral infections are frequently asymptomatic in the GI tract, isolation of virus from the throat or the stool does not allow a definitive diagnosis. Isolation or PCR identification of an enterovirus from the CSF is usually sufficient to allow a diagnosis. However, enteroviruses have been isolated from CSF that was otherwise normal (Wenner, 1982), and on occasion enterovirus has been isolated in cases of encephalitis associated with another agent (for example, Smith et al., 1974). Therefore, more diagnostic information should be gathered. The presence of an outbreak of a similar neurological disease in the community, virus identification in the CSF, and a fourfold antibody rise against the isolated virus consolidate the diagnosis.

Recent studies, including clinical trials, have demonstrated the activity of the compound pleconaril against many clinically significant enteroviruses (Pevear et al., 1999). The compound fits into a molecular pocket in the virus and interferes with attachment and uncoating. Unfortunately, it does not appear to be effective against EV-71. Pleconaril has been made available by the manufacturer on a compassionate-use basis for treatment of potentially life-threatening enterovirus infections (Rotbart et al., 2001).

Bulbar Polio

Poliovirus was the cause of severe epidemics of paralytic disease in the first half of the 20th century, and its global elimination is being actively pursued. The virus was first isolated and transmitted to monkeys by Landsteiner and Popper in 1908. It is a member of the picornavirus group, which are small RNA nonenveloped viruses 22 to 30 nm in diameter with an icosahedral shape. Three antigenically distinct strains of poliovirus exist. Similar to the other enteroviruses, the primary site of infection and multiplication of poliovirus is in the GI tract.

Pathology. Poliovirus, in the tiny minority of cases in which it infects the CNS, most commonly produces pathological changes in the spinal cord, where involvement is characteristically patchy and asymmetrical. In severe cases, in which most patients die in the acute stage of infection, the brain stem is also involved. As the name "poliomyelitis" implies, the damage is largely restricted to the gray matter. Bodian (1972) provided a detailed review of the pathology

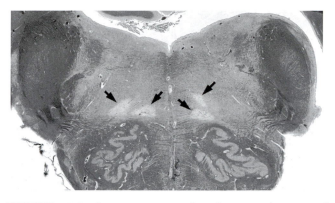

FIGURE 10.2 Low-power view of myelin-stained section of the medulla in acute bulbar poliomyelitis. Pallor of staining reflecting edema and inflammation is seen in focal regions of the reticular formation (arrows).

of polio. Molecular aspects of the biology of poliovirus are reviewed by Blondel et al. (1998). Macroscopically, congestion and edema are evident in the most severely affected areas, but the changes are not gross. In the spinal cord the most intense microscopic lesions are confined to the anterior horns of the gray matter (Fig. 10.1). Less severe changes are seen in the intermediate and posterior gray matter and in the anterior nerve roots and posterior root ganglia. The sacral anterior segments concerned with sphincter function are selectively spared (Elliott, 1947).

In the brain stem the motor nuclei of cranial nerves V, VII, IX, and X are most severely involved. There is also diffuse or patchy damage to the reticular formation of the medulla and pons (Fig. 10.2 and 10.3). In the pons and midbrain the tegmental areas and sometimes the substantia nigra are affected. Certain other brain stem nuclei, including the oculomotor nuclei and inferior olives, are spared. Above the midbrain the pathological changes are less severe, but there are frequently some inflammatory foci in the hypothalamus and subthalamic nuclei and, to a lesser extent, the thalamus, basal ganglia, and precentral motor cortex. The deep gray matter of the cerebellum is also frequently but mildly involved.

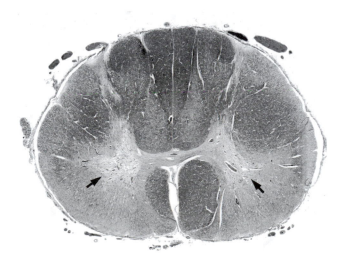

FIGURE 10.1 Low-power view of myelin-stained section of the cervical spinal cord in acute poliomyelitis. There is pallor reflecting edema and inflammation selectively affecting the anterior horns (arrows).

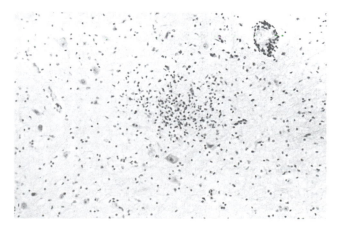

FIGURE 10.3 Focus of neuronophagia in the tegmentum of the pons in acute poliomyelitis. Lymphocytic cuffing is seen around a small vessel, top right. Hematoxylin and eosin stain.

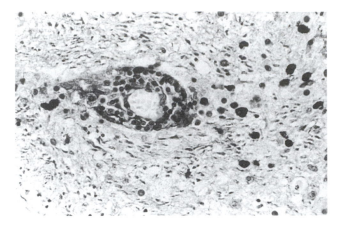

FIGURE 10.4 Perivascular cuffing in acute poliomyelitis. The section has been treated with an antibody to IgA and shows plasma containing IgA and lymphocytes in the perivascular space and neuropil. Counterstained with hematoxylin.

The earliest microscopic changes have not been observed in humans but have been studied in animals experimentally infected with poliovirus. First, infected neurons show dispersal of Nissl substance and homogenization of cytoplasm. Within a day or so, severely affected neurons die and disintegrate, giving rise to many foci of neuronophagia in which neutrophil polymorphs predominate for the first few days, to be gradually replaced by lymphocytes and macrophages. The early changes in the parenchyma are accompanied by intense congestion, endothelial hyperplasia, and in the most severe cases, petechial hemorrhages. The inflammatory response appears to require the presence of degenerating neurons as well as virus, for virus injected into the monkey thalamus deprived of neurons by prior retrograde degeneration induced by ablation of the cerebral cortex did not result in inflammation (Bodian and Howe, 1941). Neuronophagia is a prominent part of the pathology in human cases of acute polio; it is accompanied by perivascular inflammation in which lymphocytes and macrophages predominate from about 5 to 10 days. Slightly later, plasma cells are numerous within perivascular cuffs of inflammatory cells and in the surrounding parenchyma (Fig. 10.4) (Esiri, 1980). Microglial cells are increased in affected areas and show enhanced proteolytic enzyme activity. The meninges show a mild lymphocytic infiltrate. In experimental infections, poliovirus is detectable in the CNS commencing on the day before onset of weakness by isolation procedures or immunofluorescence. Thereafter, titers of virus fall rapidly to near negligible levels, where they may persist for several weeks. Neurons recovering from the infection in the second and third weeks appear chromatolytic. By 4 to 6 weeks the inflammation is still severe, but surviving motor neurons have returned to normal and the extent of the loss of motor neurons is apparent. Nodules of microglial cells and lymphocytes persist at sites of neuron destruction as well as in perivascular spaces. Reactive astrocytes are more evident at this stage than earlier. Months or years later, there is residual gliosis and loss of lower motor neurons with corresponding wasting of anterior nerve roots and longstanding denervation atrophy of skeletal muscles.

Histochemical studies of the muscles show type grouping in surviving normal-sized muscle fibers, indicating that surviving motor neurons have taken over the innervation of some of the muscle fibers that lost their nerve supply. Such extended innervation may cause motor neurons to fail decades later in the post polio syndrome (PPS) (see below). There is not usually evidence of any upper motor neuron loss at this stage, and the corticospinal tracts in the spinal cord appear intact.

Pathogenesis of Polio. The pathogenesis of polio was studied in detail in experimental infections of primates in the 1940s and 1950s (reviewed by Bodian, 1972). After oral ingestion, the virus produces an infection of the GI tract and its associated lymphoid tissue, where it multiplies. This is followed by a phase of viremia, which is thought to provide the opportunity for hematogenous spread of virus to the CNS. Certainly, cerebral endothelial cells can become infected experimentally (Blinzinger et al., 1969). Earlier experiments (Bodian and Howe, 1940, 1941) demonstrated a capacity of the virus to spread to the CNS along neural routes. Neural spread of virus in humans from gut to CNS directly along autonomic nerves to the spinal cord has not been excluded (Sabin, 1956). The possibility of neural spread from muscles is also suggested by the frequently noted tendency of the paralysis in human cases to be confined to or predominate in muscles that were injected or vigorously exercised a few days earlier. Furthermore, it is now known that the poliovirus receptor, a member of the immunoglobulin superfamily of surface glycoproteins, is expressed at muscle motor end plates (Freistadt et al., 1995). The alternative explanation offered for this occurrence is that there is a reflex increase in blood flow or altered metabolism in the anterior cord segment supplying the affected muscle, which renders these motor neurons more susceptible to infection (Nathanson and Bodian, 1962). This explanation may be convincing in the case of exercise but is less so in the case of intramuscular injections, in which the risk is increased if dirty needles are used for the injections. This observation lends weight to the view that the virus may enter the muscle and then reach the spinal cord by the neural route. Inflammation and enhanced vascular permeability in the muscle would be expected to be greater in the presence of contamination and infection at the site of injection. Support for this interpretation comes from a recent study of a mouse model of paralytic polio in which intramuscular injection of virus into gastronemius muscle provided one route of viral entry. The inoculated mice showed hind limb paralysis maximal on the side injected (Ford et al., 2002). Paralysis of injected muscles is still commonly observed in children in underdeveloped parts of the world (Wyatt, 1982).

Once virus has reached the CNS, it spreads within it along neural pathways (Bodian and Howe, 1940; Jubelt et al., 1980). The elements of the CNS that are particularly susceptible to infection are the large motor neurons of the spinal cord, cranial nerve nuclei, and motor cortex. This susceptibility of the motor neurons, the basis of which is not understood, is not absolute; other neurons, but not glial cells, can also become infected. The human polio receptor shows a wide distribution in and outside the nervous system, so its distribution does not provide an explanation for the selective vulnerability of motor neurons in polio (Freistadt et al., 1995).

Diagnosis and Management. Infection with poliovirus occurs by fecal-oral transmission. The great majority of infected individuals, about 90%, suffer no detectable symptomatology (Modlin and Coffey, 1997); 4 to 8% experience "minor illness" (Table 10.3). The incubation time to detectable non-CNS symptoms is 3 to 4 days. The symptoms are typically those of a viral syndrome, such as fever, headache, nausea and vomiting, and sore throat, which tend to clear within a few days. In the remaining 1 or 2%, the viral syndrome, termed the minor illness, is followed by more severe symptoms, termed the major illness, in which paralysis may occur. The major illness can occur following a period of well-being after the minor illness, continue directly from the minor illness, or appear in the absence of detectable minor illness. The major illness occurs 9 to 14 days following exposure to the virus. Manifestations include headache; pain and stiffness of the back, neck, and limbs; vomiting; fever; and a CSF pleocytosis. The illness may progress no further; however, if paralysis is to appear, it usually does so within the first week of the major illness.

The majority of patients with paralytic polio demonstrate a spinal cord distribution. The onset is during the febrile major illness and may progress for 2 or 3 days. The distribution of limb involvement is asymmetric, with groups of large muscles suffering the greatest burden of disease. Sensory loss is absent or minor, but sphincter control may be impaired, particularly during the acute phase. Even in the absence of bulbar involvement, respiration can be compromised through involvement of thoracic innervation of intercostal muscles and cervical innervation of the phrenic nerve. Gradual return of muscle function starts days to weeks after lysis of the fever and may continue for 18 months or more. Return of urinary sphincter function occurs subsequent to the acute phase, and continued difficulty is rare.

Brain stem involvement may occur on its own or in combination with spinal cord paralysis. It was particularly feared because of its high mortality rate, which had reached over 50%. Estimates of the overall incidence of bulbar involvement in paralytic polio vary. In a study of the large epidemic in 1946 in Minnesota, the incidence of bulbar involvement was 23% in patients under 16 years of age and 32% above that age (Baker et al., 1950). The distribution of brain stem dysfunction includes cranial nerve nuclei and centers for respiration and circulation (Baker et al., 1950). The frequency of involvement of specific cranial nerve nuclei varies. Wemstedt (cited in Merritt, 1967) found facial weakness to be most frequent, followed by pharyngeal and ocular weakness. Others have found that the 10th nerve was most frequently involved, followed by facial weakness, with significantly less involvement of oculomotor nerves (Krugman and Ward, 1968). Difficulty in swallowing, lasting about 1 week, was found in over two-thirds of a large group of patients with bulbar polio (Brahdy and Lenarsky, 1934). Dysphagia and dysarthria are manifestations of involvement of the nucleus ambiguus, which was found to be frequently involved in bulbar polio in the studies of Baker et al. (1950). The greatest danger occurs with the involvement of the medullary centers of respiration. When coupled with cervical and thoracic cord disease, respiration could be totally compromised. Involvement of medullary vasomotor centers resulting in circulatory collapse similarly poses a significant threat to life. Although mortality in the bulbar form is high, over 50% in some epidemics of polio (Merritt, 1967), recovery of function in survivors is often complete. Application of modern ICU support and respiratory care would be expected to reduce mortality.

Diagnosis of sporadic cases of polio may be difficult. The differential diagnosis is broad and includes the polyneuritis of Guillain-Barré, other enteroviruses, and other viral causes of brain stem encephalitis. The CSF in the first 2 weeks contains a pleocytosis of between 30 and 140 cells and protein between 50 and 125 mg per 100 ml (Merritt, 1967). However, normal spinal fluids may be found (Krugman and Ward, 1968). As time progresses, the cells disappear and the protein continues to rise, causing confusion with the Guillain-Barré syndrome. Stool may harbor the virus during and after the onset of neurological symptoms. CSF isolations are distinctly rare after the onset of paralytic disease.

Therapy in the acute phase should be directed toward maintenance of respiration and circulation. Respiratory function may be compromised in several ways. Excursion of the diaphragm, expansion of the chest cage by intercostal muscles, and regulation of respiratory movements by the medullary centers may be individually or simultaneously compromised. Additionally, pooling of fluids, incapacity to swallow, and spasm of the vocal cords may each obstruct respiration. Initial attempts to treat vaccine-associated and wild-type poliovirus infections with pleconaril appeared to be promising and the drug was well tolerated (Rotbart et al., 2001). Polio and its clinical complications may become a thing of the past if the global eradication effort is successful.

PPS. Decades following acute paralytic poliomyelitis, a significant proportion of patients may develop PPS, the post-polio syndrome, the core components of which are fatigue, weakness, and pain (Mulder et al., 1972). Estimates of the prevalence vary widely. For example, a population-based study in Pennsylvania found a prevalence of 28.5% (Ramlow et al., 1992), whereas one in Minnesota found 60% (Windebank et al., 1995). Because it has been estimated that there are between 300,000 and 600,000 survivors in the United States from the polio epidemics in the 1940s and 1950s (Melnick, 1996), PPS is a significant public health issue. The interval between acute polio and PPS was found by Ramlow et al. (1992) to be 30 to 34 years. Thus, there is the anomalous situation of the progressive elimination of acute poliovirus infection from the world simultaneous with the continued emergence of a neuromuscular syndrome in survivors of acute polio infection acquired decades earlier.

Diagnosis of PPS rests on four widely accepted criteria (Jubelt and Agre, 2000): a history of paralytic polio with evidence of motor neuron loss; an extended period of functional stability of at least 15 years; the onset of new weakness, atrophy, or fatigue; and the exclusion of other conditions as a cause of the signs and symptoms. Symptoms referable to the brain stem, such as swallowing and speech disorders and sleep apnea, may be seen in those who had had bulbar polio (Jubelt and Agre, 2000). When weakness is associated with atrophy, it has been termed post-polio progressive muscular atrophy (Dalakas, 1995). Respiratory difficulties may emerge in those with residual respiratory muscular weakness (Thorsteinsson, 1997). Muscle and joint pain may result from a variety of neuromuscular imbalances and attempted interventions. Generalized fatigue has been uniformly found in a high percentage of patients (Jubelt and Agre, 2000).

While it has been speculated that chronic viral infection or an immune response was the cause of the new symptoms, the consensus appears to accept excessive stress on overextended motor neurons with cell dropout as the cause. No specific viral or immune markers are diagnostically useful, and the clinical evaluation is directed toward elimination of other processes. Electromyogram (EMG)/NCV studies are useful to exclude other insults to nerve roots, plexi, nerves, or muscles, as is neuroimaging to exclude cord and root injury. The clinical absence of corticospinal tract signs and slow or little clinical progression distinguish PPS from amyotrophic lateral sclerosis. One case with pathology has been reported of late amyotrophic lateral sclerosis following childhood polio, but this is exceptional (Shimada et al., 1999).

Pharmacological intervention has not been found to be successful in PPS (Dalakas, 1999). Rather, nonfatiguing exercise appears to promote improvement, with care to avoid overuse (Jubelt and Agre, 2000). The wide range of management techniques for symptoms is considered by Thorsteinsson (1997). The prognosis in general appears to be for relative stability (Dalakas, 1995), with lifestyle changes occuring in only a minority of patients (Windebank et al., 1995).

Global Eradication. The success of the polio vaccines has been remarkable. In the United States, over 20,000 cases of paralytic polio occurred in 1952 (Centers for Disease Control and Prevention, 2000b). Following the introduction of the inactivated Salk vaccine and the oral Sabin vaccine (OPV), no indigenous wild type of poliovirus has been detected in the United States since 1979. Subsequently, only imported or vaccine-associated paralytic polio cases have been detected. As a consequence, recent immunization recommendations in the United States have shifted to the exclusive use of inactivated Salk vaccine to preclude vaccine-associated paralytic polio cases.

In 1988, the World Health Assembly set the goal of global elimination of polio by 2000 (Dowdle, 2001). While that goal has not been met, remarkable progress has been made. There were an estimated 350,000 cases worldwide annually of paralytic polio before the start of the program. By the year 2000, fewer than 3,000 cases were identified annually (Dowdle, 2001). The goal of global eradication is feasible because there are no nonhuman reservoirs, and except for immunocompromised individuals, no chronic carrier state exists in humans. It is noteworthy that chronic virus shedding has been documented in immunocompromised individuals; one individual, for example, has shed a revertant neurovirulent vaccine strain for 16 years (John, 2000). Whether the pandemic of HIV/AIDS will compromise the goal of global eradication of polio remains to be determined.

The eradication strategies were originally developed for use in the Americas, where the Pan American Health Organization in 1985 had resolved to eliminate polio by 1990 (Dowdle, 2001). These strategies included: high rates of vaccine coverage with OPV in infants less than 1 year of age; sensitive laboratory and epidemiologic surveillance; national immunization days for supplemental OPV doses for children under 5 years of age; and intense "mopping-up" campaigns of door-to-door immunization in areas at high risk of transmission (Centers for Disease Control and Prevention, 2000b). The mobilization efforts are massive; for example, approximately 300,000 health workers participated in national immunization days in west and central Africa (Centers for Disease Control and Prevention, 2001b). Cooperation by regional warring factions has temporarily suspended hostilities to allow vaccine programs on "days of tranquility" (Centers for Disease Control and Prevention, 2001b; Dowdle, 2001). An estimated 10 million people worked globally in 2000 on eradication efforts (Dowdle, 2001). Funding of the campaigns comes from a mixture of international and national health bodies, the Rotary International, nongovernmental organizations, private foundations, and corporations. Viral surveillance involves 127 national labs, 15 regional reference labs, and seven specialized reference labs (Dowdle, 2001). This system evaluates stool specimens submitted in association with aggressive surveillance of cases of acute flaccid paralysis. In 2001 fewer than 1,000 cases were found worldwide, and only 10 countries harbored endemic polioviruses (Nathanson and Fine, 2002). However, it is of concern that vaccine-derived poliovirus was documented to have caused an outbreak of paralytic polio in 2000 and 2001 in the Dominican Republic and Haiti on the island of Hispaniola (Kew et al., 2002).

EV-71

"This caused a panic in Taiwan because of publicity surrounding a small number of children who had a short febrile illness (2-day duration), decompensated suddenly, developed acute pulmonary edema and hemorrhage, and died within 12 to 24 hours." Thus do Shen et al. (1999) describe one of the most sinister expressions of EV-71 disease—neurogenic edema resulting from brain stem infection. Originally identified in California in 1969 (Schmidt et al., 1974), EV-71 has presented in a pleomorphic fashion with a large degree of variability from epidemic to epidemic. It has had a simple febrile form and both dermatotropic and neurotropic manifestations. HFM disease, herpangina, aseptic meningitis, and poliomyelitis-like disease in addition to various manifestations of brain stem infection have been widely described (Shindarov et al., 1979; J. Blomberg, E. Lyeke, K. Ahlifors, T. Johnsson, S. Wolontis, and G. von Zeipel, Letter, *Lancet* **ii:**112, 1974; Nagy et al., 1982; Ishimaru et al., 1980; Lum et al., 1998), including in Taiwan in 1998 (Ho et al., 1999) and recurrently in Australia (Kennett et al., 1974; Gilbert et al., 1988). The Centers for Disease Control and Prevention has reported that EV-71 has been endemic in the United States at least since 1977 and that a marked increase of cases occurred in 1987 (Alexander et al., 1994). However, it has not been among the most common nonpolio enterovirus isolates in the United States, ranking 15th for the period 1993 to 1996 (World Health Organization, 1998) and 13th for the period 1997 to 1999 (Centers for Disease Control and Prevention, 2000a, 2000b). It represents only 2.1% of the identified nonpolio enteroviral isolates in each time period.

The burden of EV-71 illness has fallen most heavily on children under the age of 5 years. The infection can be asymptomatic or can present as a brief febrile illness as HFM disease or as herpangina. HFM disease presents with vesicular lesions on hands, feet, mouth, and buttocks, whereas herpangina is a painful condition of the fauces and soft palate with vesicles, sore throat, and painful swallowing (Ho et al., 1999). Clinical descriptions include "... papules and vesicles accompanied by a flare on the hands and feet, and aphthae on tongue and oral mucosa" (Ishimaru et al., 1980), and "... widely dispersed fine discrete reddish violet pinpoint petechiae were noted on all extremities including both palms and soles" (Landry et al., 1995). HFM disease is also commonly caused by coxsackievirus A16, to which EV-71 is related on phylogenetic analysis (Oberste et al., 1999). However, while coxsackievirus A16 can be associated with aseptic meningitis, it has not yet been linked to epidemics of parenchymal CNS disease.

Prior to the onset of neurological illness, HFM disease, herpangina, GI symptoms, and fever separately or in aggregate last an average of slightly over 3 days, with the range being from 2 to 5 days (Huang et al., 1999). In the 1998 Taiwan epidemic, three neurological complications were observed (Huang et al., 1999). Patients with aseptic meningitis presented with headache, fever, vomiting, and stiff neck. The syndrome cleared in less than a week without sequelae. Flaccid motor weakness of the extremities was the second form observed, with good recovery in two patients and mild weakness and atrophy in two others. Fifty-two cases out of 705 were characterized as poliomyelitislike in the 1975 epidemic in Bulgaria; there were also 29 cases of isolated paresis of the facial nerve and 68 cases of the bulbar form, including 44 fatalities (Shindarov et al., 1979). Huang et al. (1999) characterized the third and predominant form in Taiwan as rhombencephalitis. Myoclonus, ataxia, and/or tremor were seen in the majority of patients. Further involvement of the brain stem included cranial nerves with ocular and/or bulbar dysfunction. Seizures and significant impairment of consciousness were not commonly found. Sequelae included persistent myoclonus when awake, facial weakness, ataxia, ocular movement disorders, and dysarthria. An earlier report (Ishimaru et al., 1980) emphasized cerebellar signs as the major component of an encephalitis syndrome. These included ataxia, myoclonus, and tremor. It is of note that Shen et al. (1999) reported 7 of 20 patients with lesions in the dentate nuclei of the cerebellum.

EV-71 brain stem encephalitis merits special attention because of its potential for abrupt onset and rapidly fatal evolution. Lum et al. (1998) reported on four children who experienced sudden cardiopulmonary arrest and died within hours of admission to the hospital. Histopathological abnormalities were found in the brain stem and spinal cord with severe gray matter inflammation, microglial nodules, and neuronophagia. Virus isolation was more readily achieved from the brain stem than from other neural sites. Lung weights were increased in the majority, pulmonary edema was present in all, and there was no inflammation in the myocardium. The authors postulated EV-71 infection of "the brain stem as the cause of neurogenic pulmonary edema and cardiac dysfunction leading to death." Subsequent reports have sustained these observations. The sudden onset of tachycardia, dyspnea, and cyanosis in 11 children was noted 1 to 3 days after the onset of disease in the Taiwan epidemic of 1998 by Chang et al. (1999). Nine of the 11 died within 12 h of intubation, and another was brain dead within 15 h. Significant correlations include CNS involvement and hyperglycemia. Huang et al. (1999) attribute the vasomotor collapse and neurogenic pulmonary edema to destruction of the vasomotor and respiratory centers in the lower brain stem.

McMinn et al. (2001) reported several types of neurological disorders in association with EV-71 infection that suggested an immune-mediated pathogenesis. These included the Guillain-Barré syndrome, acute transverse myelitis, acute cerebellar ataxia, and the opsoclonus-myoclonus syndrome. In addition, cases of aseptic meningitis, benign intracranial hypertension, and a febrile seizure were observed. Management of a putative immune-mediated illness, which often includes steroids, would require judicious treatment to avoid amplifying acute infection.

The neuropathology and virus isolation studies support a mechanism of direct infection of neural parenchyma. Virus was isolated from the medulla and spinal cord in all three cases in which this was attempted by Lum et al. (1998). In earlier studies, Shindarov et al. (1979) found loss of neurons, neuronophagia, and inflammatory infiltrates in tissue and in the perivascular space in the medulla and spinal cord. Yan et al. (2000) found prominent inflammation in the posterior two-thirds of the pons and medulla and in the anterior two-thirds of the spinal cord. Immunohistology revealed EV-71 antigens in a few neurons in the medulla and in the spinal cord.

Localization to brain stem and cervical spinal cord in 15 of 20 patients was found on T2-weighted MRI images by Shen et al. (1999). In a report from different hospitals in the same Taiwan epidemic, Huang et al. (1999) reported that 17 of 24 patients with clinical signs of rhombencephalitis demonstrated lesions in the medulla on T2-weighted images. CSF revealed findings compatible with aseptic meningitis (Ishimaru et al., 1980). Huang et al. (1999) found an average of 33 white cells in CSF of EV-71-related aseptic meningitis, 151 cells in acute flaccid paralysis, and 194 cells in rhombencephalitis. No difference in glucose, protein, or lactate levels was found. Electroencephalographic study has not produced significant diagnostic information. In 24 patients, Ishimaru et al. (1980) found 9 with dysrhythmia and 10 with sporadic synchronous high-voltage slow waves. Intermittent slow waves were reported by Huang et al. (1999) in some cases of rhombencephalitis.

Diagnosis is facilitated in children with the rash of HFM disease during an epidemic season. However, sporadic cases occur (Landry et al., 1995), adults can become symptomatic (Shindarov et al., 1979), and neurological disease can occur without dermatotrophic manifestations (Shindarov et al., 1979). Virus isolation from CSF has been notoriously difficult (Landry et al., 1995), and throat or stool isolation, while more successful, leads to concern about relevance to CNS illness. Antibodies specific for EV-71 were used during the Taiwan 1997 epidemic in a dot blot assay to identify the virus in throat, rectal, or CSF specimens (Shen et al., 1999).

Management of brain stem encephalitis subsequent to EV-71 infection requires ICU management to anticipate cardiopulmonary collapse. MRI is likely to document the localization (Huang et al., 1999; Shen et al., 1999), and hyperglycemia is a strong risk factor (Chang et al., 1999). Cardiac and respiratory monitoring is essential. Chest X rays may show pulmonary edema (Lum et al., 1998; Huang et al., 1999; Chang et al., 1999), and measures to reduce pulmonary edema are crucial. Seizure management and reduction of raised intracranial pressure have not been reported as clinical management issues in EV-71 brain stem encephalitis. Unfortunately, while there is hope that pleconaril may prove therapeutically useful in certain other enteroviral infections (Pevear et al., 1999; Rotbart et al., 2001), it has not yet proven effective against EV-71 (communication cited by McMinn et al., 2001). No vaccine is available.

ANIMAL-TO-HUMAN TRANSMISSION: NIPAH VIRUS

In 1998, Malaysia experienced the start of a highly lethal outbreak of encephalitis among adult men who worked on pig farms (Centers for Disease Control and Prevention, 1999a). Although originally thought to be Japanese encephalitis virus (JEV), a new paramyxovirus was isolated in cell culture. The epidemic struck adults whereas JEV usually strikes children in areas of endemicity; furthermore, while pigs serve as an amplifying host for JEV, they do not usually become sick (Farrar, 1999). The epidemic spread to abattoir workers in Singapore who handled pigs imported from Malaysia. No human-to-human transmission was believed to have occurred, and the outbreaks were halted by the culling of hundreds of thousands of pigs, interdiction of importation of pigs, and the closing of slaughterhouses (Centers for Disease Control and Prevention, 1999b). Flying foxes, or fruit-eating bats, appeared to be the natural reservoir, with pigs presumably becoming infected in proximity to fruit trees (Enserink, 2000). Contact with pigs served to infect humans, possibly by aerosol.

The isolate was named Nipah virus, after the village where the first known fatality occurred (Enserink, 2000). It is closely related to Hendra virus, an agent that causes severe respiratory disease in horses and that has been transmitted to humans (Murray et al., 1995). In one human case of Hendra virus infection, fatal encephalitis developed 13 months after an episode of aseptic meningitis (O'Sullivan et al., 1997). While closely related to the morbillivirus genus of the *Paramyxoviridae* family, which includes measles virus and canine distemper virus, the Nipah and Hendra viruses are sufficiently different to suggest a new genus (Chua et al., 2000). It is remarkable that morbilliviruses have emerged since 1988 as the cause of numerous epizootics of respiratory and CNS disease in aquatic mammals (Kennedy, 1998). Thus, it appears that the Nipah and Hendra viruses are part of a larger global picture of emerging paramyxovirus disease of the nervous system.

Histopathological studies in patients dying with Nipah virus encephalitis revealed disseminated microinfarctions resulting from virus-induced vasculitis (Paton et al., 1999; Chua et al., 1999, 2000; Goh et al., 2000; Wong et al., 2002).

Evidence for paramyxovirus infection of the vascular endothelium included multinucleated giant cells, endothelial cell lysis, syncytial cell formation, and viral antigen. Intranuclear and cytoplasmic inclusions were observed in neurons near vasculitic lesions. White and gray matter were each involved, as was cerebral cortex and brain stem. Surprisingly, while massive intracerebral hemorrhage was reported as a late occurrence in one patient (Goh et al., 2000), hemorrhage does not appear to be a consistent finding despite damage to vessels and areas of parenchymal rarefaction (Chua et al., 2000). Furthermore, cerebral swelling appears not to be a clinical management issue, on the evidence of autopsy examinations and negative CT reports (Goh et al., 2000).

The clinical picture is that of a rapidly evolving encephalitis with multifocal signs reflecting the pathology of diffusely distributed microinfarctions (Paton et al., 1999; Chua et al., 1999; Lee et al., 1999; Goh et al., 2000; Lim et al., 2000). Fever, headache, decreased level of consciousness, dizziness, and vomiting are early signs. The incubation period, as judged by last contact with pigs in over 90% of the cases, was 2 weeks or less (Goh et al., 2000). Once symptomatic, the disease evolution was rapid, averaging just under 7 days to the nadir. Comment has regularly been made on the presence of clinical brain stem findings including ptosis, abnormal doll's eye movements, dysphonia, dysarthria, segmental myoclonus, and vasomotor changes of hypertension and tachycardia suggesting medullary involvement. Comment has also been made on clinical signs suggesting cerebellar involvement, including dysmetria, gait ataxia, and dysdiadachokinesia (Lee et al., 1999). Seizures were found in 23% of patients (Goh et al., 2000), and 50% of patients required mechanical respiration. A remarkable pattern of clinical recovery was described in 10 comatose patients (Goh et al., 2000). Flaccid tetraplegia and areflexia initially persisted, while motor cranial nerves and cognitive functions improved. Eight of the 10 patients ultimately recovered limb strength with return of reflexes. Of 265 cases reported in Malaysia, 105 deaths occurred, almost 40% (Chua et al., 2000). In the largest individual series of 94 patients (Goh et al., 2000), 32% died, 53% recovered fully, and 15% had persistent neurological defects, including five patients in a persistent vegetative state. Three patients experienced relapses 13 to 39 days following a mild illness. MRI demonstrated diffuse and confluent involvement of the cortical gray matter in the patients suffering relapse or delayed onset. Further data have emerged concerning relapsed Nipah encephalitis and late-onset encephalitis occurring months after an acute infection without neurological symptoms (Tan et al., 2002). In contrast to acute Nipah encephalitis, in which the pathology demonstrated virus-induced vasculitis and thrombosis, delayed/recurrent Nipah encephalitis was found on clinical, imaging, and autopsy data to result from focal cortical disease. In contrast to acute cases, viral antigen was more abundant in neurons and glial cells but not present in endothelium. There was no perivenous demyelination (Wong et al., 2002). Hence, this form of the disease is thought to represent a direct viral attack.

As of 2 years follow-up, 7.5% of survivors of acute encephalitis had had a recurrent episode, and 3.4% had had a late-onset encephalitis. The relapsed/late-onset cases occurred on average 8.4 months after the acute infection and presented as an acute encephalitis. Three patients had another episode, on average 7.6 months later. The evolution of the episodes was about 3 weeks. Fever was found in 46%, headache in 42%, seizures in 50%, and focal signs in 42%. CSF revealed an average of 59 white blood cells per μl and a minimally elevated protein. MRIs revealed cortical involvement of a patchy and confluent nature, usually involving multiple areas. Diffuse slowing was found on EEGs with focal preponderance in temporal and frontal areas. As might be espected, all patients had serum immunoglobulin G (IgG) antibodies against Nipah virus, and 12 of 13 CSF samples examined had such IgG antibodies. Viral cultures of CSF, urine, and tracheal secretions were negative, as was one sample of brain tissue. Four of 22 relapsed/late-onset patients died (18%), 11 had residua, and 7 were without deficit.

Nipah virus encephalitis should be suspected in Malaysia in a patient presenting with a rapidly evolving encephalitis and a recent history of contact with pigs. However, it remains to be seen if the territory at risk expands to become that of the putative natural reservoir of species of flying foxes (Enserink, 2000). It seems likely that viruses such as Nipah virus, Hendra virus, and potentially other related viruses will emerge elsewhere. An encephalitis outbreak in Meherpur, Bangladesh, in April and May 2001 was associated with Nipah virus or a closely related virus (World Health Organization, 2002). Antibodies to viruses closely related to Nipah virus have been found in fruit bats in Cambodia (Olson et al., 2002).

CT scans have been normal, but MRI scans show multiple and widespread discrete hyperintense lesions (Goh et al., 2000; Lim et al., 2000). The latter authors note the usefulness of MRI to distinguish Nipah virus encephalitis from that of Japanese encephalitis, in which the thalamus is frequently involved bilaterally, with the basal ganglia, brain stem, and hippocampus also involved. Findings in CSF include a moderate pleocytosis, usually mononuclear, and protein elevation, although both values can be normal or highly abnormal. Goh et al. (2000) reported that there is no correlation between CSF findings and the severity of encephalitis. EEGs revealed diffuse slow wave activity, focal sharp waves, and bilateral sharp and slow wave periodic complexes in patients in deep coma. Focal abnormalities tended to localize in the temporal areas (Goh et al., 2000). General laboratory abnormalities have included thrombocytopenia, leukopenia, and elevated liver enzymes. Atypical pneumonia was found on X rays of some patients in the cases reported from Singapore (Paton et al., 1999).

Viral diagnosis by serology in the clinical reports from the 1998/1999 outbreak depended on Hendra virus antigen-based assays for IgM capture ELISA and indirect IgG ELISA (Goh et al., 2000; Paton et al., 1999). Virus isolation was achieved in cultures of Vero cells several days after inoculation (Chua et al., 1999; Goh et al., 2000).

Management merits ICU admission, particularly because assisted respiration is needed in at least half of patients. Raised intracranial pressure has not been a clinical management issue. However, strategies for management of an infection-triggered vasculitis and the resultant disseminated thrombosis are needed. Immunosuppression to arrest the immune component of the vasculitis seems unwise in light of viral lysis of cerebrovascular endothelium. Goh et al. (2000) reported the empiric use of aspirin and pentoxifylline because of thrombosis but made no comment as to effectiveness. These authors did comment, however, that antiviral treatment with ribavirin appeared to make no significant difference in outcome. In contrast, Chong et al. (2001) reported that an open-label trial of ribavirin reduced mortality by 36% in comparison to nonrandomized controls. A controlled randomized clinical trial is needed, as is development of a clearly effective antiviral agent against Nipah virus. Intravenous phenytoin was used successfully in the control of seizures (Goh et al., 2000). Because of the ultimate return of motor function, sustained physical therapy is justified. However, in light of the observation of late-onset and recurrent encephalitis, the issue of antiviral suppression may need to be addressed. Close clinical follow-up is certainly called for.

Prevention entailed breaking the chain of transmission, principally by culling hundreds of thousands of pigs (Centers for Disease Control and Prevention, 1999b). Removal of fruit trees, which attract fruit-eating flying foxes, from the environs of pig farms should also help interrupt the chain of infection. Development of a vaccine for use in swine and for pig farm workers is needed. Finally, one is left to wonder whether the chain of infection from flying fox to pig to human is the only route to infect humans. Might not sporadic cases occur on exposure of humans to bats or their excreta, and could another amplifying intermediate host other than farmed swine emerge?

UNKNOWN MEANS OF TRANSMISSION

von Economo's Encephalitis

EL remains one of the most perplexing and distressing biological puzzles of the last century. It is perplexing because we do not know what caused its intense worldwide dissemination or why it disappeared in epidemic form after a decade. Nor do we know its etiology. It is distressing because we are unprepared to halt its spread should it reappear. It raged worldwide in the decade 1916 to 1926, causing thousands of cases and deaths and leaving in its wake postencephalitic parkinsonism in a significant percentage of survivors. Although, as von Economo himself pointed out, similar disease patterns had been seen at Tubingen in 1712 and in northern Italy in the 1890s, where it was known as "Nona" (von Economo, 1917), there was no precedent for a worldwide epidemic of encephalitis.

Cases appeared first in 1915 in Romania and France, were observed by von Economo in Vienna in the winter of 1916 to 1917, and appeared in the United States and the United Kingdom in 1918. Although it spread simultaneously with the great pandemics of influenza, it had appeared before influenza. It started at the time of World War I, and its spread may have been encouraged by wartime stress, movement of troops, and poor nutrition. Principally a winter disease, the peak number of cases was in February and March. The mode of spread was not satisfactorily worked out; only about 2.5% of cases had evidence of infection from a contact (Hall, 1924). Thus, although incubation periods of 10 to 15 days have been cited (Debre, 1970), it seems difficult in retrospect to be certain of this number. Furthermore, in the absence of a serological marker of infection, it is impossible to know the ratio of inapparent to apparent infections. No epidemics of EL have been experienced since 1926. Sporadic cases that fit the clinical and histopathological pattern continue to be reported, as are studies on postencephalitic parkinsonism, in the hope of discovering the etiology of EL.

Pathology

One of the striking features of EL was the biphasic nature of the clinical disease. Pathological studies showed that the initial febrile illness was an encephalitis and the later phase of neurological disease, which developed in some survivors, was an encephalopathy.

In the initial phase there were few macroscopic abnormalities in the brain unless complications such as sagittal sinus thrombosis and cerebral venous infarction had supervened (Buzzard and Greenfield, 1919). The meninges were also normal apart from minimal cloudiness and congestion. The sliced brain showed congestion, sometimes with small petechial hemorrhages in the gray matter, especially in the basal ganglia and periaqueductal regions. Microscopically, there were features suggestive of a viral encephalitis with marked perivascular, particularly perivenular, mononuclear inflammatory cell infiltrates, neuronophagic nodules, and diffuse microglial proliferation, but inclusion bodies were not seen. These changes mainly involved the gray matter, and while none of the gray matter was exempt, they were concentrated in the midbrain, with less severe extension upwards to the subthalamic nucleus, thalamus, and hypothalamus and downwards to the pons and medulla (von Economo, 1917). In some cases the gray matter of the spinal cord was also involved. In the midbrain the worst damage was to the periaqueductal and tegmental regions, reticular formation, and substantia nigra (Fig. 10.5 and 10.6).

In the late chronic phase of the disease in which parkinsonian symptoms and oculogyric crises were clinically prominent, the site of lesions extended from the midbrain upwards into the basal ganglia and parts of the thalamus.

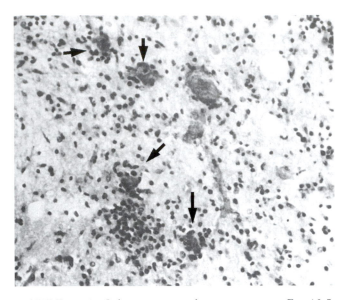

FIGURE 10.6 Substantia nigra from same case as Fig. 10.5. Degenerate pigmented neurons are surrounded by inflammatory cells (arrows). Hematoxylin and eosin stain.

The pathology at this stage consisted mainly of cell loss and gliosis. Inflammation was much reduced or absent. Some remaining neurons in affected regions contained neurofibrillary tangles (Fig. 1.7) like those seen in Alzheimer's disease (Hallevorden, 1935). The substantia nigra was the site of most severe neuron loss (Fig. 10.6 and 10.7). Much of the other pathology was secondary to loss of nigrostriatal fibers with associated gliosis.

Some, though not all, recent cases of EL-like illness have responded to immunosuppressant therapy, raising the possibility that it may represent a parainfectious disease (R. C. Dale, A. J. Church, R. A. H. Surtees, A. J. Lees, B. G. R. Neville, and G. Giovanni, *Abstr. A. B. N. Spring Meeting*, 2002).

Clinical Presentation

The clinical presentation of EL was that of a brain stem encephalitis and reflected the frequent involvement of the gray matter of the dorsal mesencephalon. The triad of delirious somnolence, fever, and dysfunction of the oculomotor nerves, particularly ptosis, constituted the core findings. The expression of the disease, however, was extremely variable, and each or all of the triad could be missing. Von Economo (1931) identified three types: somnolent-ophthalmoplegic, hyperkinetic, and amyostatic-akinetic. An early American work (Tilney and Howe, 1920) defined eight subgroups. Fever was common but not invariable. Signs of meningeal irritation, if present, were minimal. Various combinations of disordered sleep, personality disturbance, altered motor tone and spontaneous movement abnormalities, and cranial nerve and spinal cord dysfunction were found. However, it was said that particular epidemics tended to be clinically consistent. Epidemics of an unusual nature, such as epidemic hiccough, were included in the spectrum. Another distressing manifestion was algomyoclonia, in which episodes of thalamic pain were followed by the sudden onset of

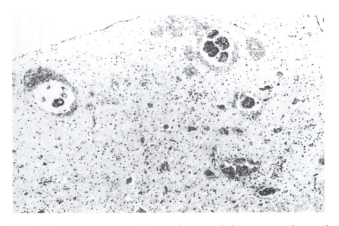

FIGURE 10.5 Case of EL with 1 week history; male aged 15 years. Periaqueductal region of midbrain with ependymal surface at top left. Intense congestion with red cell diapedesis and parenchymal inflammation. Hematoxylin and eosin.

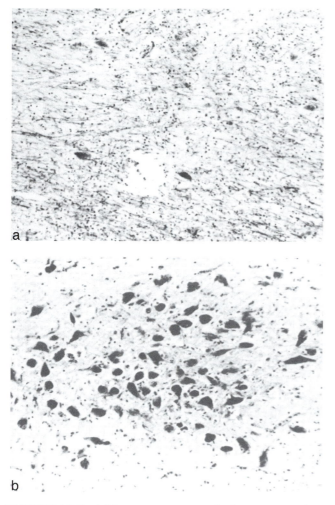

FIGURE 10.7   (a) Lower-power view of substantia nigra from the same case as Fig. 1.7. The few large neurons present represent the severely depleted neuronal population. (b) Normal substantia nigra for comparison. Luxol fast blue/cresyl violet stain.

myoclonus. Psychiatric disturbances and coma could supervene (Debre, 1970). The course of the illness was similarly variable and could run to weeks and months. It has been estimated that 25% died, 25% recovered completely, and 50% had residua or sequelae, of which 25% developed postencephalitic parkinsonism (Hall, 1924).

The disease was often characterized by the development of new manifestations after an apparently disease-free interval. Most significant among the late manifestations was postencephalitic parkinsonism. It could be distinguished from idiopathic parkinsonism by a younger age of onset and by the appearance of oculogyric crises. In such a crisis the eyes would suddenly roll up and the patient would fall backwards without warning. Personality disorders and psychiatric disturbances were a frequent outcome, particularly in children. A most appalling sequela was a state of suspended animation in which people were frozen, often for decades. In the book *Awakenings*, which has subsequently been turned into a movie, Sacks (1973) described his attempts to pharmacologically free people from such states. Choreiform movements,

sleep disorders, myoclonus, tremors, and obesity were among the sequelae (Hall, 1924).

Laboratory findings were unimpressive and nonspecific. The peripheral white blood count was not regularly unusual. The CSF often contained a few cells but was frequently acellular. The CSF protein was normal or slightly elevated and the sugar in the CSF was sometimes elevated, though not of diagnostic usefulness. The EEG and the several neuroimaging techniques were not developed at the time of the last epidemic appearance of EL. Modern descriptions of sporadic cases compatible with EL, described below, include such studies. The problem, of course, is whether such sporadic cases are representative of the epidemic form.

Among the most vexing of the questions associated with EL is the problem of etiology. Although von Economo's report of 1917 strongly endorsed a viral causation, neither consistent viral isolations nor antibody changes have been demonstrated. Several infectious causes were considered (Matheson Commission, 1939). Streptococcal isolates of Rosenow were not confirmed, nor were the isolations of herpes simplex virus (HSV) of Levaditi. Antigens of HSV were not found in preserved brain tissue using the immunoperoxidase technique (Esiri and Swash, 1984). The coincidence of the influenza pandemics has kept this virus as a candidate. Most commentators at the time of the epidemics pointed out the clinical and epidemiologic differences between influenza and EL (for example, Hall [1924] and the review of Reid et al. [2001]). The possibility has been held out that more sensitive techniques would reveal traces of influenza. However, McCall et al. (2001) applied techniques that have successfully identified RNA of influenza in stored lung samples from 1918 and failed to find influenza RNA in archived CNS samples from acute EL or postencephalitic parkinsonism cases. A systematic review of postencephalitic parkinsonism and established viruses concluded that the etiology was unknown (Casals et al., 1998).

What evidence, then, supports an infectious etiology? The presence of fever and a CSF pleocytosis, albeit both inconstant; the pathological findings of an inflammatory response in the CNS; and the epidemic nature of the disease certainly point toward an infectious agent. The identity of the agent will be of paramount importance if we are confronted with epidemics in the future. We lack a generation of physicians experienced in the recognition and management of acute cases of epidemic EL.

With the caveat that sporadic cases of EL may differ etiologically from the epidemic form, representing diverse processes attacking the same anatomic territory, clinical criteria have been considered (Rail et al., 1981; Howard and Lees, 1987). For example, Howard and Lees (1987) suggest that major criteria in cases of acute or subacute encephalitis include at least three of the following: basal ganglia dysfunction, oculogyric crises, ophthalomoplegia, obsessive-compulsive behavior, akinetic mutism, central respiratory abnormalities, and sleep disorders, including somnolence or sleep cycle inversion. Howard and Lees (1987) reported that the CSF is frequently abnormal, with slight elevations of protein and pressure, moderate pleocytosis, and oligoclonal bands of IgG. Kiley and Esiri (2001) found a high level of CSF IgG and oligoclonal bands. The postmortem revealed

CNS plasma cell infiltrates, including morula cells distended with immunoglobulin. EEG and evoked potential studies of Howard and Lees (1987) suggested a cortical component of the illness. The case report of Kiley and Esiri (2001) included an EEG with intermittent bilateral slow wave activity and repeatedly normal cerebral MRI scans.

Etiologies of sporadic cases have appeared to vary. A case termed "encephalitis lethargica-like" appeared to have the clinical pattern of parainfectious process following clinical measles infection (Mellon et al., 1991). Another "encephalitis lethargica-like" case also appeared to follow the clinical pattern of a parainfectious process following an upper respiratory infection with a fourfold rise in mycoplasma complement-fixing antibodies (Al-Mateen et al., 1988). Yet another report drew attention to the potential relationship between coxsackieviruses and cases that would have been described as EL (Peatfield, 1987). No etiologic agent was uncovered in the case of Kiley and Esiri (2001). Therapy in sporadic cases has been symptomatic. Blunt et al. (1997) used levadopa to treat akinesia and clonazepam to treat myoclonus in two cases of presumed sporadic EL. In addition, both cases responded to intravenous methylprednisolone. The case of Kiley and Esiri (2001) failed to have a therapeutic response to levadopa.

Myalgic Encephalomyelitis and the Chronic Fatigue Syndrome

The epidemic form of myalgic encephalomyelitis was first described in 1934 and had several distinctive epidemiologic and clinical features (Acheson, 1959). However, no etiologic agent was identified, characteristics of various epidemics have differed, and its standing as an infectious disease has been challenged (McEvedy and Beard, 1970). It had been known by several other names, including epidemic neuromyasthenia, Iceland disease, and Royal Free disease. No epidemics have occurred in the past few decades, but sporadic cases have been described (Leitch, 1995). A syndrome in groups of patients with similar symptoms has been termed postviral fatigue syndrome and chronic fatigue syndrome (Sharpe et al., 1991). However, the majority of patients with myalgic encephalomyelitis did not experience chronic disease.

In a review of 14 epidemics, Acheson (1959) found that 7 occurred in hospital settings, that there was a high attack rate, that young adult women were most frequently involved, and that most occurred in the summer. Many of the original outbreaks occurred in the setting of concern for polio. Transmission was thought to occur by direct contact, and the incubation period was thought to vary from 4 days to 3 weeks or longer. The onset varied from abrupt to insidious. Headache, myalgia, and neck and back stiffness were prominent features. Muscle weakness was diagnostically critical. The incidence of this symptom varied from 10 to 80% and averaged 40% in Acheson's review (1959). Often painful, it was not usually associated with clear signs of an upper or lower motor neuron lesion. Electromyography in some cases showed a reduced number of action potentials on volition; however, muscle atrophy was not a feature. Mental signs, including acute irritability, crying spells, and anxiety were seen. In convalescence, depression, impaired memory, and reduced concentration were prominent in some patients.

Other symptomatology included urinary retention, sensory phenomena, and cranial nerve dysfunction. In the majority of cases, resolution of the acute illness occurred between 1 and 2 months after onset. In some cases a chronic phase occurred; in still others exacerbations were found, but not death. Clinical and laboratory evidence for infection varied. Fever was low grade or absent. Lymphadenopathy, particularly cervical, was prominent in some epidemics and absent in others. Elevation of the peripheral white cell count was uncommon. The CSF was normal in the great majority of cases, as was the EEG. The etiology of this syndrome remained a puzzle. Acheson (1959) concluded that it was most likely an infectious disease, but others have argued that the epidemics were psychosocial phenomena (McEvedy and Beard, 1970).

The apparent disappearance of the epidemic form of myalgic encephalomyelitis leaves unresolved whether an organic basis was responsible (Editorial, 1978) or whether the outbreaks represented epidemic anxiety states (Editorial, 1970). Sporadic cases with similar symptoms are currently most frequently termed chronic fatigue syndrome. That entity represents a heterogeneous group of disorders in which comorbid conditions frequently complicate attempts at study (Natelson, 2001). Whether there is a pathogenic relationship to epidemic myalgic encephalomyelitis is not clear. Certain cases have had a relationship to viral infection, such as the fatigue associated with Epstein-Barr virus infection, or have followed viral infection, such as the postviral fatigue syndrome. In considering the potential role of viruses, Greenlee and Rose (2000) concluded that the chronic fatigue syndrome is a heterogeneous group of disorders and that "a complex relationship may exist between the physical, psychological, and social factors leading to chronic incapacitation."

REFERENCES

Acheson, E. D. 1959. The clinical syndrome variously called benign myalgic encephalomyelitis, Iceland disease and epidemic neuromyasthenia. *Am. J. Med.* **26:**569–595.

Ahmed, F., J. A. Singleton, and A. L. Franks. 2001. Influenza vaccination for healthy young adults. *N. Engl. J. Med.* **345:**1543–1547.

Aiba, H., M. Mochizuki, M. Kimura, and H. Hojo. 2001. Predictive value of serum interleukin-6 level in influenza virus associated encephalopathy. *Neurology* **57:**295–299.

Alexander, J. P., Jr., L. Baden, M. A. Pallansch, and L. J. Anderson. 1994. Enteroviral infections and neurologic disease–United States, 1977–1991. *J. Infect. Dis.* **169:**905–908.

Al-Mateen, M., M. Gibbs, R. Dietrich, W. G. Mitchell, and J. H. Menkes. 1988. Encephalitis lethargica-like illness in a girl with mycoplasma infection. *Neurology* **38:**1155–1158.

Anonymous. 1970. Laboratory reports. *Br. Med. J.* **1:**311.

Baker, A. B., H. A. Matzke, and J. R. Brown. 1950. Poliomyelitis. III. Bulbar poliomyelitis: a study of medullary function. *Arch. Neurol. Psychiatr.* **63:**257–281.

Blinzinger, K., J. Simon, D. Magrath, and L. Boulger. 1969. Poliovirus crystals within the endoplasmic reticulum of endothelial and mononuclear cells in the monkey spinal cord. *Science* **163:**1336–1337.

Blondel, B., G. Duncan, T. Couderc, F. Delpeyroux, N. Pavio, and F. Colbere-Garapin. 1998. Molecular aspects of poliovirus biology with a special focus on the interactions with nerve cells. *J. Neurovirol.* **4:**1–26.

Blunt, S. B., R. J. M. Lane, N. Turjanski, and G. D. Perkin. 1997. Clinical features and management of two cases of encephalitis lethargica. *Movement Disorders* **12:**354–359.

Bodian, D. 1972. Poliomyelitis, p. 2323–2344. *In* J. Minackler (ed.), *Pathology of the Nervous System.* McGraw-Hill, New York, N.Y.

Bodian, D., and H. A. Howe. 1940. An experimental study of the role of neurons in the dissemination of poliomyelitis virus in the nervous system. *Brain* **63:**135–162.

Bodian, D., and H. A. Howe. 1941. Experimental studies on intraneural spread of poliomyelitis virus. *Bull. Johns Hopkins Hosp.* **68:**248–267.

Brahdy, M. B., and M. Lenarsky. 1934. Difficulty in swallowing in acute epidemic poliomyelitis. *JAMA* **103:**229–234.

Buzzard, E. F., and J. G. Greenfield. 1919. Lethargic encephalitis; its sequelae and morbid anatomy. *Brain* **42:**305–308.

Cappel, R., L. Thiry, and G. Clinet. 1975. Viral antibodies in the CSF after acute CNS infections. *Arch. Neurol.* **32:**629–631.

Casals, J., J. T. S. Elizan, and M. D. Yahr. 1998. Post-encephalitic Parkinsonism–a review. *J. Neural Transm.* **105:**645–676.

Center for Disease Control. 1981. *Encephalitis Surveillance Annual Summary 1978.* Center for Disease Control, Atlanta, Ga.

Centers for Disease Control and Prevention. 1997. Nonpolio enterovirus surveillance–United States, 1993–1996. *Morb. Mortal. Wkly. Rep.* **46:**748–750.

Centers for Disease Control and Prevention. 1999a. Outbreak of Hendra-like Virus–Malaysia and Singapore, 1998–1999. *Morb. Mortal. Wkly. Rep.* **48:**265–269.

Centers for Disease Control and Prevention. 1999b. Update: outbreak of Nipah Virus–Malaysia and Singapore, 1999. *Morb. Mortal. Wkly. Rep.* **48:**335–337.

Centers for Disease Control and Prevention. 2000a. Enterovirus surveillance–United States, 1997–1999. *Morb. Mortal. Wkly. Rep.* **49:**913–916.

Centers for Disease Control and Prevention. 2000b. Poliomyelitis prevention in the United States. Updated recommendations of the Advisory Committee on Immunization Practices (ACIP). *Morb. Mortal. Wkly. Rep.* **49**(RR-5):1–22.

Centers for Disease Control and Prevention. 2001a. Enterovirus type 13–United States, 2001. *Morb. Mortal. Wkly. Rep.* **50:**777–780.

Centers for Disease Control and Prevention. 2001b. Progress toward poliomyelitis eradication–West and Central Africa, 1999–2000. *Morb. Mortal. Wkly. Rep.* **50:**481–485.

Centers for Disease Control and Prevention. 2002a. Prevention and control of influenza. Recommendations of the Advisory Committee on Immunization Practices. *Morb. Mortal. Wkly. Rep.* **51**(RR-3):1–31, plus inside and outside covers.

Centers for Disease Control and Prevention. 2002b. Enterovirus Surveillance—United States, 2000–2001. *Morb. Mortal. Wkly. Rep.* **51:**1047–1049.

Chang, L.-Y., T.-Y. Lin, K.-H. Hsu, Y.-C. Huang, K.-L. Lin, C. Hsueh, S.-R. Shih, H.-C. Ning, M.-S. Hwang, H. S. Wang, and C.-Y. Lee. 1999. Clinical features and risk factors of pulmonary edema after Enterovirus 71-related hand, foot and mouth disease. *Lancet* **354:**1682–1686.

Chong, H.-T., A. Kamarulzamen, C.-T. Tan, K.-J. Goh, T. Thayaparan, S. R. Kunjapan, N.-K. Chew, K.-B. Chua, and S.-K. Lam. 2001. Treatment of acute Nipah encephalitis with ribavirin. *Ann. Neurol.* **49:**810–813.

Chua, K. B., K. J. Goh, K. T. Wong, A. Kamarulzaman, P. S. K. Tan, T. G. Ksiazek, S. R. Zaki, G. Paul, S. K. Lam, and C. T. Tan. 1999. Fatal encephalitis due to Nipah Virus among pig-farmers in Malaysia. *Lancet* **354:**1257–1259.

Chua, K. B., W. J. Bellini, P. A. Rota, B. H. Harcourt, A. Tamin, S. K. Lam, T. G. Ksiazek, P. E. Rollin, S. R. Zaki, W.-J. Shieh, C. S. Goldsmith, D. J. Gubler, J. T. Roehrig, B. Eaton,

A. R. Gould, J. Olson, H. Field, P. Daniels, A. E. Ling, C. J. Peters, L. J. Anderson, and B. W. J. Mahy. 2000. Nipah virus: a recently emergent deadly paramyxovirus. *Science* **288:**1432–1435.

Couch, R. B. 2000. Prevention and treatment of influenza. *N. Engl. J. Med.* **343:**1778–1787.

Cox, N. J., and K. Subbarao. 1999. Influenza A. *Lancet* **354:**1277–1282.

Dalakas, M. C. 1995. The post-polio syndrome as an evolved clinical entity: definition and clinical description. *Ann. N.Y. Acad. Sci.* **753:**68–80.

Dalakas, M. C. 1999. Why drugs fail in post-polio syndrome. Lessons from another clinical trial. *Neurology* **53:**1166–1167.

Dalldorf, G., and J. L. Melnick. 1965. Coxsackie viruses, p. 474–512. *In* F. L. Horsfall and L. Tamin (ed.), *Viral and Rickettsial Infections of Man,* 4th ed. B. Lippincott Co., Philadelphia, Pa.

Davenport, F. 1982. Influenza viruses, p. 373–396. *In* A. S. Evans (ed.), *Viral Infections of Humans. Epidemiology and Control,* 2nd ed. Plenum Press, New York, N.Y.

Davis, L. E., and M. Kornfeld. 1980. Influenza A virus and Reye's Syndrome in adults. *J. Neurol. Neurosurg. Psychiatr.* **43:**516–521.

Davis, L. E., K. S. Blisard, and M. Kornfeld. 1990. The Influenza B virus mouse model of Reye's Syndrome: clinical, virologic, and morphologic studies of an encephalopathy. *J. Neurol. Sci.* **97:**221–231.

Debre, R. 1970. Lethargic encephalitis or von Economo's disease, p. 193–202. *In* R. Debre and J. Cellars (ed.), *Clinical Virology, The Evaluation and Management of Human Viral Infections.* W. B. Saunders & Co., Philadelphia, Pa.

Delorme, L., and P. J. Middleton. 1979. Influenza A virus associated with acute encephalopathy. *Am. J. Dis. Child.* **133:**822–824.

Dick, G. W. A., A. M. Best, A. J. Haddow, and K. C. Smithburn. 1948. Meningo-encephalomyelitis. A hitherto unknown virus affecting man. *Lancet* **ii:**286–289.

Dowdle, W. R. 2001. Polio eradication: turning the dream into reality. *ASM News* **67:**397–402.

Editorial. 1970. Epidemic malaise. *Br. Med. J.* **1:**1–2.

Editorial. 1978. Epidemic myalgic encephalomyelitis. *Br. Med. J.* **2:**1436–1437.

Elliott, H. C. 1947. Studies on motor cells of spinal cord; poliomyelitis lesion in spinal motor nuclei in acute cases. *Am. J. Pathol.* **23:**313–325.

Enserink, M. 2000. Malaysian researchers trace Nipah Virus outbreak to bats (News). *Science* **289:**518–519.

Esiri, M. M. 1980. Poliomyelitis: immunoglobulin containing cells in the central nervous system in acute and convalescent phases of human disease. *Clin. Exp. Immunol.* **40:**42–48.

Esiri, M. M., and M. Swash. 1984. Absence of herpes simplex virus antigen in brain in Encephalitis Lethargica. *J. Neurol. Neurosurg. Psychiatr.* **47:**1049–1050.

Farrar, J. J. 1999. Commentary. Nipah-Virus encephalitis–investigation of a new infection. *Lancet* **354:**1222–1223.

Flewett, T. H., and J. G. Hoult. 1958. Influenzal encephalopathy and post influenzal encephalitis. *Lancet* **ii:**11–15.

Ford, D. J., S. L. Ropka, G. H. Collins, and B. Jubelt. 2002. The neuropathology observed in wild-type mice inoculated with human poliovirus mirrors human paralytic poliomyelitis. *Microb. Pathog.* **33:**97–107.

Frankova, V., A. Jirasek, and B. Tumova. 1977. Type A influenza: postmortem virus isolations from different organs in human lethal cases. *Arch. Virol.* **53:**265–268.

Freistadt, M. S., D. A. Stoltz, and K. E. Eberle. 1995. Role of poliovirus receptors in the spread of the infection. *Ann. N. Y. Acad. Sci.* **753:**37–47.

Fujii, Y., M. Kuriyama, Y. Konishi, and M. Sudo. 1992. MRI and SPECT in influenzal encephalitis. *Pediatr. Neurol.* **8**:133–136.

Fujimoto, S., M. Kobayashi, O. Uemura, M. Iwasa, T. Ando, T. Katoh, C. Nakamura, N. Maki, H. Togari, and Y. Wada. 1998. PCR on spinal fluid to show influenza associated acute encephalopathy or encephalitis. *Lancet* **352**:873–875.

Furtado, D. 1958. Encephalite par grippe asiatique. *Rev. Neurol.* **98**:192–205.

Gibbs, F. A., E. L. Gibbs, P. R. Carpenter, and H. W. Spies. 1962. Electroencephalographic study of patients with acute aseptic meningitis. *Pediatrics* **29**:181–186.

Gilbert, G. L., K. E. Dickson, M.-J. Waters, M. L. Kennett, S. A. Land, and M. Sneddon. 1988. Outbreak of Enterovirus 71 infection in Victoria, Australia, with a high incidence of neurologic involvement. *Pediatr. Infect. Dis. J.* **7**:484–488.

Goh, K. J., C. T. Tan, N. K. Chew, P. S. K. Tan, A. Kamarulzaman, S. A. Sarji, K. T. Wong, B. J. J. Abdullah, K. B. Chua, and S. K. Lam. 2000. Clinical features of Nipah Virus Encephalitis among pig farmers in Malaysia. *N. Engl. J. Med.* **342**:1229–1235.

Greenlee, J. E., and J. W. Rose. 2000. Controversies in neurological infectious diseases. *Semin. Neurol.* **20**:375–386.

Grist, N. R., E. J. Bell, and F. Assaad. 1978. Enterovirus in human diseases. *Prog. Med. Virol.* **24**:114–157.

Hall, A. J. 1924. *Epidemic Encephalitis (Encephalitis Lethargica).* John Wright and Sons Ltd., Bristol, United Kingdom.

Hall, C. B. 2001. Respiratory syncytial virus and parainfluenza virus. *N. Engl. J. Med.* **344**:1917–1928. (Discussion, **345**:1132, 1133.)

Hallervorden, J. 1935. Anatomische Untersuchungen zur Pathogenese des postencephalitischen Parkinsonismus. *D. Z. Nervenheilk.* **136**:68–77.

Harada, K. 1966. Zur morphologischen Differenzierung hämorrhagischer Encephalitiden. *D. Z. Nervenheilk.* **188**:142–186.

Hayden, F. G., and P. Palese. 1997. Influenza virus, p. 911–942. *In* D. G. Richman, R. J. Whitley, and F. G. Hayden (ed.), *Clinical Virology.* Churchill Livingstone, New York, N.Y.

Haynes, R. E., H. G. Cramblett, and H. J. Kronfal. 1969. Echovirus 9 meningoencephalitis in infants and children. *JAMA* **208**:1657–1660.

Heathfield, K. W. G., R. Pilsworth, J. Wall, and J. A. N. Corseffis. 1967. Coxsackie B5 infections in Essex 1965 with particular reference to the nervous system. *Q. J. Med.* **36**:579–595.

Hirayama, K., H. Salazaki, S. Murakami, S. Yonezawa, K. Fujimoto, T. Seto, K. Tanaka, H. Hattori, O. Matsuoka, and R. Murata. 1999. Sequential MRI, SPECT and PET in respiratory syncytial virus encephalitis. *Pediatr. Radiol.* **29**:282–286.

Ho, M., E.-R. Chen, K.-H. Hsu, S.-J. Twu, K.-T. Chen, S.-F. Tsai, J.-R. Wang, and S.-R. Shih for the Taiwan Enterovirus Epidemic Working Group. 1999. An epidemic of enterovirus 71 infection in Taiwan. *N. Engl. J. Med.* **341**:929–935.

Horstmann, D. M., and N. Yamada. 1968. Enterovirus infections of the central nervous system. *Res. Publ. Assoc. Res. Nerv. Ment. Dis.* **44**:236–253.

Hoult, J. G., and T. H. Flewett. 1960. Influenzal encephalopathy and post-influenzal encephalitis. Histological and other observations. *Br. Med. J.* **1**:1847–1850.

Howard, R. S., and A. J. Lees. 1987. Encephalitis lethargica. A report of four recent cases. *Brain* **110**:19–33.

Huang, C.-C., C.-C. Liu, Y.-C. Chang, C.-Y. Chen, S.-T. Wang, and T.-F. Yeh. 1999. Neurologic complications in children with Enterovirus 71 infection. *N. Engl. J. Med.* **341**:936–942.

Hung, T.-P., S.-M. Sung, H.-C. Liang, D. Landsborough, and I. J. Green. 1976. Radiculomyelitis following acute haemorrhagic conjunctivitis. *Brain* **99**:771–790.

Ishimaru, Y., S. Nakano, K. Yamaoka, and S. Takami. 1980. Outbreak of Hand, Foot, and Mouth Disease by Enterovirus 71. High incidence of complication disorders of central nervous system. *Arch. Dis. Child.* **55**:583–588.

Ito, Y., T. Ichiyama, H. Kimura, M. Shibata, N. Ishiwada, H. Kuroki, S. Furukuwa, and T. Morishima. 1999. Detection of influenza virus RNA by reverse transcription-PCR and proinflammatory cytokines in influenza-virus-associated encephalopathy. *J. Med. Virol.* **58**:420–425.

John, T. J. 2000. The final stages of the global eradication of polio. *N. Engl. J. Med.* **343**:806–807.

Jubelt, B., and J. C. Agre. 2000. Characteristics and management of post-polio syndrome. *JAMA* **284**:412–414.

Jubelt, B., G. Gallez-Hawkins, O. Narayan, and R. T. Johnson. 1980. Pathogenesis of human poliovirus infection in mice. I. Clinical and pathological studies. *J. Neuropathol. Exp. Neurol.* **39**:138–148.

Kasai, T., T. Togashi, and T. Morishima. 2000. Encephalopathy associated with influenza epidemics. *Lancet* **355**:1558–1559.

Kennedy, S. 1998. Morbillivirus infections in aquatic mammals. *J. Comp. Pathol.* **119**:201–225.

Kennett, M. L., C. J. Birch, F. A. Lewis, A. P. Yung, S. A. Locarnini, and I. D. Gust. 1974. Enterovirus-71 infection in Melbourne. *Bull. W. H. O.* **51**:609–615.

Kew, O., V. Morris-Glasgow, M. Landaverde, C. Burns, J. Shaw, Z. Garib, J. André, E. Blackman, C. J. Freeman, J. Jorba, R. Sutter, G. Tambini, L. Venczel, C. Pedreira, F. Laender, H. Shimuzu, T. Yoneyama, T. Miyamura, H. van der Avoort, M. S. Oberste, D. Kilpatrick, S. Cochi, M. Pallansch, and C. de Quadros. 2002. Outbreak of poliomyelitis in Hispaniola associated with circulating type I vaccine-derived poliovirus. *Science* **296**:356–359.

Kiley, M., and M. M. Esiri. 2001. A contemporary case of encephalitis lethargica. *Clin. Neuropathol.* **20**:2–7.

Kimura, S., T. Kobayashi, H. Osaka, C. Shimizu, S. Uebara, and N. Ohtuki. 1995. Serial magnetic resonance imaging in postinfectious focal encephalitis due to influenza virus. *J. Neurol. Sci.* **131**:74–77.

Kono, R., A. Sasagawa, H. Kodama, N. Uchida, Y. Akao, J. Mukoyama, and T. Fujreau. 1973. Neurovirulence of acute-haemorrhagic-conjunctivitis virus in monkeys. *Lancet* **i**:61–63.

Krugman, S., and R. Ward. 1968. Enteroviral infections, p. 56–89. *In Infectious Diseases of Children,* 4th ed. CV Mosby Co., St. Louis, Mo.

Landry, M. L., S. N. S. Fonseca, S. Cohen, and C. W. Bogue. 1995. Fatal enterovirus type 71 infection: rapid diagnosis and diagnostic pitfalls. *Pediatr. Infect. Dis. J.* **14**:1095–1100.

Langmuir, A. D., D. J. Bregman, L. T. Kurland, N. Nathanson, and M. Victor. 1984. An epidemiologic and clinical evaluation of Guillain-Barré syndrome reported in association with the administration of Swine influenza vaccines. *Am. J. Epidemiol.* **119**:841–879.

Lee, K.-E., T. Umapathi, C.-B. Tan, H. T.-L. Tjia, T.-S. Cua, H. M.-L. Oh, K.-M. Fock, A. Kurup, A. K.-Y. Tan, and W.-L. Lee. 1999. The neurological manifestations of Nipah virus encephalitis, a novel paramyxovirus. *Ann. Neurol.* **46**:428–432.

Leitch, A. G. 1995. Neurasthenia, myalgic encephalitis or cryptogenic chronic fatigue syndrome? *Q. J. Med.* **88**:447–450.

Lepow, M. L., N. Coyne, L. B. Thompson, D. H. Carver, and F. C. Robbins. 1962. A clinical, epidemiological and laboratory investigation of aseptic meningitis during the four year period 1955–1958. II. The clinical disease and its sequelae. *N. Engl. J. Med.* **266**:1188–1193.

Lim, C. C. T., Y. Y. Sitoh, F. Hui, K. E. Lee, B. S. P. Ang, E. Lim, W. E. H. Lim, H. M. L. Oh, P. A. Tambyah, J. S. L. Wong, C. B. Tan, and T. S. G. Chee. 2000. Nipah viral encephalitis or Japanese encephalitis? MR findings in a new zoonotic disease. *Am. J. Neuroradiol.* **21:**455–461.

Linneman, C. C., Jr., L. Shea, J. C. Partinj, W. K. Schubert, and G. M. Schiff. 1975. Reye's syndrome: epidemiologic and viral studies 1963–74. *Am. J. Epidemiol.* **101:**517–526.

Lum, L. C. S., K. T. Wong, S. K. Lam, K. B. Chua, A. Y. T. Goh, W. W. L. Lim, B. B. Ong, G. Paul, S. AbuBakar, and M. Lambert. 1998. Fatal Enterovirus 71 encephalomyelitis. *J. Pediatr.* **133:**795–798.

Mace, S. E. 2002. Bronchiolitis: an update. *Resid. Staff Physician* **48:**50–57.

Matheson Commission. 1939. *Epidemic Encephalitis. Etiology, Epidemiology, Treatment.* Third Report of the Matheson Commission. Columbia University Press, New York, N.Y.

McCall, S., J. M. Henry, A. H. Reid, and J. K. Taubenberger. 2001. Influenza RNA not detected in archival brain tissues from acute encephalitis lethargica cases or in postencephalitic Parkinson cases. *J. Neuropathol. Exp. Neurol.* **60:**696–704.

McCullers, J. A., S. Facchinis, P. J. Chesney, and R. G. Webster. 1999. Influenza B encephalitis. *Clin. Infect. Dis.* **28:**989–900.

McEvedy, C. P., and A. W. Beard. 1970. Concept of benign myalgic encephalomyelitis. *Br. Med. J.* **1:**11–15.

McMinn, P., I. Stratov, L. Nagara, and S. Davis. 2001. Neurological manifestations of Enterovirus 71 infection in children during an outbreak of Hand, Foot, and Mouth Disease in Western Australia. *Clin. Infect. Dis.* **32:**236–242.

Mellon, A. F., R. E. Appleton, D. Gardner-Medwin, and A. Aynsley-Groen. 1991. Encephalitis lethargica-like illness in a five year old child. *Dev. Med. Child. Neurol.* **33:**158–161.

Melnick, J. L. 1996. Current status of poliovirus infections. *Clin. Microbiol. Rev.* **9:**293–300.

Merritt, H. H. 1967. Acute anterior poliomyelitis, p. 55–66. *In A Textbook of Neurology*, 4th ed. Lea and Febiger, Philadelphia, Pa.

Mizuguchi, M., J. Abe, S. Noma, K. Yoshida, T. Yamanaka, and S. Kamoshita. 1995. Acute necrotizing encephalopathy of childhood: a new syndrome presenting with multifocal symmetric brain lesions. *J. Neurol. Neurosurg. Psychiatr.* **58:**555–561.

Modlin, J. F., and D. J. Coffey. 1997. Poliomyelitis, polio vaccines, and the post-poliomyelitis syndome, p. 57–72. *In* W. M. Scheld, R. J. Whitley, and D. T. Durack (ed.), *Infections of the Central Nervous System.* Lippincott-Raven, Philadelphia, Pa.

Modlin, J. F., R. Dagan, L. E. Berlin, D. M. Virshup, R. H. Yolken, and M. Menegus. 1991. Focal encephalitis with enterovirus infections. *Pediatrics* **88:**841–845.

Muir, P., U. Mammerer, K. Korn, M. N. Mulders, T. Poyry, B. Weissbrich, R. Kandolph, G. M. Gleator, and A. M. van Loon for the European Union Concerted Action on Virus Meningitis and Encephalitis. 1998. Molecular typing of enteroviruses: current status and future requirements. *Clin. Microbiol. Rev.* **11:**202–227.

Mulder, D. W., R. A. Rosenbaum, and D. D. Layton, Jr. 1972. Late progression of poliomyelitis or forme fruste amyotrophic lateral sclerosis? *Mayo Clin. Proc.* **47:**756–761.

Murray, K., P. Selleck, P. Hooper, A. Hyatt, A. Gould, A. Gleeson, H. Westbury, L. Hiley, L. Selvey, B. Rodwell, and P. Ketterer. 1995. A morbillivirus that caused fatal disease in horses and humans. *Science* **268:**94–97.

Nagai, T., A. Yagishita, Y. Tsuchiya, S. Asumura, H. Kurokawa, and N. Matsuo. 1993. Symmetrical thalamic lesions on CT in influenza A virus infection presenting with or without Reye's syndrome. *Brain Dev.* **15:**67–73.

Nagy, G., S. Takatsy, E. Kukan, I. Mihaly, and I. Domok. 1982. Virological diagnosis of enterovirus type 71 infections: experiences gained during an epidemic of acute CNS diseases in Hungary in 1978. *Arch. Virol.* **71:**217–227.

Natelson, B. H. 2001. Chronic fatigue syndrome. *JAMA* **285:**2557–2559.

Nathanson, N., and D. Bodian. 1962. Experimental poliomyelitis following intramuscular virus injection. 3. The effect of passive antibody on paralysis and viraemia. *Bull. Johns Hopkins Hosp.* **111:**198–220.

Nathanson, N., and P. Fine. 2002. Poliomyelitis eradication—a dangerous endgame. *Science* **296:**269–270.

Ng, Y. T., C. Cox, J. Atkins, and I. J. Butler. 2001. Encephalopathy associated with respiratory syncytial virus bronchiolitis. *J. Child. Neurol.* **16:**105–108.

Oberste, M. S., K. Maher, D. R. Kilpatrick, and M. A. Pallansch. 1999. Molecular evolution of the human enteroviruses: correlation of serotype with VPI sequence and application to picornavirus classification. *J. Virol.* **73:**1941–1948.

Olson, J. G., C. Rupprecht, P. E. Rollin, U. S. An, M. Niezgoda, T. Clemins, J. Walston, and T. G. Ksiazek. 2002. Antibodies to Nipah-like virus in bats (*Pteropus lylei*). Cambodia. *Emerg. Infect. Dis.* **8:**987–991.

Oseasohn, R., L. Adelson, and M. Kaji. 1959. Clinicopathologic study of thirty-three fatal cases of Asian influenza. *N. Engl. J. Med.* **26:**509–518.

O'Sullivan, J. D., A. M. Altworth, D. L. Paterson, T. M. Snow, R. Boots, L. J. Gleeson, A. R. Gould, A. D. Hyatt, and J. Bradfield. 1997. Fatal encephalitis due to novel paramyxovirus transmitted from horses. *Lancet* **349:**93–95.

Paton, N. I., Y. S. Leo, S. R. Zaki, A. P. Auchus, K. E. Lee, A. E. Ling, S. K. Chew, B. Ang, P. E. Rollin, T. Umapathi, I. Sng, C. C. Lee, E. Lim, and T. G. Ksiazek. 1999. Outbreak of Nipah-virus infection among abattoir workers in Singapore. *Lancet* **354:**1253–1256.

Paul, J. R. 1966. *Clinical Epidemiology*, revised ed. University of Chicago Press, Chicago, Ill.

Peatfield, R. C. 1987. Basal ganglia damage and subcortical dementia after possible insidious Coxsackie Virus Encephalitis. *Acta Neurol. Scand.* **76:**340–345.

Pevear, D. C., T. M. Tull, M. E. Seipel, and J. M. Groarke. 1999. Activity of pleconaril against enteroviruses. *Antimicrob. Agents Chemother.* **43:**2109–2115.

Rail, D., C. Scholtz, and M. Swash. 1981. Post-encephalitic parkinsonism: current experience. *J. Neurol. Neurosurg. Psychiatr.* **44:**670–676.

Ramlow, J., M. Alexander, R. LaPorte, C. Kaufman, and L. Kuller. 1992. Epidemiology of the post-polio syndrome. *Am. J. Epidem.* **136:**769–786.

Reid, A. H., S. McCall, J. M. Henry, and J. K. Taubenberger. 2001. Experimenting on the past: the enigma of von Economo's encephalitis lethargica. *J. Neuropathol. Exp. Neurol.* **60:**663–670.

Rose, E., and P. Prabhakar. 1982. Influenza A Virus associated neurological disorders in Jamaica. *West Ind. Med. J.* **31:**29–33.

Rotbart, H. A. 1995. Enteroviral infections of the central nervous system. *Clin. Infect. Dis.* **20:**971–981.

Rotbart, H. 1997. Enteroviruses, p. 997–1023. *In* D. D. Richman, R. J. Whitley, and F. G. Hayden (ed.), *Clinical Virology.* Churchill Livingstone, New York, N.Y.

Rotbart, H. A., and A. D. Webster for the Pleconaril Treatment Registry Group. 2001. Treatment of potentially life-threatening enterovirus infections with pleconaril. *Clin. Infect. Dis.* **32:**228–235.

Sabin, A. B. 1956. Pathogenesis of poliomyelitis. Reappraisal in the light of new data. *Science* **123:**1151–1157.

Sacks, O. 1973. *Awakenings.* Duckworth, London, United Kingdom.

Schmidt, N. J., E. H. Lennette, and H. H. Ho. 1974. An apparently new enterovirus isolated from patients with disease of the central nervous system. *J. Infect. Dis.* **129:**304–309.

Sharpe, M. C., L. C. Archard, J. E. Banatvala, A. W. Clare, A. David, R. H. T. Edwards, K. E. H. Hawton, H. P. Lambert, R. J. M. Lane, E. M. McDonald, J. F. Mowbray, D. J. Pearson, T. E. A. Peto, V. R. Preedy, A. P. Smith, D. G. Smith, D. J. Taylor, D. A. J. Tyrell, S. Wessely, and P. D. White. 1991. A report—chronic fatigue syndrome: guidelines for research. *J. R. Soc. Med.* **84:**118–121.

Shen, W.-C., H.-H. Chiu, K.-C. Chow, and C.-H. Tsai. 1999. MR imaging findings of enteroviral encephalomyelitis: an outbreak in Taiwan. *Am. J. Neuroradiol.* **20:**1889–1895.

Shimada, A., D. J. Lange, and A. P. Hays. 1999. Amyotrophic lateral sclerosis in an adult following acute paralytic poliomyelitis in early childhood. *Acta Neuropathol.* (Berlin) **97:**317–321.

Shindarov, L. M., M. P. Chumakov, M. K. Voroshilova, S. Bojinov, S. M. Vasilenko, I. Iordanov, I. D. Kirov, E. Kamenov, E. V. Leshinskay, G. Mitov, I. A. Robinson, S. Sivchev, and S. T. Staikov. 1979. Epidemiological, clinical, and pathomorphological characteristics of epidemic poliomyelitis-like disease caused by Enterovirus 71. *J. Hyg. Epidemiol. Microbiol. Immunol.* **23:**284–295.

Simoes, E. A. F. 1999. Respiratory syncytial virus infection. *Lancet* **354:**847–852.

Smith, R., J. P. Woodall, E. Whitney, R. Deibel, M. A. Gross, V. Smith, and T. F. Bast. 1974. Powassan virus infection: a report of three human cases of encephalitis. *Am. J. Dis. Child.* **127:**691–693.

Strikas, R. A., L. J. Anderson, and R. A. Parker. 1986. Temporal and geographic patterns of isolates of nonpolio enterovirus in the United States, 1970–1983. *J. Infect. Dis.* **153:**346–351.

Sulkava, R., A. Rissanen, and R. Pyhala. 1981. Post-influenzal encephalitis during the influenza A outbreak in 1979/1980. *J. Neurol. Neurosurg. Psychiatr.* **44:**161–163.

Tan, C. T., K. J. Goh, K. T. Wong, S. A. Sarji, K. B. Chua, N. K. Chew, P. Murugasu, Y. L. Loh, H. T. Chong, K. S. Tan, T. Thayaparan, S. Kumma, and M. R. Jusoh. 2002. Relapsed and late-onset Nipah encephalitis. *Ann. Neurol.* **51:**703–708.

Thorsteinsson, G. 1997. Management of post-polio syndrome. *Mayo Clin. Proc.* **72:**627–638.

Tilney, F., and H. S. Howe. 1920. *Epidemic Encephalitis (Encephalitis Lethargica).* Paul B. Hoeber, New York, N.Y.

von Economo, C. 1917. Encephalitis lethargica. *Wien. Klin. Wschr.* **30:**581–585. Translated in **Wilkins, R. H. and I. A. Brody.** 1968. Encephalitis lethargica. *Arch. Neurol.* **18:**324–328.

von Economo, C. 1931. *Encephalitis Lethargica: Its Sequelae and Treatment.* Oxford University Press, London, United Kingdom.

Wells, C. E. C. 1971. Neurological complications of so-called "influenza." A winter study in south-east Wales. *Br. Med. J.* **1:**369–373.

Wenner, H. A. 1982. The enteroviruses: recent advances. *Yale J. Biol. Med.* **55:**277–282.

Windebank, A. J., W. J. Litchy, and J. R. Daube. 1995. Prospective cohort study of polio survivors in Olmsted County, Minnesota. *Ann. N. Y. Acad. Sci.* **753:**81–86.

Wong, K. T., W.-J. Shien, S. Kumar, K. Norain, W. Abdullah, J. Guarner, C. S. Goldsmith, K. B. Chua, S. K. Lam, C. T. Tan, K. J. Goh, H. T. Chong, R. Jusoh, P. E. Rollin, T. G. Ksiazek, and S. R. Zaki. 2002. Nipah virus infection: pathology and pathogenesis of an emerging paramyxoviral zoonosis. *Am. J. Pathol.* **161:**2153–2167.

World Health Organization. 1998. Surveillance of nonpoliomyelitis enteroviruses, 1993–1996. *Wkly. Epidemiol. Rec.* **29:**220–223.

World Health Organization. 2002. Acute neurological syndrome, Bangladesh. Followed by an account of Nipah virus. *Wkly. Epidemiol. Rec.* **77:**297–299.

Wyatt, H. V. 1982. Any questions? *Trop. Doctor* **12:**218.

Yan, J.-J., J.-R. Wang, C.-C. Liu, H.-B. Yang, and I.-J. Su. 2000. An outbreak of Enterovirus 71 infection in Taiwan 1998: a comprehensive pathological, virological, and molecular study on a case of fulminant encephalitis. *J. Clin. Virol.* **17:**13–22.

Zeichhardt, H., and H.-P. Grunert. 2000. Enteroviruses, p. 252–269. *In* S. Specter, R. L. Hodinka, and S. A. Young (ed.), *Clinical Virology Manual*, 3rd ed. ASM Press, Washington, D.C.

11

The Arboviruses

On a global scale, the public health danger posed by the arboviruses is massive. For example, in Asia alone, over 50,000 cases of Japanese encephalitis (JE) are reported annually with approximately 10,000 deaths (World Health Organization, 1998), while globally dengue fever afflicts over 50 million people annually (Rigau-Perez et al., 1998). Probably no area in virology is as daunting for the practicing clinician as are the arboviruses. Much of the problem comes from the sheer number—now over 530 known arboviruses (Karabatsos, 1985; N. Karabatsos, personal communication). Yet much information about arboviral infections can be organized into patterns that greatly facilitate diagnosis of infection by specific viruses. Another problem has been the replacement of the epidemiologically based arboviral nomenclature with one based on physical and chemical characteristics of the viruses. The term "arbo," which is a contracture of "arthropod-borne," emphasizes the importance of the arthropod vector in the natural cycle between arthropods and animals. In the present taxonomy, the most important arbovirus causes of encephalitis fall into three families: *Togaviridae*, *Flaviviridae*, and *Bunyaviridae*. Encephalitis can also complicate the systemic manifestations of Colorado tick virus, in the family *Reoviridae*. In the clinical discussions that follow, we retain the central importance of the vector. Table 11.1 is organized by the transmitting vector and the viral family.

PATHOLOGY

The neuropathology of the various human arbovirus encephalitides is sufficiently similar for them to be considered together. Variations in the topography of the pathology may suggest a particular virus as the cause of the encephalitis but do no more than that. Serology is the most convenient way of identifying the virus responsible. Macroscopic alterations are usually minimal, with congestion and edema being the most common findings in the brain, together with minimal cloudiness and congestion of the leptomeninges. Microscopic lesions are widespread, but even so some topographical predilections can be discerned. Gray matter is distinctly more affected than white matter, and in most types of arbovirus encephalitis, the main focus of the pathology lies in the diencephalon and the brain stem, particularly the upper brain stem (Osetowska, 1977). The structures most regularly involved are the thalamus, hypothalamus, midbrain, pons, and medulla. Also frequently involved are the caudate nucleus, putamen, globus pallidus, cerebral cortex, cerebellum, and cervical spinal cord. Pathological changes are generally too

163

TABLE 11.1 Taxonomic classification of the arboviruses discussed in this chapter

Mosquito-borne encephalitides
  Togaviridae
    Eastern equine encephalitis virus (EEEV)
    Western equine encephalitis virus (WEEV)
    Venezuelan equine encephalitis virus (VEEV)
  Flaviviridae
    St. Louis encephalitis virus (SLEV)
    West Nile virus (WNV)
    Japanese encephalitis virus (JEV)
    Murray Valley encephalitis virus (MVEV)
    Dengue virus
  Bunyaviridae
    La Crosse virus
    Rift Valley fever virus (RVFV)
Tick-borne encephalitides
  Flaviviridae
    Tick-borne encephalitis virus (TBEV)
      Far East Russian subtype
      Central European subtype
      Powassan fever virus
  Reoviridae
    Colorado tick fever virus

diffuse to be diagnostically useful on their own, and there are no structural abnormalities that are pathognomonic of infection by a particular virus. Nevertheless, the severity of the changes seen varies from one viral infection to another, as does the relative topographical emphasis of the damage produced. The most severe pathological changes are seen most commonly in eastern equine encephalitis (EEE) and JE; much milder pathology is characteristic of western equine encephalitis (WEE), Venezuelan equine encephalitis (VEE), and California encephalitis. Topographical localization of damage is centered on the basal ganglia in tick-borne encephalitis (TBE). In West Nile virus (WNV) encephalitis (WNVE), the brain stem, particularly the medulla, is targeted (Sampson et al., 2000). These variations are summarized in Table 11.2, in which references to pathological studies of each of the forms of arbovirus are given.

The microscopic changes that are found are edema, capillary endothelial cell swelling, neuronophagic nodules, diffuse microglial proliferation, and perivascular cuffing with inflammatory cells (Fig. 11.1). An astrocytic reaction is relatively inconspicuous. Small necrotic foci resembling microabscesses are also seen, as are acellular foci of necrosis (Fig. 11.2), some of which may be of vascular origin, though thrombotic occlusion of small vessels is infrequent (Miyake, 1964; Ravi et al., 2000) (see Table 11.2). Inclusion bodies are not seen. The leptomeninges show some infiltration with inflammatory cells, most of them lymphocytes and macrophages. In subacute cases, inflammation is less intense than in acute cases, but some perivascular cuffing with mononuclear inflammatory cells and more diffuse microglial proliferation persists. Amongst the lymphocytes present in the central nervous system (CNS), T lymphocytes, particularly CD4$^+$ T cells, predominate; only about 10% of the cells are B cells and these are confined to perivascular spaces (Iwasaki et al., 1993; Johnson et al., 1985).

Diagnosis generally depends on the results of viral culture or PCR or, more often, serological evidence of rising antibody titers to a particular arbovirus. Viral culture from blood is rarely successful because the viremic phase of the disease is more or less over by the time symptoms of encephalitis develop. Culture from the brain is relatively uncommon, partly because of the low biopsy and mortality rates and partly because by the time a patient dies and autopsy specimens are taken, the disease has entered a phase in which virus is no longer detectable in the brain. However, viral antigen has been demonstrated in neurons in fatal cases of JE (Fig. 11.1) (Desai et al., 1995a; Johnson et al., 1985; Li et al., 1988; Iwasaki et al., 1986; Garen et al., 1999) and St. Louis encephalitis (SLE) (Reyes et al., 1981), and viral particles have been seen by electron microscopy in the brain in cases of EEE (Bastian et al., 1975; Kim et al., 1985). Foci of rarefaction necrosis without inflammation but with cyst formation, surrounding gliosis, and gritty calcification are fairly frequent late features, and secondary Wallerian degeneration may be present in white matter in long-surviving cases (Zimmerman, 1946; Smadel et al., 1958; Ishii et al., 1977).

PATHOGENESIS

Little is known directly of the manner in which virus reaches the brain in human arbovirus encephalitis (Grimley, 1983). The pattern of disturbance produced by infection with many of these viruses is biphasic (Webb, 1975). In the first phase, commencing a day or two after infection and lasting over a week, nonspecific symptoms and fever may occur. Viremia occurs during this phase and is thought to afford access of virus to the brain. Next, a disease-free interval of a few days occurs, followed by the appearance of the encephalitic illness. The ratio of clinical to subclinical infection at the systemic stage is extremely variable and at the encephalitic stage it is largely unknown, though estimates for clinical:subclinical JE, for example, have ranged from 1:25 to 1:1,000 (Halstead and Grosz, 1962; Huang, 1982; Vaughn and Hoke, 1992). These ratios are similar to those for WEE but are much higher for EEE (1:2 to 1:50) (Johnson, 1998). Young children are generally more susceptible to arbovirus encephalitis than older people (see below) except for SLE (Monath and Tsai, 1987; Tsai et al., 1988).

Animal studies have shed some light on the mode of entry of virus into the nervous system. In louping ill, which is caused by a tick-borne virus that produces illness in sheep and rarely in humans in Scotland and northern England, experimental infection in sheep results in viremia within 4 to 5 days. The virus multiplies in cells of the reticuloendothelial system (Doherty and Vantsis, 1973) and reaches the brain from the blood. Different viruses probably take different routes across the blood-brain barrier. For example, studies of Semliki Forest virus and JE virus (JEV) in mice suggest that virus crosses the endothelium within pinocytotic vesicles or is phagocytosed within white blood cells (WBC) (Pathak and Webb, 1974; Liou and Hsu, 1998). Endothelial cells are themselves infected with replicating virus in experimental infection with Sindbis virus, which is related to WEE virus (WEEV) (Johnson, 1965). Astrocytic infection without preceding endothelial infection is described in experimental studies of EEE virus (EEEV) (Murphy and Whitfield, 1970). JEV has been shown to stimulate production of a low-molecular-weight macrophage-derived neutrophil chemotactic factor capable of impairing the blood-brain barrier (Mathur et al., 1992). Concomitant cysticercosis, which might be expected to lower the blood-brain barrier, has been repeatedly described in JE and tends to increase the density of JE lesions (reviewed in Ravi et al., 2000). There appears to be no predilection for replication of arboviruses in cells of the choroid plexus, a finding that is consonant with the greater tendency of these viruses to produce encephalitis than aseptic meningitis in humans. One experimental study of the virus causing SLE, in which low levels of viremia were produced in an effort to simulate conditions occurring in human infection, suggested that virus may gain access to the brain following preliminary invasion of and multiplication in olfactory neuroepithelium (Monath et al., 1983).

Once inside the CNS, multifocal lytic infection of neurons occurs. In experimental infection of mice with JEV, electron microscopy showed replication of virus in the rough endoplasmic reticulum of neurons, which became hypertrophic and displayed dilated, virion-laden cisternae. The Golgi apparatus of infected neurons was severely damaged (Hase, 1993). A similar sequence of events is seen with experimental Sindbis virus infection (Griffin and Hardwick, 1997). The contribution of the immune response to the damage produced in arbovirus infections is unclear. It would seem to be negligible in some experimental infections (e.g., louping ill) in which animals die when neurons are infected and when an immune response has scarcely begun (Doherty and Reid, 1971).

However, the pathology of some other experimental arbovirus infections has been dramatically modified and the clinical outcome has been altered by manipulating the immune state of the animals. For example, Zlotnik et al. (1970) found that administration of cyclophosphamide to monkeys infected with louping ill virus converted what was normally an inflammatory disease with no mortality into a degenerative one with prominent neuronal necrosis and spongy change and a high mortality rate. Inflammation was similarly suppressed by cyclophosphamide, but without increasing mortality, in experimental infection with WEEV and EEEV (Zlotnik et al., 1970), Sindbis virus, and Semliki Forest virus (Webb et al., 1979). In the latter case the mortality was negligible in normal adult mice unless a form of macrophage blockade was produced by administration of myocrisin (Allner et al., 1974). Persistent infection with Sindbis virus can be established in mature immunodeficient mice (Levine et al., 1991). In mice, adoptive transfer of spleen cells, especially cytotoxic T cells, from immunized mice protected adult but not young mice against lethal intracerebral challenge (Murali-Krishna et al., 1994, 1996).

In humans, too, there is evidence that immune status can influence outcome in arbovirus encephalitis. SLE is more likely to occur in human immunodeficiency virus-infected humans with impaired T-cell function (Okhuysen et al., 1993). In JE the presence of virus-specific immune complexes and high levels of tumor necrosis factor alpha in cerebrospinal fluid (CSF) in humans is associated with a fatal outcome (Desai et al., 1995b; Ravi et al., 1997). In human

TBE, lower concentrations of serum neutralizing antibodies and higher cell counts in CSF characterized those with a severe course (Kaiser and Holzmann, 2000). While there is evidence from these and similar studies that the immune response can undoubtedly modify the pathology of arbovirus infection of the brain, it appears that in general other factors such as the age of the host, the strain of the virus, and its rate of replication are even more potent in determining the outcome of these infections (Schlesinger, 1980). The capacity of Sindbis virus to produce fatal encephalitis in mice was reduced in animals infected with virus carrying the anti-apoptotic *bcl-2* gene, suggesting that neurovirulence of this virus is in part correlated with its capacity to induce neuronal apoptosis (Levine et al., 1996).

DIAGNOSIS AND MANAGEMENT

Central to the clinical suspicion of any case of arboviral encephalitis is the pattern of epidemiologic information. First, season is a key. Arboviral encephalitides have seasonal patterns of spring-summer, as with the eastern variety of TBE, or summer-early fall, as with the arboviral encephalitides found in the United States. In the absence of recent foreign travel, arboviral encephalitis is not in the differential diagnosis of a winter encephalitis. A second key is location. EEE, for example, has tended to occur in certain areas along the eastern seaboard and Gulf Coast of the United States. A call to the regional virus diagnostic laboratory is always in order to learn the current local virus activity. Third, certain climatic conditions favor the proliferation of specific vectors and increase the likelihood of certain infections. For example, a summer preceded by heavy rains or heavy snowpack melting, resulting in flooding, favors breeding of *Culex tarsalis*. This enhances the possibility of SLE in rural areas of the western United States. Fourth, certain high-risk groups exist in human populations. La Crosse virus encephalitis occurs as a yearly endemic infection in circumscribed areas of the United States and over 90% of cases are in children 15 years of age or younger. Fifth, certain arboviral outbreaks are associated with epizootics. The type of WNV that has become established in the United States is particularly lethal for crows. Hence, the clinician can develop a pattern of epidemiologic information, including season, location, atmospheric conditions, risk groups, and epizootics, that will greatly narrow the list of possible arboviral causes. For most of the arboviruses discussed below a table of the principal epidemiologic features is given.

MOSQUITO-BORNE ENCEPHALITIDES

Togaviruses-Alphaviruses

EEE

EEE is the most lethal of the principal arboviral encephalitides to affect the United States. First verified in humans in southeastern Massachusetts in 1938, mortality in the early epidemics in that state was 68% (Feemster, 1957). From 1964 to 1999, there was a median of four U.S. cases per year (Centers for Disease Control and Prevention, 2001a). Several epidemiologic features of the outbreaks in the United

TABLE 11.2 Summary of pathological features in various forms of arbovirus encephalitis

Disease	Glial nodules	Perivascular infiltrate	Foci of rarefaction necrosis without inflammation	Meningeal infiltrate	Sites of most severe damage	Vasculitis	Foci of tissue necrosis with inflammation	Neuronophagia	White matter lesions	References[c]
EEE	Yes	Neutrophils, mononuclear	Yes (may be late calcification)	Neutrophils, mononuclear	Basal ganglia, substantia nigra, cerebral cortex, hippocampus	Yes, with thrombi	Many, especially in gray matter	Yes, neutrophils, macrophages	Only near affected gray matter	8, 11, 17, 32, 48
WEE	Yes	Mononuclear	Yes	Sparse, mononuclear	Striatum, thalamus, cerebral and cerebellar cortex, base of pons	Not usually	No	Yes, macrophages	No	2, 10, 17, 32–36, 47, 48
VEE	Yes	Sparse, mononuclear	No	Sparse, mononuclear	Putamen	No	No	Rare	No	17, 32, 38, 45
SLE	Yes	Mononuclear	Rare	Mononuclear	Thalamus, basal ganglia, brain stem, especially midbrain	No	No	Rare	Mild inflammation	5, 17, 26, 29, 32, 39, 41, 44, 46
JE	Yes	Neutrophils only in fulminating cases; mononuclear	Yes (may be late calcification)	Mononuclear	Thalamus, substantia nigra, cerebral cortex, hippocampus, cerebellar cortex, spinal cord	No	Yes (may be late calcification)	Yes	Only near affected gray matter	7, 17–24, 27, 28, 31, 32, 42, 49, 50
MVE	Yes	Neutrophils only in fulminating cases; mononuclear	Yes (may be late calcification)	Mononuclear	Cerebral and cerebellar cortex, basal ganglia, brain stem	No			No	1, 12, 32, 37, 40
WNVE	Yes	Mononuclear	Yes	Mononuclear	Brainstem, especially medulla	No			Yes	4
TBE	Yes	Mononuclear	Yes	Mononuclear	Upper spinal cord, brain stem, cerebellum, thalamus, basal ganglia	Yes	Yes	Yes	No	3, 9, 13–15, 17, 25, 30, 32, 35, 43
CalE[a]	Yes	Mononuclear	No	Mononuclear	Cerebral cortex, basal ganglia, thalamus, mid-brain, pons	Yes	Few	Yes	No	24
DE[b]	No	Mononuclear	No	Mononuclear	Generalized	No	No	No	Yes (one case only)	4, 6, 16

[a]CalE, California encephalitis.
[b]DE, Dengue encephalitis.
[c]References:

1. **Anderson, S. G.** 1954. *J. Hyg.* **52:**447.
2. **Baker, A. B., and H. H. Noran.** 1942. *Arch. Neurol. Psychiatr.* **47:**565.

3. **Bednár, B.** 1961. p. 17. *In* L. Van Bogaert, J. Radermecker, J. Hozay, and A. Lowenthal (ed.), *Encephalitides.* Elsevier, Amsterdam, The Netherlands.
4. **Bhamarapravati, N.,** et. al. 1967. *Am. Trop. Med. Parasitol.* **61:**500–510.
5. **Broun, G. O.** 1958. *Neurology* **8:**883.
6. **Chimelli, L.,** et al. 1990. *Clin. Neuropathol.* **9:**157–162.
7. **Desai, A.,** et al. 1995. *Acta Neuropathol.* **89:**368–373.
8. **Farber, S.,** et al. 1940. *JAMA* **114:**1725.
9. **Fingerland, A.,** and **V. Vortel.** 1961. p. 23, 60. *In* L. Van Bogaert, J. Radermecker, J. Hozay, and A. Lowenthal (ed.), *Encephalitides.* Elsevier, Amsterdam, The Netherlands.
10. **Finley, K.,** and **A. C. Hollister.** 1951. *Cal. Med.* **74:**225.
11. **Garen, P. D.,** et al. 1999. *Mol. Pathol.* **12:**646–652.
12. **Garven, A. K.,** et al. 1952. *Med. J. Austr.* **2:**623.
13. **Greenfield, J. G.,** and **W. B. Matthews.** 1954. *J. Neurol. Neurosurg. Psychiatr.* **17:**50.
14. **Grinschgl, G.** 1955. *Bull. W.H.O.* **12:**535.
15. **Grinschgl, G.,** et al. 1961. p. 3. *In* L. Van Bogaert, J. Radermecker, J. Hozay, and A. Lowenthal (ed.), *Encephalitides.* Elsevier, Amsterdam, The Netherlands.
16. **Gubler, D. J.,** et al. 1983. *Proc. Int. Conf. Dengue Kuala Lumpur,* p. 290–306.
17. **Haymaker, W.** 1961. p. 38. *In* L. Van Bogaert, J. Radermecker, J. Hozay, and A. Lowenthal (ed.), *Encephalitides.* Elsevier, Amsterdam, The Netherlands.
18. **Haymaker, W.,** and **A. B. Sabin.** 1947. *Arch. Neurol. Psychiatr.* **57:**673.
19. **Ishii, T.,** et al. 1977. *Acta Neuropathol.* **38:**181.
20. **Iwasaki, Y.,** et al. 1986. *Acta Neuropathol.* **70:**79–81.
21. **Iwasaki, Y.,** et al. 1993. *Acta Neuropathol.* **85:**653–657.
22. **Iyer, C. G. S.,** and **G. G. Hadley.** 1957. *Ind. J. Med. Sci.* **11:**227.
23. **Johnson, R. T.,** et al. 1985. *Ann. Neurol.* **18:**567–573.
24. **Kalfayan, B.** 1983. *Proc. Clin. Biol. Res.* **123:**179.
25. **Kornyey, S.** 1978. *Acta Neuropathol.* **43:**179.
26. **Leech, R. W.,** and **J. C. Harris.** 1977. *J. Neuropathol. Exp. Neurol.* **36:**611.
27. **Li, Z. S.,** et al. 1988. *China Med. J.* **101:**768–771.
28. **Matsuyama, H.** 1955. *Keio. J. Med.* **4:**11.
29. **McCordock, H. A.,** et al. 1934. *JAMA* **103:**822.
30. **McLean, D. M.,** and **W. L. Donahue.** 1959. *Can. Med. Assoc.* **80:**708.
31. **Miyake, M.** 1964. *Bull. W.H.O.* **80:**153–160.
32. **Nieberg, K. C.,** and **J. M. Blumberg.** 1972. p. 2269. *In* J. Minckler (ed.), *Pathology of the Nervous System,* vol. 3. McGraw-Hill, New York, N.Y.
33. **Noran, H. H.,** and **A. B. Baker.** 1943. *Arch. Neurol. Psychiatr.* **49:**398.
34. **Noran, H. H.,** and **A. B. Baker.** 1945. *J. Neuropathol. Exp. Neurol.* **4:**269.
35. **Osetowska, E.** 1977. *Tissue Neuropathology of Viral and Allergic Encephalitides,* p. 93–109. National Technical Information Service, Springfield, Va.
36. **Peers, J. H.** 1942. *Arch. Pathol.* **34:**1050.
37. **Perdrau, J. R.** 1936. *J. Pathol. Bacteriol.* **42:**59.
38. **Randall, R.,** and **J. W. Mills.** 1944. *Science* **99:**225.
39. **Reyes, M. G.,** et al. 1981. *Arch. Neurol.* **38:**329.
40. **Robertson, E. G.,** and **H. McLorinan.** 1952. *Med. J. Austr.* **1:**103–107.
41. **Shinner, J. J.** 1963. *Arch. Pathol.* **75:**309.
42. **Shiraki, H.,** et al. 1963. *Rev. Neurol.* **180:**633.
43. **Silber, L. A.,** and **V. D. Soloviev.** 1946. *Am. Rev. Soviet Med.* (special suppl.).
44. **Suzuki, M.,** and **C. A. Phillips.** 1966. *Arch. Pathol.* **81:**47.
45. **Tigertt, W. D.,** and **W. G. Downs.** 1962. *Am. J. Trop. Med.* **11:**822.
46. **Weil, A.** 1934. *Arch. Neurol. Psychiat.* **31:**1139.
47. **Weil, A.,** and **P. J. Breslich.** 1942. *J. Neuropathol. Exp. Neurol.* **1:**49.
48. **Wolf, A.** 1950. p. 194. *In* J. G. Kidd (ed.), *The Pathogenesis and Pathology of Viral Diseases.* Columbia Press, New York, N.Y.
49. **Zimmerman, H. M.** 1946. *Am. J. Pathol.* **22:**965.
50. **Zimmerman, H. M.** 1948. *J. Neuropathol. Exp. Neurol.* **7:**106.

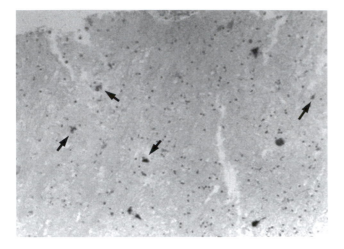

FIGURE 11.1   Section of the brain stem from a case of acute JE immunostained with an antibody to the virus. Immunostaining is seen in scattered neuronal cell bodies (arrows). Courtesy of T. Solomon.

States have emerged (Table 11.3), particularly from the studies of the Massachusetts epidemics and the New Jersey outbreak of 1959 (Goldfield and Sussman, 1968). Human cases have occurred in the late summer and early fall, preceded by heavy rainfall, which favors proliferation of the vector. The regions involved tend to be woody swamps or ponds, often adjacent to saltwater marshes. In general, the human outbreaks have been preceded by epizootics in horses and sometimes in penned pheasants as well.

From the first outbreak it was noted that the disease was explosive in onset, fulminant in course, and destructive in outcome, particularly in children. In a clinical-pathological report of eight cases, seven in children, Farber et al. (1940) described the findings from the 1938 Massachusetts epidemic. Six of the eight cases were etiologically verified by virus isolation or antibody development. The onset was

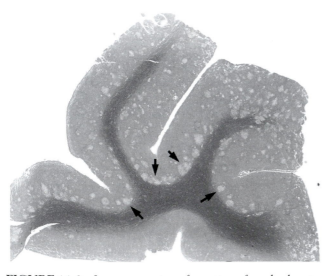

FIGURE 11.2   Low-power view of a section of cerebral cortex from a case of acute JE. Pale foci (arrows) represent foci of a cellular necrosis. PTAH stain.

TABLE 11.3   Epidemiologic features of EEE[a]

Locations in U.S.:	Atlantic and Gulf Coast states and inland foci, including upper New York State, southwestern Michigan, northeastern Indiana, south central Georgia, eastern Kansas, eastern Illinois
Season:	Late summer to early fall
Habitat:	Freshwater marshes and swamps, small lakes and ponds
Climate:	Preceding heavy rainfall
Vector	
To birds:	*Culiseta melanura*
To humans:	Species of *Aedes* and *Coquillettidia*
Reservoir:	Birds
Epizootic feature:	Preceding or concurrent epizootic in horses and penned birds
Group at risk:	Severe disease in children

[a] Tsai and Monath, 1997.

usually rapid with high fever, depression of consciousness, vomiting, and seizures. It often progressed rapidly to stiff neck, bulging fontanelle, Babinski signs, and coma. Two to four days after the start of the disease, five patients developed nonpitting edema in the periorbital areas, face, and extremities. In adults, fever and headache preceded the development of frank neurological signs such as seizures, stiff neck, and depression of level of consciousness. Five of the eight patients died, and three were left with severe sequelae. Of 36 more recent patients reviewed by Deresiewicz et al. (1997), 32 became stuporous or comatose, 18 developed seizures, and focal weakness was found in 16.

During the acute disease, a peripheral leukocytosis has been noted in most patients, with neutrophils often predominating. Initial lumbar punctures were characterized by elevated CSF pressure, protein and WBC, with neutrophils again predominating. Hyponatremia is common. The pathology has been characterized by meningeal and parenchymal inflammation, often with neutrophils, and vascular involvement. A generally gloomy outlook was found in a 9-year follow-up of survivors of the 1938 Massachusetts epidemic (Ayres and Feemster, 1949). Of eight survivors accounted for, two had died, five were severely impaired, and only one was completely well. Studies of later outbreaks, however, have demonstrated that return to normal can occur after EEE, particularly in adults (Webster, 1956; Clarke, 1961). Between 1988 and 1994 in the United States, mortality was 36%, and 35% of survivors were moderately or severely impaired (Deresiewicz et al., 1997). Of the principal arbovirus encephalitides in the United States, EEE has the lowest ratio of inapparent to apparent infection, ranging from 8:1 in young children to 50:1 in young adults (reviewed in Monath, 1978). Of interest in this regard, however, is the observation that people along the Amazon River in South America have been found to have antibodies to EEEV without any detectable clinical illness (Downs, 1982).

Consistent abnormalities have been found on neurodiagnostic tests. Elevated CSF pressure and protein with a neutrophilic pleocytosis are often found early in the disease. Electroencephalogram (EEG) abnormalities include generalized slowing and background disorganization (Deresiewicz et al., 1997). In certain cases, EEGs have mimicked the findings in herpes simplex encephalitis (HSE), namely unilateral periodic discharges and sharp waves (Fernandez and Dooling, 1982; Deresiewicz et al., 1997). Neuroimaging studies are of considerable diagnostic usefulness. Both computed tomography (CT) and magnetic resonance imaging (MRI) demonstrate abnormalities in the basal ganglia and thalami (Deresiewicz et al., 1998). Other less frequently involved areas have included the brain stem, cortex, periventricular areas, and meninges. The sensitivity of MRI was greater than that of CT; 13 of 14 studies were abnormal with the former and 21 of 32 studies were abnormal with the latter. On MRI, lesions were best seen on T2-weighted studies. Gray matter lesions were seen early in the illness and declined with clinical improvement. Virus has been isolated from an early serum sample (Clarke, 1961), from the CSF on the third day (Fernandez and Dooling, 1982), and from brain biopsy, and virus has been visualized by electron microscopic examination of a biopsy sample (Kim et al., 1985). However, confirmed diagnosis in life usually depends on the demonstration of the development of specific antibodies between acute- and convalescent-phase serum samples. Acutely, a presumptive diagnosis can be based on a positive serum immunoglobulin M (IgM) capture enzyme-linked immunosorbent assay (ELISA). A positive CSF IgM capture ELISA has been accepted as confirming the diagnosis (Deresiewicz et al., 1997).

Protection of humans is dependent on knowledge of the principal vector, *Culiseta melanura*, which feeds on wild birds in deep swamp locations. The recognition of an outbreak in horses, sentinel birds, or penned birds should alert public health officials to the threat of an outbreak in vulnerable regions. A vaccine is available for veterinary use. No specific antiviral drug therapy is available. However, the somewhat better mortality figures in more recent years may reflect advances in intensive care facilities and procedures.

WEE

Since the original observations of WEE in humans in the United States (Eklund and Blumstein, 1938; Baker and Noran, 1942), WEEV has lived up to its name. Although an analog of WEEV, Highlands J virus, is found in birds and mosquitoes in the eastern United States and infects horses in Florida (Karabatsos et al., 1988), most human cases of WEE have been found west of the Mississippi and in contiguous provinces in Canada (Table 11.4). Massive numbers of horses and humans have been infected in various outbreaks. Almost 800 human cases were reported in 1941 in Minnesota (Eklund, 1946), and almost 500 human cases were reported in 1965 in Saskatchewan (Rozdilsky et al., 1968). Such outbreaks have abated for some years, with only three cases reported in the United States in the 1990s (Centers for Disease Control and Prevention, 2001a).

Coincidental activity with SLE has been found in the United States. In the well-studied California epidemic of encephalitis in 1952, 348 cases were associated with WEEV infection and 38 cases were associated with SLE virus (SLEV) (Kokernot et al., 1953). WEEV and western epidemics of SLEV share the same vector, *Culex tarsalis*, and each has reservoirs in wild birds. Flooding, heavy rainfall, and heavy

TABLE 11.4 Epidemiologic features of WEE[a]

Locations:	States west of the Mississippi River and contiguous provinces in Canada
Season:	Summer and early fall
Habitat:	Water pools and irrigated land
Climate:	Preceding heavy rain, floods, or heavy snow pack melting
Vector:	*Culex tarsalis*
Reservoir:	Wild birds
Groups at risk:	Elderly and infants

[a]Tsai and Monath, 1997.

snowpack melts, with resultant pooling, and stagnant pools from irrigation projects, encourage multiplication of the vector and the creation of conditions for epidemics. However, WEEV can apparently replicate faster and at lower temperatures than SLEV, so its activity begins earlier in the summer and advances further north, into Canada. Clinically, the two encephalitides are difficult to distinguish. Kokernot et al. (1953), in the clinical description of the 1952 California epidemic, did not distinguish between cases shown to be SLE and those of WEE. However, extremes of age do tend to separate the illnesses. Although SLE can affect the elderly severely, no cases of SLE were found in babies under 1 year of age in the combined California epidemic (Kokernot et al., 1953). In contrast, WEE has devastating effects on babies under 1 year as well as on the elderly.

The ratio of inapparent to apparent infection has been estimated to be 58:1 in children and ca. 1,150:1 in adults (reviewed in Tsai and Monath, 1997). The incubation period has been estimated to be between 1 and 2 weeks. Transplacental infection has been reported (Finley et al., 1967). Infants develop high fever, convulsions, bulging fontanelles, generalized rigidity, and a CSF pleocytosis (Medovy, 1942). In a follow-up of 17 infants, Medovy (1942) found that 9 had recovered completely, 6 had spastic paralysis, and 2 had died. Finley et al. (1967) found that the most profound disabilities were in the youngest patients. Sequelae were cognitive and behavioral. Those that were continuous from the acute illness began as behavioral disorders, inclusive of motor and speech problems, whereas those that were delayed in onset tended to be cognitive. Disorders in the delayed category were felt to represent failures to mature, provoking the hypothesis that WEEV infection in infancy impaired cerebral differentiation.

The spectrum of illness in adults consists of febrile headache, aseptic meningitis, and encephalitis (Leech et al., 1981). By and large, a consistent pattern emerges of WEE in the adult (Adamson and Dubo, 1942; Baker and Noran, 1942; Eklund, 1946; Kokernot et al., 1953; Leech et al., 1981). Headache, impaired consciousness, and fever are found in the majority, with sudden onset being characteristic (Eklund, 1946). On examination, stiff neck, disorientation, and lethargy are common. Less frequent are tremors of the extremities, tongue, and lips. Interestingly, parkinsonism was not found to be a sequela of this illness (Earnest et al., 1971). An upgoing plantar response, nystagmus, and dysarthria have been noted. Coma, which occurs in less than 15% of patients, is usually reversed after 3 to 4 days. Seizures are not a usual manifestation of disease in the adult. The course of the acute illness is about 10 days. Prolonged convalescence attributed to weakness was noted by Eklund (1946). Although subjective symptoms have been reported (Adamson and Dubo, 1942), few if any significant neurological sequelae indisputably due to WEEV infection are found in adults (Adamson and Dubo, 1942; Earnest et al., 1971).

The CSF usually demonstrates a pleocytosis. A transition from neutrophilic to mononuclear predominance is seen in the first 2 days (Adamson and Dubo, 1942). Protein in the CSF may be normal or elevated. A moderate leukocytosis is often found in the peripheral blood during the acute illness. EEG results are usually nonspecific, and the absence of significant numbers of cases in recent decades has resulted in a paucity of neuroimaging reports. Diagnosis is made principally by serology. Demonstration of specific IgM in acute-phase serum or CSF is useful for rapid presumptive diagnosis. Virus has been isolated at autopsy from the CNS. The principal differential diagnosis is often SLE. However, Bia et al. (1980) reported a case of WEE presenting like HSE, including focal EEG slowing over the right temporal region.

No specific therapy is available; however, there is ample evidence to encourage aggressive general medical support. The multiple focal nature of the pathology (Quong, 1942) suggests that large contiguous areas of brain are not routinely destroyed. Furthermore, the appearance of coma in WEE is not necessarily an indication of a fatal outcome. A vaccine is available for veterinary use (Monath, 1978). An experimental WEEV vaccine is available for at-risk laboratory workers from the U.S. Army Medical Research Institute of Infectious Diseases (USAMRIID) at Fort Detrick, Maryland.

VEE

Massive epizootics and epidemics due to VEE virus (VEEV) have occurred in South America, Central America, and Mexico and have reached the United States in south Texas on occasion (Bowen et al., 1976). Several subtypes of VEEV exist that exhibit marked differences in epidemic behavior and in their pathogenicity for humans (Tsai and Monath, 1997). The epidemic cycles are classed as sylvatic or epizootic, producing enzootic/endemic or epizootic/epidemic disease, respectively (Table 11.5). The Florida strain (Everglades virus, subtype II), which is enzootic in southern Florida, cycles between a *Culex* species and small rodents (Monath, 1978). In some areas, positive serological reactions are found in over 50% of tested humans, and virus has been repeatedly isolated in locations in the Everglades Park (reviewed in Ehrenkranz et al., 1970). However, human disease is rare in association with this focus. Three cases of VEE in adults, all with complete recovery, were described by Ehrenkranz and Ventura (1974). In contrast to the relatively benign behavior of the Everglades type virus, other subtypes of VEEV have been associated with severe disease in horses and in people. Widespread epizootics in horses have occurred in the northern part of South America and Central America, often originating in the Guajira Peninsula shared by Colombia and Venezuela and on the Atlantic coastal plain of Colombia (Lord, 1974). A massive epizootic and epidemic reemerged in Venezuela and Colombia in 1995 (Weaver et al., 1996; Rivas et al., 1997).

TABLE 11.5 Epidemiologic features of VEE[a]

Feature	Sylvatic cycle	Epizootic cycle
Location:	South and Central America, Florida Everglades	South and Central America, Mexico, and South Texas
Vectors:		
To humans:	*Aedes taeniorhynchus*	Numerous species
To birds, small mammals, and humans:	*Culex melaviconium*	
Animal hosts:	Birds and small mammals	Horses, donkeys, and mules
Season:	Year-round in tropical and subtropical sites	Rainy season
Climate:	NA[b]	Heavy rainfall producing high vector density

[a]Tsai and Monath, 1997; Booss and Karabatsos, in press; Rivas et al., 1997.
[b]NA, not applicable.

A brief incubation period of 1 to 4 days has been found (Bowen et al., 1976), with a low inapparent to apparent infection ratio (Tsai and Monath, 1997). The clinical manifestations are an acute febrile illness of fever and chills, headache, myalgia, prostration, and vomiting of 3 to 4 days in duration (Weaver et al., 1996). Complications reported in the 1995 South America epidemic were seizures, abortions, and stillbirths, with a case fatality rate of 0.7 (Weaver et al., 1996). In addition to seizures, hemiparesis, behavioral change, and impaired consciousness have been reported (Rivas et al., 1997; Bowen et al., 1976). Neurological manifestations have developed about 4 days into the febrile illness (Rivas et al., 1997). Children were more susceptible to neurological complications in the south Texas series of Bowen et al. (1976). Mortality is higher among patients with encephalitis, but overall it is equal to or less than 1%. Systematic follow-up studies of survivors of VEE have not been found.

A peripheral leukopenia results, and the CSF contains a lymphocytic pleocytosis, elevated protein, and a moderate depression of glucose (Bowen et al., 1976). Although a case report included an EEG from a Florida Everglades case that demonstrated slowing and disorganization (Ehrenkranz et al., 1970), there is no systematic literature on the EEG and neuroimaging findings in VEE. The virological diagnosis can be made by virus isolation from serum and by serological changes, including IgM capture ELISA. Other assays include traditional seroconversion and indirect IgG ELISA testing. Weaver et al. (1996) isolated virus from throat swabs, raising the possibility of human-to-human transmission.

Vaccination of horses and donkeys, vector control, and interdiction of transport of horses, donkeys, and mules are methods used to reduce the spread of an epidemic/epizootic. No antiviral medication has proven to be effective. A veterinary vaccine is available. Laboratory workers who are likely to be exposed to VEEV should be offered the vaccine, although it is not licensed for general use in humans.

TABLE 11.6 Epidemiologic features of SLE[a]

Feature	Urban cycle (epidemic)	Rural cycle (endemic)
Locations in U.S.:	Midwest, Southeast, East	West
Season:	Summer and early fall	Summer and early fall
Vector habitat:	Stagnant streams, pools, sewage ditches	Water pools and irrigated land
Climate:	Summer drought and hot weather	Preceding heavy rain, floods, or heavy snowpack melting
Vector:	*Culex pipiens* complex (*pipiens* or *quinquefasciatus*)	*Culex tarsalis*
Reservoir:	Birds	Birds
Group at risk:	Most severe illness in the elderly	No age predilection

[a] Monath, 1978; Shope, 1980.

Flaviviruses

SLE

The thorough study of the St. Louis epidemic of 1933 rapidly established a great deal of information that has remained valid to this day (Public Health Bulletin no. 214, 1935). The virus was isolated, the neuropathology was described, and the clinical manifestations were observed. Identification of the vector, reservoir, and transmission cycles was to come later. SLEV has been the most frequent and the most widespread cause of epidemic encephalitis in the United States. From 1964 to 1999, a median of 26 cases have been reported annually in the United States (Centers for Disease Control and Prevention, 2001a). An epidemic in 1975 of 2,800 cases covered 31 states (Monath, 1980).

SLE presents two patterns in the United States: an epidemic urban-suburban cycle and an essentially rural endemic cycle (Table 11.6). They present many contrasts. Whereas the urban cycle is likely to follow a dry, hot period, the rural cycle follows a particularly wet or flooded period. The vectors for the urban cycle are found in pools of sewage water or water rich in other organic matter. The drying up of streams and rivers within cities leads to pools of stagnant water. In contrast, multiplication of the rural vector is facilitated by faulty drainage and irrigation practices. The rural cycle of SLEV shares much of its habitat as well as its vector, *Culex tarsalis*, with WEEV. It was originally stated that SLE is most severe in the elderly (Public Health Bulletin no. 214, 1935). That has remained valid for the urban cycle but not for disease consequent to the rural cycle, possibly because elderly rural residents are immune. In endemic areas an increased incidence of infection is associated with inadequate screening, open foundations, no air conditioning, and the presence of domestic fowl (reviewed in Monath, 1980). The association of risk with buildings that were poorly sealed against mosquitoes has been reconfirmed in an outbreak of the urban type (Centers for Disease Control, 1986).

The incubation period for SLE is variable and ranges from 4 to 21 days. Estimates of the ratio of inapparent to apparent disease vary from 16:1 to 425:1 (Monath, 1980). Clinically apparent illness takes one of three forms: febrile headache, aseptic meningitis, or encephalitis (Brinker and Monath, 1980). With the first description of the illness, it was recognized that there could be two modes of onset. One is abrupt with sudden headache, fever, and stiff neck, followed in 1 or 2 days by an impaired sensorium. Onset of the second type is less rapid and is associated with malaise, lassitude, myalgia, nausea, and vomiting prior to frank signs of encephalitis. In a prospectively studied group from the 1966 Dallas epidemic, Southern et al. (1969) documented the incidence and duration of various signs and symptoms. Fever was present in 94% and lasted an average of 4 days; stiff neck was found in 71% and lasted an average of 8 days; an abnormal sensorium was present in 86% and also lasted an average of 8 days. Tremor of the face, tongue, arms, and hands has been noted since the first descriptions of the disease. It was found in 67% in the 1966 Dallas epidemic and lasted an average of 8 days. Seizures were found in 10%. Lower motor neuron facial weakness was found in 18%, and an upgoing plantar response was found in 29%.

A number of unusual observations in SLEV infection deserve mention. In the study of Southern et al. (1969), urinary tract symptoms were present in 20%. An elevated blood urea nitrogen and pyuria were found in 56%. There was electromyographic evidence for lower motor neuron disease and elevated muscle enzymes in a number of patients. Finally, the syndrome of inappropriate ADH secretion has been documented (Southern et al., 1969; Brinker et al., 1979).

Overall, the course of the disease is fatal in about 17% of patients, with mortality occurring within the first 2 weeks (Monath and Tsai, 1997). Cerebral edema sufficient to cause death by herniation is rarely seen (Gardner and Reyes, 1980). However, secondary complications such as pneumonia, gastrointestinal bleeding, aspiration, and pulmonary emboli are significant causes of death (Southern et al., 1969). The disease is more severe for the elderly in urban cycle epidemics. In the 1966 Dallas epidemic, all 16 deaths occurred in persons over 41 years old (Southern et al., 1969). The reversal of impaired consciousness can be quite rapid. Although the acute disease may run a span of 2 to 3 weeks, convalescence may run up to 8 weeks. Follow-up studies have shown generally mild but consistent patterns of disability in survivors, which have tended to clear. Finley and Riggs (1980) used the term "convalescent fatigue syndrome" to cover a variety of emotional and somatic complaints. The incidence was found to be 35 to 50% and had cleared in 80% by 3 years. No intellectual changes were found. Brinker et al. (1979) on follow-up approximately 4 months after the illness found tremor in 6 of 11 survivors; however, parkinsonism is not described as a sequela. This is particularly noteworthy because neuropathological studies have indicated involvement of the substantia nigra in cases of SLE coming to autopsy (Suzuki and Phillips, 1966).

Laboratory findings are nonspecifically abnormal. Many patients have a mild peripheral leukocytosis and a moderate CSF pleocytosis with mild protein elevation. EEGs are abnormal, showing diffuse background slowing and, less frequently, periodic lateralized epileptiform discharges or status epilepticus (Wasay et al., 2000). MRI has been found to be more sensitive than CT scanning. Wasay et al. (2000) found T2 signal hyperintensity in the substantia nigra.

A definite diagnosis of SLE depends on a fourfold elevation of hemagglutination, complement fixation (CF), or neutralizing antibodies. Presumptive diagnosis can be made based on a positive IgM capture ELISA. Confirmation is required with fourfold elevations in other assays because of cross-reactivity with other flaviviruses. Virus isolation from blood has been unsuccessful after neurological symptoms have developed (Monath and Tsai, 1997).

In the absence of a vaccine for SLEV, prevention depends on several factors, including sanitary management of water courses and sewage in urban settings. The proper management of irrigation projects and flood control is necessary to prevent the rural disease. Spraying of insecticide to reduce the vector should be combined with proper management of water projects. Adequate screening and the use of air conditioning to exclude mosquitoes have been stressed.

WNVE

Originally isolated from the blood of a febrile woman in the West Nile district of Uganda in 1937 (Smithburn et al., 1940), WNV has traveled far and in various clinical guises (Table 11.7). It was isolated from human sera in Egypt in 1950 (Melnick et al., 1951) and in Israel in 1952 (Goldblum et al., 1954) and from brains of children in India in 1980 and 1981 (George et al., 1984). It has caused large epidemics in South Africa, where it occurred simultaneously with Sindbis virus infection (McIntosh et al., 1976), and in Bucharest, where it was manifest as meningoencephalitis (Ceausu et al., 1997). Remarkably, WNV turned out to be the culprit (Briese et al., 1999) in a cluster of cases of encephalitis evaluated at the Flushing Hospital in Queens, New York City, in 1999 (Asnis et al., 2000). It reappeared in 2000 in New York City, principally on Staten Island (Centers for Communicable Disease, 2001). By 2001, human cases had appeared from Connecticut to Florida. 2002 was a major epidemic year, with over 3,700 cases and over 200 deaths (Centers for Disease Control

and Prevention, 2002a). Excellent surveillance demonstrated westward movement to the West Coast, and virus was detected in 43 states and the District of Columbia. Thus, it has established itself in the New World. At the time of the New York outbreak in 1999, southern Russia experienced an outbreak of about 1,000 cases of encephalitis, of whom at least 40 patients died. WNV was isolated during this outbreak (Lvov et al., 2000; Platonov et al., 2001). Kunjin virus, which has more than 80% nucleotide identity with WNV (Berther et al., 1997), is a counterpart in Southeast Asia and Australia (Hubalek and Halouzka, 1999).

The virus that emerged in New York City is most closely related to a virus originally isolated from an Israeli goose (Lanciotti et al., 1999). Birds are the principal reservoir for WNV, and migratory birds have been suspected to be the mechanism that brings the virus to new regions in the Old World (Rappole et al., 2000). Simultaneous with the outbreak in humans in Queens, New York, there was an outbreak in exotic birds at the Bronx Zoo (Steele et al., 2000) and a die-off of crows in and around New York City. Horses too were afflicted on the north fork of Long Island in association with the New York City outbreak. Equine encephalomyelitis outbreaks associated with WNV have occurred in and near the Camargue in France and have been reported from Tuscany in Italy (Cantile et al., 2000). The vector is most commonly a culicine species mosquito. Risk factor evaluation of the 1996 Bucharest epidemic implicated household mosquitoes, often as a consequence of flooded basements (Han et al., 1999). Vigorous spraying for mosquito control was undertaken in New York. During the 2002 U.S. epidemic, WNV was transmitted to four organ recipients from a single donor (Centers for Disease Control and Prevention, 2002b), and concern has arisen about transmission through the blood supply. In the United States, the Food and Drug Administration (FDA) issued recommendations concerning blood donors, blood, and blood products with respect to WNV infection [http://www.fda.gov/cber/gdlns/wnvguid.html]. Intrauterine infection and breast milk transmission have been reported (Centers for Disease Control and Prevention, 2002c).

After an incubation period of 3 to 14 days (Petersen and Martin, 2002), the clinical onset of uncomplicated WNVE has often been characterized as abrupt, with a brief duration of 3 to 6 days (Goldblum et al., 1954). Typical symptoms in the 1953 Israeli epidemic included fever, lymph node swelling, and rash (Marbert et al., 1956). Southam and Moore (1954) reported that the Egypt 101 isolate used as cancer therapy induced fever alone in 89% of patients, but that 11% showed clinical signs of encephalitis. Pruzanski and Altman (1962) established encephalitis as a component of the Israeli outbreaks; all but one of the reported seven patients recovered quickly. Meningitis, meningoencephalitis, and encephalitis occurred at a high rate in the 1996 Bucharest outbreak (Tsai et al., 1998). The onset of fever was typically abrupt, with headache, neck stiffness, and vomiting. Encephalitis was manifest by disorientation, confusion, weakness, and impaired consciousness. The case fatality rate was 4.3%. All deaths were in patients over 50 years of age and increased with advancing age. Full function had not been achieved in over half of patients at discharge, and residual abnormalities, including fatigue, memory loss,

TABLE 11.7   Epidemiologic features of WNVE[a]

Locations:	Africa, Middle East, Europe, Russia, India, Indonesia, and North America
Season:	Summer
Reservoir:	Birds
Vector:	Mosquitoes, principally *Culex* species
Population at risk:	Mortality most likely in those over 50 years of age

[a] Hubalek and Halouzka, 1999; Asnis et al., 2000.

difficulty walking, weakness, and depression, were found in 38 to 67% of survivors at 1 year (reviewed in Petersen and Marfin, 2002). The ratio of clinically inapparent to apparent infections ranged from 140:1 to 320:1.

In the 1999 New York City outbreak, fever, weakness, gastrointestinal symptoms, headache, altered mental status, stiff neck, and rash were found. Encephalitis was found in 63%, meningitis in 29%, and febrile headache in 8% (Nash et al., 2001). Diffuse flaccid weakness was found in 10 patients, and motor axonopathy was found in eight on electrophysiological testing. Flaccid paresis has previously been reported (Gadoth et al., 1979). Another critical neurological feature is the capacity to attack the brain stem. Nichter et al. (2000) described a 15-year-old boy with bifacial weakness, tongue fasiculations, and bilateral extremity and trunkal ataxia. Neuropathological examination of four cases in the New York City outbreak confirmed the involvement of the brain stem, particularly the medulla (Sampson et al., 2000). Taken together, the propensity to cause an axonopathy and the involvement of the medulla require clinical vigilance for the need for ventilatory assistance. Overall, the mortality in the 1999 New York City outbreak was 7 of 62 cases, or 11%, again targeting the elderly (Asnis et al., 2000).

The syndrome of acute flaccid paralysis was further studied during the 2002 epidemic (Centers for Disease Control and Prevention, 2002d). Electromyography and nerve conduction studies supported an asymmetric involvement of anterior horn cells and/or their axons. This poliolike syndrome is important to distinguish from the Guillain-Barré syndrome because interventions for the latter would be of no benefit in the former. However, the need for vigilance to institute assisted respiration is common to both conditions.

Examination of the spinal fluid reveals findings characteristic of encephalitis, with a moderate mononuclear pleocytosis and moderate protein elevation (Asnis et al., 2000). The mononuclear pleocytosis can be preceded by polymorphonuclear predominance. Peripheral lymphopenia has been found. EEGs have revealed slow high-voltage theta waves and no alpha rhythm (Ceausu et al., 1997). No acute changes were found on CT scanning, but 31% of MRIs showed leptomeningeal and/or periventricular enhancement, without significant focal parenchymal abnormalities (Nash et al., 2001). While parenchymal changes can be found on MRI, they do not appear to be characteristic.

As a practical matter, the presumptive diagnosis of WNVE relies heavily on IgM capture ELISA methodology. When samples from both serum and CSF are available, the CSF may show a response first (Tardei et al., 2000). Laboratory studies must confirm suspected positives because of cross-reactivity with related flaviviruses. Fourfold increases in antibody between acute and convalescent samples, as measured by plaque reduction neutralization tests, are diagnostic, and virus isolation or demonstration of viral antigen or genomes in tissues, CSF, or serum can be attempted. A PCR for rapid detection of the virus in CSF has been developed (Briese et al., 1999).

Management of the acute encephalitis demands stay in the intensive care unit (ICU). A low-level threshold for instituting ventilatory support is needed because of the virus's propensity to involve the medulla (Sampson et al., 2000) or to cause a motor axonopathy (Asnis et al., 2000) or an

acute flaccid paralysis syndrome (Centers for Disease Control and Prevention, 2002b). Neither significant cerebral swelling nor recalcitrant seizures are reported as common clinical features. Ribavirin (Jordan et al., 2000; Anderson and Rahal, 2002) and alpha 2b interferon (Anderson and Rahal, 2002) have been reported to inhibit WNV replication in vitro, and reports of controlled clinical trials would be welcomed. The U.S. FDA approved a clinical trial of alpha interferon at the time of the 2002 epidemic in the United States.

A human vaccine is currently in development, and a vaccine to protect horses has been developed. Prevention efforts for humans are directed toward vector control, elimination of vector breeding sites, and personal protection. Full screening for households, avoidance of outdoor activities at dusk and dawn, full-length clothing, avoidance of mosquito habitats, and application of insect repellents are recommended (Tsai, 1992; Fradin, 1998).

MVE

At the time that much of the rest of the world was experiencing winter epidemics of von Economo's encephalitis, Australia experienced four summer epidemics of an encephalitis termed "Australian X" disease. The cases occurred principally in the region of the Murray River and its tributaries. Clinically, it was associated with an abrupt onset, a rapid evolution, and a high mortality. Virus was isolated in monkeys. After 1925, no further epidemics occurred in that region until 1951. The 1951 disease was termed "Murray Valley encephalitis" (MVE), and virus was isolated (French, 1952). Because the Australian X disease isolates were not sustained in passage, no virological comparisons could be performed. However, based on epidemiologic, clinical, histopathological, and host spectrum evidence, Anderson (1954) concluded that the diseases were in fact the same. The term "Australian encephalitis," which incorporates both MVE and the closely related Kunjin virus encephalitis, was introduced following an epidemic in 1974 (Mackenzie and Broom, 1995).

Most of the cases of MVE have occurred in association with the Murray River and Darling River systems (Table 11.8). The epidemics have tended to follow in the wake of conditions that encourage high densities of the vector

TABLE 11.8 Epidemiologic features of MVE[a]

Locations:	Australia, Papua New Guinea
	Enzootic: northern and western Australia northern islands
	Epidemic: Murray and Darling River valleys
Reservoir:	Birds, particularly waterfowl
Vector:	*Culex annulirostris*
Habitat:	Freshwater ponds and pools
Season:	Summer
Climatic features:	Mild winter followed by wet spring or early summer
Epidemic features:	Postulated southward spread by waterfowl from enzootic regions subsequent to flooding conditions
Group at risk:	More severe disease in children

[a] Anderson, 1954; Kay, 1980; Monath and Tsai, 1997.

Culex annulirostris. Conditions that favor the vector are a mild winter followed by a wet and flooded spring and early summer (Kay, 1980). The principal reservoir is in birds, particularly waterfowl. Under favorable climatic conditions, the virus is believed to be transported south from northern areas of enzootic concentration to southern and eastern portions of Australia (Anderson, 1954). This could be achieved by more southerly breeding of the vector, coupled with carriage of the virus by migrations of infected waterfowl. The role of interepidemic persistence of the virus has also been raised (noted in Kay, 1980). Areas of high prevalence of antibodies to MVE virus (MVEV) have been found in New Guinea (Mackenzie et al., 1994). Serological surveys have suggested that the ratio of inapparent to apparent disease varies from 800:1 to 1,000:1 (Anderson, 1954; Mackenzie et al., 1994). During a serological survey of neurological disease in the 1974 epidemic, the only positive results were in cases of encephalitis (Bennett, 1976). However, Mackenzie et al. (1993) described a patient with mild infection manifested by headache alone. The data suggest a greater occurrence in males than females (Mackenzie et al., 1993).

The prodrome usually lasts 2 days or less and consists of fever, malaise, headache, and nausea and vomiting; however, it is not always present (Mackenzie et al., 1993). Depression of consciousness, ranging from drowsiness to coma, and disordered thinking, also ranging in severity, are common findings. In mild disease, nuchal rigidity and generalized tremors can be found (Bennett, 1976). Mackenzie et al. (1993) found an altered mental state, neck stiffness, or convulsions in moderate disease. In severe and fatal disease, coma and spastic quadraparesis were found and the need for respiratory support was critical. Progression to death or stabilization usually occurs within 2 weeks of onset. Children may evolve more rapidly, are more likely to develop seizures, and may demonstrate a rash (Robertson and McLorinan, 1952; Doherty et al., 1972). Ataxia, dysarthria, and dysphasia have been noted. By and large, the clinical configuration is not sufficiently characteristic to distinguish MVE from other types of encephalitis.

Mortality has ranged from 18 to 42.5%. The lower figure may reflect the more recent use of respiratory support. In survivors, 7 of 11 patients with mild disease in Bennett's series (1976) made complete recoveries, with 4 demonstrating mild emotional, intellectual, or coordination difficulties. In the severe disease group, all seven patients had marked physical or intellectual sequelae. Similarly, of the two young patients described by Doherty et al. (1972), at follow-up one had severe retardation of development, hypotonia, and athetoid movements. The second was discharged with hypotonia, and the level of response was to painful stimuli or simple command. Neurological sequelae have been estimated at 40% following mild disease and 100% following severe disease (Monath and Tsai, 1997).

It is common to find a mild elevation of the peripheral white cell count. The lumbar puncture almost always reveals a pleocytosis, usually mononuclear in type, although Mackenzie et al. (1993) reported several patients in whom neutrophils predominated. A normal or somewhat elevated protein content is found. EEGs show diffuse slow-wave activity, but spikes have been described (Mackenzie et al.,

TABLE 11.9 Epidemiologic features of JE[a]

Locations:	Asia and Oceana, particularly Southeast Asia, China, and India
Season:	Late summer epidemics in temperate regions such as Japan
	Year-round sporadic occurrence in tropical regions such as Malaysia
Reservoir:	Birds and mammals, particularly herons, egrets, and pigs
Vector:	Culicine species, particularly *Culex tritaeniorhynchus* in Japan, *Culex vishnui* complex in India and Nepal
Habitat:	In rural areas, *Culex tritaeniorhynchus* inhabits rice paddies
	In cities, close association with infected pigs may enhance risk for human infection by mosquitoes
Population at risk:	Higher incidence of cases, more severe disease, higher mortality, and significant sequelae in children

[a]Clarke and Casals, 1965; Monath and Tsai, 1997; World Health Organization, 1998.

1993). There is a paucity of neuroimaging data. Head CT scans have been reported as showing areas of reduced attenuation from the thalami to the brain stem in one fatal case and edema and hydrocephalus in another fatal case (Mackenzie et al., 1993).

Virological diagnosis during life depends on demonstrating changes in antibody titer. Specific IgM antibody is useful in the acute stage. Virus isolation attempts from serum, CSF, and throat washings are unsuccessful during life, but isolation attempts have been successful at postmortem within the first 2 weeks of illness (Lehmann et al., 1976). No specific antiviral drug is available, nor is there a vaccine. Improved survival is likely dependent on ICU management with respiratory support in severe cases.

JE

JEV is remarkable for the colossal sweep of territory it involves, the damage it inflicts on the CNS, and its regular recurrence. The territory sweeps eastward from Pakistan to the arctic regions of Siberia and reaches southward to Australia (Table 11.9) where it abuts territory that hosts MVEV. JEV's territory continues to enlarge. Some epidemic years have been particularly devastating. In 1958 there were 1,800 cases with 519 deaths in Japan and 5,700 cases with 1,322 deaths in Korea (Clarke and Casals, 1965). It is estimated that there are 50,000 cases with 10,000 deaths annually (World Health Organization, 1998).

Whereas the most significant amount of disease occurs in epidemic form, endemic disease accounts for sporadic cases, particularly in tropical regions. In Japan, close association of humans and infected pigs has been thought to amplify the risk of infection. The disease is transmitted principally by species of culicine mosquitoes. In rural areas the mosquitoes can multiply on flooded rice paddies. The virus may be transported to urban areas by birds. Insecticide spraying for vector eradication is a formidable task, but JEV has virtually disappeared from Japan coincident with use of agricultural insecticides and other interventions. The greater susceptibility of children has encouraged a program of vaccination of children in Japan, Korea, Taiwan, and China as a means to reduce disease.

Estimates of the ratio of inapparent to clinically apparent infection have varied widely, but a representative figure from an endemic region is 270:1 (Gajanana et al., 1995). As with many other arboviral infections, febrile headache and meningitic forms are produced in addition to encephalitis (Shiraki, 1970). Incubation of the encephalitis varies from 6 to 16 days. The onset may be associated with a prodrome of 2 to 3 days, in which headache, fever, nausea, and vomiting are prominent. Nuchal rigidity and other signs of a meningitic response are common. An altered sensorium is particularly prominent. The illness may present with confusion, disorientation, or hyperkinetic activity. However, lethargy and apathy can be observed, with progression to coma. Seizures are more often a part of the clinical picture in children. In a review of 65 confirmed cases in American servicemen in Korea in 1950, Dickerson et al. (1952) emphasized a masklike facies resembling parkinsonism, slow thick speech, ocular tremor, and neurogenic paresis, in addition to changes in the sensorium.

Weakness of the neck and upper extremities is common (Rose et al., 1983). This is often lower motor neuron in type and may be associated with residual wasting. Unilateral facial weakness of the lower motor neuron type has been described (Dickerson et al., 1952). Upper motor neuron weakness of the extremities, although more frequent than lower motor neuron weakness, is more likely to resolve completely. Sensory changes, which are remarkable for their segmental character (Dickerson et al., 1952; Rose et al., 1983), usually improve by concentric diminution but may partially persist. Rigidity has been found in 40% of patients, and a coarse tremor of fingers, tongue, or eyelids has been found in 98% of patients (Gatus and Rose, 1983).

The reported outcomes of the acute illness and the percentage of survivors with sequelae have varied widely. Fatality has varied from 5 to 50% and sequelae are found in 3 to 32% (Gatus and Rose, 1983). Both mortality and sequelae are greater in children. The sequelae are complicated both in type and evolution. Postrecovery psychosis is not uncommon (Shiraki, 1970; Gatus and Rose, 1983). Various psychiatric, intellectual, and movement disorders have been thoroughly studied in the Japanese survivors (Shiraki, 1970). Motor disorders include lower motor neuron wasting, spasticity, paralysis, and disorders of motor tone. Persistent movement disorders, including generalized dystonia in children and parkinsonism in adults, each seen in two patients, were reported by Murgod et al. (2001). Problems in social adaptation, particularly school adjustment in children, are described (Shiraki, 1970).

During the acute illness, general and neurodiagnostic laboratory studies are abnormal. Peripheral leukocytosis, principally of neutrophils, and an elevated sedimentation rate may occur. Pleocytosis in the spinal fluid peaks during the first week, but pleocytosis may continue for weeks (Dickerson et al., 1952). The CSF protein is usually only slightly elevated. EEGs have been reported as showing diffuse delta slowing, delta waves and spikes, or alpha pattern coma (Kalita and Misra, 1998). CT scanning demonstrates involvement of the thalamus in most patients (Misra et al.,

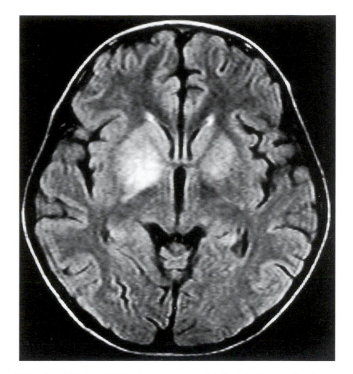

FIGURE 11.3 MRI of acute JE. Axial FLAIR image discloses hyperintensity of the basal ganglia bilaterally, right greater than left, with mild mass effect. Courtesy of Minh Dung and Bridget Wills, University of Oxford Clinical Research Unit, Hospital for Tropical Diseases, Ho Chi Minh City, Vietnam.

1998). The basal ganglia, midbrain, and pons may also be involved (Fig. 11.3). Involvement of the substantia nigra on MRI has been associated with parkinsonian sequelae (Pradham et al., 1999).

Provisional viral diagnosis during life depends on IgM capture ELISA during acute illness or on elevations in other antibody titers. Isolation of the virus from CSF or blood is rarely achieved. Isolation from the brain at autopsy may be successful within the first 5 days of illness and is unlikely to be positive after day 10. IgM capture ELISA has high sensitivity in serum and CSF (Burke et al., 1985). In regions where other flaviviruses are present, care must be taken in the interpretation of serological results. Most prominent among other possibilities will be dengue virus, WNV, and MVEV. The CF, ELISA, and hemagglutination inhibition assays have commonly been used. Six weeks or more may be required to demonstrate a rise in CF antibody.

No specific antiviral therapy is available. A controlled trial of alpha 2a interferon did not improve the outcome (Solomon et al., 2003). Differences in general medical care, particularly in mechanical respiratory assistance and management of cerebral swelling, likely explain differences of survival. Steroids have been used but have not been shown to be clinically beneficial (Hoke et al., 1992). Prevention through national vaccination programs for schoolchildren, vector eradication, and modern farming methods and animal husbandry have been successful in Japan. Because of adverse reactions, travelers are not advised to be vaccinated against JEV unless they are to spend significant time in endemic areas.

TABLE 11.10   Epidemiologic features of dengue fever and DHF, including DSS[a]

Distribution:	Worldwide in the tropics, reflecting the distribution of *Aedes aegypti*
Transmission cycles:	Vector to human in endemic, hyperendemic (cocirculation of multiple serotypes), and epidemic patterns
Principal host:	Humans
Principal vector:	*Aedes aegypti*, a household mosquito
Populations most at risk:	
Dengue fever	Older children and adults
DHF/DDS	Children under 15
Risk factor for DHF/DSS:	Previous exposure to a different serotype

[a] Gubler, 1998; Solomon and Mallewa, 2001.

Dengue Fever and DHF

Dengue virus produces massive numbers of human infections. Its more benign form, classic dengue fever, probably occurs in 50 to 100 million people worldwide annually. Its more severe form, dengue hemorrhagic fever (DHF), occurs in 250,000 to 500,000 people worldwide annually (Rigau-Perez et al., 1998). The most severe form of DHF, dengue shock syndrome (DSS), can be lethal in 20% to more than 40% of cases if inadequately treated. Neurological complications have long been recognized. Dengue virus as a cause of encephalopathy was reported by Wulur et al. (1978). Several causes for encephalopathy in DHF as well as hemorrhagic complications in the CNS were described by Nimmannitya et al. (1987), including some cases compatible with Reye's syndrome. Postinfectious disseminated encephalomyelitis with perivenous demyelination has been documented (Chimelli et al., 1990). Furthermore, encephalopathy as part of classic dengue fever has been documented (Row et al., 1996). There has been dispute as to whether dengue virus can infect the CNS, and the entity of dengue encephalitis has been challenged in part because the CSF is usually bland and many factors causing encephalopathy are often present. However, evidence of virus in CSF by virus isolation, PCR (Lum et al., 1996), and antiviral IgM has been detected (Chen et al., 1991). Prospective studies of acute encephalitis and encephalopathy have demonstrated dengue virus, many of the cases without clear diagnostic features of dengue fever (Solomon et al., 2000; Kankirawatana et al., 2000). Hence, a wide spectrum of neurological disorders in this significant vector-borne disease of humans, while relatively infrequent, must be anticipated.

There appears to be agreement among dengue scholars that the first unambiguous clinical description of dengue fever was that of the 1780 epidemic in Philadelphia of "breakbone fever" described by Benjamin Rush (Innes, 1995; Gubler, 1998; Solomon and Mallewa, 2001). Ambiguity of previous descriptions arose from similar presentations by other epidemic fevers. The more ominous history of dengue, the appearance of DHF, begins in Southeast Asia in 1954. The presentation of fever, shock, and hemorrhage was most commonly seen in children and had mortality of more than 10% (Innes, 1995).

Four serotypes of dengue virus exist. Types 1 and 2 were isolated from cases of dengue fever by Sabin in 1944 and types 3 and 4 were isolated by Hammon and coworkers in 1956 in the Philippines during an outbreak of hemorrhagic disease (Hayes and Gubler, 1992). The growth of dengue as a worldwide public health problem subsequent to World War II is attributed to several factors, including explosive growth of urban centers in the tropics; abatement of programs to control the principal vector, *Aedes aegypti* (Table 11.10); the household location and habits of that vector; markedly expanded travel; and the absence of a vaccine. An empirical model of climate and population changes raised the possibility of even greater expansion of the population at risk (Hales et al., 2002).

Aedes aegypti is a household mosquito with elusive feeding and hiding patterns. The extrinsic incubation cycle, the period between a blood meal and development of the capacity for a mosquito to transmit infectious virus, is 8 to 12 days (Gubler, 1998). The factors facilitating the development of DHF/DSS are thought to include both viral genetic variation and antibody enhancement of infection (Halstead, 1988). Enhancement is thought to be dependent on the ingestion of complexes formed by the newly infecting serotype with cross-reacting antibody from a previous infection with a different serotype. The complex, which insufficiently neutralizes the virus, is picked up and internalized by macrophages, where it is released and undergoes replication (Halstead, 1988). Cocirculation of multiple serotypes, hyperendemicity, facilitates immune enhancement. While there is a forest/enzootic cycle sustained by other *Aedes* vectors and primates, and a rural/epidemic cycle involving *Aedes aegypti*, other *Aedes* vectors, and humans, the most important transmission cycle, by far, is urban endemic/hyperendemic/epidemic (Gubler, 1998).

The incubation period for dengue fever is usually between 4 and 7 days, although it can range from 3 to 14 days (Rigau-Perez et al., 1998). The ratio of apparent to inapparent infections is not well defined, but it has been noted that the majority of infections in children under 15 are asymptomatic or minimally symptomatic (Rigau-Perez et al., 1998). Thus, young children may manifest only nonspecific fever, or fever with respiratory symptoms. In older children and adults, symptoms include the abrupt onset of fever, bodily pains, retro-orbital pain, and photophobia, rash, and lymphadenopathy (Solomon and Mallewa, 2001). The febrile period ranges from 2 to 7 days, may be associated with a bradycardia, and in some instances can be biphasic or "saddlebacked" (Gubler, 1998). Skin manifestations are commonly seen. The initial eruptions are found in half of patients and are characterized as "... a transient mottling, flushing, or maculopapular rash" (Solomon and Mallewa, 2001). One-third of patients will demonstrate a positive tourniquet test, in which a blood pressure cuff inflated midway between diastolic and systolic pressures for 5 min results in 20 or more petechiae in a 2.5-by-2.5-cm area on the forearm (Solomon and Mallewa, 2001). A maculopapular rash can occur during recovery, lasting 2 to 3 days. Skin peeling can also be observed during this time.

Laboratory abnormalities in dengue fever include leukopenia and some thrombocytopenia. The clinical picture is usually insufficiently distinctive in any given case to establish an unambiguous diagnosis. Virus isolation from blood for diagnosis can be achieved at the start of the illness, and viremia may be detectable into the second week (Gubler, 1998). Serological diagnosis requries care because of cross-reactivity among the dengue virus serotypes and with other flaviviruses. Commercially available ELISA kits for antibody determinations should facilitate presumptive diagnosis (Solomon and Mallewa, 2001). In most instances the course of dengue fever is self-limited and benign. Fluid intake is to be encouraged, and aspirin use is to be avoided because of the risk of Reye's syndrome. A prolonged period of lethargy and depression following defervescence may occur.

Of major concern is that what appears to be classic dengue fever may, in days 3 to 7, emerge as DHF. The underlying pathological change is plasma leakage into tissues and serous spaces due to loss of vascular integrity. Hemoconcentration is found because of the loss of intravascular fluid, despite the concomitant thrombocytopenia and coagulopathy with bleeding of varying degrees. The World Health Organization (WHO) has established a grading system for DHF in which grades III and IV are classified as DSS (World Health Organization, 1997). The diagnosis and management of DHF/DSS are considered in a WHO monograph and in other authoritative sources (World Health Organization, 1997; Rigau-Perez et al., 1998; Solomon and Mallewa, 2001). The importance of early recognition and expert management of fluid extravasation, thrombocytopenia, hemorrhage and hypotension, and shock is great. Mortality in DSS can be as high as 44%, but in experienced institutions it can be below 1% (Rigau-Perez et al., 1998).

The literature on CNS effects of dengue virus infection of the past three decades reveals considerable controversy. In 1978 Wulur et al. reported four cases of encephalopathy with virologically confirmed dengue virus infection. However, a report in 1987 by Nimmannitya et al. including 10 autopsied cases found no pathological evidence for encephalitis and emphasized multifactoral systemic causes such as shock, metabolic acidosis, coagulation disorders, hyponatremia, liver dysfunction, and toxic effects of medication for the CNS dysfunction. A 1996 report by Lum et al. of six cases in children presenting clinically as encephalitis included four in whom virus was isolated from CSF and a fifth in whom CSF and blood PCR were positive. The issue gained clarity from prospective studies of encephalitis published in 2000 that confirmed dengue virus as a cause of encephalitis (Solomon et al., 2000; Kankirawatana et al., 2000). The potential neurovirulence of particular serotypes has also received attention. Lum et al. (1996), in a study from Kuala Lumpur, Malaysia, postulated that types 2 and 3 could cross the blood-brain barrier to cause encephalitis, whereas Chimelli et al. (1990) reported the neuropathology of five fatal cases from Rio de Janeiro, Brazil, associated with serotype 1.

TABLE 11.11   Cerebral complications in dengue virus infection

Encephalopathy associated with systemic factors, including:
  Liver failure
  Hypoperfusion/hypoxia
  Hyponatremia
  Renal failure
Encephalopathy associated with cerebral vasogenic changes
Reye's syndrome
Encephalitis with evidence of virus in CSF or CNS
Parainfectious encephalomyelitis
Intracranial hemorrhage
Cranial nerve palsy

CNS complications of dengue virus infection will present in several different clinical settings (Table 11.11). Most commonly, perhaps, in dengue endemic and epidemic areas, patients will develop fever, headache, and obtundation associated with DHF/DSS. Five of the six patients reported by Lum et al. (1996) had DHF or DSS. Evaluation and management require attention to systemic disorders such as fluid extravasation, bleeding disorders, hypotension, and renal and liver failure (World Health Organization, 1997). Head CT to evaluate the possibilities of intracranial hemorrhage and cerebral swelling will play an important role in management to protect brain tissue from raised intracranial pressure. CSF examination may be indicated to exclude other treatable infections, but due concern for bleeding from the puncture site and complications from raised intracranial pressure is required.

Another clinical setting is the patient who develops encephalitis or encephalopathy in an area endemic/epidemic for dengue but in whom DHF or DHF/DSS does not emerge, or emerges after the evaluation of encephalitis is under way. In the 21 patients evaluated by Solomon et al. (2000), 12 had no features specific for dengue on admission and 8 had not developed such characteristics by discharge. One developed DHF during hospitalization, and most interestingly, three developed the late, or recovery, rash prior to discharge. The clinical features of these patients included fever in all, impaired consciousness in 18, spastic paraparesis in 2, and severe headache, meningism, and vomiting in 1. Of the 21 cases, 9 were characterized as encephalitis, 5 as hepatic encephalopathy, 4 as encephalopathy, 2 as myelitis, and 1 as meningism.

Postinfectious complications of dengue virus infection, i.e., acute disseminated encephalomyelitis (ADEM), have also been documented. One of the two cases of transverse myelitis reported by Solomon et al. (2000) had a dengue-like illness 2 weeks earlier. Of the five fatal cases for which Chimelli et al. (1990) reported the neuropathology, one developed neurological signs 5 days following improvement of symptoms of infection. Perivenous demyelination, lipid-laden macrophages, and perivenous mononuclear cell infiltrates were found in hemispheric white matter.

Finally, travelers who have recently returned from dengue endemic areas are at risk of developing the CNS complications of unrecognized dengue virus infection. Jannsen et al. (1998) described a fatal case in a Dutch woman who had recently returned from Thailand. CT revealed massive cerebral edema, and the patient died 30 h following hospital admission. The brain was positive for dengue virus by reverse transcriptase PCR and had no inflammation but did reveal complement complexes on capillaries and diffuse capillary endothelial swelling. The full spectrum of dengue infection-related conditions must be suspected in travelers returning from the tropics: dengue fever and DHF/DSS and their concomitant CNS complications.

Evaluation of CNS complications of dengue will usually produce findings compatible with encephalopathy. CSF, if examined, will often be within normal limits, but some cases will demonstrate an elevated protein and/or a pleocytosis. Remarkably, elevated levels of red blood cells are not commonly reported. CT scans have been reported as showing cerebral edema (Lum et al., 1996; Solomon et al., 2000; Janssen et al., 1998; Kankirawatana et al., 2000) or as being normal (Solomon et al., 2000). Scattered reports of EEG examinations do not allow an overall summary. Generalized slow waves (Lum et al., 1996), high-amplitude periodic slow waves (Solomon et al., 2000), isoelectric in brain death (Janssen et al., 1998), and normal tracings following recovery from acute illness that included convulsions (Solomon et al., 2000) have each been described. Virus isolation, PCR positivity, and identification of anti-dengue virus antibody have each been achieved in CSF (e.g., Solomon et al., 2000). Such findings are useful in cases in which the acute systemic manifestations of dengue are missing.

Management of DHF and DHF/DSS requires highly skilled experienced clinicians. There is no antiviral medication for dengue virus infection. The greatest challenge with respect to the brain is the management of edema to maintain cerebral perfusion pressure. Seizures in the acute phase have been treated with standard intravenous anticonvulsant medication. Despite hemorrhagic manifestations elsewhere in the body, massive intracranial hemorrhage appears to be unusual. Focal cerebral hemorrhages were found in three of five cases examined neuropathologically by Chimelli et al. (1990). They were characterized as small and perivascular. Hemorrhage found at autopsy by Nimmannitya et al. (1987) included cases in which heparin had been given. Patey et al. (1993) reported a patient with focal subarachnoid hemorrhage who had mild meningismus but no focal signs or impairment of consciousness. The hemorrhage resolved spontaneously. There is insufficient reported experience with the ADEM following dengue virus infection to generalize on its complications, treatment, and outcome.

In DHF/DSS the outcome will depend primarily on the management of systemic vascular leak, hemorrhage, and hypotension/shock. Thus one of six patients with documented CNS infection reported by Lum et al. (1996) died of multiorgan failure, one experienced residual paralysis, and four were listed as well on outcome. Seven of eight patients with CNS presentations studied prospectively by Kankirawatana et al. (2000) developed DHF, but all eight recovered completely. Of the 21 patients reported by Solomon et al. (2000), none died, 15 recovered fully, and 6 had sequelae. The latter included both patients with myelitis who had residua of mild spastic paraparesis.

Absent antiviral therapy or a licensed vaccine, vector control and avoidance are the best weapons against infection

TABLE 11.12   Endemic characteristics of La Crosse virus encephalitis of the Cal serogroup[a]

Locations in U.S.:	Upper Midwest to West Virginia
Season:	June to the start of October
Habitat:	Rolling woodlands, coulees
Mosquitoes:	*Aedes triseriatus*
Breeding sites:	Basal holes of hardwood trees, old tires
Reservoir:	Small woodland mammals, for example, squirrels and chipmunks
Population at risk:	Children under 15 years of age in endemic areas

[a]Rust et al., 1999.

with dengue virus. Effective interventions to control cerebral vasogenic edema are needed. Several efforts to develop a vaccine are at various stages of progress (Clarke, 2002).

Bunyaviruses

La Crosse virus

First isolated from mosquitoes in 1943, a California (Cal) serogroup virus was not isolated from a human case until 1964. The Cal serogroup viruses belong to the *Bunyaviridae* family. These are small RNA viruses composed of a three-segmented, single-stranded genome that is capable of genetic reassortment (Rust et al., 1999). Of the 14 separate viruses of the Cal serogroup, 6 are known to cause encephalitis in humans, and the great majority of cases have been caused by the La Crosse virus. From 1964 to 1999, a median of 66 cases were reported each year in the U.S. (Centers for Disease Control and Prevention, 2001a). In those years, it was the most commonly identified arbovirus in the United States. It remains to be seen whether West Nile fever will usurp that distinction in the years to come.

The occurrence of La Crosse virus encephalitis is endemic (Table 11.12), with cases found from Minnesota and Wisconsin in the upper Midwest to West Virginia and New York in the east (McJunkin et al., 1998). The vector is *Aedes triseriatus*, a woodland mosquito that breeds in basal tree holes and abandoned tires. The usual cycle in nature involves small woodland animals. Seasonally, the disease occurs from the start of June until the start of October. The habitat is often one of rolling woodland or wooded coulees. Over 90% of cases of La Crosse virus encephalitis occur in children 15 years or under, with the greatest concentration between the ages of 4 and 10 years. Those at risk live in rural or suburban wooded areas, with serological positivity closely tied to specific geographic areas (Balfour et al., 1973). Huang et al. (1997), in a study of fatal cases, suggest that neurovirulence may be associated with a particular genotype.

Estimates of the ratio of inapparent to apparent disease vary greatly. Disease can take the form of a febrile illness, headache, respiratory symptoms, or aseptic meningitis, in addition to encephalitis. The incubation period is 3 to 7 days (Balfour et al., 1973). The encephalitis is remarkable for its rapid onset, evolution, and frequent rapid reversal. In 50 cases reviewed by Hilty et al. (1972), the period from onset of the illness to significant neurological dysfunction was 2 to 4 days. Reversal and resolution of dysfunction occurred within the following week, so that the whole period of acute illness lasted 7 to 10 days. The onset is characterized by fever, headache, nausea, and vomiting (McJunkin et al., 2001). The findings of meningeal irritation have varied from one-quarter (McJunkin et al., 2001) to the majority of patients (Chun et al., 1968). Rapidly developing neurological signs include disorientation, depression of level of consciousness, focal motor signs, and seizures. Approximately half of the reported cases have had seizures, often generalized, but one-third may have focal seizures (Chun et al., 1968). Rapid reversal of fever and neurological dysfunction with few lasting sequelae is the general experience. Mortality has been reported to be 0.3% (Kappus et al., 1983).

The convalescent period can take 2 to 3 months, during which time headache, emotional lability, and irritability may be present (Hilty et al., 1972). In follow-up studies of 35 cases, Chun et al. (1968) found minimal motor and coordination problems in 14 patients but only a few significant sequelae. Seizures were present in two, hemiparesis was present in one, and an intelligence quotient below 90 was present in two but without premorbid testing. Significant EEG abnormalities were found in 10, of which five were epileptiform. In contrast, no lasting sequelae were found in 50 children reported by Hilty et al. (1972). In this context Balfour et al. (1973) commented that there are mild and severe forms of the disease. The more recent studies of McJunkin et al. (2001) suggest that cognitive impairment and neurobehavioral disorders may be significantly more prevalent in survivors than previously suspected.

Of general diagnostic studies, the peripheral WBC count and the percentage of neutrophils are usually elevated. The CSF contains a moderate lymphocytic pleocytosis, and the protein may be moderately elevated, particularly after 5 days. The EEG is usually abnormal with generalized slowing, sometimes with paroxysmal features, which may be focal, such as periodic lateralizing epileptiform discharges. A significant percentage of the abnormal EEGs will suggest HSE (McJunkin et al., 2001). CT scans have been abnormal in 12%, often showing generalized edema. MRIs can show focal gadolinium enhancement or be normal (McJunkin et al., 2001). Virus diagnostic studies rely heavily on serological changes because the virus is difficult to isolate from clinical specimens. Virus isolation attempts from the CSF are usually negative (Beaty et al., 1983; McJunkin et al., 2001). Neutralizing and hemagglutinating antibody develop within the first 2 weeks, while CF antibody requires 3 to 4 weeks (Balfour et al., 1973). Because of the rapid and often focal evolution of La Crosse virus encephalitis, rapid serological diagnosis is of great urgency to differentiate it from HSE. An indirect immunofluorescence assay allows a presumptive diagnosis (McJunkin et al., 1998), and an IgM antibody capture enzyme immunoassay is available (Dykers et al., 1985).

There is as yet no clinically demonstrated antiviral agent effective against La Crosse virus. However, ribavirin reduces virus replication in vitro (Cassidy and Patterson, 1989), and a clinical trial has been reported to be under way (McJunkin et al., 2001). ICU management is indicated for acute deterioration in level of consciousness and for recurrent seizures. Prospective treatment of HSE is indicated until the diagnosis of La Crosse virus encephalitis is established. Control of raised intracranial pressure, which may require monitoring, is needed to sustain cerebral perfusion. Management of seizures, including status epilepticus, is often required.

The endemic distribution and the breeding sites of *Aedes triseriatus* offer the potential for disease control. Within defined endemic areas, vector control can be accomplished in both usual and novel ways. The filling of tree holes, elimination or drainage of water-collecting tires, and placement of drain holes in tire swings and in tires used to hold down haystack tarps may reduce breeding sites (Rust et al., 1999). The vector is an aggressive daytime feeder, so breeding sites need to be avoided. A vaccine, if developed, could be given to children living in endemic areas.

RFV

Rift Valley fever (RVF) virus (RVFV), previously limited to the African continent, moved into Saudi Arabia and Yemen on the Arabian peninsula in 2000 (Centers for Disease Control and Prevention, 2000a, 2000b). It hospitalized hundreds and killed 17%, according to one report (Centers for Disease Control and Prevention, 2000c). An arbovirus of the *Bunyaviridae* family, it is transmitted by mosquitoes and directly to humans handling infected animals, their carcasses, or abortuses, or during slaughter. While blood can be highly infectious on direct contact, RVFV can apparently also be transmitted by aerosol from infected animals (Hoogstraal et al., 1979).

RVF was first described as an enzootic hepatitis affecting sheep, cattle, and humans in East Africa in 1930 (Daubney and Hudson, 1931). Symptoms of a brief febrile illness in humans were described, and the likely transmission by mosquitoes was demonstrated. Neurological signs were described in humans during an epizootic in South Africa in 1975 (Van Velden et al., 1977). Outbreaks had been limited to sub-Saharan Africa until 1977, when a large outbreak occurred in the Nile Delta in animals and humans (Meegan et al., 1979). Four forms of human disease were described: simple febrile, ocular, CNS, and a more lethal hemorrhagic form (Laughlin et al., 1979). The ocular form, although previously described, was verified serologically, described clinically, and well illustrated (Siam et al., 1980). RVFV reappeared in Egypt in 1978 and 1993 (Abu-Elyazeed et al., 1996) and in East Africa in 1997 to 1998 (Centers for Disease Control and Prevention, 1998) before spreading to the Arabian peninsula in 2000 (Centers for Disease Control and Prevention, 2000a, 2000b).

As early as the first report of RVF, it was observed that outbreaks tended to follow heavy rainfall and the consequent proliferation of mosquitoes (Daubney and Hudson, 1931) (Table 11.13). This characteristic has allowed the prediction of outbreaks using remote sensors for climate and satellite indicators (Linthicum et al., 1999; Beck et al., 2000). Transmission to humans is achieved either by handling infected animals or through vector transmission by any of numerous species of mosquitoes. *Aedes caspius*, which was the most effective vector in the 1993 Egyptian outbreak (Turell et al., 1996), was suspected along with *Culex tritaeniorrhynchus* in preliminary evaluation of the 2000 outbreak in Saudi Arabia (Centers for Disease Control and Prevention, 2000c). From the first, the association of human disease with epizootics, including aborted sheep fetuses and death in lambs, was

TABLE 11.13   Epidemiologic features of RFV[a]

Geographic areas:	Africa and Arabian peninsula
Climate:	Following heavy rains, which facilitate vector proliferation
Reservoir:	Epidemics occur in association with epizootics involving sheep, cattle, goats, and camels
Exposure:	Mosquito vectors of many species Sick animals, abortuses, carcasses, and slaughter

[a] Daubney and Hudson, 1931; Centers for Disease Control and Prevention, 2000a.

noted (Daubney and Hudson, 1931). These authors and Hoogstraal et al. (1979) recorded febrile infection of themselves during investigations of epizootics. Buffalo, camels, goats, donkeys, and dogs can also serve as amplifying hosts. Hoogstraal et al. (1979) suspected that camels from the Sudan may have been the mechanism to introduce RVFV into southern Egypt.

The uncomplicated febrile disease occurs 3 to 6 days following exposure to the virus with the abrupt onset of fever, malaise, headaches, myalgia, and anorexia (Laughlin et al., 1979). Fever breaks by 4 days and most patients are altogether well within 2 weeks. The majority of infections are uncomplicated; however, ocular, neurological, and hemorrhagic complications occur in a variable percentage of cases, depending on the particular outbreak. Ocular complications include lesions of the macula and paramacular regions as well as other regions of the retina (Siam et al., 1980). Permanent loss of visual acuity has been found in half of the patients with the ocular form. The Arabian peninsula outbreak included a large number of patients with a hemorrhagic form (Centers for Disease Control and Prevention, 2000c). The disease was rapidly evolving, with hospitalization occurring on average 3.3 days after disease onset, and death occurring on average 6.3 days after disease onset in 17% of hospitalized patients. Reversible renal failure was observed in mild and moderate cases of RVFV infections, whereas dialysis was required in 18% of severe disease cases (Centers for Disease Control and Prevention, 2000c).

The neurological form, which is less fatal than the hemorrhagic form and may occur in about 1% of cases (World Health Organization, 2000), is not yet well characterized. Van Velden et al. (1977) described neurological complications, often occurring in a biphasic pattern after the initial febrile period. Of 12 patients, meningeal irritation was noted in 6, confusion in 4, stupor and coma in 4, and hypersalivation with grinding of teeth in 3. Visual hallucinations, the locked-in syndrome, and choreoform movements were listed in one patient each. CSF revealed 20 or fewer polymorphonuclear cells and up to 300 mononuclear cells. Protein was elevated, with normal glucose values. Brain biopsy in one patient showed perivascular infiltration of lymphocytes. Autopsy examination of the CNS in one patient revealed areas of focal necrosis with cellular infiltrates of lymphocytes and macrophages. Pathological examination in two other cases revealed only perivascular cuffing. Laughlin et al.

(1979) described five patients, all with meningismus and a CSF pleocytosis of 20 to 600 cells per mm³, mostly lymphocytic. Neurological signs developed 5 to 10 days after systemic symptoms, except in one case in which the delay was 30 days. Clinical symptoms included vertigo, hallucinations, and disorientation. Four of the five patients had lethargy or coma on admission, two had hemiparesis, and one who died at 2 months had signs of decerebration. Hemiparesis remained in the two patients at 3 months. Riou et al. (1989) observed two groups of neurological complications, acute and subacute, in 17 of 348 patients in Mauritania. The acute cases were of brief duration and could end in death, whereas the subacute cases were of longer duration and had sequelae. We have not found case series reports of neuroimaging or EEG studies.

Diagnosis of RVF is facilitated by the simultaneous presence of an epizootic in cattle, sheep, and goats and an epidemic manifested by the abrupt onset of fever, headache, and myalgia. Laboratory confirmation employs virus isolation, viral antigen detection, PCR, or IgM capture (Centers for Disease Control and Prevention, 2000b; Niklasson et al., 1984). Acute- and convalescent-phase hemagglutination inhibition antibody determinations have been used in studies of early outbreaks (e.g., Meegan et al., 1979). There are insufficient clinical reports to determine whether cerebral swelling and acute seizure disorders are management issues in RVFV encephalitis. Animal models suggest that ribavirin should be tested as an antiviral therapy, and the feasibility of such a study was noted (Centers for Disease Control and Prevention, 2000a).

The association of human disease with epizootics in domestic animals suggests that vaccination of cattle, insecticide-impregnated bed nets, and caution in handling animals should be employed along with restriction of animal shipping and migration during epizootic periods. Vaccine for protection of at-risk workers, such as laboratory personnel, is available from USAMRIID, Fort Detrick, Maryland (Karak et al., 1982; World Health Organization, 2000).

TBEs

Flaviviruses

There are several medically important viruses carried by ticks in the *Flaviviridae* family. Certain of these viruses have been regularly associated with encephalitis. The two most important viruses are the closely related Central European and Far Eastern (Russian spring-summer) subtypes of TBE virus (TBEV). Other illnesses of importance include Powassan fever, Kyasanur Forest disease, and louping ill.

TBEV

There are two subtypes of TBEV which differ in a variety of ways. Medically, the Far Eastern subtype has been associated with much higher mortality and higher frequency of severe sequelae than the Central European subtype. Epidemiologically, the subtypes have been associated with different distributions in Europe and Asia and are carried by different ticks (Table 11.14). Antigenically, the structural glycoproteins of the viruses, though quite similar, have been demonstrated to differ and to be associated with different virus-antibody

TABLE 11.14 Epidemiologic features of TBE[a]

Feature	European	Eastern
	Central European encephalitis	Russian spring-summer encephalitis
Regions:	Central Europe, Western Russia	Far East Russia, China (Mongolia)
Season:	Late spring to early autumn	Spring and early summer
Vector:	*Ixodes ricinus*	*Ixodes persulcatus*
Habitat:	Endemic woodland foci	
Climatic conditions:	Temperature and humidity favoring tick development	
Reservoirs:	Birds and mammals, particularly small rodents; ticks	
Mode of infection:	Tick bite, ingestion of infected goats' milk	
Groups at risk:	Woodland vacationers, forest workers, users of raw goats' milk	

[a]Monath and Tsai, 1997.

interactions (Heinz et al., 1983). Protein E, the envelope glycoprotein, induces antibody formation (Heinz and Mandl, 1993).

Far Eastern Subtype

Severe forms of encephalitis recognized in far eastern portions of Russia in the 1930s were originally thought to be Japanese B encephalitis. However, a state scientific expedition in 1937 defined the cases as a new disease, isolated the agent, and identified the vector (Silber and Soloviev, 1946; Smorodintsev, 1958). A virus pathogenic for mice was isolated at autopsy and from the tick *Ixodes persulcatus*. Study of the ecology of the infection led to the development of Pavlovsky's concept of natural nidality (Pavlovsky, 1966). According to this concept, disease results from people's intrusion into a system in which the topography and climate support specific animals and arthropods, which in turn support certain infectious agents. In the case of Far Eastern TBE, the system involved the taiga, vast tracts of virgin forest.

It was recognized early that the outbreaks of encephalitis were closely associated with the proliferation of ticks (Silber and Soloviev, 1946). The cases peaked in May and June and resulted in the name Russian spring-summer encephalitis. Peak tick activity was found prior to the hottest and driest times of the year. Although other ticks have also been implicated, the principal vector is *Ixodes persulcatus* (Grascenkov, 1964). The original studies found that infections were associated with the villages of the taiga. Subsequently, ingestion of raw goats' milk has also been found to result in infection.

The incubation period was found to be 10 to 14 days, after which there was the abrupt onset of headache, fever, nuchal rigidity, hyperesthesia, and vomiting. Evolution was often rapid; in fact, coma was recorded in 12% on the first day (Silber and Soloviev, 1946). Sleepiness and dullness were found in two-thirds of cases. Seizures were found in 13% on the first day. Cases demonstrating no focal features, even in the presence of coma, were felt to have the best prognosis for recovery. However, other clinical syndromes were found. Hemiparetic forms were associated with varying degrees of weakness, which often developed on the second or third day of the illness. The most distinctive manifestation, if not the most common, was a combination of high cervical cord and lower bulbar involvement resulting in muscle weakness and atrophy. Lower motor neuron weakness of the

shoulder girdle, upper extremities, neck, palate, and face resulted in characteristic appearances.

The course of the disease was described as consisting of a brief febrile period and a prolonged convalescence (Silber and Soloviev, 1946). Mortality ranged from 20 to 30%. Death usually occurred in the first week of illness, often in the second to the fourth day. In those destined to survive, fever usually lasted for 5 to 7 days. However, survivors often remained bed-bound for a month and out of work for 6 months. Residual disabilities were noted in 20 to 30% and most frequently involved atrophy and weakness of arm, shoulder, girdle, neck, or jaw muscles. Other residual findings included cranial nerve palsies, tremors, irritability, and impaired memory.

Laboratory studies demonstrated a moderate leukocytosis and an elevated erythrocyte sedimentation rate (Silber and Soloviev, 1946). The spinal fluid was reported to have elevated pressure, pleocytosis, some protein elevation, and a positive reaction for globulin. Virus was recovered from the CNS, blood, CSF, liver, and spleen in the first week of illness. It was isolated in mice and was found to replicate in cultures of chicken embryo. Neutralizing antibody developed after a month or more. There appears to be a lack of documentation of neuroimaging and the clinical neurophysiology of Russian spring-summer encephalitis. Recent clinical reports in English or English translation appear to be unavailable.

Chronic and/or late-developing sequelae have been demonstrated or suspected. Continuous focal seizures, Kozhevnikov's epilepsy, has been observed in some survivors. Silber and Soloviev (1946) reported, however, that parkinsonism was not seen as a sequela. A late-developing chronic progressive encephalitis, 13 years after an acute episode of TBE with serological evidence of TBEV infection, has been reported (Ogawa et al., 1973).

Several strategies for prevention of the disease exist. A formalized vaccine was developed in 1938/1939 by Smorodintsev (Clarke and Casals, 1965). Spraying with the pesticide DDT to eliminate the vector has been suggested, as has control of small woodland mammals. Careful skin cover and avoidance of tick infestation are sensible.

Central European Subtype

In the 1940s and 1950s, it became apparent that a TBE separate from the Far Eastern/Russian spring-summer encephalitis disease was present in several foci in central Europe and

European Russia. The disease was less severe and frequently diphasic. Although carried by a different tick and associated with a longer season, infection was also found to be closely associated with woodland exposure. The disease is of great public health importance, with cases appearing from Germany to European Russia and from Scandinavia to the Baltic Sea. Despite the multiplicity of sites and times of isolation, the virus subtype appears to be stable (Heinz et al., 1983).

Infection can be acquired by tick bite or by ingesting infected goats' milk. Disease associated with tick bites occurs from April to October and is transmitted by *Ixodes ricinus*. Reservoirs for virus in addition to ticks include rodents, hares, mice, wild rats, cows, and goats (Osetowska, 1970). Infection occurs at woodland sites and can result from habitation, work, or holiday excursions such as woodland picnics. A study found that 91% of cases were among people who lived in villages and 9% were among town dwellers (Kmet et al., 1955). Infection by raw goats' milk is not confined to woodland villages. A well-studied outbreak of goats' milk infection occurred in 1957 in Roznava, Czechoslovakia (Bailey, 1958). All 660 patients consumed raw goats' milk from a single source. Approximately 50% of the cases were diphasic, and no fatalities occurred. Awareness of the risks of raw goats' milk has resulted in a reduction of cases transmitted by this means.

The incubation period after tick bite ranges from 4 to 20 days but is usually around 10 days (Bedjanic et al., 1955), similar to the incubation period of 10 to 14 days following the ingestion of contaminated goats' milk (Bailey, 1958). The prevalence of a biphasic course has varied in recent reports from 33% (Anic et al., 1998) to 87% (Gunther et al., 1997). The first or viremic phase is flulike, with fever, headache, and myalgia. After about 2 to 7 days, the fever falls, followed by an afebrile period ranging from 4 to 20 days but on average about 10 days (Bedjanic et al., 1955). This is followed by the phase of neurological involvement, which may take any of several forms. In a study of about 300 hospitalized patients at Graz, Austria, Grinschgl (1955) found that more than 50% were meningeal in form without focal neurological signs, in agreement with the more recent studies of Gunther et al. (1997) but at variance with the roughly 10% reported by Anic et al. (1998). As with Far Eastern forms, cervical spinal cord involvement can produce atrophic weakness of the arms, shoulder, girdle, and neck. Other types of spinal cord involvement and an ascending paralysis have been described. Bulbar involvement alone or in combination with dysfunction of the cervical cord is also found. Encephalitic involvement can result in a reduced level of consciousness. Approximately 14% of cases reported by Radsel-Medvescek et al. (1980) displayed somnolence, and 10% of cases reported by Bedjanic et al. (1955) developed coma. Tremor was seen in 246 of 315 cases of the Radsel-Medvescek series. Seizures, including focal continuous seizures, are also described in a low percentage of cases. Gunther et al. (1997) found impaired consciousness, concentration, and memory; ataxia; tremor; dysesthesia; and dysphasia to be common symptoms. The acute course of the neurological phase usually lasts 2 to 10 days.

Convalescence can be considerably prolonged, with headache, irritability, and impaired concentration (Bedjanic et al., 1955).

Mortality is variable but considerably lower than in the Far Eastern type. None was found in the Roznava outbreak (Bailey, 1958), and in the recent Swedish prospective study (Gunther et al., 1997), 0.95% was reported from Ljubljana, Slovenia (Radsel-Medvescek et al., 1980), 3.3% was reported from eastern Croatia (Anic et al., 1998), and 4.6% was reported from Graz, Austria (Grinschgl, 1955). Sequelae are also much less frequent than in the Far East Russian type. Characteristic atrophy of the arms, shoulder girdle, or neck is reported from most centers. Facial weakness is also described. Approximately 7% of the Ljubljana patients demonstrated some form of weakness on follow-up at 1 month (Radsel-Medvescek et al., 1980). Myeloradiculitic forms can result in bulbar and cervical cord dysfunction and residua (Schellinger et al., 2000). Also reported is Kozhevnikov's continuous partial epilepsy. Gunther et al. (1997) found impaired memory and concentration, ataxia, dysphasia, and tremor to be the most common symptoms at 1-year follow-up. The percentage with residua varied from 28% after mild encephalitis to 67% after severe encephalitis.

During the first phase of the illness there may be a depression of the peripheral white blood cell count. This is often reversed with a slight leukocytosis in the second phase, during which an elevated sedimentation rate can also be found. The spinal fluid is said to be normal in the first phase but contains a pleocytosis in the second phase. Variable percentages of polymorphonuclear cells and mononuclear cells have been found. The pressure is sometimes elevated. The protein is normal or slightly elevated with evidence of intrathecal IgG synthesis (Gunther et al., 1997). The CSF findings may remain abnormal into the convalescence period (Bedjanic et al., 1955; Gunther et al., 1997). EEG findings have been unremarkable—"diffuse, minor, and non-specific" abnormalities—and they have been normal in about 37% of cases (Anic et al., 1998). Neither of the more recent series (Anic et al., 1998; Gunther et al., 1997) reported neuroimaging data. Viral diagnosis can be made by virus isolation from the blood during the first phase. However, the usual method of diagnosis is by the development of serum antibody. Traditionally, the combined use of hemagglutination-inhibition, CF, and neutralizing antibody has been recommended. An IgM ELISA capture can be used for presumptive diagnosis (Heinz et al., 1981).

Vaccines are in wide use and have been remarkably effective (Heinz and Mandl, 1993). Prevention includes the use of protective clothing to prevent tick infestation, particularly at peak seasons in regions of endemic disease. No specific antiviral therapy exists, and no special medical management procedures have been advocated.

Powassan Fever

First described in Canada in 1959, Powassan virus has been found in Canada and the United States (Gholam et al., 1999) and can cause sporadic cases of severe encephalitis, sometimes resembling HSE (Embil et al., 1983). Four cases of Powassan encephalitis in Maine and Vermont from 1999 to 2001 have heightened the need for clinical suspicion and diagnostic testing, particularly in the northeastern United States (Centers for Disease Control and Prevention, 2001c). Gray matter is involved at all levels of the CNS, so no characteristic clinical picture has emerged. As with TBE, spinal cord involvement and atrophy can be found. A related deer tick virus can also cause human disease (Kuno et al., 2001). Kyasanur Forest disease in India (Pavri, 1989) and louping ill, a disease of sheep in Scotland (Davidson et al., 1991), are other tick-borne causes of encephalitis that can afflict humans.

Reoviruses

Colorado Tick Fever

Characterized by the sudden onset of fever, malaise, headaches, and muscular aches, Colorado tick fever is a relatively common systemic illness in much of the western United States (Silver et al., 1961). It can occasionally be complicated by aseptic meningitis, meningoencephalitis, or encephalitis (Spruance and Bailey, 1973). Common features that help to distinguish it from Rocky Mountain spotted fever (RMSF) are a biphasic, or saddlebacked, fever pattern in about 50% of patients and leukopenia in Colorado tick fever (Goodpasture et al., 1978). Rash is uncommon in Colorado tick fever—Goodpasture et al. (1978) found it in only 5% of 228 cases. However, it is found in the majority of RMSF patients. The distinction between Colorado tick fever and RMSF is crucial, of course, because of the response to antibiotics of RMSF.

Colorado tick fever virus is in the *Coltivirus* genus of the *Reoviridae* family. Coltiviruses transmitted by mosquitoes have also been associated with encephalitis in China (Tsai, 1997). Colorado tick fever virus is transmitted by *Dermacentor andersoni*, and the incidence of disease corresponds to the areas in the United States and Canada in which these ticks are found (Eklund et al., 1955). Symptoms develop a mean of 4.3 days following the tick bite (Spruance and Bailey, 1973). The illness is remarkable for a sustained viremia. Goodpasture et al. (1978) demonstrated virus isolation from blood in 46% of patients examined in a prospective study. Antigenemia was found in association with erythrocytes in 42% at 8 weeks into the illness. Virological changes can be achieved by virus isolation from blood, positive PCR, or diagnostic rises in serum antibody. Virus can be isolated from the CSF, even in the absence of CNS signs (Florio et al., 1952).

Neurological symptoms have been described by Eklund (1958) as somnolence that may lapse into coma, or restlessness and delirium. Delusions and convulsions were noted to occur. Muscle tenderness was also noted, as was hyperesthesia. Nuchal rigidity can be absent, present on its own, or found in combination with depressed level of consciousness (Spruance and Bailey, 1973). EEGs can reveal diffuse or generalized abnormalities. The CSF usually reveals a mononuclear pleocytosis but can on occasion be acellular or have a neurophilic predominance, particularly early in the course of the illness (Spruance and Bailey, 1973). Resolution of the illness can be prompt, although death and sequelae have been recorded (Spruance and Bailey, 1973).

REFERENCES

Abu-Elyazeed, R., S. El-Sharkawy, J. Olson, B. Botros, A. Soliman, A. Salib, C. Cummings, and R. Arthur. 1996. Prevalence of anti-Rift-Valley-Fever IgM antibody in abattoir workers in the Nile Delta during the 1993 outbreak in Egypt. *Bull. W. H. O.* **74:**155–158.

Adamson, J. D., and S. Dubo. 1942. Clinical findings in encephalitis (western equine). *Can. Public Health J.* **33:**288–300.

Allner, K., C. L. Bradish, R. Fitzgeorge, and N. Nathanson. 1974. Modification by sodium aurothiomalate of the expression of virulence in mice by defined strains of Semliki Forest virus. *J. Gen. Virol.* **24:**221–228.

Anderson, J. F., and J. J. Rahal. 2002. Efficacy of interferon alpha 2-b and ribavirin against West Nile virus in vitro. *Emerg. Infect. Dis.* **8:**107–108.

Anderson, S. G. 1950. Murray Valley encephalitis: epidemiological aspects. *Med. J. Aust.* **1:**97–100.

Anderson, S. G. 1954. Murray Valley encephalitis and Australian X disease. *J. Hyg.* **52:**447–468, *plus four plates.*

Anic, K., I. Soldo, L. Peric, I. Karner, and B. Barac. 1998. Tick-borne encephalitis in Eastern Croatia. *Scand. J. Infect. Dis.* **30:**509–512.

Asnis, D. S., R. Conetta, A. A. Teixeira, G. Waldman, and B. A. Sampson. 2000. The West Nile Virus outbreak of 1999 in New York: the Flushing Hospital experience. *Clin. Infect. Dis.* **30:**413–418.

Ayres, J. C., and R. F. Feemster. 1949. The sequelae of eastern equine encephalitis. *N. Engl. J. Med.* **240:**960–962.

Bailey, P. 1958. VII. Czechoslovakian tick encephalitis. *Neurology* **8:**890–896. [This is a résumé of a report by K. Henner, and F. Hanzals, (1957) in *Rev. Neurol.* **96:**384–408.]

Baker, A. B., and H. H. Noran. 1942. Western variety of equine encephalitis in man. A clinicopathological study. *Arch. Neurol. Psychiatr.* **47:**565–587.

Balfour, H. H., Jr., R. A. Siem, H. Bauer, and P. G. Quie. 1973. California arbovirus (La Crosse) infections. I. Clinical and laboratory findings in 66 children with meningoencephalitis. *Pediatrics* **52:**680–691.

Bastian, F. O., R. D. Wende, D. B. Singer, and R. S. Zeller. 1975. Eastern equine encephalomyelitis. Histopathologic and ultrastructure changes with isolation of the virus in a human case. *Am. J. Clin. Pathol.* **64:**10–13.

Beaty, B. H., T. L. Jamnback, S. W. Hildreth, and K. L. Brown. 1983. Rapid diagnosis of La Crosse virus infections: evaluation of serologic and antigen detection techniques for clinically relevant diagnosis of La Crosse encephalitis, p. 293–302. In C. H. Calisher and W. H. Thompson (ed.), *California Serogroup Viruses.* Alan R. Liss, Inc., New York, N.Y.

Beck, L. R., B. M. Lobitz, and B. L. Wood. 2000. Remote sensing and human health: new sensors and new opportunities. *Emerg. Infect. Dis.* **6:**217–227.

Bedjanic, M., S. Rus, J. Kmet, and J. Vesenjak-Zmijanac. 1955. Virus meningoencephalitis in Slovenia. 2. Clinical observations. *Bull. W. H. O.* **12:**503–512.

Bennett, N. M. 1976. Murray Valley encephalitis, 1974. Clinical features. *Med. J. Aust.* **2:**446–450.

Berther, F.-X., H. G. Zeller, M.-T. Drouer, J. Rauzier, H.-P. Digoutte, and V. Deube. 1997. Extensive nucleotide changes and deletions within the envelope glycoprotein gene of Euro-African West Nile viruses. *J. Gen. Virol.* **78:**2293–2297.

Bia, F. J., G. F. Thornton, A. J. Main, C. K. Y. Fong, and G. D. Hsiung. 1980. Western equine encephalitis mimicking herpes simplex encephalitis. *JAMA* **244:**367–369.

Booss, J., and N. Karabatsos. Arthropod-borne virus encephalitis. *In* A. Nath and J. R. Berger (ed.), *Clinical Neurovirology*, in press. Marcel-Dekker, New York, N.Y.

Bowen, C. S., T. R. Fashinell, P. B. Dean, and M. B. Gregg. 1976. Clinical aspects of human Venezuelan equine encephalitis in Texas. *PAHO Bull.* **10:**47–57.

Briese, T., X.-Y. Jia, C. Huang, L. J. Grady, and W. I. Lipkin. 1999. Identification of a Kunjin/West Nile-like flavivirus in brains of patients with New York encephalitis. *Lancet* **354:**1261–1262.

Brinker, K. R., and T. P. Monath. 1980. The acute disease, p. 503–534. *In* T. P. Monath (ed.), *St. Louis Encephalitis.* American Public Health Assoc., Washington, D.C.

Brinker, K. R., G. Paulson, T. P. Monath, G. Wise, and R. J. Fass. 1979. St. Louis encephalitis in Ohio, September 1975. *Arch. Intern. Med.* **139:**561–566.

Burke, D. S., A. Nisalak, M. A. Ussery, T. Laorakpongse, and L. Chantavibul. 1985. Kinetics of IgM and IgG responses to Japanese encephalitis virus in human serum and cerebrospinal fluid. *J. Infect. Dis.* **151:**1093–1099.

Cantile, C., G. DiGuardo, C. Eleni, and M. Arispic. 2000. Clinical and neuropathological features of West Nile Virus equine encephalomyelitis in Italy. *Equine Vet. J.* **32:**31–35.

Cassidy, L. F., and J. L. Patterson. 1989. Mechanism of LaCrosse virus inhibition by ribavirin. *Antimicrob. Agents Chemother.* **33:**2009–2011.

Ceausu, E., P. Ersciou, P. Calistru, D. Ispas, O. Dorobat, M. Homos, C. Barbulescu, I. Cojocaru, C. V. Simion, C. Cristea, C. Oprea, C. Dumitrescu, D. Duiculescu, I. Marcu, C. Mociornita, T. Stoicev, I. Zolotusca, C. Calomfirescu, R. Rusu, R. Hodrea, S. Geamai, and L. Paun. 1997. Clinical manifestations in the West Nile virus outbreak. *Rom. J. Virol.* **48:**3–11.

Centers for Disease Control. 1986. St. Louis encephalitis—Baytown and Houston, Texas. *Morb. Mortal. Wkly. Rep.* **33:**693–695.

Centers for Disease Control and Prevention. 1998. Rift Valley fever—East Africa, 1997–1998. *Morb. Mortal. Wkly. Rep.* **47:**261–264.

Centers for Disease Control and Prevention. 2000a. Outbreak of Rift Valley fever—Yemen, August–October 2000. *Morb. Mortal. Wkly. Rep.* **49:**1065–1066.

Centers for Disease Control and Prevention. 2000b. Outbreak of Rift Valley fever—Saudi Arabia, August–October, 2000. *Morb. Mortal. Wkly. Rep.* **49:**905–908.

Centers for Disease Control and Prevention. 2000c. Update: outbreak of Rift Valley fever—Saudi Arabia, August–November 2000. *Morb. Mortal. Wkly. Rep.* **49:**982–985.

Centers for Disease Control and Prevention. 2001a. Summary of notifiable diseases. United States. 1999. *Morb. Mortal. Wkly. Rep.* **48:**1–101.

Centers for Disease Control and Prevention. 2001b. Serosurveys for West Nile Virus infection—New York and Connecticut counties, 2000. *Morb. Mortal. Wkly. Rep.* **50:**37–39.

Centers for Disease Control and Prevention. 2001c. Outbreak of Powassan encephalitis—Maine and Vermont, 1999–2001. *Morb. Mortal. Wkly. Rep.* **50:**761–764.

Centers for Disease Control and Prevention. 2002a. West Nile virus activity—United States, November 21–26, 2002. *Morb. Mortal. Wkly. Rep.* **51:**1072–1073.

Centers for Disease Control and Prevention. 2002b. West Nile infection in organ donor and transplant recipients—Georgia and Florida. *Morb. Mortal. Wkly. Rep.* **51:**790.

Centers for Disease Control and Prevention. 2002c. Intrauterine West Nile virus infection, New York, 2002. *Morb. Mortal. Wkly. Rep.* **51:**1135–1136.

Centers for Disease Control and Prevention. 2002d. Acute flaccid paralysis syndrome associated with West Nile virus infection—Mississippi and Louisiana, July–August 2002. *Morb. Mortal. Wkly. Rep.* **51:**825–828.

Chen, W.-J., K.-P. Hwang, and A.-H. Fang. 1991. Detection of IgM antibodies from cerebrospinal fluid and sera of dengue fever patients. *Southeast Asian J. Trop. Med. Public Health* **22:**660–663.

Chimelli, L., M. Dumas-Hahn, M. B. Netto, R. G. Ramos, M. Dias, and F. Gray. 1990. Dengue: Neuropathological findings in 5 fatal cases from Brazil. *Clin. Neuropathol.* **9:**157–162.

Chun, R. W. M., W. H. Thompson, J. D. Grabow, and C. G. Matthews. 1968. California arbovirus encephalitis in children. *Neurology* **18:**369–375.

Clarke, D. H. 1961. Two non-fatal human infections with the virus of eastern encephalitis. *Am. J. Trop. Med. Hyg.* **10:**67–70.

Clarke, D. H., and J. Casals. 1965. Arboviruses; group B, p. 606–658. *In* F. L. Horsfall and I. Tamm (ed.), *Viral and Rickettsial Infections of Man*, 4th ed. J. B. Lippincott Co., Philadelphia, Pa.

Clarke, T. 2002. Break-bone fever. *Nature* **416:**672–674.

Daubney, R., and J. R. Hudson. 1931. Enzootic hepatitis or Rift Valley fever. An undescribed virus disease of sheep, cattle, and man from East Africa. *J. Pathol. Bacteriol.* **34:**545–579.

Davidson, M. M., H. Williams, and J. A. Macleod. 1991. Louping ill in man: a forgotten disease. *J. Infect.* **23:**241–249.

Deresiewicz, R. L., S. L. Thaler, L. Hsu, and A. A. Zamani. 1997. Clinical and neuroradiographic manifestations of eastern equine encephalitis. *N. Engl. J. Med.* **336:**1867–1874.

Desai, A., S. K. Sanker, V. Ravi, A. Chandramaki, and M. Gourie-Devi. 1995a. Japanese encephalitis virus antigen in human brain and its topographic distribution. *Acta Neuropathol.* **89:**368–373.

Desai, A., V. Ravi, A. Chandramuki, and M. Gourie-Devi. 1995b. Detection of immune complexes in the CSF of Japanese encephalitis patients: correlation of findings with outcome. *Intervirology* **37:**352–355.

Dickerson, R. B., J. R. Newton, and J. E. Hanson. 1952. Diagnosis and immediate prognosis of Japanese B encephalitis. *Am. J. Med.* **12:**277–288.

Doherty, P. C., and A. W. Reid. 1971. Experimental louping ill in sheep and lambs. 2. Neuropathology. *J. Comp. Pathol.* **81:**331–337.

Doherty, P. C., and J. T. Vantsis. 1973. Louping ill encephalomyelitis in the sheep. 7. Influence of immune status on neuropathology. *J. Comp. Pathol.* **83:**481–491.

Doherty, R. L., J. G. Carley, M. R. Cremer, J. T. Rendle-Short, L. J. Hopkins, D. H. Herbert, A. J. Caro, and W. B. Stephens. 1972. Murray Valley encephalitis in eastern Australia, 1971. *Med. J. Aust.* **2:**1170–1173.

Downs, W. G. 1982. The Rockefeller Foundation virus program: 1951–1971 with update to 1981. *Annu. Rev. Med.* **33:**1–29.

Dykers, T. I., K. L. Brown, C. B. Gunderson, and B. J. Beatty. 1985. Rapid diagnosis of specific immunoglobulin M in cerebrospinal fluid. *J. Clin. Microbiol.* **22:**740–744.

Earnest, M. P., H. A. Goolishian, J. R. Calverly, R. O. Hayes, and H. R. Hill. 1971. Neurologic, intellectual, and psychologic sequelae following western encephalitis. A follow-up study of 35 cases. *Neurology* **21:**969–974.

Ehrenkranz, N. J., M. C. Sinclair, E. Buff, and D. O. Lyman. 1970. The natural occurrence of Venezuelan equine encephalitis in the United States. First case and epidemiologic investigations. *N. Engl. J. Med.* **282:**298–302.

Ehrenkranz, N. J., and A. K. Ventura. 1974. Venezuelan equine encephalitis in man. *Annu. Rev. Med.* **25:**9–14.

Eklund, C. M. 1946. Human encephalitis of the western equine type in Minnesota in 1941. Clinical and epidemiological study of serologically positive cases. *Am. J. Hyg.* **43:**171–193.

Eklund, C. 1958. VI. Colorado tick fever. *Neurology* **8:**889.

Eklund, C. M., and A. Blumstein. 1938. The relation of human encephalitis to encephalomyelitis in horses. *JAMA* **111:**1734–1735.

Eklund, C. M., G. M. Kohls, and J. M. Brennan. 1955. Distribution of Colorado tick fever and virus-carrying ticks. *JAMA* **157:**335–337.

Embil, J. A., P. Camfield, H. Artsob, and D. P. Chase. 1983. Powassan virus encephalitis resembling herpes simplex encephalitis. *Arch. Intern. Med.* **143:**341–343.

Farber, S., A. Hill, M. L. Connerly, and J. H. Dingle. 1940. Encephalitis in infants and children caused by the virus of the eastern variety of equine encephalitis. *JAMA* **114:**1725–1731.

Feemster, R. F. 1957. Equine encephalitis in Massachusetts. *N. Engl. J. Med.* **257:**701–704.

Fernandez, R. J., and E. C. Dooling. 1982. Eastern equine encephalitis mimicking herpes simplex encephalitis. *Neurology* **32**(2):A178.

Finley, K. H., and N. Riggs. 1980. Convalescence and sequelae, p. 535–550. *In* T. P. Monath (ed.), *St. Louis Encephalitis.* American Public Health Assoc., Washington, D.C.

Finley, K. H., L. H. Fitzgerald, R. W. Richter, N. Riggs, and J. T. Shelton. 1967. Western encephalitis and cerebral ontogenesis. *Arch. Neurol.* **16:**140–164.

Florio, L., M. S. Miller, and E. R. Mugrage. 1952. Colorado tick fever: recovery of virus from human spinal fluid. *J. Infect. Dis.* **91:**285–289.

Fradin, M. S. 1998. Mosquitoes and mosquito repellants: a clinician's guide. *Ann. Intern. Med.* **128:**931–940.

French, E. L. 1952. Murray Valley encephalitis: isolation and characterization of the etiological agent. *Med. J. Aust.* **1:**100–103.

Gadoth, N., S. Weitzman, and E. E. Lehmann. 1979. Acute anterior myelitis complicating West Nile fever. *Arch. Neurol.* **36:**172–173.

Gajanana, A., V. Thenmozhi, P. P. Samuel, and R. Reuben. 1995. A community-based study of subclinical flavivirus infections in an area of Tamil Nadu, India where Japanese encephalitis in endemic. *Bull. W.H.O.* **73:**237–244.

Gardner, J. J., and M. G. Reyes. 1980. Pathology, p. 551–569. *In* T. P. Monath (ed.), *St. Louis Encephalitis.* American Public Health Assoc., Washington, D.C.

Garen, P. D., T. F. Tsai, and J. M. Powers. 1999. Human eastern equine encephalitis: immunohistochemistry and ultrastructure. *Mol. Pathol.* **12:**646–652.

Gatus, B. J., and M. R. Rose. 1983. Japanese B encephalitis: epidemiological, clinical, and pathological aspects. *J. Infect.* **6:**213–218.

George, S., M. Gourie-Devi, J. A. Rao, S. R. Prasad, and K. M. Pavri. 1984. Isolation of West Nile virus from the brains of children who had died of encephalitis. *Bull. W. H. O.* **62:**879–882.

Gholam, B. I. A., S. Puksa, and J. P. Provias. 1999. Powassan encephalitis: a case report with neuropathology and literature review. *Can. Med. Assoc. J.* **161:**1419–1422.

Goldblum, N., V. V. Sterk, and B. Paderski. 1954. West Nile fever. The clinical features of the disease and the isolation of West Nile virus from the blood of nine human cases. *Am. J. Hyg.* **59:**89–103.

Goldfield, M., and O. Sussman. 1968. The 1959 outbreak of eastern encephalitis in New Jersey. I. Introduction and description of outbreak. *Am. J. Epidemiol.* **87:**1–10.

Goodpasture, H. C., J. D. Poland, D. B. Francy, G. S. Bowen, and K. A. Horn. 1978. Colorado tick fever: clinical, epidemiologic, and laboratory aspects of 228 cases in Colorado in 1977–1974. *Ann. Intern. Med.* **88:**303–310.

Grascenkov, N. I. 1964. Tick-borne encephalitis in the USSR. *Bull. W. H. O.* **30:**187–196.

Griffin, D. E., and J. M. Hardwick. 1997. Regulators of apoptosis on the road to persistent alphavirus infection. *Annu. Rev. Microbiol.* **51:**565–592.

Grimley, P. M. 1983. Arbovirus encephalitis: which road traveled by makes all the difference? *Lab. Invest.* **48:**369–371.

Grinschgl, G. 1955. Virus meningo-encephalitis in Austria. 2. Clinical features, pathology, and diagnosis. *Bull. W. H. O.* **12:**535–564.

Gubler, D. J. 1998. Dengue and dengue hemorrhagic fever. *Clin. Microbiol. Rev.* **11:**480–496.

Gunther, G., M. Haglund, L. Lindquist, M. Forsgren, and B. Skoldenberg. 1997. Tick-borne encephalitis in Sweden in relation to aseptic meningoencephalitis of unknown etiology: a prospective study of clinical course and outcome. *J. Neurol.* **244:**230–238.

Hales, S., N. de Wet, J. Maindonald, and A. Woodward. 2002. Potential effect of population and climate changes on global distribution of Dengue fever: an empirical model. *Lancet* **360:**830–834.

Halstead, S. B. 1988. Pathogenesis of dengue: challenges to molecular biology. *Science* **239:**476–481.

Halstead, S. B., and C. R. Grosz. 1962. Subclinical Japanese encephalitis. I. Infection of Americans with limited residence in Korea. *Am. J. Hyg.* **75:**190–201.

Han, L. L., F. Popovici, J. P. Alexander, Jr., V. Laurentia, L. A. Tengelsen, C. Cernescu, H. E. Gary Jr., N. Ion-Nedelcu, G. L. Campbell, and T. F. Tsai. 1999. Risk factors for West Nile virus infection and meningoencephalitis, Romania, 1996. *J. Infect. Dis.* **179:**230–233.

Hase, T. 1993. Virus-neuron interactions in the mouse brain infected with Japanese encephalitis virus. *Virchows Arch. B Cell Pathol. Incl. Mol. Pathol.* **64:**162–170.

Hayes, E. B., and D. J. Gubler. 1992. Dengue and dengue hemorrhagic fever. *Pediatr. Infect. Dis. J.* **11:**311–317.

Heinz, F. X., and C. W. Mandl. 1993. The molecular biology of tick-borne encephalitis virus. *APMIS* **101:**735–745.

Heinz, F. S., M. Roggendorf, H. Hofmann, C. Kunz, and F. Deinhardt. 1981. Comparison of two different enzyme immunoassays for detection of immunoglobulin M antibodies against tick borne encephalitis virus in serum and cerebrospinal fluid. *J. Clin. Microbiol.* **14:**141–146.

Heinz, F. X., R. Berger, W. Tuma, and C. Kunz. 1983. A topological and functional model of epitopes on the structural glycoprotein of tick-borne encephalitis virus defined by monoclonal antibodies. *Virology* **126:**525–537.

Hilty, M. D., R. E. Hayes, P. H. Azimi, and H. G. Cramblett. 1972. California encephalitis in children. *Am. J. Dis. Child.* **124:**530–533.

Hoke, C. H., Jr., D. W. Vaughn, A. Nisalak, P. Intralawan, S. Poolsuppasit, V. Jongsawas, U. Titsyakorn, and R. T. Johnson. 1992. Effect of high dose dexamethasone on the outcome of acute encephalitis due to Japanese encephalitis virus. *J. Infect. Dis.* **165:**631–637.

Hoogstraal, H., J. M. Meegan, and G. M. Khalil. 1979. The Rift Valley fever epizootic in Egypt 1977–1978. 2. Ecological and entomological studies. *Trans. R. Soc. Trop. Med. Hyg.* **73:**624–629.

Huang, C. H. 1982. Studies of Japanese encephalitis in China. *Adv. Virus Res.* **27:**71–101.

Huang, C., W. H. Thompson, N. Karabatsos, L. Grady, and W. P. Campbell. 1997. Evidence that fatal human infections with La Cross virus may be associated with a narrow range of genotypes. *Virus Res.* **481**:143–148.

Hubalek, Z., and J. Halouzka. 1999. West Nile fever—a reemerging mosquito-borne viral disease in Europe. *Emerg. Infect. Dis.* **5**:643–650.

Innes, B. L. 1995. Dengue and dengue hemorrhagic fever, p. 103–146. *In* J. S. Porterfield (ed.), *Exotic Viral Infections.* Chapman and Hall Medical, London, United Kingdom.

Ishii, T., M. Matsushita, and S. Hamada. 1977. Characteristic residual neuropathological features in Japanese B encephalitis. *Acta Neuropathol.* **38**:181–186.

Iwasaki, Y., J. X. Zhao, T. Yamamoto, and H. Konno. 1986. Immunohistochemical demonstration of viral antigens in Japanese encephalitis. *Acta Neuropathol.* **70**:79–81.

Iwasaki, Y., K. Sako, I. Tsumoda, and Y. Ohara. 1993. Phenotypes of mononuclear cell infiltrates in human central nervous system. *Acta Neuropathol.* **85**:653–657.

Janssen, H. L. A., H. P. Bienfait, C. L. Jansen, S. G. van Duinen, R. Vriesendorp, R. J. Schimsheimer, J. Groen, and A. D. M. E. Osterhaus. 1998. Fatal cerebral-edema associated with primary dengue infection. *J. Infect.* **36**:344–346.

Johnson, R. T. 1965. Virus invasion of the central nervous system. A study of *Sindbis* virus infection in the mouse using fluorescent antibody. *Am. J. Pathol.* **46**:929–943.

Johnson, R. T. 1998. *Viral Infections of the Nervous System*, 2nd ed., p. 109–125. Lippincott-Raven, Philadelphia, Pa.

Johnson, R. T., D. S. Burke, M. Elwell, C. J. H. Leake, A. Nisalak, C. H. Hoke, and W. Lorsomrudee. 1985. Japanese encephalitis: immunocytochemical studies of viral antigen and inflammatory cells in fatal cases. *Ann. Neurol.* **18**:567–573.

Jordan, I., T. Briese, N. Fischer, J. Y.-L. Lau, and W. I. Lipkin. 2000. Ribavirin inhibits West Nile virus replication and cytopathic effect in neural cells. *J. Infect. Dis.* **182**:1213–1217.

Kaiser, R., and H. Holzmann. 2000. Laboratory findings in tick-borne encephalitis—correlation with clinical outcome. *Infection* **28**:78–84.

Kalita, J., and U. K. Misra. 1998. EEG in Japanese encephalitis: a clinicoradiological correlation. *Electroenceph. Clin. Neurophysiol.* **106**:238–243.

Kankirawatana, P., K. Chokephaibulkit, P. Puthavathana, S. Yoksan, S. Apintanapong, and V. Pongthapisit. 2000. Dengue infection presenting with central nervous system manifestation. *J. Child Neurol.* **15**:544–547.

Kappus, K. D., T. P. Monath, R. M. Kaminski, and C. H. Calisher. 1983. Reported encephalitis associated with California serogroup virus infections in the United States 1963–1981, p. 31–41. *In* C. H. Calisher and W. H. Thompson (ed.), *California Serogroup Viruses.* Alan R. Liss Inc., New York, N.Y.

Karabatsos, N. (ed.). 1985. *International Catalogue of Arboviruses Including Certain Other Viruses of Vertebrates*, 3rd ed. American Society of Tropical Medicine and Hygiene, San Antonio, Tex.

Karabatsos, N., A. L. Lewis, C. H. Calisher, A. R. Hunt, and J. T. Roehrig. 1988. Identification of highlands J virus from a Florida horse. *Am. J. Trop. Med. Hyg.* **39**:603–606.

Karak, J. D., Y. Aynor, and C. J. Peters. 1982. A Rift Valley fever vaccine trial. I. Side effects and serologic response over a six-month follow up. *Am. J. Epidemiol.* **116**:808–820.

Kay, B. H. 1980. Towards prediction and surveillance of Murray Valley encephalitis activity in Australia. *Aust. J. Exp. Biol. Med. Sci.* **58**:67–76.

Kim, J. H., J. Booss, E. E. Manuelidis, and C. C. Duncan. 1985. Human eastern equine encephalitis: electron microscopic study of a brain biopsy. *Am. J. Clin. Pathol.* **84**:223–227.

Kmet, J., J. Vesenjak-Zmijanac, M. Bedjanic, and S. Rus. 1955. Virus meningoencephalitis in Slovenia. 1. Epidemiological observations. *Bull. W.H.O.* **12**:491–501.

Kokernot, R. H., H. R. Shinefield, and W. A. Longshore, Jr. 1953. The 1952 outbreak of encephalitis in California. Differential diagnosis. *Cal. Med.* **79**:73–77.

Kuno, G., H. Artsob, N. Karabatsos, K. R. Tsuchiya, and G. J. J. Chang. 2001. Genomic sequencing of deer tick virus and the phylogeny of the Powassan-related viruses of North America. *Am. J. Trop. Med.* **65**:671–676.

Lanciotti, R. S., J. T. Roehrig, V. Deubel, J. Smith, M. Parker, K. Steele, B. Crise, K. E. Volpe, M. B. Crabtree, J. H. Scherret, R. A. Hall, J. S. MacKenzie, C. B. Cropp, B. Panigrahy, E. Ostlund, B. Schmitt, M. Malkinson, C. Banet, J. Weissman, N. Komar, H. M. Savage, W. Stone, T. McNamara, and D. J. Gubler. 1999. Origin of the West Nile virus responsible for an outbreak of encephalitis in the Northeastern United States. *Science* **286**:2333–2337.

Laughlin, L. W., J. M. Meegan, L. J. Strausbaugh, D. M. Morens, and R. H. Watten. 1979. Epidemic Rift Valley fever in Egypt: observations of the spectrum of human illness. *Trans. R. Soc. Trop. Med. Hyg.* **73**:630–633.

Leech, R. W., J. C. Harris, and R. W. Johnson. 1981. 1975 encephalitis epidemic in North Dakota and western Minnesota. An epidemiological, clinical and neuropathologic study. *Minn. Med.* **64**:545–548.

Lehmann, N. I., I. D. Gust, and R. Doherty. 1976. Isolation of Murray Valley encephalitis virus from the brain of three patients with encephalitis. *Med. J. Aust.* **2**:450–454.

Levine, B., J. M. Hardwick, B. D. Trapp, T. O. Crawford, R. C. Bolinger, and D. E. Griffin. 1991. Antibody-mediated clearance of alphavirus infection from neurons. *Science* **254**:856–860.

Levine, B., J. E. Goldman, H. H. Jiang, D. E. Griffin, and J. M. Hardwick. 1996. Bcl-2 protects mice against fatal alphavirus encephalitis. *Proc. Natl. Acad. Sci. USA* **93**:4810–4815.

Li, Z. S., S. F. Hong, and N. L. Ghong. 1988. Immunohistochemical study of Japanese B encephalitis. *China Med. J.* **101**:768–771.

Linthicum, J. J., A. Anyamba, C. J. Tucker, P. W. Kelley, M. F. Myers, and C. J. Peters. 1999. Climate and satellite indicators to forecast Rift Valley fever epidemics in Kenya. *Science* **285**:397–400.

Liou, M.-L., and C. Y. Hsu. 1998. Japanese encephalitis virus is transported across the cerebral blood vessels by endocytosis in mouse brain. *Cell Tissue Res.* **293**:389–394.

Lord, R. D. 1974. History and geographic distribution of Venezuelan equine encephalitis. *Bull. Pan Am. Health Org.* **8**:100–110.

Lum, L. C. S., S. K. Lam, Y. S. Choy, R. George, and F. Harun. 1996. Dengue encephalitis: a true entity? *Am. J. Trop. Med. Hyg.* **54**:256–259.

Lvov, D. K., A. M. Butenko, V. L. Gromashevsky, V. P. Larichev, S. Y. Gaidamovich, O. I. Vyshemirsky, A. N. Zhukov, V. V. Lazorenko, V. M. Salko, A. I. Kovtunov, K. M. Galimzyanov, A. E. Platonov, T. N. Morozova, N. V. Khutoretskaya, E. O. Shishkina, and T. M. Skvortsova. 2000. Isolation of two strains of West Nile virus during an outbreak in southern Russia. *Emerg. Infect. Dis.* **6**:373-376.

Mackenzie, J. S., and A. K. Broom. 1995. Australian X Disease, Murray Valley encephalitis and the French connection. *Vet. Microbiol.* **46**:75–90.

Mackenzie, J. S., D. W. Smith, A. K. Brown, and M. R. Bucens. 1993. Australian encephalitis in Western Australia, 1978–1991. *Med. J. Aust.* **158**:591–595.

Mackenzie, J. S., M. D. Lindsay, R. J. Coelen, A. K. Broom, R. A. Hall, and D. W. Smith. 1994. Arboviruses causing human disease in the Australasian zoographic region. *Arch. Virol.* **136:**447–467.

Marbert, K., N. Goldblum, V. V. Sterk, W. Jasinska-Klingberg, and M. A. Klingberg. 1956. The natural history of West Nile fever. I. Clinical observations during an epidemic in Israel. *Am. J. Hyg.* **64:**259–269.

Mathur, A., N. Khanna, and U. C. Chaturvedi. 1992. Breakdown of blood-brain barrier by virus-induced cytokine during Japanese encephalitis virus infection. *Int. J. Exp. Pathol.* **73:**603–611.

McIntosh, B. M., P. G. Jupp, I. Dos Santos, and G. M. Meenehan. 1976. Epidemics of West Nile and Sindbis viruses in South Africa with *Culex (Culex) univittatus* theobald as vector. *S. Afr. J. Sci.* **72:**295–300.

McJunkin, J. E., R. R. Khan, and T. F. Tsai. 1998. California-LaCrosse encephalitis. *Infect. Dis. Clin. N. Am.***12:**83–93.

McJunkin, J. E., E. C. DeLos Reyes, J. E. Irazuzta, M. J. Caceres, R. R. Khan, L. L. Minnich, K. D. Fu, G. D. Lovett, T. Tsai, and A. Thompson. 2001. LaCrosse encephalitis in children. *N. Engl. J. Med.* **344:**801–807.

Medovy, H. 1942. Western equine encephalitis in infants. *Can. Public Health J.* **33:**307–312.

Meegan, J. M. 1979. The Rift Valley fever epizootic in Egypt 1977–78. I. Description of the epizootic and virological studies. *R. Soc. Trop. Med. Hyg.* **73:**618–623.

Meegan, J. M., H. Hoogstraal, and M. I. Moussa. 1979. An epizootic of Rift Valley fever in Egypt in 1977. *Vet. Rec.* **105:**124–125.

Melnick, J. L., J. R. Paul, J. T. Riordan, V. H. Barnett, N. Goldblum, and E. Zabin. 1951. Isolation from human sera in Egypt of a virus apparently identical to West Nile Virus. *Proc. Soc. Exp. Biol. Med.* **77:**661–665.

Misra, U. K., J. Kalita, and M. Srivastava. 1998. Prognosis of Japanese encephalitis: a multivariate analysis. *J. Neurol. Sci.* **161:**143–147.

Miyake, M. 1964. The pathology of Japanese encephalitis: a review. *Bull. W.H.O.* **30:**153–160.

Monath, T. P. 1978. Central nervous system infections (Acute), p. 261–294. *In* G. D. Hsiung and R. H. Green (ed.), *Virology and Rickettsiology*, vol. I, part 2. CRC Press, West Palm Beach, Fla.

Monath, T. P. 1980. Epidemiology, p. 239–312. *In* T. P. Monath (ed.), *St. Louis Encephalitis.* American Public Health Assoc., Washington, D.C.

Monath, T. P., and T. F. Tsai. 1987. St Louis encephalitis: lessons from the last decade. *Am. J. Trop. Med. Hyg.* **37**(3 Suppl.)**:**40S–59S.

Monath, T. P., and T. F. Tsai. 1997. Flaviviruses, p. 1133–1185. *In* D. D. Richman, R. J. Whitley, and F. G. Hayden (ed.), *Clinical Virology.* Churchill Livingstone, New York, N.Y.

Monath, T. P., B. C. Cropp, and A. K. Harrison. 1983. Mode of entry of a neurotropic arbovirus into the central nervous system. *Lab. Invest.* **48:**399–410.

Murali-Krishna, K., V. Ravi, and R. Manjunath. 1994. Cytotoxic T lymphocytes against Japanese encephalitis virus: effector cell phenotype, target specificity and in vitro clearance. *J. Gen. Virol.* **75:**799–807.

Murali-Krishna, K., V. Ravi, and R. Manjumath. 1996. Protection of adult but not newborn mice against intra cerebral challenge with Japanese encephalitis virus by adoptively transferred virus-specific T lymphocytes: requirement of LST4+ cells. *J. Gen. Virol.* **77:**705–714.

Murgod, U. A., U. B. Muthane, V. Ravi, S. Radhesh, and A. Desai. 2001. Persistent movement disorders following Japanese encephalitis. *Neurology* **57:**2313–2315.

Murphy, F. A., and S. G. Whitfield. 1970. Eastern equine encephalitis virus infection: electron microscopic studies of mouse central nervous system. *Exp. Mol. Pathol.* **13:**131–146.

Nash, D., F. Mostashari, A. Fine, J. Miller, D. O'Leary, K. Murray, A. Huang, A. Rosenberg, A. Greenberg, M. Sherman, S. Wong, and M. Layton for the 1999 West Nile Outbreak Response Working Group. 2001. The outbreak of West Nile virus infection in the New York City area in 1999. *N. Engl. J. Med.* **344:**1807–1814.

Nichter, C. A., S. G. Pavlakis, U. Shaikh, K. A. Cherian, J. Dobrosyzcki, M. E. Porricola, and I. Chatturvedi. 2000. Rhombencephalitis caused by West Nile Fever virus. *Neurology* **55:**153.

Niklasson, B., C. J. Peters, M. Grandien, and O. Wood. 1984. Detection of human immunoglobulins G and M antibodies to Rift Valley Fever virus by enzyme-linked immunosorbent assay. *J. Clin. Microbiol.* **19:**225–229.

Nimmannitya, S., U. Thisyakorn, and V. Hemsrichart. 1987. Dengue haemorrhagic fever with unusual manifestations. *Southeast Asian J. Trop. Med. Public Health* **18:**399–406.

Ogawa, M., H. Okubu, Y. Tsunji, N. Yasui, and K. Someda. 1973. Chronic progressive encephalitis occurring 13 years after Russian spring-summer encephalitis. *J. Neurol. Sci.* **19:**363–373.

Okhuysen, P. C., J. K. Crane, and J. Pappas. 1993. St Louis encephalitis in patients with human immunodeficiency virus infection. *Clin. Infect. Dis.* **17:**140–141.

Osetowska, E. 1970. Tick-borne encephalitides, p. 182–193. *In* R. Debre and J. Celers (ed.), *Clinical Virology. The Evaluation and Management of Human Viral Infections.* W. B. Saunders Co., Philadelphia, Pa.

Osetowska, E. 1977. *Tissue Neuropathology of Viral and Allergic Encephalitides*, p. 93–109. National Technical Information Service, Springfield, Va.

Patey, O., L. Ollivaud, J. Breuil, and C. Lafaix. 1993. Unusual neurologic manifestations occurring during dengue fever infection. *Am. J. Trop. Med. Hyg.* **48:**793–802.

Pathak, S., and H. E. Webb. 1974. Possible mechanism for the transport of Semliki Forest virus into and within mouse brain. An electron microscopic study. *J. Neurol. Sci.* **23:**175–184.

Pavlovsky, E. N. 1966. *Natural Nodality of Transmissible Disease, with Special Reference to the Landscape Epidemiology of Zooanthroponoses.* (Translated by F. K. Plous, Jr.; English translation edited by N. D. Levine.) University of Illinois Press, Urbana, Ill.

Pavri, K. 1989. Clinical, clinicopathologic, and hematologic features of Kyasanur Forest disease. *Rev. Infect. Dis.* **11:**S854–S859.

Petersen, L. R., and A. A. Martin. 2002. West Nile virus: a primer for the clinician. *Ann. Intern. Med.* **137:**173–179.

Platonov, A. E., G. A. Shipulin, O. Yu. Shipulina, E. N. Tyutyunnik, T. I. Frolochkina, R. S. Lanciotti, S. Yazyshina, O. V. Platinov, I. L. Obukhov, A. N. Zhukov, Y. Ya. Vengerov, and V. I. Pokrovskii. 2001. Outbreak of West Nile virus infection, Volgograd region, Russia. 1999. *Emerg. Infect. Dis.* **1:**128–132.

Pradham, S., N. Pandey, S. Shashank, R. K. Gupta, and A. Mathur. 1999. Parkinsonism due to predominant involvement of substantia nigra in Japanese encephalitis. *Neurology* **53:**1781–1786.

Pruzanski, W., and R. Altman. 1962. Encephalitis due to West Nile fever virus. *World Neurol.* **3:**524–527.

Public Health Service. 1935. *Report on the St. Louis Outbreak of Encephalitis.* Public Health Bulletin 214. Public Health Service, U.S. Department of the Treasury. U.S. Government Printing Office, Washington, D.C.

Quong, T. L. 1942. The pathology of western equine encephalitis. 18 human cases, Manitoba epidemic, 1941. *Can. Public Health J.* **33**:300–306, *with fold-out chart following p. 306.*

Radsel-Medvescek, A., M. Marolt-Gomiscek, and M. Gajsek-Zima. 1980. Clinical characteristics of patients with TBE treated at the University Medical Center Hospital for Infectious Diseases in Ljubljana during the years 1974 and 1977, p. 277–280. In J. Vesenjak-Hirjan, J. S. Porterfield, and E. Arslanagaic (ed.), *Arboviruses in Mediterranean Countries.* Gustav Fischer Verlag, Stuttgart, Germany.

Rappole, J. H., S. R. Derrickson, and Z. Hubalek. 2000. Migratory birds and spread of West Nile virus in the western hemisphere. *Emerg. Infect. Dis.* **6**:319–328.

Ravi, V., S. Parida, A. Chandramuki, M. Gourie-Devi, and G. E. Grau. 1997. Correlation of TNF levels in the serum and CSF in Japanese encephalitis patients. *J. Med. Virol.* **51**:132–136.

Ravi, V., A. Desai, S. K. Shankar, and M. Gourie-Devi. 2000. Japanese encephalitis, p. 231–257. In L. E. Davis and P. G. E. Kennedy (ed.), *Infectious Diseases of the Nervous System.* Butterworth-Heinemann, Oxford, United Kingdom.

Reyes, M. G., J. J. Gardner, J. D. Poland, and T. P. Monath. 1981. St. Louis encephalitis: quantitative histologic and immunofluorescent studies. *Arch. Neurol.* **38**:329–334.

Rigau-Perez, R. G., G. G. Clark, D. J. Gubler, P. Reiter, E. J. Sanderes, and A. V. Vorndam. 1998. Dengue and dengue hemorrhagic fever. *Lancet* **352**:971–977.

Riou, O., B. Philippe, A. Jouan, I. Coulibaly, M. Mondo, and J. P. Digoutte. 1989. Neurologic and neurosensory forms of Rift Valley fever (in French). *Bull. Soc. Path. Exot. Ses Filiales* **82**:605–610.

Rivas, F., L. A. Diaz, V. M. Cardenas, E. Daza, L. Bruaon, A. Alcala, O. DelaHoz, F. M. Caceres, G. Aristizabal, J. W. Martinez, D. Revelo, F. DelaHoz, J. Boshell, T. Camacho, L. Calderon, V. A. Olano, L. I. Villareal, D. Roselli, G. Alverez, G. Ludwig, and T. Tsai. 1997. Epidemic Venezuelan equine encephalitis in LaGuajira, Columbia, 1995. *J. Infect. Dis.* **175**:828–832.

Robertson, E. G., and H. McLorinan. 1952. Murray Valley encephalitis: clinical aspects. *Med. J. Aust.* **1**:103–107.

Rose, M. R., S. M. Hughes, and B. J. Gatus. 1983. A case of Japanese B encephalitis imported into the United Kingdom. *J. Infect.* **6**:261–265.

Row, D., P. Weinstein, and S. Murray-Smith. 1996. Dengue fever with encephalopathy in Australia. *Am. J. Trop. Med. Hyg.* **54**:253–255.

Rozdilsky, B., H. E. Robertson, and J. Chorney. 1968. Western encephalitis: report of eight fatal cases: Saskatchewan epidemic, 1965. *Can. Med. Assoc. J.* **98**:79–86.

Rust, R. S., W. H. Thompson, C. G. Matthews, B. J. Beaty, and R. W. M. Chun. 1999. LaCrosse and other forms of encephalitis. *J. Child. Neurol.* **14**:1–14.

Sampson, B. A., C. Ambrosi, A. Charlot, K. Reiber, J. F. Veress, and V. Armbrustmacher. 2000. The pathology of human West Nile virus infection. *Hum. Pathol.* **31**:527–531.

Schellinger, P. D., E. Schmutzhard, J. B. Fiebach, B. Pfausler, H. Maier, and S. Schwab. 2000. Poliomyelitic-like illness in Central European encephalitis. *Neurology* **55**:299–302.

Schlesinger, R. W. 1980. *The Togaviruses; Biology, Structure and Replication.* Academic Press, New York, N.Y.

Shiraki, H. 1970. Japanese Encephalitis, p. 155–175. In R. Debre and J. Celers (ed.), *Clinical Virology. The Evaluation and Management of Human Viral Infections.* W. B. Saunders Co., Philadelphia, Pa.

Shope, R. E. 1980. Arbovirus-related encephalitis. *Yale J. Biol. Med.* **53**:93–99.

Siam, A. L., J. M. Meegan, and K. F. Garbawi. 1980. Rift Valley Fever ocular manifestations: observations during the 1977 epidemic in Egypt. *Br. J. Ophthalmol.* **64**:366–374.

Silber, L. A., and V. D. Soloviev. 1946. Far Eastern tick-borne spring-summer (spring) encephalitis. *Am. Rev. Soviet Med.* **(special suppl.).**

Silver, H. K., G. Meiklejohn, and C. H. Kempe. 1961. Colorado tick fever. *Am. J. Dis. Child.* **101**:30–36.

Smadel, J. E., P. Bailey, and A. B. Baker. 1958. Sequelae of the arthropod-borne encephalitides. *Neurology* **8**:878–896.

Smithburn, K. C., T. P. Hughes, A. W. Burke, and J. H. Paul. 1940. A neurotropic virus isolated from the blood of a native of Uganda. *Am. J. Trop. Med.* **20**:471–492.

Smorodintsev, A. A. 1958. Tick-borne spring-summer encephalitis. *Prog. Med. Virol.* **1**:210–248.

Solomon, T., and M. Mallewa. 2001. Dengue and other emerging flaviviruses. *J. Infect.* **42**:104–115.

Solomon, T., N. M. Dung, D. W. Vaughn, R. Kneen, L. T. T. Thao, B. Raengsakulrach, H. T. Loan, N. P. J. Day, J. Farrar, K. S. A. Myint, M. J. Warrell, W. S. James, A. Nisalak, and N. J. White. 2000. Neurological manifestations of dengue infection. *Lancet* **355**:1053–1059.

Solomon, T., N. M. Dung, B. Wills, R. Kneen, M. Gainsborough, T. V. Diet, T. T. N. Thuy, H. T. Loan, V. C. Khanh, D. W. Vaughn, N. J. White, and J. J. Farrar. 2003. Interferon alfa-2a in Japanese encephalitis: a randomized double-blind placebo controlled trial. *Lancet* **361**:821–826.

Southam, C. M., and A. E. Moore. 1954. Induced virus infections in man by the Egypt isolates of West Nile virus. *Am. J. Trop. Med. Hyg.* **3**:19–50.

Southern, P. M., Jr., J. W. Smith, J. P. Luby, J. A. Barnett, and J. P. Sanford. 1969. Clinical and laboratory features of epidemic St. Louis encephalitis. *Ann. Intern. Med.* **71**:681–689.

Spruance, S. L., and A. Bailey. 1973. Colorado tick fever. A review of 115 laboratory-confirmed cases. *Arch. Intern. Med.* **131**:288–293.

Steele, K. E., M. J. Linn, R. J. Schoepp, N. Komar, T. W. Geisbert, R. M. Manduca, P. P. Calle, B. L. Raphael, N. A. Panella, and T. S. McNamara. 2000. Pathology of fatal West Nile virus infections in native and exotic birds during the 1999 outbreak in New York City, New York. *Vet. Pathol.* **37**:208–224.

Suzuki, M., and C. A. Phillips. 1966. St. Louis encephalitis. A histopathologic study of the fatal cases from the Houston epidemic in 1964. *Arch. Pathol.* **81**:47–54.

Tardei, G., S. Ruta, V. Chitu, C. Rossi, T. F. Tsai, and C. Cernescu. 2000. Evaluation of immunoglobulin M (IgM) and IgG enzyme immunoassays in serologic diagnosis of West Nile virus encephalitis. *J. Clin. Microbiol.* **38**:2232–2239.

Tsai, T. F. 1992. Arboviral infections: general considerations for prevention, diagnosis, and treatment in travelers. *Semin. Pediatr. Infect. Dis.* **3**:62–69.

Tsai, T. F. 1997. Coltivirus Colorado tick fever, p. 1209–1211. In S. S. Long, L. K. Pickering, and C. G. Prober (ed.), *Principles and Practice of Pediatric Infectious Diseases.* Churchill Livingstone, New York, N.Y.

Tsai, T. F., and T. P. Monath. 1997. Alphaviruses, p. 1217–1255. In D. D. Richman, R. J. Whitley, and F. G. Hayden (ed.), *Clinical Virology.* Churchill Livingstone, New York, N.Y.

Tsai, T. F., M. A. Canfield, C. M. Reed, V. L. Flannery, K. H. Sullivan, G. R. Reeve, R. E. Bailey, and J. D. Poland. 1988. Epidemiological aspects of a St Louis encephalitis outbreak in Harris County, Texas, 1986. *J. Infect. Dis.* **157**:351–356.

Tsai, T. F., F. Popovici, C. Cernescu, G. L. Campbell, and N. I. Nedelcu. 1998. West Nile encephalitis epidemic in Southeastern Romania. *Lancet* **352**:767–771.

Turell, M. J., S. M. Presley, A. M. Gad, S. E. Cope, D. J. Dohm, J. C. Morrill, and R. R. Arthur. 1996. Vector competence of Egyptian mosquitoes for Rift Valley fever virus. *Am. J. Trop. Med. Hyg.* **54:**136–139.

Van Velden, D. J. J., J. D. Meyer, J. Olivier, J. H. S. Gear, and B. McIntosh. 1977. Rift Valley fever affecting humans in South Africa. A clinicopathological study. *S. Afr. Med. J.* **51:**867–871.

Vaughn, D. W., and C. H. Hoke. 1992. The epidemiology of Japanese encephalitis: prospects for prevention. *Epidemiol. Rev.* **14:**197–221.

Wasay, M., R. Diaz-Arrastia, R. A. Suss, S. Kojan, A. Haq, D. Burns, and P. V. Ness. 2000. St. Louis encephalitis. A review of 11 cases in a 1995 Dallas, Tex. epidemic. *Arch. Neurol.* **57:**114–118.

Weaver, S. C., R. Salas, R. Rico-Hesse, G. V. Ludwi, M. S. Oberste, J. Boshell, and R. B. Tesh. 1996. Re-emergence of epidemic Venezuelan equine encephalomyelitis in South America. *Lancet* **348:**436–440.

Webb, H. E. 1975. The arbovirus encephalitides, p. 1–18. In L. S. Illis (ed.), *Viral Diseases of the Nervous System.* Bailliere Tindall, London, United Kingdom.

Webb, H. E., M. Chew-Lim, S. Jagelman, S. W. Oaten, S. Pathak, A. J. Suckling, and A. Mackenzie. 1979. Semliki Forest virus infections in mice as a model for studying acute and chronic central nervous system virus infections in man, p. 369–390. In F. C. Rose (ed.), *Clinical Neuroimmunology.* Blackwell Scientific Publications, Oxford, United Kingdom.

Webster, H. D. 1956. Eastern equine encephalomyelitis in Massachusetts. Report of two cases, diagnosed serologically, with complete clinical recovery. *N. Engl. J. Med.* **255:**267–270.

World Health Organization. 1983. The use of veterinary vaccines for prevention and control of Rift Valley fever: memorandum from a WHO/FAO meeting. *Bull. W. H. O.* **61:**261–268.

World Health Organization. 1997. Dengue haemorrhagic fever. *Diagnosis, Treatment, Prevention and Control,* 2nd ed. World Health Organization, Geneva, Switzerland.

World Health Organization. 1998. Japanese encephalitis vaccines. World Health Organization Position Paper. *Wkly. Epidemiol. Rec.* **73:**337–344.

World Health Organization. 2000. *Rift Valley Fever.* Fact Sheet Number 207, 1–4. World Health Organization, Geneva, Switzerland.

Wulur, S. H., E. Jahja, D. J. Gubler, T. S. Sutomenggolo, and J. S. Saroso. 1978. Encephalopathy associated with dengue infection. *Lancet* **i:**449–450.

Zimmerman, H. M. 1946. The pathology of Japanese B encephalitis. *Am. J. Pathol.* **22:**965–975.

Zlotnik, I., C. E. Smith, D. P. Grant, and S. Peacock. 1970. The effect of immunosuppression in viral encephalitis with special reference to cyclophosphamide. *Br. J. Exp. Pathol.* **51:**434–439.

SUBACUTE AND CHRONIC ENCEPHALITIS AND PRION DISEASES

12

HIV/AIDS

F ive cases of pneumocystis pneumonia in previously healthy homosexual men seen at the University of California at Los Angeles Medical Center and reported in the June 5, 1981, *Morbidity and Mortality Weekly Report* launched the public recognition of AIDS (Gottlieb, 2001). Over 20 years later, the global impact of the causative agent, human immunodeficiency virus (HIV), is enormous and escalating. An estimated 56 million people have been infected, with 20 million deaths and 5.3 million new infections acquired annually (Piot et al., 2001). Michael Gottlieb, the clinician who recognized the first reported cluster of cases, wrote 20 years later "…I still find it unnerving that in 1981 in Los Angeles, I stumbled onto a decades-old African zoonosis that had settled into an ecological niche in the New World." In the same essay, he also echoed the sentiments of many AIDS health care providers in working with persons living with AIDS: "treating patients with AIDS has enabled me to recapture a large measure of the empathy that led me into medicine in the first place" (Gottlieb, 2001).

In retrospect, progress in the understanding of the illness has been rapid. The cellular immune defect was published in the same year as the recognition of the syndrome, the virus was isolated 2 years later, an assay to detect HIV was licensed within 4 years, and the first antiretroviral compound (zidovudine [AZT]) was approved by the Food and Drug Administration within 6 years (Weiss, 2001; Sepkowitz, 2001). From the beginning, it was recognized that AIDS had multiple significant consequences for the nervous system (Snider et al., 1983; Booss and Harris, 1987). The virus was shown to be the cause of a condition then known as AIDS encephalopathy (Shaw et al., 1985). Despite the advances, the first 15 years of the epidemic were witness to great sorrow for the afflicted: frustration with governmental and other agencies and burnout and disillusionment for health care providers.

The period from 1994 to 1996, however, was in many ways a turning point for AIDS care in the western world, with significantly increased survival resulting (Sepkowitz, 2001). Treatment to prevent mother-to-child transmission; the introduction of a powerful class of antiretroviral drugs, the protease inhibitors; the recognition of continued high-level HIV replication throughout the course of the infection; the importance of the plasma viral load for prognosis; and the effectiveness of highly active antiretroviral therapy (HAART), which combined classes of antiretrovirals, all emerged during this time (Weiss, 2001; Sepkowitz, 2001). However, the numbers of persons with the infection in the year 2000 in North America (920,000) and in western Europe (540,000) were miniscule compared to sub-Saharan Africa, where 25.3 million people were infected, and to south and Southeast Asia, where 5.8 million were infected (Piot et al., 2001). A vaccine, simple inexpensive therapy, and political will are badly needed.

While first reported in 1981, evidence for clinical conditions compatible with AIDS in the United States was observed as early as 1979. Virus was present in U.S. donors of plasma for factor VIII from 1977, and antibodies were detected in stored serum from 1959 from the Belgian Congo (Gottlieb, 2001). Molecular studies demonstrated the close relationship to simian retroviruses prevalent in west equatorial Africa. HIV type 2 (HIV-2) and the simian immundeficiency virus from sooty mangabey monkeys have the same genome structure, and the major epidemic form of HIV-1 appears to have arisen from the chimpanzee subspecies *Pan troglodytes troglodytes* (Hahn et al., 2000). Cross-species transmission may have occurred during slaughter of subhuman primates for bush meat. The worldwide dissemination of the human infection has been facilitated by social-political turmoil in Africa, movement of village peoples to the cities of Africa, and greatly expanded international air travel. Korber et al. (2000) estimated that the last common ancestor of the epidemic form of HIV-1 emerged in the period from 1915 to 1941.

THE PATHOGENESIS AND PATHOLOGY OF AIDS

There are two recognized variants of HIV: HIV-1 and HIV-2. Both belong to the lentivirus subgroup of retroviruses, which are, by definition, single-stranded RNA viruses that catalyze the production of a DNA strand complementary to their viral RNA. Some of the proviral DNA then becomes integrated into host cell DNA, though some may also remain unintegrated. The lentivirus subgroup of retroviruses contains viruses that have been known since the mid-20th century to cause disease in sheep and, more recently, in cats and cattle by infecting monocytes and macrophages and causing immunodeficiency. In sheep the lentiviruses also cause the central nervous system (CNS) demyelinating disease visna maedi. The diseases they cause are associated with unusually long incubation periods measured in months or years (Atwood et al., 1993). HIV-1 is responsible for the vast majority of cases of AIDS worldwide. We shall refer to it here as HIV. There are subtypes of HIV that differ markedly in prevalence throughout the world. These are referred to as clades designated by uppercase letters. Thus, clade B is common in North American and European infections, and non-B clades are common in sub-Saharan African infections. HIV-2 seems to be less pathogenic than HIV-1 and is much less common, causing infections largely limited to West and Central Africa.

HIV is acquired through person-to-person contact with infected body fluids that are rich in inflammatory cells—blood, semen, and breast milk—or through mucosal surfaces, broken skin, or intravenous (i.v.) inoculation. In practice, most infection is acquired through sexual contact, i.v. drug use, or blood transfusion, but substantial infection also occurs vertically from mother to infant either during birth or through breast milk. This is the most important cause of pediatric AIDS. In developed countries, male homosexual sex has been a particularly prominent means of transmission of HIV, but in women and in the developing parts of the world, heterosexual sex is the major route of transmission. I.v. drug use, the third most common risk factor for AIDS, accounts for one-fifth of new cases in the United States. In America, men are infected more frequently than women; they account for 70% of new adult cases. However, in sub-Saharan Africa, women are more frequently affected.

The target cells for infection with HIV are lymphocytes and macrophages. Entry of virus into these cells is effected by binding of one of the two envelope proteins of the virus, gp120, to the CD4 receptor on helper lymphocytes and macrophages (Dalgleish et al., 1984; Klatzmann et al., 1984). This step requires the additional presence of chemokine receptors—β chemokine receptor CXCR4 for infection of $CD4^+$ lymphocytes and, principally, the CCR5 cytokine receptor, whose normal ligands are the β chemokines macrophage inflammatory proteins 1α and β and RANTES ("regulation upon activation normal T expressed")—for infection of macrophages (Alkhatib et al., 1996; Deng et al., 1996; Dragic et al., 1996; Feng et al., 1996; Samson et al., 1996). There are distinct strains of HIV that are either T lymphocyte or macrophage tropic, differing in the amino acid sequence of the hypervariable V3 loop of the gp120 protein (De Jong et al., 1992a, 1992b; Fouchier et al., 1992). There are also dual T-cell- and macrophage-tropic strains (Doranz et al., 1996). The macrophage-tropic strains are important in CNS disease. At the time of the primary infection, the virus is usually macrophage tropic, but later on, it is usually T-cell tropic. This switch is thought to reflect the influence both of changes in the virus—mutations allowing survival in the face of CD8-mediated, epitope-specific cytotoxicity—and host factors, including the expression and density of the chemokine receptors mentioned above. Host gene polymorphisms and deletions in genes coding for the chemokine coreceptors for HIV can influence susceptibility to infection and rate of progression to AIDS (Berger et al., 1999).

HIV's genome contains nine different genes: two structural (*gag* and *env*), one enzymatic (*pol*), two regulatory (*tat* and *ref*), and four accessory (*vif, vpu, vpr*, and *ref*). After binding of the virus to the surface of the cell, the outer coat of the virus fuses with that of the cell and the virus enters the cell. The capsid is uncoated, and proviral DNA is synthesized by the action of the reverse transcriptase enzyme (coded by the *pol* gene) and some host components. The DNA is incorporated into the host genome and acts as a template for viral RNA, which can act as mRNA for the synthesis of Gag and Gag-Pol precursor proteins or accessory proteins that are proteolytically cleaved in the cell cytoplasm and are assembled, together with more viral RNA, at the cell membrane (Ratner, 1996). The host cell membrane contributes to the outer coat of the released viral particles. Infection of host cells with HIV leads to production of chemokines, which can attract further uninfected cells into the vicinity, thus supplying a ready source of further host cells.

After initial infection, a viremia rapidly develops, peaking at 3 weeks (Little et al., 1999), during which the virus is distributed to virtually all tissues, particularly important of which are the lymphoid tissue and possibly the brain (Haase, 1999). The viremia then declines and almost disappears as a result of a strong CD8$^+$ T-cell response, which leads to inhibition of viral replication, partly through a direct cytotoxic effect of the CD8$^+$ cells and partly through the stimulation of cytokine and chemokine production, some of the products of which include chemokines that are ligands for the HIV chemokine co-receptors and can substantially inhibit HIV replication in vitro (Chun et al., 2001; Cocchi et al., 1995; Kannagi et al., 1990; Smith et al., 2000; Walker et al., 1986, 1991). There follows a prolonged period of clinical latency in which viral DNA, transcribed from the infecting RNA, is integrated into the DNA of latently infected CD4$^+$ T cells, chiefly in lymph nodes, with probably a small amount of productive infection at these sites in some CD4$^+$ cells in which unintegrated viral DNA can be detected (Ball et al., 1999; Chun et al., 1997a; Hosmalin et al., 2001). Virions at this stage are concentrated in follicular dendritic cells of lymph nodes, which are, however, not productively infected, at least in animal models (Haase, 1999). They are nevertheless capable of transferring virions to uninfected CD4$^+$ T cells. Some of the infected cells in lymph nodes are long-lived CD4$^+$ memory cells with a life span of several years. Because they express only very low levels of viral antigens, they escape immune surveillance. Any T-cell death occurring is initially balanced by further production of T cells. Nevertheless, sooner or later, the CD4$^+$ T-cell population starts to decline, which, in the absence of treatment, ushers in the symptomatic AIDS phase of the infection.

The mechanisms of CD4$^+$ T-cell depletion are complex but include the cytopathic effect of viral replication and apoptosis, which occurs in both infected and uninfected cells (Finkel et al., 1995). Activation of T cells not only enhances replication of HIV in infected cells but may be particularly important in promoting apoptosis (activation-induced cell death), which can occur in CD8$^+$ T cells as well as CD4$^+$ T cells and can probably involve a number of different mechanisms (Badley et al., 1996, 1997; Banda et al., 1992; Gougeon et al., 1993; Hanabuchi et al., 1994; Katsikis et al., 1995; Yang et al., 1997). The destruction of CD8$^+$ T cells, which includes the cells that have been responsible for controlling HIV replication during the presymptomatic phase of infection, coupled with impaired function of CD8$^+$ T cells (Shankar et al., 2000) and depletion of CD4$^+$ T cells (needed to promote CD8$^+$ T-cell function) enables HIV viremia to reappear and increase, leading to yet more CD4$^+$ cell depletion.

This pathogenetic scenario can be considerably modified by anti-HIV therapy. Initial treatment with the single antiretroviral drug AZT, a reverse transcriptase inhibitor, was shown to decrease mortality and opportunistic infections in AIDS (Fischl et al., 1987) but had relatively short-term effectiveness owing to the emergence of resistant strains of HIV under selection pressure from the presence of the antiviral agents. It is effective, however, in reducing the risk of infection to infants of HIV-positive women (Brenner and Wainberg, 2000). The use of two nucleoside reverse transcriptase inhibitors (NRTIs) is more effective than one alone (Hammer et al., 1996), but multidrug resistance is still liable to emerge.

There followed the development of a different type of antiretroviral drug, the non-NRTIs, which inhibited reverse transcriptase by a different mechanism from the earlier drugs. One of these new drugs, combined with two of the conventional reverse transcriptase inhibitors, showed improved efficacy (Floridia et al., 1999; Montaner et al., 1998), which was further enhanced when a compound from a third group of drugs, the protease inhibitors (PIs), was added. Current commonly recommended therapy consists of three drugs of any class in what is termed HAART (highly active antiretroviral therapy) (Hammer et al., 1997) (see section on treatment below). Even in the presence of HAART some viral replication seems to occur, as evidenced by unintegrated HIV DNA in resting T cells (Chun et al., 1997b; Zhang et al., 1999). However, this drug regimen is associated with a more prolonged decline in morbidity and mortality due to AIDS and arrested decline in CD4$^+$ T-cell counts, reduction in plasma HIV load, and immune activation (Detels et al., 1998; Palella et al., 1998). Additional immunological interventions such as administration of interleukin-2 (IL-2) have been attempted (Davey et al., 2000), but the fact remains that despite the improvements in therapy seen in the last decade, eradication of the virus is still not achievable.

SYSTEMIC PATHOLOGY OF AIDS

There are two aspects to the systemic pathology of AIDS in untreated cases. The first reflects the direct and indirect destructive effects of HIV on lymphoid tissue, and the second reflects the diseases that are a consequence of this destruction. These are considered only in outline here. Free-radical damage indicated by low plasma levels of reduced glutathione may also contribute to the manifestations of the disease (Halliwell and Gutteridge, 1999). In untreated cases, lymphoid tissue is severely atrophic and depleted of lymphocytes and follicular dendritic cells. The spleen shows white pulp depletion, hemosiderin deposition, spindle cell proliferation, and perivascular hyalinization and may show infections or malignant complications. There is usually evidence of at least one opportunistic infection, which may be viral, bacterial, fungal, or protozoal. Of the extra-CNS infections, the most common is the lung infection *Pneumocystis carinii* pneumonia. Other common infections are with *Candida* spp. (esophagitis), *Mycobacteria avium-intracellulare* and *Mycobacterium tuberculosis* (lung and lymph nodes), *Cryptococcus neoformans*, cytomegalovirus (CMV) (pneumonitis, hepatitis, adrenalitis), and varicella-zoster virus (VZV) (shingles). Gastrointestinal infections occur with a host of different organisms (e.g., microsporidia, *Cyclospora, Isospora,* cryptosporidia, enteropathogenic bacteria, *Cryptococcus, Leishmania,* and adenovirus). These opportunistic infections display considerable geographic variation, which reflects the local prevalence of the organisms (Lucas, 2002).

Two systemic neoplastic conditions also occur with greatly increased prevalence in AIDS. They are both associated with and probably caused by viral infections. The first is the skin condition Kaposi's sarcoma, which is associated with infection with human herpesvirus 8 (Chang et al., 1994), and the second is B-cell lymphoma, which is associated with another herpesvirus, Epstein-Barr virus (EBV). In HAART-treated cases of AIDS the opportunistic infections can be less evident. Prevalence in cases autopsied in the United States from 1996 to 2000 was lower for many viral, fungal, and parasitic diseases, M. avium-intracellulare, and Kaposi's sarcoma compared to earlier autopsied cases of AIDS (Morgello et al., 2002). A similar pattern of change has been seen in Europe (Jellinger et al., 2000).

NEUROPATHOLOGY OF HIV INFECTION

CNS involvement with HIV was recognized from the start of the epidemic (Snider et al., 1983). Despite the presence of the blood-brain barrier, HIV is capable of reaching the CNS, and in many cases this apparently occurs during the first wave of viremia following primary infection. This was directly demonstrated in a case in which HIV was isolated from the brain 15 days after iatrogenic infection (Davis et al., 1992) and is more indirectly indicated by the demonstration of HIV RNA in cerebrospinal fluid (CSF) in presymptomatic HIV infection (Ellis et al., 2000).

PRE-AIDS NEUROPATHOLOGY IN UNTREATED INDIVIDUALS: LYMPHOCYTIC MENINGITIS

By the time of seroconversion, 8 to 24% of those infected develop acute aseptic meningitis (Boufassa et al., 1995; Schacker et al., 1996). It is thought likely that HIV reaches the CNS and leptomeninges in infected leukocytes, although this has not been conclusively demonstrated. Antibodies to HIV can be detected in CSF in such cases (Janssen et al., 1989). The pathological correlate of this meningitis may be the lymphocytic meningitis reported in up to 74% of HIV-positive, pre-AIDS drug users at autopsy (Bell et al., 1993) (Fig. 12.1). A mild lymphocytic meningitis may also occur in AIDS, but it is less commonly seen then than earlier in the course of HIV infection (Kibayashi et al., 1996). Most of the infiltrating cells are CD8 lymphocytes (Bell

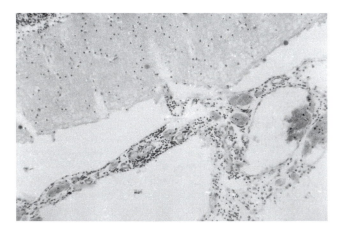

FIGURE 12.1 Sparse lymphocytic cuffing of meningeal veins overlying the cerebellum in a case of pre-AIDS HIV infection in a hemophiliac.

et al., 1993; Tomlinson et al., 1999). However, no clear relationship has been established between this lymphocytic meningitis and HIV or with an opportunistic infection (Budka, 1991; Budka et al., 1991).

Apart from the aseptic meningitis, HIV does not usually cause further neurological problems referable to the CNS until the onset of AIDS. However, peripheral nerve disorders may be manifest in the pre-AIDS phase, most commonly a Guillain-Barré type disorder that probably represents an autoimmune demyelinating polyneuritis triggered by the initial infection (Cornblath et al., 1987; Lipkin et al., 1985). Polymyositis may also rarely occur (Gherardi, 1994). Dorsal root ganglia and nerve roots from subjects with AIDS and/or presymptomatic HIV infection show enhanced expression of major histocompatibility complex (MHC) class II antigens and lymphocytic infiltration (Esiri et al., 1993). A multiple sclerosis (MS)-like illness has also been described (Graber et al., 2000). Some pre-AIDS sufferers show the diffuse pallor of myelin staining described in the section below on HIV encephalitis. Most studies have failed to detect HIV in peripheral nerves in those suffering from neuropathies.

AIDS NEUROPATHOLOGY

CNS disease clinically affected up to two-thirds of cases of AIDS presenting before treatment was available. The proportion of cases with neuropathological changes was even higher—up to 80% or more (Anders et al., 1986; Burns et al., 1991; Lantos et al., 1989).

Opportunistic Infections of the CNS

Approximately half the neuropathology was accounted for by opportunistic infections and lymphoma (which probably results from EBV infection [see above and below]). The infections may be bacterial, fungal, protozoal, or viral. The prevalence of these infections varies geographically and reflects the prevalence of infection generally in the local population. The most common of these infections is toxoplasmosis, which produces a multifocal necrotizing encephalitis with an incidence of 3.9 cases per 100 person-years before the introduction of HAART (Abgrall et al., 2001). Also relatively common are cryptococcal meningitis and, until recently, CMV encephalitis. In all these infections the key diagnostic feature is the presence of the infecting organism. Sensitivity in the search for these organisms is considerably aided by use of PCR, antibodies, and immunocytochemistry. Because of the severe immunodeficiency in AIDS, the lymphocytic infiltrate expected to accompany these infections is mild or absent. Another important CNS infection seen in AIDS is progressive multifocal leukoencephalopathy (PML), whose pathology is described in the following chapter. A general neuropathology textbook should be consulted for the pathology of nonviral CNS infections (e.g., Graham and Lantos, 2002). The other viral infections are described in other chapters in this volume.

Tumors

Primary CNS Lymphoma

Primary CNS lymphoma is a malignant B-cell lymphoma that is 3,600 times more frequent in cases of AIDS (and to a lesser extent in transplant recipients) than in normal subjects (Camilleri-Broet et al., 1997; Cote et al., 1996). As a consequence of the AIDS epidemic, the incidence of this neoplasm has risen more than 10-fold in the United States from 2.5 cases per 10 million population in 1973 to 30 per 10 million population in 1991/1992 (Corn et al., 1997). It is thought to be related to infection with EBV, the genome of which is detectable in 95% of tumors in immunocompromised subjects but in only 0 to 20% of tumors in otherwise normal subjects (Camilleri-Broet et al., 1997; Morgello, 1995; Rooney et al., 1997). Recent treatment with HAART has reduced the prevalence of primary CNS lymphoma in AIDS sufferers (Gates and Kaplan, 2002).

The tumor is usually supratentorial in position and can be multifocal. Lymphomas are often deeply situated and have extensive areas of necrosis and sometimes hemorrhage within them. The border with the surrounding brain is variably well delineated. Histologically, the tumor cells are arranged in diffuse sheets and in perivascular spaces. They are pleomorphic lymphoid cells with frequent mitoses. Ninety-eight percent of primary CNS lymphomas in AIDS patients express B-cell markers, and many express immunoglobulins (Igs). The remainder are T-cell or other rare lymphomas. The conundrum of why a B-cell neoplasm showing close genetic similarities to B cells in lymph node germinal centers grows, usually exclusively within the brain, is as yet unsolved. Secondary lymphomas infiltrating diffusely within the meninges and nerve roots are also relatively common in AIDS patients. These lymphomas infiltrating the meninges do not usually penetrate into the brain itself.

Leiomyoma

Leiomyomas, angioleiomyomas, and leiomyosarcomas are rare smooth-muscle tumors encountered from time to time in the leptomeninges. Several cases of such tumors have been described in people with AIDS, and as with CNS lymphomas, EBV is thought to play a role in their etiology (Brown et al., 1999).

Other HIV-Related CNS Disorders

The other HIV-related CNS conditions to be considered here are HIV encephalitis (HIVE), other nonspecific but related brain pathology (white matter abnormalities, neuronal pathology, vascular pathology), and HIV-associated myelopathy and myelitis.

HIVE

The term "HIV encephalitis" (HIVE) is a morphological one that describes the pathology in the brain that correlates most closely with cognitive impairment in AIDS and is directly attributable to the presence of HIV in the brain (Bell et al., 1996; Wiley and Achim, 1994). However, the clinicopathological correlation of HIVE with dementia in AIDS is not very high. The prevalence of HIVE in untreated AIDS varies in different medical centers, probably reflecting the selection of cases, for example, 28% in New York (Petito et al., 1986), 25% in the United Kingdom (Davies et al., 1997) and 40% in Vancouver (Cornford et al., 1992). In Edinburgh it is more common in i.v. drug users than homosexuals with AIDS (Bell et al., 1996), a point we shall return to later.

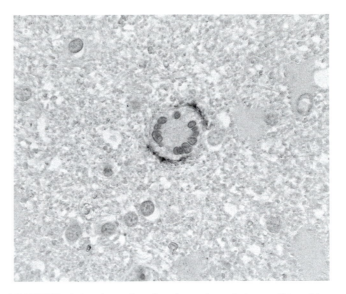

FIGURE 12.2 An isolated multinucleated giant cell in white matter from a case of HIVE. Sparse HIV p24 antigen is visible at the periphery of the cytoplasm. Immunostain for p24 HIV core protein, counterstained with hematoxylin.

No diagnostic features of HIVE are visible macroscopically. The brain may appear slightly swollen, show a mottled gray appearance in the cerebral white matter, or be slightly atrophic, but these are nonspecific changes. The key histological hallmark of HIVE is the presence of multinucleated giant cells expressing macrophage immune markers that can be shown to contain HIV antigens using immunocytochemistry (Fig. 12.2). According to a consensus report (Budka et al., 1991), the term "HIVE" can also be used in the absence of such multinucleated cells if macrophages and microglial cells can be shown immunocytochemically or by in situ hybridization to contain HIV. Multinucleated cells and infected macrophages and microglial cells are found most frequently in cerebral white matter, followed by subcortical gray matter and cerebral cortex. The multinucleated cells may occur in relative isolation (Fig. 12.2), but more often they are accompanied by microglial cells and macrophages forming loose microglial nodules. Multinucleated cells are commonly found in perivascular spaces. Astrocytes show reactive changes and the nonspecific white matter abnormalities described below. Lymphocytic infiltration is absent or mild. Modest neuron loss accompanies HIVE (see below).

It has been difficult to establish the dynamics of HIV infection in the brain during the time course of systemic HIV infection, but it seems likely that any viral presence in the brain remains very slight until the AIDS phase develops. HIVE represents an end point of seemingly relatively unhampered HIV infection of microglial cells and macrophages (Fig. 12.3). In simian immunodeficiency virus infection, it has been shown that perivascular macrophages are infected and allow viral replication in the early stage of infection but that later on replication in the CNS is suppressed until immunodeficiency develops (Williams et al., 2001). HIV proviral DNA has been demonstrated in the brain in presymptomatic HIV infection, but it is very limited in extent in

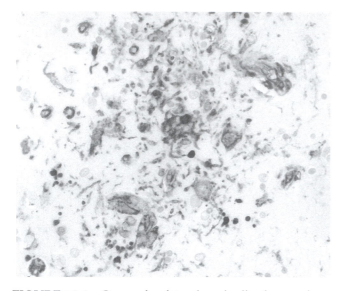

FIGURE 12.3   Group of multinucleated cells of macrophage origin in the basal ganglia of a case of HIVE. *Ricinus communis* agglutinin I immunostain, counterstained with hematoxylin.

comparison with the abundance of virus in HIVE (Gray et al., 1996). In end-stage HIV infection there are many infected monocytes in the circulation that can probably pass relatively easily through a blood-brain barrier that is significantly impaired, thus sowing the seeds for HIVE. The passage of infected leukocytes through the blood-brain barrier is probably assisted by the expression of the adhesion molecules E-selectin and vascular cell adhesion molecule (V-CAM), as these molecules have been detected on infected monocytes in vitro. Furthermore, a soluble factor produced by infected monocytes can induce expression of adhesion molecules on endothelial cells in vitro (Nottet et al., 1996). Disruption of the tight junctions of endothelial cells has been demonstrated in HIVE (Boven et al., 2000; Dallasta et al., 1999), and matrix metalloproteinases capable of degrading components of the blood-brain barrier have been found in CSF in HIVE (Liuzzi et al., 2000).

The pathology of HIVE supports the view that macrophage-tropic virus is essential for HIVE to develop (Power et al., 1995). Some macrophage-tropic variants with alterations in the amino acid sequence of the hypervariable region of the V3 loop of the gp120 protein seem to thrive particularly well in cultured microglial cells in vitro. The presence of such variants in the CNS in AIDS may determine whether HIVE and its clinical correlate, HIV-associated dementia (see below), will develop (Smith et al., 2000; Strizki et al., 1996). Infection of lymphocytes seems to have little direct relevance to HIVE. There is no very convincing evidence that other cells of the CNS are productively infected with HIV, although HIV nucleic acid has been demonstrated in neurons (Bagasra et al., 1996; Nuovo et al., 1994; Torres-Munoz et al., 2001) and astrocytes. Astrocytes can be transiently, but not productively, infected in vitro (Brengel-Pesce et al., 1997; Fiala et al., 1996; Gorry et al., 1998), and the presence of the HIV regulatory genes in astrocytes has been demonstrated in

vivo (Thompson et al., 2001; Tornatore et al., 1994), but it is not clear that they play a role in HIVE.

The observation that HIVE was more prevalent in i.v. drug users than in homosexuals with AIDS (Bell et al., 1993, 1996) has been followed up by studies seeking an explanation for this finding (Arango-Viano, 2001). A higher prevalence of the apolipoprotein E ε2 allele and a lower prevalence of the apolipoprotein E ε3 allele were found in drug users than in homosexuals with AIDS or normal subjects. The drug users with AIDS also had fewer opportunistic infections and higher blood CD4[+] cell counts than homosexuals with AIDS. The explanation for these differences is unclear. The presence of opiate drugs is thought to favor the development of HIVE through enhancement of microglial cell activation, which has been demonstrated in the presence of opiates both in vivo and in vitro (Chao et al., 1994; Peterson et al., 2001; Sharp et al., 2001; Tomlinson et al., 1999).

Nonspecific White Matter Abnormalities

The most frequent abnormality seen in the brain in AIDS is a diffuse alteration of cerebral white matter (Navia et al., 1986a) (Fig. 12.4). This has several components to it: pallor of myelin staining and, in some cases, myelin loss, reactive microglial cells and astrocytes, and vacuolar swelling of myelin (Fig. 12.5). In some cases there is damage to axons with axonal swellings and transections well shown with immunocytochemistry using an antibody to the axonally

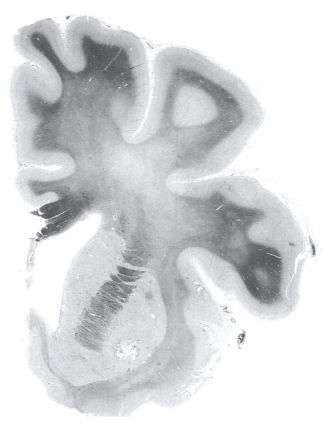

FIGURE 12.4   Diffuse pallor of myelin staining of cerebral white matter in HIVE.

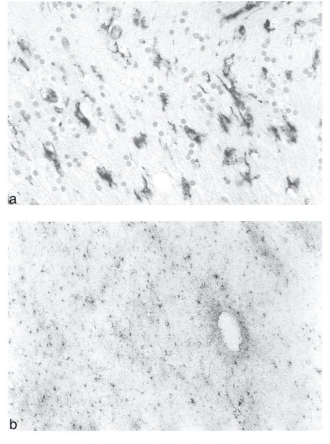

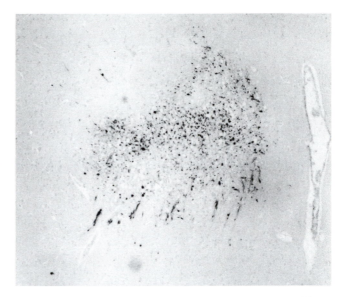

FIGURE 12.6   Focus of β-amyloid precursor-positive (damaged) axons in deep white matter from a case of HIVE. Counterstained with hematoxylin.

FIGURE 12.5   Reactive microglia (a) and astrocytes (b) in HIVE. (a) *Ricinus communis* agglutinin I, (b) GFAP immunostain, both counterstained with hematoxylin.

transported protein β-amyloid precursor protein (Fig. 12.6) (An et al., 1996; Raja et al., 1997). There is indirect evidence of blood-brain barrier abnormalities with extravasation of plasma proteins (Budka et al., 1991; Everall et al., 1999; Power et al., 1993) (Fig. 12.7). These changes show a significant correlation with HIVE, although this condition does not always accompany them.

NEURONAL PATHOLOGY AND ITS PATHOGENESIS

Introduction

Reduced neuronal density of varying extent has been described in HIV infection and AIDS, particularly in frontal cortex (Everall et al., 1991, 1993; Ketzler et al., 1990; Oster et al., 1995; Weis et al., 1993). Pyramidal neurons are most affected. Calbindin and somatostatin-immunoreactive neurons are among those affected (Fox et al., 1997; Masliah et al., 2000). A stereological study of the hippocampus failed to confirm neuron loss there (Korbo and West, 2000). Reduced density of cortical dendrites and synapses in AIDS has also been reported (Everall et al., 1999; Masliah et al., 1997). Neuronal loss and reduced synaptic density as well as HIV viral load and HIVE have been shown to correlate with cognitive impairment in AIDS (Bell et al., 1998; Everall et al.,

1999). Although some of the cognitive difficulties experienced in AIDS are thought to represent subcortical functional impairment in keeping with the predominantly subcortical location of pathology in HIVE (Peavy et al., 1994), the neuronal and synaptic alterations are thought likely to contribute as well.

Much investigation has been devoted to trying to explain how infection of macrophages and microglial cells with HIV leads to synaptic and neuronal loss in AIDS. Apoptosis of neurons is thought to be an important mechanism. Thus, using various immunological or in situ hybridization techniques to detect apoptosis, this form of cell death has been described in neurons and astrocytes in various brain regions in HIV infection (Adamson et al., 1996; Adle-Biassette et al., 1995, 1997, 1999; An et al., 1996; Gelbard et al., 1995; Petito and Roberts, 1995; Thompson et al., 2001). It has been noted in some studies that DNA fragmentation or apoptosis was located near perivascular infiltrates of inflammatory cells (Gelbard et al., 1995) or multinucleated cells (Adle-Biassette et al., 1999; Wiley et al., 2000). However, the fact that neuronal loss affects cortical neurons particularly prominently while most of the other pathology associated with HIV infection is located subcortically suggests that at least some of the mechanisms responsible can operate at a distance.

Studies have established that some HIV proteins— gp120, Tat, and Vpr—can trigger neuronal apoptosis in vitro (Kruman et al., 1998; Muller et al., 1992). The other major class of apoptosis-promoting soluble factors is cytokines and metabolites of arachidonic acid derived from infected and uninfected macrophages and from astrocytes. Likely candidates include tumor necrosis factor alpha (TNF-α) (Talley et al., 1995; Perry et al., 1998), gamma interferon, quinolic acid, and prostaglandins (Achim et al., 1993; Griffin et al., 1994b; Nath et al., 1999; Seilhean et al., 1997; Vitkovic et al., 1995; Wesselingh et al., 1993, 1997; Wilt et al., 1995;

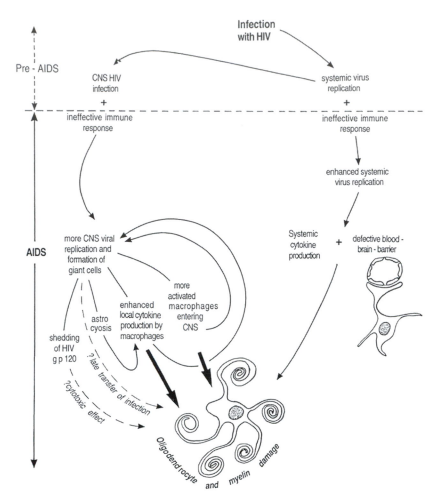

FIGURE 12.7 The suggested pathogenic cascade leading to oligodendrocyte and myelin damage in the CNS in AIDS.

Yeung et al., 1995). Some of these effectors of apoptosis involve excitotoxic mechanisms as well. Reactive oxygen species also likely to play a role include superoxide and nitric oxide, although the evidence for the involvement of the latter is conflicting (Achim et al., 1993; Bagasra et al., 1997; Boven et al., 1999; Griffin et al., 1994b; Nath et al., 1999; Seilhean et al., 1997; Vitkovic et al., 1995; Wesselingh et al., 1993, 1997; Wilt et al., 1995; Yeung et al., 1995). The chemoattractant β chemokines produced by macrophages have a supportive role in recruiting monocytes, which, on activation, produce more of the apoptosis-inducing chemicals. Some recent studies have found correlations between high levels of β chemokines in CSF and cognitive impairment in AIDS (Kelder et al., 1998; Letendre et al., 1999). β-Chemokine receptors that assist entry of HIV into cells are abundantly expressed on microglial cells and macrophages (He et al., 1997; Kitai et al., 2000).

Apart from evidence of neuronal apoptosis, there is evidence of neuronophagia in HIV infection. This suggests that neuronal necrosis also occurs. Whether this is effected by some of the apoptotic mechanisms mentioned above, many of which can produce necrosis as well in vitro, is unclear. In one recent study neuronophagia was detected in 40% of

78 AIDS cases. It was mainly found in the hippocampus, basal ganglia, substantia nigra, and inferior olivary nuclei and was significantly associated with HIVE (Arango-Viano, 2001). It has been suggested that some neuronal populations may be selectively vulnerable to the neurotoxic damage inflicted in HIVE. Some selectivity for cortical pyramidal neurons has already been noted. Other sites of selective damage that have been suggested are the hippocampus (Petito et al., 2001) and the substantia nigra (Itoh et al., 2000)—interestingly, two of the five sites where neuronophagia was relatively commonly noted.

Clinicopathological Correlation in HIV/AIDS Dementia

Although HIVE is generally regarded as the best pathological correlate for HIV/AIDS dementia, the correlation remains a relatively poor one. Quite a number of AIDS sufferers develop dementia in the absence of HIVE or any other pathology to account for it, while others are found at autopsy to have HIVE without having developed dementia (Achim et al., 1994; Glass et al., 1993; Navia et al., 1986a). The severity of HIVE is not readily quantifiable, which may be part of the difficulty in obtaining a good correlation between it and dementia severity, but there may be other factors that are not yet sufficiently taken into account when assessing the full impact of AIDS and HIVE on the brain.

VASCULAR PATHOLOGY

In adults, cerebrovascular pathology has been described in 8 to 34% of autopsy series of AIDS cases (Anders et al., 1986; Berger et al., 1990; Lantos et al., 1989; Mizusawa et al., 1988). The range of vascular pathology seen is wide: sub-arachnoid hemorrhage, subdural hematoma, cerebral infarction, intracerebral hemorrhage, vasculitis, and calcification of the walls of blood vessels. Some subgroups of AIDS sufferers have an increased prevalence of vascular pathology that is often associated with additional disease, such as intracranial hemorrhages in HIV-positive hemophiliacs and drug users (Esiri et al., 1989; Pinto, 1996) and those with thrombocytopenia or CNS lymphoma. Cerebral infarcts, which are usually small and most frequently involve the basal ganglia, are associated with opportunistic infections and nonbacterial endocarditis (Pinto, 1996). Vasculitis is suspected to be immunologically mediated or associated with the presence of VZV.

AIDS-ASSOCIATED MYELOPATHY AND HIV MYELITIS

A myelopathy in those with AIDS was first described in 1985 (Petito et al., 1985). The pathology bears a close resemblance to that of subacute combined degeneration of the cord caused by vitamin B$_{12}$ deficiency. The condition varies widely in reported prevalence in pretreatment autopsy series of AIDS cases: 3% in California (Anders et al., 1986), 17% in Paris (Henin et al., 1992), 20% in Edinburgh (Shepherd et al., 1999), 29% in New York (Petito et al., 1986), and 46% in Baltimore (Dal Pan et al., 1994). It produces progressive spastic leg weakness, ataxic sensory disturbance, and incontinence (see below).

The pathological features of AIDS-associated myelopathy are vacuolation and loss of myelin in the white matter tracts of the posterior and lateral white matter columns with macrophage infiltration of the same regions. The change is maximal at the thoracic level of the cord. Severe cases show axonal degeneration as well. Astrocytosis is occasionally present. The relationship of this condition to HIV infection is not clear; some cases show HIV-containing macrophages and multinucleated cells in the spinal cord, but most do not, and there is no relationship between the abundance of detectable HIV and the severity of the vacuolar changes (Henin et al., 1992; Shepherd et al., 1999; Tan et al., 1995, 1996). When HIV antigens, nucleic acid, or multinucleated cells are present, the term used to describe these features is HIV myelitis. Like HIVE, HIV myelitis was more common in drug users than homosexuals with AIDS in Edinburgh (Shepherd et al., 1999). It is thought likely that products of infiltrating macrophages, whether infected with HIV or not, play a role in the development of AIDS-associated myelopathy. TNF-α levels in CSF are elevated in the condition (Geraci et al., 2000; Tan et al., 1996). The similarity

of HIV myelopathy to subacute combined degeneration of the spinal cord due to vitamin B$_{12}$ deficiency supports the view that a secondary metabolic deficiency involving methyl group metabolism may also play a part. Some metabolites in the transmethylation pathway—S-adenosylmethionine in CSF and methionine in serum—have recently been found to be reduced in HIV myelitis (Di Rocco et al., 2002).

INFLUENCE OF ANTIRETROVIRAL TREATMENT ON THE NEUROPATHOLOGY OF AIDS

There is evidence that the incidence of major neurological disease has declined since the introduction of HAART (Maschke et al., 2000; Sacktor et al., 2001a), and reduced prevalence of HIVE has been found in some (Gray et al., 2001), although not all (Masliah et al., 2000; Ives et al., 2001), recent, antiretroviral drug-treated AIDS cases compared to untreated ones. Clinical remission of AIDS-associated myelopathy after HAART has also been documented (Staudinger and Henry, 2000). Some opportunistic brain infection rates have been reduced during the period of HAART (Abgrall et al., 2001; Masliah et al., 2000). However, there is concern that during the extended life span of those on HAART, there may still be opportunities for other subtle pathological changes to be expressed in more minor but nevertheless troublesome neurological disease (Rausch and Davis, 2001).

CLINICAL FEATURES OF EARLY HIV DISEASE IN THE CNS

Overview

The general medical care of persons with HIV requires knowledge of the protean manifestations of the illness; the complex and evolving patterns of antiretroviral therapy, including side effects, complications, and adherence issues; and prophylaxis, treatment, and suppression of opportunistic infections. Risk factor determination, including candid substance abuse and sexual practices history, with subsequent counseling, is an important part of the management (Table 12.1). Many persons with HIV are also victims of serious mental illness and/or substance addictions, so that they carry double or triple diagnoses. Such individuals are often marginalized by society, with employment and home ownership made difficult. Many end up homeless.

The neurological diagnostic process is based on two fundamental questions, namely, what is the localization, and what is the disease process? Localization depends on the neurological exam, supplemented by neuroimaging and electrodiagnostic testing. In HIV-associated illness, two further major questions are asked concerning the disease process (Table 12.2). First, what is the stage of the HIV disease process as reflected by clinical manifestations, plasma RNA viral load, and CD4 lymphocyte count? Second, what is the nature of the HIV-related pathogenesis: HIV induced, opportunistic process, or medication effect?

TABLE 12.1 HIV risk factors

Sex
  Male sex with males
  Commercial sex workers
  Partners of i.v. drug abusers
  Heterosexual activity, particularly in Africa
Blood and blood products
  i.v. drug abuse
  Transfusion prior to or without HIV screening of blood supply
  Nonsterile instruments and procedures contaminated
    with blood
  Needlestick injuries of health care workers
Birth and infancy
  Peripartum
  Breast-feeding

The clinical stage of the illness is of considerable value in predicting which neurological illnesses the HIV-infected individual will manifest (Table 12.3). While "latency" is inaccurate as a virological characterization, it is a useful term for the clinical stage between the acute HIV syndrome with seroconversion and the emergence of opportunistic infections.

Acute HIV Infection

Acute viral infections can be characterized by definition of the incubation period between exposure and onset of illness, ratio of apparent to inapparent illness, and duration of the acute viral syndrome. HIV is no exception. However, the emphasis on late-stage complications and the complexities of management of antiretroviral therapy have tended to divert attention from the acute illness. Variously called acute HIV-1 infection, seroconversion illness, primary HIV infection, or the acute retroviral syndrome, the illness of acute infection with HIV requires that the clinician have incorporated questions concerning HIV risk behaviors and factors into the evaluation of persons presenting with a "viral syndrome." Neurologically, aseptic meningitis is a common component of the acute syndrome (Schacker et al., 1996). Complications of the acute syndrome include encephalopathy (Carne et al., 1985), neuropathy (Piette et al., 1986), and myelopathy (Denning et al., 1987). Neuropathological review supports an immunopathological mechanism (see above and Gray et al., 1993). However, the issue of

TABLE 12.2 Neurological diagnosis in HIV-related disease

Localization
  Neurological exam
  Neuroimaging
  Electrodiagnostic testing
Nature of disease process
  CSF evaluation
  Clinical stage of HIV infection
    Symptomatic/asymptomatic
    CD4 lymphocyte count
    Serum RNA viral load
  Pathogenesis
    HIV itself
    Opportunistic process
    Medication effect

TABLE 12.3 Clinical stages of HIV infections and representative neurological illnesses

Acute HIV syndrome
  Headache and aseptic meningitis common
  Complex parainfectious processes uncommon
    Probable host-mediated illnesses in the presence of infectious
      virus
    Encephalopathy, leukoencephalopathy, myelopathy, and a
      variety of neuropathies
Clinical latency
  Guillain-Barré-like syndrome
  Mononeuritis multiplex
  Myopathy/myositis
  MS-like illness
Significant immunosuppression (≤200 CD4 lymphocytes)
  Opportunistic processes
    Cryptococcal meningitis
    Cerebral toxoplasmosis
    Primary CNS lymphoma
    PML
    CMV encephalitis and radiculomyelitis
    Neurosyphilis (in all HIV clinical stages)
    CNS TB
    Numerous other organisms
  HIV itself
    Minor cognitive motor complex
    AIDS dementia complex
    Vacuolar myelopathy
    HIV myelitis
    Distal symmetric sensory neuropathy
  Treatment related
    AZT/HIV myopathy
    Nucleoside neuropathy: ddI, ddC, ddT
    Other treatment causes of neuropathy, e.g., dapsone,
      thalidomide, vincristine, and isoniazid
    Myopathy of cholesterol-lowering agents
    Efavirenz-associated confusion
Immune reconstitution
  Syndromes occur secondary to immune restoration with
    HAART, with resultant inflammation
  CNS examples
    Cryptococcal meningitis
    PML
    VZV

pathogenesis is complicated by the presence of replicating virus following infection (Vergis and Mellors, 2000).

Acute HIV infection has been characterized as abrupt in onset and resembling acute mononucleosis (Quinn, 1997). The onset is usually from 2 to 6 weeks following exposure, with 50 to 90% of patients becoming symptomatic (Quinn, 1997). Symptoms include fever, sore throat, nausea, vomiting, diarrhea and weight loss, myalgia and arthralgia, headache, and skin rash (Schacker et al., 1996; Quinn, 1997). Physical findings include pharyngitis, thrush, mucocutaneous ulcerations, adenopathy, postural hypotension, and rashes including macular, maculopapular, vesicular, or pustular types (Schacker et al., 1996; Quinn, 1997). Hecht et al. (2002) found fever and rash to be the most common clinical symptoms. No pathognomic finding or cluster of findings characterizes the acute syndrome to differentiate it from other acute viral syndromes, and the diagnosis is not commonly suspected. Thus, it has been estimated that 90% of acute HIV infections are undiagnosed, of the more than 40,000 new cases that occur annually in the United States (Flanigan and Tashima, 2001).

The diagnosis of the acute retroviral syndrome is established by the finding of viral RNA or p24 antigen in the blood in the absence of antibodies as tested for by enzyme-linked immunosorbent assay (ELISA) and Western blot (Kahn and Walker, 1998; Hecht et al., 2002). Leukopenia with a subsequent increase in the CD8 lymphocyte subset and decrease of the CD4 lymphocyte subset and, on occasion, atypical lymphocytes are found. Whether to treat the acute infection, with which antiretroviral agents, and for what duration remain under investigation (Centers for Disease Control and Prevention, 2002a). In favor of treatment are protection of the developing immune response to facilitate long-term host control mechanisms and lowering the viral set point—that level of sustained viral replication following the acute viral syndrome. However, the duration of therapy with the development of resistance to antiretroviral treatment and the burden of side effects of long-term treatment give cause for concern. Untreated, the syndrome is usually self-limited, resolving in 1 to 2 weeks.

HIV meningitis is commonly found in acute HIV infection. Schacker et al. (1996) found signs and symptoms of aseptic meningitis in 24% (10 of 41) of patients in their study of primary HIV infection. Of 24 patients who had agreed to lumbar puncture, HIV was isolated in 12, and 15 had more than five leukocytes in the CSF. Hence, aseptic meningitis appears to be a component of the acute HIV syndrome in one-half to a majority of patients. In contrast, other neurological syndromes at the time of seroconversion or soon thereafter, while affecting all levels of the nervous system, are rare, and because of their infrequency, general statements of pathogenesis and intervention cannot be made reliably. Review of the original reports of encephalopathy (Carne et al., 1985), myelopathy (Denning et al., 1987), and neuropathy (Piette et al., 1986) each reveal multifocality, compatible with a parainfectious pathogenesis. Thus, case 1 of Carne et al. (1985) had features suggesting cerebral and spinal cord localization; the first described case of Piette et al. (1986) had features of neuropathy and encephalopathy; and the case of myelopathy described by Denning et al. (1987) included comment on mental slowing. Thus, possible multifocal presentations were described in each of these reports, which focused on separate sites of dysfunction in the nervous system.

White Matter Disorders

Jones et al. (1988) described a fatal fulminating leukoencephalopathy in a 31-year-old woman with what appeared to be acute HIV infection. Zones of myelin pallor were seen on pathological examination, with scant cellular reaction and no multinucleated cells, microglial nodules, or necrotic vessels. Occasional nonprominent petechial hemorrhages were observed. The patient was negative to ELISA and Western blot antibody determinations, but CSF obtained at autopsy yielded HIV. Hence, it would appear that the fatal leukoencephalopathy occurred in the setting of acute HIV disease.

Treatment of such cases raises the dilemma of therapeutic immunosuppression to treat a putative immune-mediated complication of an immunosuppressing illness.

Several authors, beginning with Berger et al. (1989), have described MS-like white matter disease occurring in close association to seroconversion. Graber et al. (2000) described the treatment of an aggressive relapsing MS-like illness that developed in an HIV-positive woman who had been seronegative 4 months previously and whose CD4 count was 554/μl. Dexamethasone and methylprednisolone were used in successive attacks, in which remissions occurred. A subsequent attack was treated with high-dose steroid and plasma exchange, followed by daily prednisone and azathioprine therapy, then by azathioprine only. The patient remained in full remission 3 years following the last exacerbation. In a case of acute disseminated encephalomyelitis encountered during primary HIV infection, Narciso et al. (2001) found improvement following the introduction of HAART after high-dose steroids, acyclovir, and Igs had failed. The cases of Graber et al. (2000) and Narciso et al. (2001) offer striking contrasts, one interpreted as MS-like and as having responded to immunotherapy, the other interpreted as acute disseminated encephalomyelitis and as having responded to antiretroviral therapy. In cases with more advanced immunosuppression, the clinician who is considering a course of steroid therapy must be alert to accelerating the immunosuppression associated with HIV infection and the risk of opportunistic infections. Consequently, the antiretroviral regimen and prophylaxis of opportunistic infections would be considered.

Clinical Latency

Since the demonstration of high rates of viral replication and erosion of immune cells' regenerative capacity, there has been an avoidance of characterizing the period of no or minimal symptoms as latent. The periods of evolution of HIV pathogenesis are described in terms of the CD4 count (Vergis and Mellors, 2000). In early disease, the CD4 count is above 500 cells/μl and the only clinical manifestation may be a persistent generalized lymphadenopathy. Patients with midstage disease have CD4 counts of 200 to 500 cells/μl and may be asymptomatic. They may have a variety of non-life-threatening constitutional and/or dermatological complaints or bacterial infections similar to those of immunocompetent individuals (Vergis and Mellors, 2000). Taken together, these two CD4 characterized periods, from over 500 CD4 cells/μl and from 500 to 200 CD4 cells/μl, can be usefully characterized as clinically latent. These periods are certainly not virologically latent. The high rate of HIV replication, with the host attempting control but losing ground at about 75 cells/μl per year (Vergis and Mellors, 2000), has implicit the notion of latent clinical disease awaiting the ultimate weakening of host control. As the CD4 count gradually erodes and the viral load increases, the strategies of antiretroviral therapy are crucial to maintaining immunocompetence and holding life-threatening clinical disease at bay. Mellors et al. (1997) demonstrated that prognosis can be predicted by viral load and CD4 count taken together.

Neurologically, the diseases that emerge during the period of clinical latency, both in the peripheral nervous system and the CNS, resemble those that are immune-mediated rather than those resulting from immunodeficiency. Bell's palsy can be observed. A Guillain-Barré-like syndrome, or acute inflammatory demyelinating polyneuropathy, may be the first indication that HIV is afoot. In the acute form, the Guillain-Barré syndrome is much the same as in non-HIV patients, except that a pleocytosis of 10 to 50 cells/μl is often found (Wulff and Simpson, 1999). Hence, the appellation "cyto-albumino dissociation" does not apply here. There is a relatively rapid evolution of muscle weakness in the extremities with loss of tendon reflexes. The weakness can affect the facial muscles. As in the non-HIV-associated illness, the potential role of CMV must be kept in mind, although this is more likely in the later stages of the HIV-associated illness. Therapy has focused on immunomodulation such as i.v. Ig or plasmapheresis in HIV-associated acute inflammatory demyelinating polyneuropathy (Wulff and Simpson, 1999).

Chronic inflammatory demyelinating polyneuropathy, either progressive or relapsing in form, can also emerge in this stage of HIV infection. Although electrophysiological abnormalities are more prominent than in the acute form (Wulff and Simpson, 1999), the chronic form can present more diagnostic and therapeutic challenges, particularly in association with more advanced CD4 loss. In that setting, immunomodulating therapy with steroids carries the risk of opportunistic infections, so precautions need to be taken (Brew, 2001a). Mononeuritis multiplex may be seen in this clinical stage. It is usually clinically focal but may appear as symmetric with multifocal involvement. Diagnosis rests on electrophysiological demonstration of uni- or multifocality and biopsy demonstration of neural inflammation and/or vasculitis. Hepatitis B (Duffy et al., 1976) or C (Tembl et al., 1999) virus is a potential cause of a vasculitis underlying mononeuritis multiplex. In the presence of more advanced immunosuppression, the role of CMV directly infecting the nerves must be considered. Therapy in the less advanced form may be unnecessary, as spontaneous remissions occur. Absent a spontaneous remission, if the nerve biopsy reveals vasculitis, a short course of prednisone can be considered (Brew, 2001a). Otherwise, modulation of immune function in less advanced disease, as with i.v. Ig, may be attempted.

Yet another perturbation leading to disorders of the peripheral nervous system in this stage of illness is a diffuse infiltrative lymphocytosis syndrome (DILS), in which a CD8 lymphocytosis results in multiple visceral infiltration, including the peripheral nerves (Moulignier et al., 1997). The clinical presentation can mimic other neuropathies seen in HIV-infected persons, that is, often symmetric sensorimotor in type. The typical onset of the neuropathy is subacute in a patient with parotid swelling and sicca syndrome, with a peripheral CD8 count of greater than 1,000 cells/μl (Price, 1998). Treatment consists of HAART and consideration of a course of steroids.

CNS white matter is vulnerable to attack throughout the course of HIV infection. We noted above the rare occurrence of white matter disorders in the acute HIV infection syndrome. The AIDS dementia complex is associated with myelin pallor, and the JC virus (JCV) in PML (progressive multifocal leukoencephalopathy) directly attacks the CNS myelin-producing cell, the oligodendrocyte (see following chapter). Using antibodies to enzymes enriched in oligodendrocytes, Esiri et al. (1991) found an increase in the number of oligodendrocytes associated with evidence of mild damage to myelin, suggesting a reactive response during HIV infection.

Clinically and pathologically, two forms of white matter damage are seen in the clinically latent stage of HIV infection. Berger et al. (1989) reported an MS-like illness occurring early in HIV infection in the presence of positive HIV serology and normal CD4 lymphocyte counts. Thorough study of a biopsy in case 1 of that report revealed demyelination, foamy macrophages, and perivenular lymphocytic infiltrates. No evidence for JCV or HIV-1 was detected in the biopsy. Gray et al. (1991) described two patients with uniphasic neurological illnesses ending fatally 1 or 2 months after onset. Autopsies revealed histopathological features compatible with MS. Brew et al. (1989) commented that they had seen two similar cases and that this complication occurred relatively early in HIV infection. In a more recent case, Geddes et al. (J. F. Geddes, R. T. Flynn, G. H. Vowles, and H. Wheeler, Abstr., *Neuropathol. Appl. Neurobiol.*, **27**:416, 2001) described a 31-year-old HIV-positive man with a CD4 count of 394 cells/μl who presented with multifocal signs of neurological dysfunction. Magnetic resonance imaging (MRI) scans revealed a progressive increase in the number of white matter lesions. Death ensued slightly over 7 weeks into the illness. At autopsy the findings were compatible with either a fulminant form of acute disseminated encephalomyelitis (ADEM) or an acute first attack of MS.

The diagnosis of MS-like leukoencephalitis in HIV rests on the clinical presentation of disability attributable to white matter, often but not necessarily multifocal, discrete white matter lesions on MRI in a patient with evidence of HIV infection. After the acute HIV infection stage, this will include positive HIV serology and variable numbers of CD4 lymphocytes. Counts may be normal, as in case 1 of Berger et al. (1989), somewhat depressed, as in the case of Geddes et al. (2001), or significantly suppressed, such as the 60 CD4 cells/μl recorded in the case of Silver et al. (1997).

Therapy must be tailored to the individual case. The initiation of monotherapy with AZT was associated with disappearance of neurological deficits in the case of Luer et al. (1994). Because the pathogenesis may involve an immune response generated as a result of systemic and/or CNS HIV infection, it would be prudent to maximize antiretroviral therapy and to use a regimen with optimal CNS penetration. Immunosuppressive steroid therapy will need to be considered in severe acute MS-like attacks or in progressive leukoencephalopathic forms. Such therapy must be closely monitored in patients with any degree of immunocompromise, and prophylaxis against opportunistic infections must be considered. For example, methylprednisolone therapy, which had resulted in clinical improvement in case 7 of Berger et al. (1989), had to be discontinued in the face of gram-negative pneumonia. Although we have considered the use of immunomodulatory therapy in HIV-associated relapsing-remitting MS-like disease, the immunomodulatory roles of beta interferon and copolymer 1 in the MS-like illness in HIV infection are unknown (Brew, 2001c).

ANTIRETROVIRAL THERAPY

Following the remarkable clinical, immunological, and virological success of protease inhibitors and HAART regimens in 1996, there has been the realization that HIV cannot be eliminated from the body. This results from virus being "archived" in lymphocytes and sequestered in "sanctuary" compartments, such as CNS, in which antiretroviral penetration is restricted, and from the development of resistant virus. These factors are compounded by the adverse effects of the drugs, inconvenience of the therapy regimens ("pill fatigue"), and drug toxicities leading to impaired adherence on the part of the patient and the need for the provider to find alternative regimens. Hence the "hit hard and early" therapy principle has given way to a search for the best time to treat, that which ideally would give durable virological suppression, maintain immunological function, increase the disease-free interval, improve the quality of life including relative freedom from adverse drug effects, and preserve future treatment options.

Certain guideposts are accepted by many clinicians to start therapy in established HIV infection. First, clinical disease such as thrush or unexplained fever merits initiation of therapy, as does a CD4 count at or below 200 cells/mm^3. Viral loads above 55,000 to 100,000 RNA copies per mm^3 will lead many clinicians to treat. Baseline viral loads at or above 100,000 copies per ml have been shown to be associated with a higher risk for disease progression (Egger et al., 2002). Yet many of the antiretroviral therapy decisions are influenced by patient wishes and understanding and provider experience and preferences. Suffice it to say that the significant treatment decisions should be made by or in close consultation with physicians experienced in the treatment of HIV.

Two HIV treatment guides were updated in 2002 by U.S. panels with some overlapping membership. The updated recommendations of the International AIDS Society-U.S.A. panel (IAS-USA) concisely address the four questions of when to start therapy, which drugs to use, when to change therapy, and which drugs to switch to (Yeni et al., 2002). The Panel on Clinical Practices for Treatment of HIV convened by the U.S. Department of Health and Human Services and the Henry J. Kaiser Family Foundation (HHS-KFF) has published updated recommendations in print (Centers for Disease Control and Prevention, 2002a) and electronic form (http://www.aidsinfo.nih.gov). The electronic source includes access to recommendations for pediatric therapy and prevention of opportunistic infections. Neither the IAS-USA nor the HHS-KFF updated guidelines explicitly address the goal of suppressing HIV replication in the brain or constructing antiviral regimens with optimal CNS penetration. The HHS-KFF panel report includes a series of useful tables dealing with predictions of progression, assays, therapy recommendations, drug characteristics and adverse effects, drug interactions, and perinatal transmission, among other topics. The HHS-KFF panel report also contains comprehensive discussions of HAART-associated

adverse events including abnormalities of fat distribution, bone maintenance, hyperglycemia, hyperlipidemia, lactic acidosis, hepatic stestosis, hepatic toxicity, and skin rashes.

Three types of triple therapy regimens are generally recommended. They are based on two NRTIs (nucleoside reverse transcriptase inhibitors) to which are added a PI, a non-NRTI, or a third NRTI. PIs can be used with low-dose ritonavir, another PI, for its pharmacological boosting effect. These regimens serve to spare one or two drug classes for future use. Use of one drug from each class is reserved for patients with advanced disease at proximate risk of death and/or patients in whom resistance testing indicates that such a regimen is necessary. Because the first regimen has the greatest likelihood of success, adherence reinforcement and therapy monitoring are essential. Repeated contact, such as at weekly intervals, will assist the establishment of a consistent pattern of daily dosing. CD4 and viral load measurements should be performed at 4 weeks, 8 to 12 weeks, and 16 to 24 weeks. Once suppression of virus has occurred, viral load and CD4 counts should be determined every 8 to 12 weeks. The initial response usually results in a reduction of viral load by 90% (1 log$_{10}$) in 4 to 8 weeks with an increase of CD4 cells by 50 cells/mm^3. Once the CD4 count has been sustained at over 200/mm^3 for 3 to 6 months, the risk of opportunistic infections declines and discontinuation of prophylaxis can be considered (Centers for Disease Control and Prevention, 2002b). The duration of viral suppression relates to the degree of viral suppression in the first 8 weeks of therapy. In the case of drug toxicity, not treatment failure, single drug substitutions can be attempted.

Therapy failure can be clinical and/or immunological and/or virological and will require the careful design of an alternative regimen. Drug resistance testing and a thorough drug history will be necessary to construct a regimen with two or three active drugs. On some occasions therapy intensification can be tried by adding one or more drugs, including "mega HAART," in which six or more antiretrovirals are used. Structured treatment interruptions are not recommended outside of clinical trials. Similarly, adjuvant therapy such as IL-2 is advised only in the context of clinical trials.

CLINICAL FEATURES OF AIDS IN THE CNS

Most of the life-threatening conditions in HIV infections occur when the CD4 lymphocyte count has fallen below 200 cells/μl. These include, among numerous other conditions, *P. carinii* pneumonia, toxoplasma cerebritis/abscess, primary CNS lymphoma, PML, *M. avium* complex infection, cryptococcal meningitis, and tuberculosis (TB). This is a phase when the management of the antiretroviral regimen and decisions concerning initiating, discontinuing, or reinitiating prophylactic and suppressive therapy for opportunistic infections requires a well-informed and experienced HIV clinician. Neurological complications are common at all levels of the nervous system (Table 12.4) and reflect all types of pathogenesis—opportunistic infections and neoplasms, direct effects of HIV itself, toxic complications of therapy, and the secondary effects of malnutrition and neural trauma. See chapter 13

TABLE 12.4   Sites of neurological complications during AIDS

Neuropathy
   Distal symmetric sensory neuropathy
   Toxic (treatment-related) neuropathy
   Inflammatory demyelinating polyradiculopathy
   Mononeuritis multiplex
   Nutritional neuropathy
   Pressure palsies
Subacute and chronic meningitis
   Cryptococcal
   TB
   Syphilis
   Other agents
Spinal cord disorders
   Vacuolar myelopathy
   HIV myelitis
   CMV radiculomyelitis
   Other viral (e.g., HSV-2, VZV, HTLV-1) myelitis
   Compression by infection or tumor
   ALS-like disorder
Intracranial space-occupying lesions
   Toxoplasmosis
   Primary intracerebral lymphoma (EBV associated)
   Abscesses of various organisms
Viral disorders of the brain
   HIV cognitive impairment, including the AIDS
      dementia complex
   JCV-PML
   CMV encephalitis and radiculomyelitis
   Other viruses, such as VZV and human herpesvirus 6
Episodic intracranial events
   Seizures
   Vascular events, e.g., meningovascular syphilis

for discussions of CMV encephalitis, radiculomyelitis, and PML. Varicella-zoster infections in AIDS are covered in chapter 9.

It is worth noting that the two conditions that first brought HIV/AIDS to public awareness (Gottlieb, 2001), *P. carinii* pneumonia and Kaposi's sarcoma, are very uncommonly found in the CNS. The five principal intracranial complications in this phase of HIV illness have been AIDS dementia and the minor cognitive/motor complex, cryptococcal meningitis, toxoplasma cerebritis/abscess, PML, and primary CNS lymphoma. Distal symmetric polyneuropathy (DSPN) is common in this phase of the illness (Marra et al., 1998; Schifitto et al., 2002). The clinical finding of brisk knee jerks with absent ankle jerks raises the suspicion that the combination of distal symmetric polyneuropathy and mild vacuolar myelopathy is not uncommon. Immune restoration subsequent to the implementation of HAART has resulted in a significant reduction of intracranial complications of late-stage HIV infection, including toxoplasmosis, cryptococcus, HIV dementia, PML, lymphoma, and CMV (Sacktor et al., 2001a; Kovacs and Masur, 2000). In the following discussions we will focus on certain diagnostic problems in the CNS as they present clinically in adults: subacute meningitis, myelopathy, space-occupying lesions, focal and multifocal cerebral disease, and diffuse cerebral dysfunction. While it might be questioned why certain of these conditions are covered in a work devoted to viral encephalitis, it seemed clinically artificial to limit discussion to viral conditions.

Subacute and Chronic Meningitis

A wide range of infectious agents are associated with subacute or chronic meningitis in non-HIV-infected individuals. The laboratory evaluation of subacute or chronic meningitis is extensive (Coyle, 1999) and may prove to be frustrating in its failure to identify a causative agent. In HIV-infected individuals, *Cryptococcus* infection, TB, and syphilis assume particular importance. Remarkably, while the non-tuberculous M. *avium* complex produces significant disseminated disease in end-stage AIDS, it is a rare cause of chronic meningitis or other CNS disease (Flor et al., 1996). The diagnosis of neurosyphilis is often difficult in the non-HIV-infected patient. In persons coinfected with HIV, the diagnosis may be made even more difficult because syphilis and HIV each cause a mild mononuclear CSF pleocytosis. Katz et al. (1993) studied hospitalized patients with neurosyphilis and found that syphilitic meningitis was more common in HIV-infected patients than in non-HIV-infected patients. The HIV-infected group frequently demonstrated other signs of secondary syphilis, including uveitis and rash. Marra et al. (1996) found that slower resolution of abnormalities in CSF and serum occurred in HIV-infected patients with neurosyphilis treated with standard therapy, in comparison to HIV-negative patients.

TB itself or in coinfection with HIV is a massive global problem, particularly where the public health system has not been established or has broken down. Multiple-drug-resistant strains are a worrisome feature, especially in societies without the resources to implement directly observed therapy with a range of antituberculous medications to prevent resistance. CNS involvement in the HIV-infected individual coinfected with TB is most commonly manifested as tuberculous meningitis. In HIV-infected adults, the majority of patients with TB meningitis have fever, headache, and signs of meningeal irritation (Garcia-Monco, 1999). The disease can be complicated by stroke resulting from vasculitic damage to vessels traversing the subarachnoid space, by hydrocephalitis, or by parenchymal injury, including granulomata and abscesses. Nonetheless, Yechoor et al. (1996) found that the clinical presentations, laboratory abnormalities, and response to therapy in patients with HIV did not differ significantly from TB meningitis in the non-HIV-infected population.

The most common form of subacute meningitis in advanced HIV disease in many regions of the world is cryptococcal. It can cause diffuse cerebral dysfunction. In the pre-HAART era, cryptococcal meningitis developed in 6 to 10% of AIDS patients (Powderly, 1993). Even in the face of therapy, mortality had ranged from 14 to 25%. More recent therapeutic regimens have brought that figure down to slightly under 10% (van der Horst et al., 1997). Cryptococcal meningitis is a basilar meningitis that induces a remarkably mild inflammatory reaction. However, raised intracranial pressure is one of the principal factors associated with mortality (Graybill et al., 2000). Fever, headache, and malaise are common presenting symptoms; however, photophobia and neck stiffness are much less common symptoms (Powderly, 1993). Also less commonly found are symptoms of parenchymal involvement such as lethargy and obtundation, irritability, and behavioral change. Focal signs and seizures are uncommon. Evidence of pulmonary and cutaneous involvement is common. Significant immunosuppression is the rule, with CD4 lymphocyte counts usually below 100 cells/μl.

Presentation of headache and fever in an AIDS patient with a low CD4 count should prompt an urgent evaluation. In the case of cryptococcal meningitis, symptoms may have been present for 2 to 4 weeks. Serum cryptococcal antigen is extremely useful and has been found to be positive in the vast majority of AIDS patients with cryptococcal meningitis (Chuck and Sande, 1989). Neuroimaging, such as CT scanning, prior to lumbar puncture (LP) is advisable to exclude a mass lesion, evidence of raised intracranial pressure, and shift of intracranial contents. The CSF is often bland with minimal or no pleocytosis, elevation of protein, or depression of glucose levels. Opening pressure on LP should be recorded. Specific assays should include cryptococcal culture and antigen determinations, as well as India ink preparations. The latter are more frequently positive than in the non-HIV-infected population (Marra, 1999). The details of therapy of the subacute/chronic meningitides are beyond the scope of this work, and the reader is referred to regularly updated handbooks of HIV management such as that by Bartlett and Gallant (2001). However, it should be emphasized that aggressive management of raised intracranial pressure is crucial in the prevention of mortality.

Myelopathy and Myelitis

Casual observations in clinic waiting rooms and in long-term care facilities for persons with HIV/AIDS reveal gait disorders ranging from limping to the need for a wheelchair. The causes are multiple, including generalized wasting with weakness, musculoskeletal disorders, and neurological conditions, including cerebral, cerebellar, spinal cord, and peripheral nerve disorders. It is not uncommon for two or more disorders causing gait impairment to coexist.

Nonetheless, subacutely or acutely developing spinal cord signs and symptoms merit prompt evaluation for reversible illness. These include localized infection, compressive masses due to infection or tumor, herniated discs, and parenchymal inflammation associated with infection, inflammation, and immune-mediated processes. Evaluation by MRI or myelography will localize masses and reveal thickened meninges or roots and acute cord swelling. MRI with contrast enhancement will allow demonstration of areas of inflammation. In the absence of an anatomic explanation revealed by MRI or myelography, clinical clues for viral myelitis include CMV retinitis and neutrophils in the CSF in the case of CMV radiculomyelitis (see following chapter), shingles within weeks or months preceding VZV myelitis, and anogenital lesions associated with herpes simplex virus type 2 (HSV-2) sacral radiculitis and myelitis. While culture of CSF may occasionally reveal CMV or HSV-2, PCR should be performed. Human T-cell leukemia virus type 1 (HTLV-1) can be a coinfection and cause a subacute/chronic myelopathy. The spectrum of infection-related spinal cord

disease will vary by geographic locality. A prospective study of myelopathy in South Africa revealed coinfection with HTLV-1 in 36% and TB in 18%, as well as VZV, HSV, syphilis, and bilharziasis (Bhigjee et al., 2001).

Vacuolar Myelopathy and HIV Myelitis

In isolation, the clinical picture of vacuolar myelopathy in a patient with advanced HIV is that of a slowly progressive paraparesis with proprioceptive sensory impairment but no spinal cord level for loss of pin sensation. In practice, the condition often merges with the motor difficulties of the AIDS dementia complex and the proprioceptive abnormalities of distal symmetric peripheral neuropathy. Vacuolar myelopathy resembles subacute combined degeneration of the spinal cord but is not associated with decreased serum vitamin B_{12} levels. However, the resemblance has suggested that the vacuolar myelopathy of AIDS may result from a defect of methionine and transmethylation metabolism (Di Rocco et al., 2002). Pathologically, vacuolar myelopathy of AIDS has been distinguished from productive HIV infection of the spinal cord with multinucleated giant cells (Rosenblum et al., 1989), which has been termed HIV myelitis. Clinically and pathologically much less common than vacuolar myelopathy, HIV myelitis is more likely to be associated with a pin sensation loss presenting as a spinal cord level (Brew, 2001b). Measurement of central conduction times in somatosensory evoked potential studies has been advocated to evaluate progression of the vacuolar myelopathy (Tagliati et al., 2000).

The evaluation of the AIDS patient with progressive spinal cord dysfunction is undertaken to find treatable causes of myelopathy. Despite the absence of a clear motor and sensory spinal cord level, as noted above, neuroimaging with MRI or myelography must be performed to exclude spinal cord compression or swelling. Serum studies should include vitamin B_{12} to exclude subacute combined degeneration of the cord and studies for HTLV-1 to seek tropical spastic paraparesis/HTLV-1-associated myelopathy. Studies of the CSF include cytology for malignancy and PCR for CMV, HSV-2, and VZV. Tests to rule out tabes dorsalis, such as fluorescent treponemal antibody absorption in CSF, should be run. The presence of HIV RNA in the spinal fluid provides no discriminative help.

The natural history of vacuolar myelopathy has not been well defined. The general experience has been that of a subacute onset over weeks to months and stabilization after a variable period, again measured in weeks to months (Brew, 2001b). Most clinicians have failed to find a response to antiretroviral therapy or to dietary B_{12} supplements. Based on abnormal transmethylation (Di Rocco et al., 2002), a pilot investigation of treatment with L-methionine has found it to be safe (Di Rocco et al., 1998), and a controlled trial is under way.

ALS-Like Disorder

Starting with Hoffman et al. (1985), occasional cases of amyotrophic lateral sclerosis (ALS)-like presentations have been reported. Review of 1,700 patients with neurological complications of HIV by Moulignier et al. (2001) revealed six cases of ALS-like syndromes. The patients had a mean

TABLE 12.5   Features to assist evaluation of cerebral toxoplasmosis and PCNSL

Feature	Toxoplasmosis	PCNSL
Number of lesions	Often multiple	Often single
Lesions cross midline	Rare	Common
SPECT uptake	Similar to background	Enhanced
CSF PCR for EBV	Negative	Positive

CD4 lymphocyte count of 86/mm^3. Electromyogram evaluation supported the diagnosis, and multifocal conduction block was excluded. Remarkably, clinical stabilization or improvement occurred on HAART, in contrast to the usual inexorable course of ALS. While the pathogenesis is unknown and HIV does not productively infect neurons, the observation is important both as a treatable neurological complication of HIV infection and for potential insights into common pathways in the pathogenesis of motor neuron disease.

Mass Lesions

Space-occupying mass lesions in the CNS can present with headache, altered mental status, varying degrees of depression of level of consciousness, seizures, and focal neurological defects. In AIDS, despite a plethora of potential infectious etiologies (Ammassari et al., 2000; Masliah et al., 2000), the differential diagnosis breaks down to toxoplasma cerebritis/abscess versus primary lymphoma versus other considerations if the first two are excluded. Prompt evaluation begins with neuroimaging. Computed tomography (CT) or MRI with contrast is essential to identify a mass with or without a shift of intracranial contents, to seek evidence of inflammation, and to determine if hydrocephalus is present. If a mass is defined, certain laboratory evaluations will help to distinguish between toxoplasmosis and primary CNS lymphoma (Table 12.5).

In an immunosuppressed AIDS patient with a positive toxoplasma serology, a mass lesion is considered to be toxoplasma until proven otherwise. A therapeutic trial of antitoxoplasma medication for 10 days to 2 weeks is usually attempted. If the patient improves and the lesion is reduced in size, therapy is continued and a presumptive diagnosis is accepted. Without improvement, stereotactic biopsy can be considered for a definitive etiology. Recently, the demonstration that primary CNS lymphomas (PCNSLs) are associated with EBV and that they preferentially take up thalium-201 (Tl-201) in contrast to toxoplasmosis has led some clinicians to advocate a less invasive approach to the diagnosis of intracranial lesions in AIDS. Antinori et al. (1999) found that the combined studies of CSF PCR for EBV and Tl-201 single photon emission CT (SPECT) are highly diagnostic for PCNSL. This approach allows immediate therapy for PCNSL if indicated, supports empiric therapy for toxoplasmosis when PCNSL is not demonstrated, and reserves brain biopsy for those patients who fail empiric antitoxoplasmosis therapy or who have discordant PCR and SPECT results. However, some investigators have not found Tl-201 SPECT to accurately distinguish lymphoma from infections (Licho et al., 2002). While brain biopsy is required in certain cases to provide specific therapy, it is not risk free in HIV-infected individuals. Antinori et al. (2000) found

morbidity of 7.5% and mortality of 3.1%, with a diagnostic sensitivity of 87%. Therapy and suppression of toxoplasmosis is outside the scope of this chapter. The reader is referred to authoritative reviews such as that of Cohen (1999), regularly updated handbooks such as that of Bartlett and Gallant (2001), and the updated recommendations on prophylaxis and suppression of opportunistic infections (Centers for Disease Control and Prevention, 2002b). The approaches to therapy of PCNSL, their outcomes, and problems of interpreting treatment effectiveness are reviewed by Ciacci et al. (1999). Data have been presented indicating that HAART-associated immune recovery enhances survival of AIDS patients with PCNSL (Hoffman et al., 2001).

HIV/AIDS Dementia and the Minor Cognitive Motor Complex

In the day-to-day practice of medicine, there are few diseases that so thoroughly assault a human being as HIV/AIDS. Diarrheal illnesses, pneumonia, skin and mucous membrane conditions, systemic infections, generalized malaise, and wasting may act separately or in concert, on top of which are added the attacks on the nervous system of processes such as cryptococcosis and toxoplasmosis. While many of the conditions can be treated, prevented by prophylaxis, or suppressed, the toxicities, side effects, and sheer number of pills that must be taken on a daily basis are daunting. This occurs for some in the setting of other conditions such as serious mental illness and/or drug abuse, which markedly impair the life skills necessary to cope. Further, some of the conditions under which HIV infection is acquired, such as men having sex with men, or i.v. drug abuse, result in social marginalization. The final indignity, and the one which removes any residual capacity or desire to cope, is the insidious and progressive development of a subcortical dementia. It is a direct effect of HIV infection of the brain and starts with a loss of motivation, slowness of thought, and an incapacity to maintain attention and stay focused. It brings with it slowness and awkwardness in the performance of routine motor tasks such as signing one's name.

The unfolding history of the definition, understanding, and treatment of HIV/AIDS dementia is in itself fascinating. It was recognized from the early days of the AIDS epidemic that a subacute encephalitis occurred in a significant percentage of advanced AIDS patients in the absence of the regular identification of an infectious agent. In contrast to cryptococcal meningitis, cerebral toxoplasmosis, PCNSL, PML, and CMV encephalitis, for which there was precedent, there was no precedent for the dementing subacute encephalitis seen in AIDS. It was logically thought at the start of the epidemic that it too was the result of an opportunistic infection. CMV was viewed by Snider et al. (1983) as a prime candidate based on disseminated CMV found at general postmortem and on microglial nodules, sometimes associated with inclusion-bearing cells, on pathological examination of the brain. However, HIV, then called HTLV-3, was identified in the brains of 15 children and adults with AIDS encephalopathy by Shaw et al. (1985). They pointed out the relationship to visna virus, a lentivirus that causes a chronic infection of lymphocytes and the brain, and suggested that HTLV-3 be further evaluated as the cause of AIDS encephalopathy.

TABLE 12.6 Clinical staging of AIDS dementia complex[a]

Stage	Symptoms
Stage 0	Normal
Stage 0.5	Subclinical. No impairment of activities of daily living (ADLs) or work. "Soft signs" may include positive snout reflex or slowed ocular or extremity movements.
Stage 1	Mild. Some impairment of complex work or ADLs. Neuropsychological testing demonstrates functional impairment.
Stage 2	Moderate. Cannot work or handle the more difficult ADLs, but still manages basic self-care.
Stage 3	Severe. Marked cognitive and/or motor incapacity.
Stage 4	End stage. Nearly vegetative, nearly mute with double incontinence, paraparesis, or quadraparesis.

[a] Adapted from Price and Brew, 1988.

That was accomplished in the laboratory of R. W. Price by Navia et al. (1986a, 1986b). They defined the syndrome as a subcortical dementia in which psychomotor slowing was characteristic, in contrast to cortical dementias in which aphasia and apraxia dominated (Navia et al., 1986b). A complex of cognitive, motor, and behavioral abnormalities was sufficiently distinct to permit clinical recognition. In the companion neuropathology paper (Navia et al., 1986a), they demonstrated that although evidence for CMV was present in almost one-quarter of the specimens, it did not correlate with clinical dementia. Rather, white matter pallor with perivascular infiltrates was found in early cases, and clusters of macrophages and multinucleated giant cells with white matter rarefaction were found in most advanced cases. Thus, using classical clinical and pathological study of a sufficiently large group of patients, Navia et al. (1986a, 1986b) were able to define the clinical and histopathological features of AIDS dementia, and in conjunction with the viral studies of Shaw et al. (1985), establish it as a new entity caused by direct retroviral infection of the brain. Koenig et al. (1986) demonstrated that macrophages and their derivative, multinucleated giant cells, were the cells productively infected with HIV in the CNS.

A word about nosology and clinical scales is in order here, particularly in relation to an understanding of pathogenesis, interventions, and the changing manifestations of the HIV/AIDS epidemic in the HAART era. Snider et al. (1983) referred to a subacute encephalopathy, and Navia et al. (1986a, 1986b) established the term "AIDS dementia complex" based on their clinical-pathological studies. Subsequently, the AIDS Task Force of the American Academy of Neurology (AAN) proposed nomenclature for CNS disorders associated with HIV infection (American Academy of Neurology, 1991). These included HIV-1-associated dementia complex and HIV-associated minor cognitive motor disorder. In the same year, terminology was proposed for the neuropathology of HIV infection of the CNS (Budka et al., 1991). The interchangeability of the terms subacute encephalitis and encephalopathy in the early years was understandable in light of the paucity of inflammation and the fluctuation of the clinical course in some cases. The term "AIDS dementia complex" was adopted by Navia et al. (1986b) to specify the features of the distinctive syndrome that they characterized. The proposed 1991 terminology of the AAN took into account mild and severe manifestations of an HIV-1-associated cognitive and motor disorder. The recognition that a less severe dementing process can occur, so as not to be an AIDS-defining illness, and that it can

occur prior to a diagnosis of AIDS, is important. The argument against splitting the terminology rests most convincingly on the apparent continuity of the pathogenic process. There are clinical scales for the implementation of clinical trials and for the clinical care of individual patients. The reader is referred to the review of Navia and Price (1998) and to that of McArthur and Grant (1998) for complementary perspectives of these issues. The crucial clinical issues are to exclude other treatable conditions, document the presence of acquired abnormalities that have lasted for at least a month, and ascertain that impairment has been present in at least two areas of cognitive function. Those criteria satisfied, progression is assessed from subclinical to end stage (Table 12.6).

Since its recognition in the early days of the epidemic, the incidence and prevalence of AIDS dementia have varied depending on whether clinical or pathological criteria were used and whether the minor cognitive motor disorder was included. Many experts estimated the prevalence of dementia to be 20 to 30% prior to HAART (Brew, 2001d) with an annual incidence rate of 7% (McArthur et al., 1993). That incidence has declined significantly since the introduction of HAART (Maschke et al., 2000; Brew, 2001d). It is of note that the average number of CD4 lymphocytes in patients with AIDS dementia is apparently higher since the HAART era began than before it (Dore et al., 1999; Maschke et al., 2000; Sacktor et al., 2002). Furthermore, Dore et al. (1999) found that there was a proportional increase in AIDS dementia as the AIDS-defining illness relative to other initial AIDS-defining illnesses. These findings suggest that cognitive impairment in AIDS remains a significant problem, a conclusion supported by the findings of Sacktor et al. (2002). Close tracking of the incidence of AIDS dementia will be important for public health planning purposes (Booss, 2000). Antiretroviral therapy may allow sustained improvement and protection of systemic immune function so that opportunistic infections may be held at bay. However, the "slow viral" nature of HIV CNS infection and the associated cognitive impairment may be more resistant to antiviral therapy and result in significant medical management, long-term care, and public health challenges.

Subjectively, the onset of AIDS dementia is usually seen in retrospect by patients as having been insidious in onset. There may be a loss of focus, a loss of interest, or difficulty in completing tasks or following a line of thought. Depression is often considered in the differential diagnosis, as is the malaise associated with systemic infections. Chronic meningitis and other processes in noneloquent regions in the brain should be considered. The early symptoms fall into cognitive, behavioral, and motor categories. The latter can be manifested as a certain clumsiness as well as slowed motor function and some concern about gait. There may be precious little found on neurological exam—perhaps some slowing of finger snapping or tapping, slightly abnormal tracking on extraocular movement evaluation, and discomfort with and poor performance of tandem gait. Occasionally, AIDS dementia may be heralded by the onset of seizures, a movement disorder, florid psychiatric symptoms, or rarely by cerebellar dysfunction. Each of these presentations must be evaluated for a space-occupying lesion and other etiologies on their own merits. For example, a cerebellar degenerative disorder separate from AIDS dementia, clinically manifested by unsteady gait, clumsiness, and slurred speech, has been described in association with HIV infection (Tagliati et al., 1998).

There is a range of patterns in the natural history of cognitive impairment in HIV/AIDS, from apparent stability of mild cognitive impairment through rapid cognitive and motor decline of the AIDS dementia complex over a matter of months. Advanced AIDS dementia may result in global cognitive loss, psychosis, incontinence, and quadraparesis or paraparesis. Prior to the HAART era, Bouwman et al. (1998) found variable progression, including rapidly progressing patients in whom the median survival was 3.3 months but also a significant group with prolonged survival and no progressive deterioration. The advent of HAART is likely to significantly change the long-term course of AIDS dementia with respect to severity, progression, and survival. Hence, it is useful to stage the progression of AIDS dementia, not only for clinical trial purposes, but also for the clinical management of individual cases and for public health and policy purposes. Price and Brew (1988) recommended a scale based on functional disability, commonly identified as the Memorial Sloan Kettering dementia severity scale (Table 12.6), that has found wide acceptance.

There is no single definitive test for HIV/AIDS dementia. One must include the usual strategies for evaluating an early-onset dementia as well as those related to HIV. Causes of chronic encephalopathy secondary to compromised organs such as liver, lungs, and kidneys should be considered. Depression as a cause of pseudodementia or a complication of dementia or depression being mimicked by the subcortical dementia of HIV/AIDS (Brew, 2001d) requires evaluation. Serological tests for syphilis, thyroid function tests, and hemoglobin, B_{12}, and folate analyses should be performed. Chronic medication effect causing blunting of cognition is a risk, particularly in multiply diagnosed and treated individuals. Substance abuse including chronic alcoholism and habitual use of mood-altering drugs complicates the evaluation of HIV/AIDS dementia and may mimic it. Baseline and follow-up neuropsychological testing is essential to define the nature and evolution of the illness and to evaluate the need for supportive services.

CT scans will reveal atrophy in HIV/AIDS dementia, and the MRI will often demonstrate poorly defined white matter changes on T2-weighted scans. More importantly, neuroimaging will serve to exclude space-occupying lesions. The MRI has the distinct advantage of demonstrating the status of the white matter (Fig. 12.8). Although low-intensity

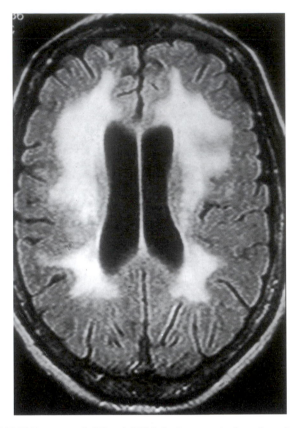

FIGURE 12.8   MRI of HIV leukoencephalopathy. Axial FLAIR image shows symmetric hyperintense diffuse white matter lesions. (Courtesy of Judith Donovan Post, University of Miami School of Medicine.)

lesions on T1-weighted images may differentiate PML (Post et al., 1999), on occasion confusion will arise over the appearance of white matter changes compatible with confluent lesions of PML. In these cases, CSF PCR for JCV is advisable. Despite the considerable contributions of magnetic resonance spectroscopy (MRS) and of functional MRI to the understanding of the pathogenesis of HIV/AIDS dementia, they do not yet have a role in the routine clinical diagnosis and management of HIV/AIDS dementia. Examination of the CSF is important to exclude chronic meningitis such as cryptococcosis and, as noted, to obtain CSF PCR studies for JCV of PML. Because the CSF of neurologically normal HIV-infected persons can contain the virus as well as a mild mononuclear pleocytosis, oligoclonal bands of IgG, and slight protein elevation, these findings must be viewed with caution in the evaluation of neurological abnormalities in the HIV-infected individual (Marshall et al., 1991). Immune activation markers in the CSF, such as beta-2 microglobulin, may help follow progress (Marshall et al., 1991). The place of CSF HIV viral load in routine management is under investigation. Ellis et al. (2002) found that elevated CSF viral load predicted neuropsychological impairment. Because seizures can occur in a low percentage of patients with HIV/AIDS dementia, an electroencephalogram (EEG) may be useful, particularly if there is ambiguity about the nature of episodic alteration of consciousness. Nuwer et al. (1992) found that EEG abnormalities were not simply related to serostatus. Hence abnormalities, particularly focal abnormalities, need to be investigated. Diffuse slowing was found to be related to abnormalities on neuropsychological testing.

There are three categories of therapy for HIV/AIDS dementia: antiretrovirals, symptomatic therapy, and CNS adjunctive treatments. The latter are as yet investigational interventions to block putative toxic factors (Lipton and Gendleman, 1995). As described above, the recommendations of two expert panels in the United States were updated in 2002 (Centers for Disease Control and Prevention, 2002a; Yeni et al., 2002). Neither of the guidelines considered CNS penetration as a criterion for selection of antiretroviral therapy. Whether an antiretroviral regimen should be chosen based on its capacity to penetrate the CNS is an unresolved question (C. M. Marra and J. Booss, Editorial, *Sex. Transm. Infect.* **76**:1–5, 2000). The ultimate answer will depend in large measure on the degree to which endogenous host defenses in the CNS, including microglia, astrocytes, and neurons, can eliminate or suppress HIV replication in the brain, and whether there is a point at which CNS endogenous and non-CNS invasive (lymphocytes and circulating monocytes) immunity is overwhelmed. Where alternative regimens are available to a particular patient, it makes sense to maximize CNS antiretroviral penetration to reduce CNS infection by HIV and thereby reduce the likelihood of developing an HIV dementia or minor cognitive motor disorder.

The onset of HIV/AIDS dementia suggests that a sufficient virus threshold in the brain has been exceeded and/or that a virus-related mechanism has triggered the cascade of toxic mechanisms underlying HIV/AIDS dementia (Lipton and Gendleman, 1995). Nottet et al. (1995) demonstrated that the overexpression of neurotoxins by macrophages can be regulated by astrocytes. Viral control in the CNS, as well as an antiviral barrier function to prevent further delivery of virus to the brain, is needed. AZT achieves CNS penetration, and it has been shown to improve neuropsychological function in the AIDS dementia complex, albeit at high doses (Sidtis et al., 1993). Hence use of the highest tolerable dose of AZT has been recommended as a component of therapy for HIV/AIDS dementia. There is significant variability among the other antiretrovirals in CNS penetration (Enting et al., 1998). That is particularly the case for the protease inhibitors, of which only indinivir achieves satisfactory levels. Consequently, Brew (2001d) recommended that at least two of the following antiretrovirals and preferably more be included in the regimen to treat HIV/AIDS dementia: AZT, stavudine, abacavir, lamivudine, nevirapine, efavirenz, and indinavir.

There is accumulating evidence for the effectiveness of HAART in preventing (e.g., Ferrando et al., 1998; Maschke et al., 2000) and reversing HIV/AIDS dementia. Chang et al. (1999) demonstrated with proton MRS that HAART reverses brain metabolite abnormalities in mild HIV dementia and that some of these changes correlate with the degree of clinical improvement. In a subsequent study, Chang and her colleagues (L. Chang, M. Witt, E. Miller, J. Jovich, N. Amers, W. Zhu, M. Gaiefsky, and T. Ernst, Abstr. *Neurology* 56[Suppl. 3]:A474, 2001). found that CD4 lymphocyte counts and CSF and plasma viral loads improved prior to improvement in neuropsychological tests

and cerebral metabolite concentrations. However, the relative importance of CNS penetration of the antiretrovirals remains moot. Sacktor et al. (2001b) found that HAART regimens containing one or multiple CNS-penetrating antiretroviral agents were equivalent in the treatment of psychomotor slowing. It was pointed out that injury to the blood-brain barrier by HIV may result in greater penetration of the CNS by antiretroviral drugs than would be anticipated.

It remains to consider CNS adjuvant treatments and symptomatic treatment. The pathogenesis of HIV/AIDS dementia is based neither on cell lysis, as in herpes simplex encephalitis, nor on cell- and antibody-mediated tissue injury, as in parainfectious encephalomyelitis, but rather on the toxic effects of viral components and what might be termed the "bystander effects" of host products released in response to viral stimulation. As a consequence, many factors and mechanisms are potential targets of therapeutic intervention, such as blocking the N-methyl-D-aspartate receptors and glutamate-mediated excitotoxic injury. Memantine is under study for this purpose in a double-blind controlled trial of the AIDS Clinical Trials Group (B. A. Navia, C. T. Yiannoutsos, L. Change, C. M. Marra, E. Miller, A. Nath, J. Berger, D. Kolson, G. Schifitto, R. Ellis, D. Simpson, S. Swindells, R. Price, and N. Rajicvc for ACTG 301 Protocol Team, Abstr., *Neurology*, **56**[Suppl. 3]:A474-A475, 2001). Clinical implementation of this or other adjuvant medications such as specific toxic factor antagonists or neuroprotectants will await the results of clinical trials.

With respect to symptomatic treatment, a few general observations can be offered. First, the antiretroviral drugs are characterized by significant drug interactions, particularly the PIs, which are metabolized in the liver by the cytochrome P450 enzymes. Hence, addition of any therapy to an established regimen requires investigation of drug interactions, anticipated changes in blood levels, and potential amplified side effects or toxicity. One of the updated guidelines for HIV treatment has particularly informative tables concerning drug interactions (Centers for Disease Control and Prevention, 2002a). Second, patients with clinical HIV involvement of CNS tend to be exquisitely sensitive to CNS-active medications such as sedatives, antidepressants, and neuroleptics. Consequently, such drugs should be started at low doses and titrated slowly, and careful monitoring should be instituted. Neuroleptics should be chosen for which the risk of extrapyramidal complications are minimized. Psychostimulants such as methylphenidate or dextroamphetamine have been reported to provide improvement in higher cortical functions (Fernandez et al., 1998). While they appear not to have been generally accepted in the treatment of cognitive slowing in HIV/AIDS dementia, they have found a place in the armamentaria of some HIV care providers.

PEDIATRIC AIDS

The discussions above have focused on HIV infections in adults. From the start of the epidemic, it has been recognized that HIV infection of neonates and children presents special features. For a comprehensive consideration of pediatric AIDS, the interested reader is referred to the text of

Pizzo and Wilfert (1998). Pediatric AIDS neuropathology is reported by Dickson et al. (1989). Clinical neurological reviews are given by Belman (1997) and Mintz (1999), and the relationship of cognitive impairment, motor dysfunction, and cortical atrophy to disease progression is reported by Pearson et al. (2000). See also several relevant chapters in Gendleman et al. (1998). Updated treatment recommendations can be found on the U.S. National Institutes of Health AIDS website (http://www.aidsinfo.nih.gov).

REFERENCES

Abgrall, S., C. Rabaud, and D. Costagliola. 2001. Incidence and risk factors for toxoplasmic encephalitis in human immunodeficiency virus-infected patients before and during the highly active antiretroviral therapy era. *Clin. Infect. Dis.* **33:**1747–1755.

Achim, C. L., M. P. Heyes, and C. A. Wiley. 1993. Quantitation of human immunodeficiency virus, immune activation factors, and quinolinic acid in AIDS brains. *J. Clin. Invest.* **91:**2769–2775.

Achim, C. L., R. Wang, D. K. Miners, and C. A. Wiley. 1994. Brain viral burden in HIV infection. *J. Neuropathol. Exp. Neurol.* **53:**284–294.

Adamson, D. C., T. M. Dawson, M. C. Zink, J. E. Clements, and V. L. Dawson. 1996. Neurovirulent simian immunodeficiency virus infection induces neuronal, endothelial, and glial apoptosis. *Mol. Med.* **2:**417–428.

Adle-Biassette, H., Y. Levy, M. Colombel, F. Poron, S. Natchev, C. Keohane, and F. Gray. 1995. Neuronal apoptosis in HIV infection in adults. *Neuropathol. Appl. Neurobiol.* **21:**218–227.

Adle-Biassette, H., L. Wingertsmann, F. J. Authier, H. Kondo, F. Poron, C. Hery, J. Bell, M. Tardieu, R. Gherardi, and F. Gray. 1997. [Neuronal apoptosis in the central and peripheral nervous system in HIV infection.] *Arch. Anat. Cytol. Pathol.* **45:**86–93.

Adle-Biassette, H., F. Chretien, L. Wingertsmann, C. Hery, T. Ereau, F. Scaravilli, M. Tardieu, and F. Gray. 1999. Neuronal apoptosis does not correlate with dementia in HIV infection but is related to microglial activation and axonal damage. *Neuropathol. Appl. Neurobiol.* **25:**123–133.

Alkhatib, G., C. Combadiere, C. C. Broder, Y. Feng, P. E. Kennedy, P. M. Murphy, and E. A. Berger. 1996. CC CKR5: a RANTES, MIP-1alpha, MIP-1beta receptor as a fusion cofactor for macrophage-tropic HIV-1. *Science* **272:**1955–1958.

American Academy of Neurology AIDS Task Force. 1991. Nomenclature and research case definitions for neurologic manifestations of human immunodeficiency virus-type 1 (HIV-1) infection. *Neurology* **41:**778–785.

Ammassari, A., A. Cingolani, P. Pezzotti, A. DeLuca, R. Murri, M. L. Giancola, L. M. Larocca, and A. Antinori. 2000. AIDS-related focal brain lesions in the era of highly active antiretroviral therapy. *Neurology* **55:**1194–1200.

An, S. F., B. Giometto, T. Scaravilli, B. Tavolato, F. Gray, and F. Scaravilli. 1996. Programmed cell death in brains of HIV-1-positive AIDS and pre-AIDS patients. *Acta Neuropathol.* **91:**169–173.

Anders, K. H., W. F. Guerra, U. Tomiyasu, M. A. Verity, and H. V. Vinters. 1986. The neuropathology of AIDS. UCLA experience and review. *Am. J. Pathol.* **124:**537–558.

Antinori, A., G. DeRossi, A. Ammassari, A. Cingolani, R. Murri, D. DiGuida, A. DeLuca, F. Pierconti, T. Tartaglione, M. Scerrati, L. M. Larocca, and L. Ortona. 1999. Value of a combined approach with thallium-201 single-photon emission computed tomography and Epstein-Barr virus DNA polymerase chain reaction in CSF for the diagnosis of AIDS-related primary CNS lymphoma. *J. Clin. Oncol.* **17:**554–560.

Antinori, A., A. Ammassari, R. Luzzati, A. Castagna, R. Maserati, G. Rizzardini, A. Ridolfo, M. Fasan, E. Vaccher, G. Landonio, M. Scerrati, A. Rocca, G. Butti, A. Nicolato, A. Lazzarin, and U. Tirelli for the Gruppo Italiano Cooperative AIDS & Tumori. 2000. Role of brain biopsy in the management of focal brain lesions in HIV infected patients. *Neurology* **54:**993–997.

Arango-Viano, J. C. 2001. The influence of drug use and apolipoprotein E on HIV related disease of the central nervous system. Edinburgh, United Kingdom.

Atwood, W. J., J. R. Berger, R. Kaderman, C. S. Tornatore, and E. O. Major. 1993. Human immunodeficiency virus type 1 infection of the brain. *Clin. Microbiol. Rev.* **6:**339–366.

Badley, A. D., J. A. McElhinny, P. J. Leibson, D. H. Lynch, M. R. Alderson, and C. V. Paya. 1996. Upregulation of Fas ligand expression by human immunodeficiency virus in human macrophages mediates apoptosis of uninfected T lymphocytes. *J. Virol.* **70:**199–206.

Badley, A. D., D. Dockrell, M. Simpson, R. Schut, D. H. Lynch, P. Leibson, and C. V. Paya. 1997. Macrophage-dependent apoptosis of CD4[+] T lymphocytes from HIV-infected individuals is mediated by FasL and tumor necrosis factor. *J. Exp. Med.* **185:**55–64.

Bagasra, O., E. Lavi, L. Bobroski, K. Khalili, J. P. Pestaner, R. Tawadros, and R. J. Pomerantz. 1996. Cellular reservoirs of HIV-1 in the central nervous system of infected individuals: identification by the combination of in situ polymerase chain reaction and immunohistochemistry. *AIDS* **10:**573–585.

Bagasra, O., L. Bobroski, A. Sarker, A. Bagasra, P. Saikumari, and R. J. Pomerantz. 1997. Absence of the inducible form of nitric oxide synthase in the brains of patients with the acquired immunodeficiency syndrome. *J. Neurovirol.* **3:**153–167.

Ball, J. K., R. Curran, W. L. Irving, and A. A. Dearden. 1999. HIV-1 in semen: determination of proviral and viral titres compared to blood, and quantification of semen leukocyte populations. *J. Med. Virol.* **59:**356–363.

Banda, N. K., J. Bernier, D. K. Kurahara, R. Kurrle, N. Haigwood, R. P. Sekaly, and T. H. Finkel. 1992. Crosslinking CD4 by human immunodeficiency virus gp120 primes T cells for activation-induced apoptosis. *J. Exp. Med.* **176:**1099–1106.

Bartlett, J. G., and J. E. Gallant. 2001. *2001–2002 Medical Management of HIV Infection.* Johns Hopkins University, Baltimore, Md.

Bell, J. E., A. Busuttil, J. W. Ironside, S. Rebus, Y. K. Donaldson, P. Simmonds, and J. F. Peutherer. 1993. Human immunodeficiency virus and the brain: investigation of virus load and neuropathologic changes in pre-AIDS subjects. *J. Infect. Dis.* **168:**818–824.

Bell, J. E., Y. K. Donaldson, S. Lowrie, C. A. McKenzie, R. A. Elton, A. Chiswick, R. P. Brettle, J. W. Ironside, and P. Simmonds. 1996. Influence of risk group and zidovudine therapy on the development of HIV encephalitis and cognitive impairment in AIDS patients. *AIDS* **10:**493–499.

Bell, J. E., R. P. Brettle, A. Chiswick, and P. Simmonds. 1998. HIV encephalitis, proviral load and dementia in drug users and homosexuals with AIDS. Effect of neocortical involvement. *Brain* **121:**2043–2052.

Belman, A. L. 1997. Infants, children, and adolescents, p. 223–253. *In* J. R. Berger and R. M. Levy (ed.), *AIDS and the Nervous System*, 2nd ed. Raven Publishers, Philadelphia, Pa.

Berger, J. R., W. A. Sheremata, L. Resnick, S. Atherton, M. A. Fletcher, and M. Norenberg. 1989. Multiple sclerosis-like illness occurring with human immunodeficiency virus infection. *Neurology* **39:**324–329.

Berger, J. R., J. O. Harris, J. Gregorios, and M. Norenberg. 1990.

Cerebrovascular disease in AIDS: a case-control study. *AIDS* **4:**239–244.

Berger, E. A., P. M. Murphy, and J. M. Farber. 1999. Chemokine receptors as HIV-1 coreceptors: roles in viral entry, tropism, and disease. *Annu. Rev. Immunol.* **17:**657–700.

Bhigjee, A. I., S. Madurai, P. L. A. Bill, V. Patel, P. Corr, M. N. Naidoo, W. M. Gopaul, A. Smith, and D. York. 2001. Spectrum of myelopathies in HIV seropositive South African patients. *Neurology* **57:**348–351.

Booss, J. 2000. Chronic-treated HIV: a neurologic disease. *J. Urban Health* **77:**204–212.

Booss, J., and S. A. Harris. 1987. Neurology of AIDS virus infection: a clinical classification. *Yale J. Biol. Med.* **60:**537–543.

Boufassa, F., C. Bachmeyer, N. Carre, C. Deveau, A. Persoz, C. Jadand, D. Sereni, and D. Bucquet. 1995. Influence of neurologic manifestations of primary human immunodeficiency virus infection on disease progression. SEROCO Study Group. *J. Infect. Dis.* **171:**1190–1195.

Bouwman, F. H., R. L. Skolasky, D. Hes, O. A. Selnes, J. D. Glass, T. E. Nance-Sproson, W. Royal, G. J. Dal Pan, and J. C. McArthur. 1998. Variable progression of HIV-associated dementia. *Neurology* **50:**1814–1820.

Boven, L. A., L. Gomes, C. Hery, F. Gray, J. Verhoef, P. Portegies, M. Tardieu, and H. S. Nottet. 1999. Increased peroxynitrite activity in AIDS dementia complex: implications for the neuropathogenesis of HIV-1 infection. *J. Immunol.* **162:**4319–4327.

Boven, L. A., J. Middel, E. C. Breij, D. Schotte, J. Verhoef, C. Soderland, and H. S. Nottet. 2000. Interactions between HIV-infected monocyte-derived macrophages and human brain microvascular endothelial cells result in increased expression of CC chemokines. *J. Neurovirol.* **6:**382–389.

Brengel-Pesce, K., P. Innocenti-Francillard, P. Morand, B. Chanzy, and J. M. Seigneurin. 1997. Transient infection of astrocytes with HIV-1 primary isolates derived from patients with and without AIDS dementia complex. *J. Neurovirol.* **3:**449–454.

Brenner, B. G., and M. A. Wainberg. 2000. The role of antiretrovirals and drug resistance in vertical transmission of HIV-1 infection. *Ann. N.Y. Acad. Sci.* **918:**9–15.

Brew, B. J. 1991. MS-like leukoencephalopathy in HIV-1. *Neurology* **41:**1166.

Brew, B. J. 2001a. Peripheral nerve involvement in early and moderately advanced HIV disease, p. 183–193. *In HIV Neurology.* Oxford University Press, New York, N.Y.

Brew, B. J. 2001b. Common spinal cord diseases, p. 165–173. *In HIV Neurology.* Oxford University Press, New York, N.Y.

Brew, B. J. 2001c. Focal brain disorders in moderately advanced HIV disease: tuberculosis and multiple sclerosis-like illness, p. 111–116. *In HIV Neurology.* Oxford University Press, New York, N.Y.

Brew, B. J. 2001d. AIDS dementia complex, p. 53–90. *In HIV Neurology.* Oxford University Press, New York, N.Y.

Brew, B. J., M. Perdices, P. Darveniza, P. Edwards, B. Whyte, W. J. Burke, R. Garrick, D. O'Sullivan, R. Penny, and D. A. Cooper. 1989. The neurological features of early and "latent" human immunodeficiency virus infection. *Aust. N.Z. J. Med.* **19:**700–705.

Brown, H. G., P. C. Burger, A. Olivi, A. K. Sills, P. A. Barditch-Crovo, and R. R. Lee. 1999. Intracranial leiomyosarcoma in a patient with AIDS. *Neuroradiology* **41:**35–39.

Budka, H. 1991. Neuropathology of human immunodeficiency virus infection. *Brain Pathol.* **1:**163–175.

Budka, H., C. A. Wiley, P. Kleihues, J. Artigas, A. A. Asbury, E.-S. Cho, D. R. Cornblath, M. C. DalCanto, U. DeGirolami, D. Dickson, L. G. Epstein, M. M. Esiri, F. Giangaspero, G.

Gosztonyi, F. Gray, J. W. Griffin, D. Henin, Y. Iwasaki, R. S. Janssen, R. T. Johnson, P. L. Lantos, W. D. Lyman, J. C. McArthur, K. Nagashima, N. Peress, C. K. Petito, R. W. Price, R. H. Rhodes, M. Rosenblum, G. Said, F. Scaravalli, L. R. Sharer, and H. V. Vinters. 1991. HIV associated disease of the nervous system: review of nomenclature and proposal for neuropathology based terminology. *Brain Pathol.* **1:**143–152.

Burns, D. K., R. C. Risser, and C. L. White III. 1991. The neuropathology of human immunodeficiency virus infection. The Dallas, Texas, experience. *Arch. Pathol. Lab. Med.* **115:**1112–1124.

Camilleri-Broet, S., F. Davi, J. Feuillard, D. Seilhean, J. F. Michiels, P. Brousset, B. Epardeau, E. Navratil, K. Mokhtari, C. Bourgeois, L. Marelle, M. Raphael, and J. J. Hauw. 1997. AIDS-related primary brain lymphomas: histopathologic and immunohistochemical study of 51 cases. The French Study Group for HIV-Associated Tumors. *Hum. Pathol.* **28:**367–374.

Carne, C. A., A. Smith, S. G. Elkington, F. E. Preston, R. S. Tedder, S. Sutherland, H. M. Daly, and J. Craske. 1985. Acute encephalopathy coincident with seroconversion for anti-HTLV III. *Lancet* **i:**1206–1208.

Centers for Disease Control and Prevention. 2002a. Guidelines for using antiretroviral agents among HIV-infected adults and adolescents: recommendation of the Panel on Clinical Practices for Treatment of HIV. *Morb. Mortal. Wkly. Rep.* **51(RR-7):**1–56 plus inside covers. Electronic version including additional information and updates at http://www.aidsinfo.nih.gov.

Centers for Disease Control and Prevention. 2002b. Guidelines for preventing opportunistic infections among HIV-infected persons–2002 recommendations of the U.S. Public Health Service and the Infectious Diseases Society of America. *Morb. Mortal. Wkly. Rep.* **51(RR–8):**1–52, plus inside covers. Electronic version including additional information and updates at http://www.aidsinfo.nih.gov.

Chang, Y., E. Cesarman, M. S. Pessin, F. Lee, J. Culpepper, D. M. Knowles, and P. S. Moore. 1994. Identification of herpesvirus-like DNA sequences in AIDS-associated Kaposi's sarcoma. *Science* **266:**1865–1869.

Chang, L., T. Ernst, M. Leonido-Yee, M. Witt, O. Speck, I. Walot, and E. N. Miller. 1999. Highly active antiretroviral therapy reverses brain metabolic abnormalities in mild HIV dementia. *Neurology* **53:**782–789.

Chao, C. C., G. Gekker, W. S. Sheng, S. Hu, M. Tsang, and P. K. Peterson. 1994. Priming effect of morphine on the production of tumor necrosis factor-alpha by microglia: implications in respiratory burst activity and human immunodeficiency virus-1 expression. *J. Pharmacol. Exp. Ther.* **269:**198–203.

Chuck, S. L., and M. A. Sande. 1989. Infections with cryptococcus neoformans in the acquired immunodeficiency syndrome. *N. Engl. J. Med.* **321:**794–799.

Chun, T. W., L. Carruth, D. Finzi, X. Shen, J. A. DiGiuseppe, H. Taylor, M. Hermankova, K. Chadwick, J. Margolick, T. C. Quinn, Y. H. Kuo, R. Brookmeyer, M. A. Zeiger, P. Barditch-Crovo, and R. F. Siliciano. 1997a. Quantification of latent tissue reservoirs and total body viral load in HIV-1 infection. *Nature* **387:**183–188.

Chun, T. W., L. Stuyver, S. B. Mizell, L. A. Ehler, J. A. Mican, M. Baseler, A. L. Lloyd, M. A. Nowak, and A. S. Fauci. 1997b. Presence of an inducible HIV-1 latent reservoir during highly active antiretroviral therapy. *Proc. Natl. Acad. Sci. USA* **94:**13193–13197.

Chun, T. W., J. S. Justement, S. Moir, C. W. Hallahan, L. A. Ehler, S. Liu, M. McLaughlin, M. Dybul, J. M. Mican, and A. S. Fauci. 2001. Suppression of HIV replication in the resting CD4$^+$ T cell reservoir by autologous CD8$^+$ T cells: implications for the development of therapeutic strategies. *Proc. Natl. Acad. Sci. USA* **98**:253–258.

Ciacci, J. D., C. Tellez, J. Von Roenn, and R. M. Levy. 1999. Lymphoma of the central nervous system in AIDS. *Semin. Neurol.* **19**:213–221.

Clifford, D. B. 1999. Opportunistic viral infections in setting of human immunodeficiency virus. *Semin. Neurol.* **19**:185–192.

Cocchi, F., A. L. DeVico, A. Garzino-Demo, S. K. Arya, R. C. Gallo, and P. Lusso. 1995. Identification of RANTES, MIP-1 alpha, and MIP-1 beta as the major HIV-suppressive factors produced by CD8+ T cells. *Science* **270**:1811–1815.

Cohen, B. A. 1999. Neurologic manifestations of toxoplasmosis in AIDS. *Semin. Neurol.* **19**:201–211.

Corn, B. W., S. M. Marcus, A. Topham, W. Hauck, and W. J. Curran, Jr. 1997. Will primary central nervous system lymphoma be the most frequent brain tumor diagnosed in the year 2000? *Cancer* **79**:2409–2413.

Cornblath, D. R., J. C. McArthur, P. G. Kennedy, A. S. Witte, and J. W. Griffin. 1987. Inflammatory demyelinating peripheral neuropathies associated with human T-cell lymphotropic virus type III infection. *Ann. Neurol.* **21**:32–40.

Cornford, M. E., J. K. Holden, M. C. Boyd, K. Berry, and H. V. Vinters. 1992. Neuropathology of the acquired immune deficiency syndrome (AIDS): report of 39 autopsies from Vancouver, British Columbia. *Can. J. Neurol. Sci.* **19**:442–452.

Cote, T. R., A. Manns, C. R. Hardy, F. J. Yellin, and P. Hartge. 1996. Epidemiology of brain lymphoma among people with or without acquired immunodeficiency syndrome. AIDS/Cancer Study Group. *J. Natl. Cancer Inst.* **88**:675–679.

Coyle, P. K. 1999. Overview of acute and chronic meningitis. *Neurol. Clin.* **17**:691–710.

Dal Pan, G. J., J. D. Glass, and J. C. McArthur. 1994. Clinicopathologic correlation of HIV-1 associated vacuolar myelopathy: an autopsy based case-control study. *Neurology* **44**:2159–2164.

Dalgleish, A. G., P. C. Beverley, P. R. Clapham, D. H. Crawford, M. F. Greaves, and R. A. Weiss. 1984. The CD4 (T4) antigen is an essential component of the receptor for the AIDS retrovirus. *Nature* **312**:763–767.

Dallasta, L. M., L. A. Pisarov, J. E. Esplen, J. V. Werley, A. V. Moses, J. A. Nelson, and C. L. Achim. 1999. Blood-brain barrier tight junction disruption in human immunodeficiency virus-1 encephalitis. *Am. J. Pathol.* **155**:1915–1927.

Davey, R. T., Jr., R. L. Murphy, F. M. Graziano, S. L. Boswell, A. T. Pavia, M. Cancio, J. P. Nadler, D. G. Chaitt, R. L. Dewar, D. K. Sahner, A. M. Duliege, W. B. Capra, W. P. Leong, M. A. Giedlin, H. C. Lane, and J. O. Kahn. 2000. Immunologic and virologic effects of subcutaneous interleukin 2 in combination with antiretroviral therapy: a randomized controlled trial. *JAMA* **284**:183–189.

Davies, J., I. P. Everall, S. Weich, J. McLaughlin, F. Scaravilli, and P. L. Lantos. 1997. HIV-associated brain pathology in the United Kingdom: an epidemiological study. *AIDS* **11**:1145–1150.

Davis, L. E., B. L. Hjelle, V. E. Miller, D. L. Palmer, A. L. Llewellyn, T. L. Merlin, S. A. Young, R. G. Mills, W. Wachsman, and C. A. Wiley. 1992. Early viral brain invasion in iatrogenic human immunodeficiency virus infection. *Neurology* **42**:1736–1739.

De Jong, J. J., J. Goudsmit, W. Keulen, B. Klaver, W. Krone, M. Tersmette, and A. de Ronde. 1992a. Human immunodeficiency virus type 1 clones chimeric for the envelope V3 domain differ in syncytium formation and replication capacity. *J. Virol.* **66**:757–765.

De Jong, J. J., A. De Ronde, W. Keulen, M. Tersmette, and J. Goudsmit. 1992b. Minimal requirements for the human

immunodeficiency virus type 1 V3 domain to support the syncytium-inducing phenotype: analysis by single amino acid substitution. *J. Virol.* **66**:6777–6780.

Deng, H., R. Liu, W. Ellmeier, S. Choe, D. Unutmaz, M. Burkhart, P. Di Marzio, S. Marmon, R. E. Sutton, C. M. Hill, C. B. Davis, S. C. Peiper, T. J. Schall, D. R. Littman, and N. R. Landau. 1996. Identification of a major co-receptor for primary isolates of HIV-1. *Nature* **381**:661–666.

Denning, D. W., J. Anderson, P. Rudge, and H. Smith. 1987. Acute myelopathy associated with primary infection with human immunodeficiency virus. *Br. Med. J.* **294**:143–144.

Detels, R., A. Munoz, G. McFarlane, L. A. Kingsley, J. B. Margolick, J. Giorgi, L. K. Schrager, and J. P. Phair. 1998. Effectiveness of potent antiretroviral therapy on time to AIDS and death in men with known HIV infection duration. Multicenter AIDS Cohort Study Investigators. *JAMA* **280**:1497–1503.

Dickson, D. W., A. L. Belman, Y. D. Park, C. Wiley, D. S. Horoupian, J. Llena, K. Kure, W. D. Lyman, R. Morecki, and S. Mitsudo. 1989. Central nervous system pathology in pediatric AIDS: an autopsy study. *APMIS* **97**(Suppl. 8):40–57.

Di Rocco, A., M. Tagliati, F. Danisi, D. Dorfman, J. Moise, and D. M. Simpson. 1998. A pilot study of L-Methionine for the treatment of AIDS-associated myelopathy. *Neurology* **51**:266–268.

Di Rocco, A., T. Bottiglieri, P. Werner, A. Geraci, D. Simpson, J. Godbold, and S. Morgello. 2002. Abnormal cobalamin-dependent transmethylation in AIDS-associated myelopathy. *Neurology* **58**:730–735.

Doranz, B. J., J. Rucker, Y. Yi, R. J. Smyth, M. Samson, S. C. Peiper, M. Parmentier, R. G. Collman, and R. W. Doms. 1996. A dual-tropic primary HIV-1 isolate that uses fusin and the beta-chemokine receptors CKR-5, CKR-3, and CKR-2b as fusion cofactors. *Cell* **85**:1149–1158.

Dore, G. J., P. K. Correll, Y. Li, J. M. Kaldor, D. A. Cooper, and B. J. Brew. 1999. Changes to AIDS dementia complex in the era of highly active antiretroviral therapy. *AIDS* **13**:1249–1253.

Dragic, T., V. Litwin, G. P. Allaway, S. R. Martin, Y. Huang, K. A. Nagashima, C. Cayanan, P. J. Maddon, R. A. Koup, J. P. Moore, and W. A. Paxton. 1996. HIV-1 entry into CD4+ cells is mediated by the chemokine receptor CC-CKR-5. *Nature* **381**:667–673.

Duffy, J., M. D. Lidsky, J. T. Sharp, J. S. Davis, D. A. Person, F. B. Hollinger, and K.-W. Min. 1976. Polyarthritis, polyarteritis and hepatitis B. *Medicine* **55**:19–37.

Egger, M., M. May, G. Chene, A. N. Phillips, B. Ledergerber, F. Dabis, D. Costagliola, A. D'Armino Monforte, F. de Wolf, P. Reiss, J. D. Lundgren, A. C. Justice, S. Staszewski, C. Leport, R. S. Hogg, C. A. Sabin, M. J. Gill, B. Salzberger, J. A. C. Sterne, and the ART Cohort Collaboration. 2002. Prognosis of HIV-infected patients starting highly active antiretroviral therapy: a collaborative analysis of prospective studies. *Lancet* **360**:119–129.

Ellis, R. J., A. C. Gamst, E. Capparelli, S. A. Spector, K. Hsia, T. Wolfson, I. Abramson, I. Grant, and J. A. McCutchan. 2000. Cerebrospinal fluid HIV RNA originates from both local CNS and systemic sources. *Neurology* **54**:927–936.

Ellis, R. J., D. J. Moore, M. E. Childers, S. Letendre, J. A. McCutchan, T. Wolfson, S. A. Spector, K. Hsia, R. K. Heaton, and I. Grant for the HNRC Group. 2002. Progression to neuropsychological impairment in human immunodeficiency virus infection predicted by elevated cerebrospinal fluid levels of human immunodeficiency virus RNA. *Arch. Neurol.* **59**:923–928.

Enting, R. H., R. M. W. Hoetelmans, J. M. A. Lange, D. M.

Burger, J. H. Beijnen, and P. Portegies. 1998. Antiretroviral drugs and the central nervous system. *AIDS* **12:**1941–1955.

Esiri, M. M., F. Scaravilli, P. R. Millard, and J. N. Harcourt-Webster. 1989. Neuropathology of HIV infection in haemophiliacs: comparative necropsy study. *Br. Med. J.* **299:**1312–1315.

Esiri, M. M., C. S. Morris, and P. R. Millard. 1991. Fate of oligodendrocytes in HIV-1 infection. *AIDS* **5:**1081–1088.

Esiri, M. M., C. S. Morris, and P. R. Millard. 1993. Sensory and sympathetic ganglia in HIV-1 infection: immunocytochemical demonstration of HIV-1 viral antigens, increased MHC class II antigen expression and mild reactive inflammation. *J. Neurol. Sci.* **114:**178–187.

Everall, I. P., P. J. Luthert, and P. L. Lantos. 1991. Neuronal loss in the frontal cortex in HIV infection. *Lancet* **337:**1119–1121.

Everall, I., P. Luthert, and P. Lantos. 1993. A review of neuronal damage in human immunodeficiency virus infection: its assessment, possible mechanism and relationship to dementia. *J. Neuropathol. Exp. Neurol.* **52:**561–566.

Everall, I. P., R. K. Heaton, T. D. Marcotte, R. J. Ellis, J. A. McCutchan, J. H. Atkinson, I. Grant, M. Mallory, and E. Masliah. 1999. Cortical synaptic density is reduced in mild to moderate human immunodeficiency virus neurocognitive disorder. HNRC Group. HIV Neurobehavioral Research Center. *Brain Pathol.* **9:**209–217.

Feng, Y., C. C. Broder, P. E. Kennedy, and E. A. Berger. 1996. HIV-1 entry cofactor: functional cDNA cloning of a seventransmembrane, G protein-coupled receptor. *Science* **272:**872–877.

Fernandez, F., F. Adams, J. K. Levy, V. F. Holmes, M. Neidhart, and P. W. A. Mansell. 1998. Cognitive impairment due to AIDS related complex and its response to psychostimulants. *Psychosomatics* **29:**38–46.

Ferrando, S., W. van Gorp, M. McElhiney, K. Goggin, M. Sewell, and J. Rabkin. 1998. Highly active antiretroviral treatment in HIV infection: benefits for neuropsychological function. *AIDS* **12:**F65–F70.

Fiala, M., R. H. Rhodes, P. Shapshak, I. Nagano, O. Martinez-Maza, A. Diagne, G. Baldwin, and M. Graves. 1996. Regulation of HIV-1 infection in astrocytes: expression of Nef, TNF-alpha and IL-6 is enhanced in coculture of astrocytes with macrophages. *J. Neurovirol.* **2:**158–166.

Finkel, T. H., G. Tudor-Williams, N. K. Banda, M. F. Cotton, T. Curiel, C. Monks, T. W. Baba, R. M. Ruprecht, and A. Kupfer. 1995. Apoptosis occurs predominantly in bystander cells and not in productively infected cells of HIV- and SIV-infected lymph nodes. *Nat. Med.* **1:**129–134.

Fischl, M. A., D. D. Richman, M. H. Grieco, M. S. Gottlieb, P. A. Volberding, O. L. Laskin, J. M. Leedom, J. E. Groopman, D. Mildvan, R. T. Schooley, G. C. Jackson, D. T. Durack, D. King, and the AZT Collaborative Working Group. 1987. The efficacy of azidothymidine (AZT) in the treatment of patients with AIDS and AIDS-related complex. A double-blind, placebo-controlled trial. *N. Engl. J. Med.* **317:**185–191.

Flanigan, T., and K. T. Tashima. 2001. Diagnosis of acute HIV infection: it's time to get moving. *Ann. Intern. Med.* **134:**75–77.

Flor, A., J. A. Capdevila, N. Martin, J. Gavalda, and A. Pahissa. 1996. Nontuberculous mycobacterial meningitis: report of two cases and review. *Clin. Infect. Dis.* **23:**1266–1273.

**Floridia, M., R. Bucciardini, D. Ricciardulli, V. Gragola, M. F. Pirillo, L. E. Weimer, C. Tomino, G. Giannini, C. M. Galluzzo, M. Andreotti, A. Cargnel, F. Alberici, B. De Rienzo, F. Leoncini, F. Fiaccadori, D. Francisci, W. Grillone, L. Ortona, M. Piazza, A. Scalzini, E. Nigra, F. Tumietto, and

S. Vella. 1999. A randomized, double-blind trial on the use of a triple combination including nevirapine, a nonnucleoside reverse transcriptase HIV inhibitor, in antiretroviral-naïve diaeresis patients with advance disease. *J. Acquir. Immune Defic. Syndr. Hum. Retrovirol.* **20:**11–19.

Fouchier, R. A., M. Groenink, N. A. Kootstra, M. Tersmette, H. G. Huisman, F. Miedema, and H. Schuitemaker. 1992. Phenotype-associated sequence variation in the third variable domain of the human immunodeficiency virus type 1 gp120 molecule. *J. Virol.* **66:**3183–3187.

Fox, L., M. Alford, C. Achim, M. Mallory, and E. Masliah. 1997. Neurodegeneration of somatostatin-immunoreactive neurons in HIV encephalitis. *J. Neuropathol. Exp. Neurol.* **56:**360–368.

Garcia-Monco, J. D. 1999. Central nervous system tuberculosis. *Neurol. Clin.* **17:**737–759.

Gates, A. E., and L. D. Kaplan. 2002. AIDS malignancies in the era of highly active antiretroviral therapy. *Oncology* **16:**441–451, 456, 459.

Gelbard, H. A., H. J. James, L. R. Sharer, S. W. Perry, Y. Saito, A. M. Kazee, B. M. Blumberg, and L. G. Epstein. 1995. Apoptotic neurons in brains from paediatric patients with HIV-1 encephalitis and progressive encephalopathy. *Neuropathol. Appl. Neurobiol.* **21:**208–217.

Gendleman, H. E., S. A. Lipton, L. Epstein, and S. Swindells. 1998. *The Neurology of AIDS.* Chapman and Hall, New York, N.Y.

Geraci, A., A. Di Rocco, M. Liu, P. Werner, M. Tagliati, J. Godbold, D. Simpson, and S. Morgello. 2000. AIDS myelopathy is not associated with elevated HIV viral load in cerebrospinal fluid. *Neurology* **55:**440–442.

Gherardi, R. K. 1994. Skeletal muscle involvement in HIV-infected patients. *Neuropathol. Appl. Neurobiol.* **20:**232–237.

Glass, J. D., S. L. Wesselingh, O. A. Selnes, and J. C. McArthur. 1993. Clinical-neuropathologic correlation in HIV-associated dementia. *Neurology* **43:**2230–2237.

Gorry, P., D. Purcell, J. Howard, and D. McPhee. 1998. Restricted HIV-1 infection of human astrocytes: potential role of nef in the regulation of virus replication. *J. Neurovirol.* **4:**377–386.

Gottlieb, M. S. 2001. AIDS–past and future. *N. Engl. J. Med.* **344:**1788–1791.

Gougeon, M. L., A. G. Laurent-Crawford, A. G. Hovanessian, and L. Montagnier. 1993. Direct and indirect mechanisms mediating apoptosis during HIV infection: contribution to in vivo CD4 T cell depletion. *Semin. Immunol.* **5:**187–194.

Graber, P., A. Rosemund, A. Probst, and W. Zimmerli. 2000. Multiple sclerosis-like illness in early HIV infection. *AIDS* **14:**2411–2413.

Graham, D. I., and P. L. Lantos. 2002. *Greenfield's Neuropathology.* Arnold, London, United Kingdom.

Gray, F., L. Chimelli, M. Mohr, P. Clavelou, F. Scaravilli, and J. Poirier. 1991. Fulminating multiple sclerosis-like leukoencephalopathy revealing human immunodeficiency virus infection. *Neurology* **41:**105–109.

Gray, F., M. Hurtrel, and B. Hurtrel. 1993. Early central nervous system changes in human immunodeficiency virus (HIV) infection. *Neuropathol. Appl. Neurobiol.* **19:**3–9.

Gray, F., F. Scaravilli, I. Everall, F. Chretien, S. An, D. Boche, H. Adle-Biassette, L. Wingertsmann, M. Durigon, B. Hurtrel, F. Chiodi, J. Bell, and P. Lantos. 1996. Neuropathology of early HIV-1 infection. *Brain Pathol.* **6:**1–15.

Gray, F., H. Adle-Biassette, F. Chretien, G. Lorin de la Grandmaison, G. Force, and C. Keohane. 2001. Neuropathology and neurodegeneration in human immunodeficiency virus infection. Pathogenesis of HIV-induced lesions of the brain, correlations with HIV-associated disorders and modifications according to treatments. *Clin. Neuropathol.* **20:**146–155.

Graybill, J. R., J. Sobel, M. Saag, C. van der Horst, W. Powderly, G. Cloud, L. Riser, R. Hamill, W. Dismukes, and the NIAID Mycoses Study Group and AIDS Cooperative Treatment Group. 2000. Diagnosis and management of increased intracranial pressure in patients with AIDS and cryptococcal meningitis. *Clin. Infect. Dis.* **30:**47–54.

Griffin, J. W., S. L. Wesselingh, D. E. Griffin, J. D. Glass, and J. C. McArthur. 1994a. Peripheral nerve disorders in HIV infection. Similarities and contrasts with CNS disorders. *Res. Publ. Assoc. Res. Nerv. Ment. Dis.* **72:**159–182.

Griffin, D. E., S. L. Wesselingh, and J. C. McArthur. 1994b. Elevated central nervous system prostaglandins in human immunodeficiency virus-associated dementia. *Ann. Neurol.* **35:**592–597.

Haase, A. T. 1999. Population biology of HIV-1 infection: viral and CD4+ T cell demographics and dynamics in lymphatic tissues. *Annu. Rev. Immunol.* **17:**625–656.

Hahn, B. H., G. M. Shaw, K. M. DeCock, and P. M. Sharp. 2000. AIDS as a zoonosis: scientific and public health implications. *Science* **287:**607–614.

Halliwell, B., and J. M. C. Gutteridge. 1999. *Free Radicals in Biology amd Medicine.* Oxford University Press, Oxford, United Kingdom.

Hammer, S. M., D. A. Katzenstein, M. D. Hughes, H. Gundacker, R. T. Schooley, R. H. Haubrich, W. K. Henry, M. M. Lederman, J. P. Phair, M. Niu, M. S. Hirsch, and T. C. Merigan. 1996. A trial comparing nucleoside monotherapy with combination therapy in HIV-infected adults with CD4 cell counts from 200 to 500 per cubic millimeter. AIDS Clinical Trials Group 175 Study Team. *N. Engl. J. Med.* **335:**1081–1090.

Hammer, S. M., K. E. Squires, M. D. Hughes, J. M. Grimes, L. M. Demeter, J. S. Currier, J. J. Eron Jr., J. E. Feinberg, H. H. Balfour Jr., L. R. Deyton, J. A. Chodakewitz, and M. A. Fischl. 1997. A controlled trial of two nucleoside analogues plus indinavir in persons with human immunodeficiency virus infection and CD4 cell counts of 200 per cubic millimeter or less. AIDS Clinical Trials Group 320 Study Team. *N. Engl. J. Med.* **337:**725–733.

Hanabuchi, S., M. Koyanagi, A. Kawasaki, N. Shinohara, A. Matsuzawa, Y. Nishimura, Y. Kobayashi, S. Yonehara, H. Yagita, and K. Okumura. 1994. Fas and its ligand in a general mechanism of T-cell-mediated cytotoxicity. *Proc. Natl. Acad. Sci. USA* **91:**4930–4934.

He, J., Y. Chen, M. Farzan, H. Choe, A. Ohagen, S. Gartner, J. Busciglio, X. Yang, W. Hofmann, W. Newman, C. R. Mackay, J. Sodroski, and D. Gabuzda. 1997. CCR3 and CCR5 are co-receptors for HIV-1 infection of microglia. *Nature* **385:**645–649.

Hecht, F. M., M. P. Busch, B. Rawal, M. Webb, E. Rosenberg, M. Swanson, M. Chesney, J. Anderson, J. Levy, and J. O. Kahn. 2002. Use of laboratory tests and clinical symptoms for identification of primary HIV infection. *AIDS* **16:**1119–1129.

Henin, D., T. W. Smith, U. De Girolami, M. Sughayer, and J. J. Hauw. 1992. Neuropathology of the spinal cord in the acquired immunodeficiency syndrome. *Hum. Pathol.* **23:**1106–1114.

Hoffman, P. M., B. W. Festoff, L. T. Giron, L. C. Hollenbeck, R. M. Garruto, and F. W. Ruscetti. 1985. Isolation of LAV/HTLV III from a patient with amyotrophic lateral sclerosis. *N. Engl. J. Med.* **313:**324–325.

Hoffman, C., S. Tabrizian, E. Wolf, C. Eggers, A. Stoeha, A. Plettenberg, T. Buhk, H.-J. Stellbrink, H.-A. Horst, H. Jager, and T. Rosenkranz. 2001. Survival of AIDS patients with primary central nervous system lymphoma is dramatically improved by HAART-induced immune recovery. *AIDS* **5:**2119–2127.

Hosmalin, A., A. Samri, M. J. Dumaurier, Y. Dudoit, E. Oksenhendler, M. Karmochkine, B. Autran, S. Wain-Hobson, and R. Cheynier. 2001. HIV-specific effector cytotoxic T lymphocytes and HIV-producing cells colocalize in white pulps and germinal centers from infected patients. *Blood* **97:**2695–2701.

Itoh, K., P. Mehraein, and S. Weis. 2000. Neuronal damage of the substantia nigra in HIV-1 infected brains. *Acta Neuropathol.* (Berlin) **99:**376–384.

Ives, N. J., B. G. Gazzard, and P. J. Easterbrook. 2001. The changing pattern of AIDS-defining illnesses with the introduction of highly active antiretroviral therapy (HAART) in a London clinic. *J. Infect.* **42:**134–139.

Janssen, R. S., D. R. Cornblath, L. G. Epstein, J. McArthur, and R. W. Price. 1989. Human immunodeficiency virus (HIV) infection and the nervous system: report from the American Academy of Neurology AIDS Task Force. *Neurology* **39:**119–122.

Jellinger, K. A., U. Setinek, M. Drlicek, G. Bohm, A. Steurer, and F. Lintner. 2000. Neuropathology and general autopsy findings in AIDS during the last 15 years. *Acta Neuropathol.* (Berlin) **100:**213–220.

Jones, J. R., Jr., D. H. Ho, P. Forgacs, L. S. Adelman, M. L. Silverman, R. A. Baker, and P. Locuratolo. 1988. Acute fulminating fatal leucoencephalopathy as the only manifestation of human immunodeficiency virus infection. *Ann. Neurol.* **23:**519–522.

Kahn, J. O., and B. D. Walker. 1998. Acute immunodeficiency virus Type I infection. *N. Engl. J. Med.* **339:**33–39.

Kannagi, M., T. Masuda, T. Hattori, T. Kanoh, K. Nasu, N. Yamamoto, and S. Harada. 1990. Interference with human immunodeficiency virus (HIV) replication by CD8+ T cells in peripheral blood leukocytes of asymptomatic HIV carriers in vitro. *J. Virol.* **64:**3399–3406.

Katsikis, P. D., E. S. Wunderlich, C. A. Smith, and L. A. Herzenberg. 1995. Fas antigen stimulation induces marked apoptosis of T lymphocytes in human immunodeficiency virus-infected individuals. *J. Exp. Med.* **181:**2029–2036.

Katz, D. A., J. R. Berger, and R. C. Duncan. 1993. Neurosyphilis. A comparative study of the effects of infection with human immunodeficiency virus. *Arch. Neurol.* **50:**243–249.

Kelder, W., J. C. McArthur, T. Nance-Sproson, D. McClernon, and D. E. Griffin. 1998. Beta-chemokines MCP-1 and RANTES are selectively increased in cerebrospinal fluid of patients with human immunodeficiency virus-associated dementia. *Ann. Neurol.* **44:**831–835.

Ketzler, S., S. Weis, H. Haug, and H. Budka. 1990. Loss of neurons in the frontal cortex in AIDS brains. *Acta Neuropathol.* **80:**92–94.

Kibayashi, K., A. R. Mastri, and C. S. Hirsch. 1996. Neuropathology of human immunodeficiency virus infection at different disease stages. *Hum. Pathol.* **27:**637–642.

Kitai, R., M. L. Zhao, N. Zhang, L. L. Hua, and S. C. Lee. 2000. Role of MIP-1beta and RANTES in HIV-1 infection of microglia: inhibition of infection and induction by IFNbeta. *J. Neuroimmunol.* **110:**230–239.

Klatzmann, D., E. Champagne, S. Chamaret, J. Gruest, D. Guetard, T. Hercend, J. C. Gluckman, and L. Montagnier. 1984. T-lymphocyte T4 molecule behaves as the receptor for human retrovirus LAV. *Nature* **312:**767–768.

Koenig, S., H. E. Gendleman, J. M. Orenstein, M. C. DalCanto, G. H. Pezeshkpour, M. Yungbluch, F. Janotta, A. Aksamit, M. A. Martin, and A. S. Fauci. 1986. Detection of AIDS virus in macrophages in brain tissue from AIDS patients with encephalopathy. *Science* **233:**1089–1093.

Korber, B., M. Muldoon, J. Theiler, F. Gao, R. Gupta, A. Lapedes, B. H. Hah, S. Wolinsky, and T. Bhattacharya. 2000. Timing the ancestor of the HIV pandemic strains. *Science* **288:**1789–1796.

Korbo, L., and M. West. 2000. No loss of hippocampal neurons in AIDS patients. *Acta Neuropathol.* (Berlin) **99:**529–533.

Kovacs, J. A., and H. Masur. 2000. Prophylaxis against opportunistic infections in patient with human immunodeficiency virus infection. *N. Engl. J. Med.* **342:**1416–1429.

Kruman, I. I., A. Nath, and M. P. Mattson. 1998. HIV-1 protein Tat induces apoptosis of hippocampal neurons by a mechanism involving caspase activation, calcium overload, and oxidative stress. *Exp. Neurol.* **154:**276–288.

Lantos, P. L., J. E. McLaughlin, C. L. Schoitz, C. L. Berry, and J. R. Tighe. 1989. Neuropathology of the brain in HIV infection. *Lancet* **i:**309–311.

Letendre, S. L., E. R. Lanier, and J. A. McCutchan. 1999. Cerebrospinal fluid beta chemokine concentrations in neurocognitively impaired individuals infected with human immunodeficiency virus type 1. *J. Infect. Dis.* **180:**310–319.

Licho, R., N. S. Litofsky, M. Senitko, and M. George. 2002. Inaccuracy of Tl-2001 brain SPECT in distinguishing cerebral infections from lymphoma in patients with AIDS. *Clin. Nucl. Med.* **27:**81–86.

Lipkin, W. I., G. Parry, D. Kiprov, and D. Abrams. 1985. Inflammatory neuropathy in homosexual men with lymphadenopathy. *Neurology* **35:**1479–1483.

Lipton, S. A., and H. E. Gendleman. 1995. Dementia associated with the acquired immunodeficiency syndrome. *N. Engl. J. Med.* **332:**934–940.

Little, S. J., A. R. McLean, C. A. Spina, D. D. Richman, and D. V. Havlir. 1999. Viral dynamics of acute HIV-1 infection. *J. Exp. Med.* **190:**841–850.

Liuzzi, G. M., C. M. Mastroianni, M. P. Santacroce, M. Fanelli, C. D'Agostino, V. Vullo, and Riccio. 2000. Increased activity of matrix metalloproteinases in the cerebrospinal fluid of patients with HIV-associated neurological diseases. *J. Neurovirol.* **6:**156–163.

Lucas, S. 2002. The pathology of HIV infection. *Lepr. Rev.* **73:**64–71.

Luer, W., J. Gerhards, S. Poser, T. Weber, and K. Felgenhauer. 1994. Acute diffuse leukoencephalitis in HIV-1 infection. *J. Neurol. Neurosurg. Psychiatr.* **57:**105–107.

Marra, C. M. 1999. Bacterial and fungal infections in AIDS. *Semin. Neurol.* **19:**177–184.

Marra, C. M., W. T. Longstreth Jr., C. L. Maxwell, and S. A. Lukehart. 1996. Resolution of serum and cerebrospinal fluid abnormalities after treatment of neurosyphilis. Influence of concomitant human immunodeficiency virus infection. *Sex. Transm. Dis.* **23:**184–189.

Marra, C. M., P. Boutin, and A. C. Collier. 1998. Screening for distal sensory peripheral neuropathy in HIV-infected persons in research and clinical settings. *Neurology* **51:**1678–1681.

Marshall, D. W., R. L. Brey, C. A. Butzin, D. R. Lucey, S. M. Abbadessa, and R. N. Boswell. 1991. CSF changes in a longitudinal study of 124 neurologically normal HIV-1-infected US Air Force personnel. *J. Acquir. Immune Defic. Syndr.* **4:**777–781.

Maschke, M., O. Kastrup, S. Esser, B. Ross, U. Hengge, and A. Hufnagel. 2000. Incidence and prevalence of neurological disorders associated with HIV since the introduction of highly active antiretroviral therapy (HAART). *J. Neurol. Neurosurg. Psychiatr.* **69:**376–380.

Masliah, E., R. K. Heaton, T. D. Marcotte, R. J. Ellis, C. A. Wiley, M. Mallory, C. L. Achim, J. A. McCutchan, J. A. Nelson, J. H. Atkinson, and I. Grant. 1997. Dendritic injury is a pathological substrate for human immunodeficiency virus-related cognitive disorders. HNRC Group. The HIV Neurobehavioral Research Center. *Ann. Neurol.* **42:**963–972.

Masliah, E., R. M. DeTeresa, M. E. Mallory, and L. A. Hansen. 2000. Changes in pathological findings at autopsy in AIDS cases for the last 15 years. *AIDS* **14:**69–74.

McArthur, J. C., and I. Grant. 1998. HIV neurocognitive disorders, p. 499–523. *In* H. E. Gendleman, S. A. Lipton, L. Epstein, and S. Swindells (ed.), *The Neurology of AIDS.* Chapman and Hall, New York, N.Y.

McArthur, J. C., D. R. Hoover, H. Bacellar, E. N. Miller, B. A. Cohen, J. T. Becker, N. M. H. Graham, J. H. McArther, O. A. Selnes, L. P. Jacobson, B. R. Vissher, M. Concha, and A. Saah for The Multicenter AIDS Cohort Study. 1993. Dementia in AIDS patients: incidence and risk factors. Multicenter AIDS cohort study. *Neurology* **43:**2245–2252.

Mellors, J. W., A. Munoz, J. V. Giorgi, J. B. Margolick, C. J. Tassolini, P. Gupta, L. A. Kingsley, J. A. Todd, A. J. Saah, R. Detels, J. P. Phair, and C. R. Rinaldo Jr. 1997. Plasma viral load and CD4 lymphocytes as prognostic markers of HIV-1 infection. *Ann. Intern. Med.* **126:**946–954.

Mintz, M. 1999. Clinical features and treatment interventions for human immunodeficiency virus-associated neurologic disease in children. *Semin. Neurol.* **19:**165–176.

Mizusawa, H., A. Hirano, J. F. Llena, and M. Shintaku. 1988. Cerebrovascular lesions in acquired immune deficiency syndrome (AIDS). *Acta Neuropathol.* **76:**451–457.

Montaner, J. S., P. Reiss, D. Cooper, S. Vella, M. Harris, B. Conway, M. A. Wainberg, D. Smith, P. Robinson, D. Hall, M. Myers, and J. M. Lange. 1998. A randomized, double-blind trial comparing combinations of nevirapine, didanosine, and zidovudine for HIV-infected patients: the INCAS Trial. Italy, The Netherlands, Canada and Australia Study. *JAMA* **279:**930–937.

Morgello, S. 1995. Pathogenesis and classification of primary central nervous system lymphoma: an update. *Brain Pathol.* **5:**383–393.

Morgello, S., R. Mahboob, T. Yakoushina, S. Khan, and K. Hague. 2002. Autopsy findings in a human immunodeficiency virus-infected population over 2 decades: influences of gender, ethnicity, risk factors, and time. *Arch. Pathol. Lab. Med.* **126:**182–190.

Moulignier, A., F.-J. Authier, M. Baudrimont, G. Pialoux, L. Belec, M. Polivka, B. Clair, F. Gray, J. Mikol, and R. K. Gherardi. 1997. Peripheral neuropathy in human immunodeficiency virus-infected patients with the diffuse infiltrative lymphocytosis syndrome. *Ann. Neurol.* **41:**438–445.

Moulignier, A., A. Moulonguet, G. Pialoux, and W. Rozenbaum. 2001. Reversible ALS-like disorder in HIV infection. *Neurology* **57:**995–1001.

Muller, W. E., H. C. Schroder, H. Ushijima, J. Dapper, and J. Bormann. 1992. gp120 of HIV-1 induces apoptosis in rat cortical cell cultures: prevention by memantine. *Eur. J. Pharmacol.* **226:**209–214.

Narciso, P., S. Galgani, B. DelGrosso, M. DeMarco, A. DeSantis, P. Balestra, V. Ciapparoni, and V. Tozzi. 2001. Acute disseminated encephalomyelitis as manifestation of primary HIV infection. *Neurology* **57:**1493–1496.

Nath, A., K. Conant, P. Chen, C. Scott, and E. O. Major. 1999. Transient exposure to HIV-1 Tat protein results in cytokine production in macrophages and astrocytes. A hit and run phenomenon. *J. Biol. Chem.* **274:**17098–17102.

Navia, B. A., E.-S. Cho, C. K. Petito, and R. W. Price. 1986a. The AIDS dementia complex: II. Neuropathology. *Ann. Neurol.* **19:**525–535.

Navia, B. A., B. D. Jordan, and R. W. Price. 1986b. The AIDS dementia complex: I. Clinical features. *Ann. Neurol.* **19:**517–524.

Navia, B. A., and R. W. Price. 1998. Clinical and biological features of the AIDS dementia complex, p. 229–240. *In* H. E. Gendelman, J. A. Lipton, L. Epstein, and S. Swindells (ed.), *The Neurology of AIDS.* Chapman and Hall, New York, N.Y.

Nottet, H. S. L. M., M. Jett, C. R. Flanagan, Q.-H. Zhai, Y. Persidsky, A. Rizzino, E. W. Bernton, P. Genis, T. Baldwin, J. Schwartz, C. J. LaBenz, and H. E. Gendelman. 1995. A regulatory role for astrocytes in HIV 1 encephalitis. An overexpression of eicosanoids, platelet activating factor, and tumor necrosis factor by activated HIV-1 infected monocytes is attenuated by primary human astrocytes. *J. Immunol.* **154:**3567–3581.

Nottet, H. S., Y. Persidsky, V. G. Sasseville, A. N. Nukuna, P. Bock, Q.-H. Zhai, L. R. Sharer, R. D. McComb, S. Swindells, C. Soderland, and H. E. Gendelman. 1996. Mechanisms for the transendothelial migration of HIV-1-infected monocytes into brain. *J. Immunol.* **156:**1284–1295.

Nuovo, G. J., J. Becker, M. W. Burk, M. Margiotta, J. Fuhrer, and R. T. Steigbigel. 1994. In situ detection of PCR-amplified HIV-1 nucleic acids in lymph nodes and peripheral blood in patients with asymptomatic HIV-1 infection and advanced-stage AIDS. *J. Acquir. Immune Defic. Syndr.* **7:**916–923.

Nuwer, M. R., E. N. Muller, B. R. Visscher, E. Niedermeyer, J. W. Packwood, L. G. Carlson, P. Satz, W. Jankel, and J. C. McArthur. 1992. Asymptomatic HIV infection does not cause EEG abnormalities: results from the Multicenter AIDS Cohort Study (MACS). *Neurology* **42:**1213–1219.

Oster, S., P. Christoffersen, H. J. Gundersen, J. O. Nielsen, C. Pedersen, and B. Pakkenberg. 1995. Six billion neurons lost in AIDS. A stereological study of the neocortex. *APMIS* **103:**525–529.

Palella, F. J., Jr., K. M. Delaney, A. C. Moorman, M. O. Loveless, J. Fuhrer, G. A. Satten, D. J. Aschman, and S. D. Holmberg. 1998. Declining morbidity and mortality among patients with advanced human immunodeficiency virus infection. HIV Outpatient Study Investigators. *N. Engl. J. Med.* **338:**853–860.

Pearson, D. A., N. M. McGrath, M. Nozyce, S. L. Nichols, C. Raskino, P. Brouwers, M. C. Lifschitz, C. J. Baker, and J. A. Englund. 2000. Predicting HIV disease progression in children using measures of neuropsychological and neurological functioning. Pediatric AIDS Clinical Trials 152 Study Team. *Pediatrics* **106:**E76. Full text at http://www.pediatrics.org.

Peavy, G., D. Jacobs, D. P. Salmon, N. Butters, D. C. Delis, M. Taylor, P. Massman, J. C. Stout, W. C. Heindel, D. Kirson, J. H. Alkinson, J. L. Chandler, I. Grant, and the HNRC Group. 1994. Verbal memory performance of patients with human immunodeficiency virus infection: evidence of subcortical dysfunction. The HNRC Group. *J. Clin. Exp. Neuropsychol.* **16:**508–523.

Perry, S. W., J. A. Hamilton, L. W. Tjoelker, G. Dbaibo, K. A. Dzenko, L. G. Epstein, Y. Hannun, J. S. Whittaker, S. Dewhurst, and H. A. Gelbard. 1998. Platelet-activating factor receptor activation. An initiator step in HIV-1 neuropathogenesis. *J. Biol. Chem.* **273:**17660–17664.

Peterson, P. K., G. Gekker, J. R. Lokensgard, J. M. Bidlack, A. C. Chang, X. Fang, and P. S. Portoghese. 2001. Kappa-opioid receptor agonist suppression of HIV-1 expression in CD4$^+$ lymphocytes. *Biochem. Pharmacol.* **61:**1145–1151.

Petito, C. K., and B. Roberts. 1995. Evidence of apoptotic cell death in HIV encephalitis. *Am. J. Pathol.* **146:**1121–1130.

Petito, C. K., B. A. Navia, E. S. Cho, B. D. Jordan, D. C. George, and R. W. Price. 1985. Vacuolar myelopathy pathologically resembling subacute combined degeneration in patients with the Acquired Immunodeficiency Syndrome. *N. Engl. J. Med.* **312:**874–879.

Petito, C. K., E. S. Cho, W. Lemann, B. A. Navia, and R. W. Price. 1986. Neuropathology of acquired immunodeficiency syndrome (AIDS): an autopsy review. *J. Neuropathol. Exp. Neurol.* **45:**635–646.

Petito, C. K., B. Roberts, J. D. Cantando, A. Rabinstein, and R. Duncan. 2001. Hippocampal injury and alterations in neuronal chemokine co-receptor expression in patients with AIDS. *J. Neuropathol. Exp. Neurol.* **60:**377–385.

Piette, A. M., F. Tusseau, D. Vignon, A. Chapman, G. Parrot, J. Leibowitch, and L. Montagnier. 1986. Acute neuropathy concidents with seroconversion for anti-LAV/HTLV-III. *Lancet* **i:**852.

Pinto, A. N. 1996. AIDS and cerebrovascular disease. *Stroke* **27:**538–543.

Piot, P., M. Bartos, P. D. Ghys, N. Walker, and B. Schwartlander. 2001. The global impact of HIV/AIDS. *Nature* **410:**968–973.

Pizzo, P. A., and M. Wilfert (ed.). 1998. *Pediatric AIDS: the Challenge of HIV Infection in Infants, Children, and Adolescents.* Williams & Wilkins, Baltimore, Md.

Post, M. J. D., C. Yiannoutsos, D. Simpson, J. Booss, D. B. Clifford, B. Cohen, J. K. McArthur, C. D. Hall, and the AIDS Clinical Trials Group, 243 Team. 1999. Progressive multifocal leukoencephalopathy in AIDS: are there any MR findings useful to patient management and predictive of patient survival? *Am J. Neuroradiol.* **20:**1896–1906.

Powderly, W. G. 1993. Cryptococcal meningitis and AIDS. *Clin. Infect. Dis.* **17:**837–842.

Power, C., P. A. Kong, T. O. Crawford, S. Wesselingh, J. D. Glass, J. C. McArthur, and B. D. Trapp. 1993. Cerebral white matter changes in acquired immunodeficiency syndrome dementia: alterations of the blood-brain barrier. *Ann. Neurol.* **34:**339–350.

Power, C., J. C. McArthur, R. T. Johnson, D. E. Griffin, J. D. Glass, R. Dewey, R., and B. Chesebro. 1995. Distinct HIV-1 env sequences are associated with neurotropism and neurovirulence. *Curr. Top. Microbiol. Immunol.* **202:**89–104.

Price, R. W. 1998. Neuropathy complicating diffuse infiltrative lymphocytosis. *Lancet* **352:**592–594.

Price, R. W., and B. J. Brew. 1988. The AIDS dementia complex. *J. Infect. Dis.* **158:**1079–1083.

Quinn, T. C. 1997. Acute primary HIV infection. *JAMA* **278:**58–62.

Raja, F., F. E. Sherriff, C. S. Morris, L. R. Bridges, and M. M. Esiri. 1997. Cerebral white matter damage in HIV infection demonstrated using beta-amyloid precursor protein immunoreactivity. *Acta Neuropathol.* (Berlin) **93:**184–189.

Ratner, L. 1996. Genetic organization of HIV. *In* S. Gupta (ed.), *Immunology of HIV.* Plenum, New York, N.Y.

Rausch, D. M., and M. R. Davis. 2001. HIV in the CNS: pathogenic relationships to systemic HIV disease and other CNS diseases. *J. Neurovirol.* **7:**85–96.

Rooney, C. M., C. A. Smith, and H. E. Heslop. 1997. Control of virus-induced lymphoproliferation: Epstein-Barr virus-induced lymphoproliferation and host immunity. *Mol. Med. Today* **3:**24–30.

Rosenblum, M., A. C. Scheck, K. Cronin, B. J. Brew, A. Khan, M. Paul, and R. W. Price. 1989. Dissociation of AIDS-related vacuolar myelopathy and productive HIV-1 infection of the spinal cord. *Neurology* **39:**892–896.

Sacktor, N., R. H. Lyles, R. Skolasky, C. Kleeberger, O. A. Selnes, E. N. Miller, J. T. Becker, B. Cohen, J. C. McArthur, and the Multicenter AIDS Cohort Study. 2001a. HIV-associated neurologic disease incidence changes: multicenter AIDS cohort study, 1990–1998. *Neurology* **56:**257–260.

Sacktor, N., P. M. Tarwater, R. L. Skolasky, J. C. McArthur, O. A. Selnes, J. Becker, B. Cohen, and E. N. Miller for the

Multicenter AIDS Cohort Study (MACS). 2001b. CSF antiretroviral drug penetrance and the treatment of HIV-associated psychomotor slowing. *Neurology* **53**:782–789.

Sacktor, N., M. P. McDermott, K. Marder, G. Schifitto, O. A. Selnes, J. C. McArthur, Y. Stern, S. Albert, D. Palumbo, K. Kieburtz, J. A. DeMarcaida, B. Cohen, and K. L. Epstein. 2002. HIV associated cognitive impairment before and after the advent of combination therapy. *J. Neurovirol.* **8**:136–142.

Samson, M., O. Labbe, C. Mollereau, G. Vassart, G., and M. Parmentier. 1996. Molecular cloning and functional expression of a new human CC-chemokine receptor gene. *Biochemistry* **35**:3362–3367.

Schacker, T., A. C. Collier, J. Hughes, T. Shea, and L. Corey. 1996. Clinical and epidemiologic features of primary HIV infection. *Ann. Intern. Med.* **125**:257–264.

Schifitto, G., M. P. McDermott, J. C. McArthur, K. Marder, N. Sacktor, L. Epstein, K. Kieburtz, and the Dana Consortium on the Therapy of HIV Dementia and Related Cognitive Disorders. 2002. Incidence of and risk factors for HIV-associated distal sensory polyneuropathy. *Neurology* **58**:1764–1768.

Seilhean, D., K. Kobayashi, Y. He, T. Uchihara, O. Rosenblum, C. Katlama, F. Bricaire, C. Duyckaerts, and J. J. Hauw. 1997. Tumor necrosis factor-alpha, microglia and astrocytes in AIDS dementia complex. *Acta Neuropathol.* (Berlin) **93**:508–517.

Sepkowitz, K. A. 2001. AIDS–the first 20 years. *N. Engl. J. Med.* **344**:1764–1772.

Shankar, P., M. Russo, B. Harnisch, M. Patterson, P. Skolnick, and J. Lieberman. 2000. Impaired function of circulating HIV-specific CD8$^+$ T cells in chronic human immunodeficiency virus infection. *Blood* **96**:3094–3101.

Sharp, B. M., K. McAllen, G. Gekker, N. A. Shahabi, and P. K. Peterson. 2001. Immunofluorescence detection of delta opioid receptors (DOR) on human peripheral blood CD4$^+$ T cells and DOR-dependent suppression of HIV-1 expression. *J. Immunol.* **167**:1097–1102.

Shaw, G. M., M. E. Harper, B. H. Hahn, L. G. Epstein, D. C. Gajduske, R. W. Price, B. A. Navia, C. K. Petito, C. J. O'Hara, J. E. Groopman, E. S. Cho, J. M. Oleske, F. Wong-Saal, and R. C. Gallo. 1985. HTLV III infection in brains of children and adults with AIDS encephalopathy. *Science* **227**:177–182.

Shepherd, E. J., R. P. Brettle, P. P. Liberski, A. Aguzzi, J. W. Ironside, P. Simmonds, and J. E. Bell. 1999. Spinal cord pathology and viral burden in homosexuals and drug users with AIDS. *Neuropathol. Appl. Neurobiol.* **25**:2–10.

Sidtis, J. J., C. Gatsonis, R. W. Price, E. J. Singer, A. C. Collier, D. R. Richman, M. S. Hirsch, F. W. Schaerf, M. A. Fischl, K. Kieburtz, D. Simpson, M. A. Koch, J. Feinberg, U. Dafni, and The AIDS Clinical Trials Group. 1993. Zidovudine treatment of the AIDS dementia complex: results of a placebo controlled trial. *Ann. Neurol.* **33**:343–349.

Silver, B., K. McAvoy, S. Mikesell, and T. W. Smith. 1997. Fulminating encephalopathy with perivenular demyelination and vacuolar myelopathy as the initial presentation of human immunodeficiency virus infection. *Arch. Neurol.* **54**:647–650.

Smith, P. R., J. D. Cavenagh, T. Milne, D. Howe, S. J. Wilkes, P. Sinnott, G. E. Forster, and M. Helbert. 2000. Benign monoclonal expansion of CD8$^+$ lymphocytes in HIV infection. *J. Clin. Pathol.* **53**:177–181.

Snider, W. D., D. M. Simpson, S. Nielson, J. W. M. Gold, C. E. Metroka, and J. B. Posner. 1983. Neurological complications of acquired Immune Deficiency Syndrome. Analysis of fifty patients. *Ann. Neurol.* **14**:403–418.

So, Y. T., and R. K. Olney. 1994. Acute lumbosacral polyradiculopathy in acquired immunodeficiency syndrome: experience in 23 patients. *Ann. Neurol.* **135**:53–58.

Staudinger, R., and K. Henry. 2000. Remission of HIV myelopathy after highly active antiretroviral therapy. *Neurology* **54**:267–268.

Strizki, J. M., A. V. Albright, H. Sheng, M. O'Connor, L. Perrin, and F. Gonzalez-Scarano. 1996. Infection of primary human microglia and monocyte-derived macrophages with human immunodeficiency virus type 1 isolates: evidence of differential tropism. *J. Virol.* **70**:7654–7662.

Tagliati, M., D. Simpson, S. Morgello, D. Clifford, R. L. Schwartz, and J. R. Berger. 1998. Cerebellar degeneration associated with human immunodeficiency virus infection. *Neurology* **50**:244–251.

Tagliati, M., A. Di Rocco, F. Danisi, and D. Simpson. 2000. The role of somatosensory evoked potentials in the diagnosis of AIDS associated myelopathy. *Neurology* **51**:266–268.

Talley, A. K., S. Dewhurst, S. W. Perry, S. C. Dollard, S. Gummuluru, S. M. Fine, D. New, L. G. Epstein, H. E. Gendelman, and H. A. Gelbard. 1995. Tumor necrosis factor alpha-induced apoptosis in human neuronal cells: protection by the antioxidant N-acetylcysteine and the genes *bcl-2* and *crmA*. *Mol. Cell. Biol.* **15**:2359–2366.

Tan, S. V., R. J. Guiloff, and F. Scaravilli. 1995. AIDS-associated vacuolar myelopathy. A morphometric study. *Brain* **118**:1247–1261.

Tan, S. V., R. J. Guiloff, D. C. Henderson, B. G. Gazzard, and R. Miller. 1996. AIDS-associated vacuolar myelopathy and tumor necrosis factor-alpha (TNF alpha). *J. Neurol. Sci.* **138**:134–144.

Tembl, J. I., J. M. Ferrer, M. T. Sevilla, A. Lago, F. Mayordomo, and J. J. Vilchez. 1999. Neurologic complications associated with hepatitis C virus infection. *Neurology* **53**:861–864.

Thompson, K. A., J. C. McArthur, and S. L. Wesselingh. 2001. Correlation between neurological progression and astrocyte apoptosis in HIV-associated dementia. *Ann. Neurol.* **49**:745–752.

Tomlinson, G. S., P. Simmonds, A. Busuttil, A. Chiswick, and J. E. Bell. 1999. Upregulation of microglia in drug users with and without pre-symptomatic HIV infection. *Neuropathol. Appl. Neurobiol.* **25**:369–379.

Tornatore, C., R. Chandra, J. R. Berger, and E. O. Major. 1994. HIV-1 infection of subcortical astrocytes in the pediatric central nervous system. *Neurology* **44**:481–487.

Torres-Munoz, J., P. Stockton, N. Tacoronte, B. Roberts, R. R. Maronpot, and C. K. Petito. 2001. Detection of HIV-1 gene sequences in hippocampal neurons isolated from postmortem AIDS brains by laser capture microdissection. *J. Neuropathol. Exp. Neurol.* **60**:885–892.

Van der Horst, C. M., M. S. Saag, G. A. Cloud, R. J. Hamill, J. R. Graybill, J. D. Sobel, P. C. Johnson, C. U. Tuazon, T. Kerkering, B. L. Moskovitz, W. G. Powderly, W. E. Dismukes, and the National Institute of Allergy and Infectious Diseases Mycoses Study Group and AIDS Clinical Trials Group. 1997. Treatment of cryptococcal meningitis associated with the Acquired Immunodeficiency Syndrome. *N. Engl. J. Med.* **337**:15–21.

Vergis, E. N., and J. W. Mellors. 2000. Natural history of HIV-I infection. *Infect. Dis. Clin. North Am.* **14**:809–825.

Vitkovic, L., J. J. Chatham, and A. da Cunha. 1995. Distinct expressions of three cytokines by IL-1-stimulated astrocytes in vitro and in AIDS brain. *Brain Behav. Immun.* **9**:378–388.

Walker, C. M., D. J. Moody, D. P. Stites, and J. A. Levy. 1986. CD8$^+$ lymphocytes can control HIV infection in vitro by suppressing virus replication. *Science* **234**:1563–1566.

Walker, C. M., A. L. Erickson, F. C. Hsueh, and J. A. Levy. 1991. Inhibition of human immunodeficiency virus replication in acutely infected CD4$^+$ cells by CD8$^+$ cells involves a non-cytotoxic mechanism. *J. Virol.* **65**:5921–5927.

Weis, S., H. Haug, and H. Budka. 1993. Neuronal damage in the cerebral cortex of AIDS brains: a morphometric study. *Acta Neuropathol.* **85**:185–189.

Weiss, R. 2001. AIDS: unbeatable 20 years on. *Lancet* **357**:2073–2074.

Wesselingh, S. L., C. Power, J. D. Glass, W. R. Tyor, J. C. McArthur, J. M. Farber, J. W. Griffin, and D. E. Griffin. 1993. Intracerebral cytokine messenger RNA expression in acquired immunodeficiency syndrome dementia. *Ann. Neurol.* **33**:576–582.

Wesselingh, S. L., K. Takahashi, J. D. Glass, J. C. McArthur, J. W. Griffin, and D. E. Griffin. 1997. Cellular localization of tumor necrosis factor mRNA in neurological tissue from HIV-infected patients by combined reverse transcriptase/polymerase chain reaction in situ hybridization and immunohistochemistry. *J. Neuroimmunol.* **74**:1–8.

Wiley, C. A., and C. Achim. 1994. Human immunodeficiency virus encephalitis is the pathological correlate of dementia in acquired immunodeficiency syndrome. *Ann. Neurol.* **36**:673–676.

Wiley, C. A., C. L. Achim, R. Hammond, S. Love, E. Masliah, L. Radhakrishnan, V. Sanders, and G. Wang. 2000. Damage and repair of DNA in HIV encephalitis. *J. Neuropathol. Exp. Neurol.* **59**:955–965.

Williams, K. C., S. Corey, S. V. Westmorelaand, D. Pauley, H. Knight, C. deBakker, X. Alvarez, and A. A. Lackner. 2001. Perivascular macrophages are the primary cell type productively infected by simian immunodeficiency virus in the brains of macaques: implications for the neuropathogenesis of AIDS. *J. Exp. Med.* **193**:905–915.

Wilt, S. G., E. Milward, J. M. Zhou, K. Nagasato, H. Patton, R. Rusten, D. E. Griffin, M. O'Connor, and M. Dubois-Dalcq.

1995. In vitro evidence for a dual role of tumor necrosis factor-alpha in human immunodeficiency virus type 1 encephalopathy. *Ann. Neurol.* **37**:381–394.

Wulff, E. A., and D. M. S. Simpson. 1999. Neuromuscular complications of the human immunodeficiency virus type 1 infection. *Semin. Neurol.* **19**:157–164.

Yang, Y., Z. H. Liu, C. F. Ware, and J. D. Ashwell. 1997. A cysteine protease inhibitor prevents activation-induced T-cell apoptosis and death of peripheral blood cells from human immunodeficiency virus-infected individuals by inhibiting upregulation of Fas ligand. *Blood* **89**:550–557.

Yechoor, V. K., W. X. Shandera, P. Rodriguez, and T. R. Cate. 1996. Tuberculous meningitis among adults with and without HIV infection. Experience in an urban public hospital. *Arch. Intern. Med.* **156**:1710–1716.

Yeni, P. G., S. M. Hammer, C. C. J. Carpenter, D. A. Cooper, M. A. Fischl, J. M. Gatell, B. G. Gazzard, M. S. Hirsch, D. M. Jacobsen, D. A. Katzenstein, J. S. G. Montaner, D. D. Richman, M. S. Saag, M. Schechter, R. T. Schooley, M. A. Thompson, S. Vella, and P. A. Volberding. 2002. Antiretroviral treatment for adult HIV infection in 2002. Updated recommendations of the International AIDS Society-U.S.A. Panel. *JAMA* **288**:222–235.

Yeung, M. C., L. Pulliam, and A. S. Lau. 1995. The HIV envelope protein gp120 is toxic to human brain-cell cultures through the induction of interleukin-6 and tumor necrosis factor-alpha. *AIDS* **9**:137–143.

Zhang, L., B. Ramratnam, K. Tenner-Racz, Y. He, M. Vesanen, S. Lewin, A. Talal, P. Racz, A. S. Perelson, B. T. Korber, M. Markowitz, and D. D. Ho. 1999. Quantifying residual HIV-1 replication in patients receiving combination antiretroviral therapy. *N. Engl. J. Med.* **340**:1605–1613.

Encephalitis in Immunocompromised Patients

Compromised immunological function exposes the host to an increased risk of infectious diseases. Among the infecting agents, those that are usually not pathogenic in the intact host, such as various fungi and viruses, become significant threats. The central nervous system (CNS) may suffer as a consequence of widespread systemic infection, such as in disseminated zoster. Alternatively, the CNS may be affected in the absence of systemic viral disease, such as in progressive multifocal leukoencephalopathy (PML). Certain of the diseases discussed here tend to have courses that are subacute, measured in months rather than days. Others present acutely. Several different viruses must be considered. The immunological defects are also variable and include B-cell failure in X-linked agammaglobulinemia and helper T-cell ablation in AIDS. In other cases, such as allograft recipients, the defects are rather more generalized. In all entities considered in this chapter the clinician must balance management of the CNS disease with the underlying, or associated, systemic disease.

PML

Described by Astrom, Mancall, and Richardson in 1958, PML was an exceedingly rare disease prior to the AIDS epidemic. Soon after the start of the human immunodeficiency virus (HIV) epidemic, Brooks and Walker (1984) reviewed 230 published and unpublished cases of PML. Originally associated with lymphoproliferative conditions such as Hodgkin's disease or chronic leukemia, evidence for what was then termed papovaviral infection was first presented by Zu Rhein and Chou (1965). Isolation of the virus termed JC virus (JCV), after the patient from whom it was derived, was achieved by Padgett et al. (1971). The histopathology is characterized by large bizarre-looking astrocytes, oligodendroglia with large inclusion-bearing nuclei, and multifocal demyelination, often subcortical in location. On electron microscopy the oligodendroglia can be seen to contain virions, often in crystalline arrays. Zu Rhein and Chou (1965) pointed out that "...the demyelination is produced by the metabolic and eventually cytocidal effect of the virus on oligodendroglial cells and that this demyelination follows massive intranuclear replication." Clinically, Brooks and Walker (1984) found motor weakness, mental symptoms, visual defects, and speech deficits to be most common, compatible with the multifocal nature of the process. Eighty percent of the patients died by 9 months after the onset of PML. Based on experience with PML in patients in whom immunosuppression was induced by therapy, Brooks and Walker observed, "Reduction in immunosuppressive therapy was associated with stabilization of PML, although neurologic recovery was not dramatic" (Brooks and Walker, 1984). That observation foreshadows the experience of PML in AIDS patients who have had immune reconstitution due to highly active antiretroviral therapy (HAART) (Gasnault et al., 1999).

The AIDS epidemic brought with it a dramatic increase in the number of cases of PML. In our own experience in southern Connecticut, for example, no cases of PML were seen in the 5 years prior to the onset of the AIDS epidemic. In contrast, in the AIDS era in the context of a therapy trial (Hall et al., 1998), more than a dozen cases were evaluated for biopsy in slightly over a year's time. The first AIDS-associated case of PML was reported in a homosexual man with a progressive disorder referable to the cerebellum and brain stem, in whom the diagnosis was established by biopsy of the cerebellum (Miller et al., 1982). Prevalence of PML in AIDS has varied depending on the source of the data. In a report of 390 autopsied AIDS cases over 15 years in southern California, Masliah et al. (2000) found a frequency of PML of 3.4%.

Pathology and Pathogenesis

PML is caused by a polyomavirus, one of two varieties of papovaviruses, the other being papillomaviruses. The polyomavirus almost universally recovered in PML is one designated JCV. Another related virus, BK, occasionally causes CNS disease. Polyomaviruses are nonenveloped icosahedral viruses containing double-stranded circular DNA that codes for six proteins. The cell receptors for the virus have not been identified. Recent reviews of the pathology and pathogenesis of PML can be found in Hon et al. (2000), Love and Wiley (2002), and Johnson (1998).

PML is, as its rather cumbersome name implies, a multifocal demyelinating disease that can affect any part of the CNS but in which lesions are most commonly found in the cerebral hemispheres. The external appearance of the brain is usually normal. Lesions are visible in slices of the brain and vary in size from less than a millimeter to several centimeters across. The larger lesions are formed by coalescence between and enlargement of the smaller ones. Small, early lesions are particularly commonly seen at or near the junction between cerebral cortex and white matter (Fig. 13.1). Sometimes the lesions appear yellowish and necrotic. Alternatively, they are gray and slightly gelatinous in texture. If the lesions are extensive, there may be associated cerebral or cerebellar atrophy and compensatory ventricular dilation.

Microscopically, the main abnormalities lie in or immediately around the foci of demyelination (Fig. 13.2). In these areas myelin sheaths are absent, but axons are at least partially preserved. The demyelinated foci show no clear relationship to vessels, in contrast to the demyelinated foci of perivenous encephalitis (chapter 7) and multiple sclerosis. Davies et al. (1973) drew attention to a relative sparing of tissue adjacent to pial and ventricular surfaces, again in contradistinction to multiple sclerosis. The cellular content within the foci varies depending on the age of the lesions. In relatively fresh lesions there are frequently some microglial

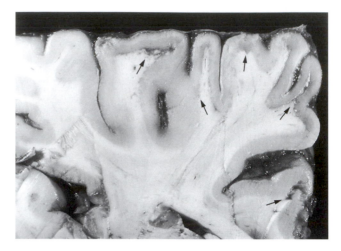

FIGURE 13.1   Close-up view of coronal slice through the brain from a case of PML. The characteristic lesions are present at the junction between cerebral cortex and white matter (arrows).

cells present, containing sudanophilic lipid. There may also be a few lymphocytes and plasma cells in and around the lesions, but in most cases these are not at all conspicuous. Old lesions are sparsely cellular and gliotic. They display a notable absence of typical oligodendrocyte nuclei in the center. Nearer the margins, oligodendrocyte nuclei may be seen, together with some abnormal, round hyperchromatic nuclei (Fig. 13.3). The latter are rather larger than typical oligodendrocyte nuclei. Some show margination of chromatin, and a few may contain basophilic or, less commonly, eosinophilic inclusion bodies. They are surrounded by little, if any, visible cytoplasm. Most authors consider these to be altered oligodendrocytes. The relatively oligodendrocyte-specific marker carbonic anhydrase isoenzyme II is intensely expressed in

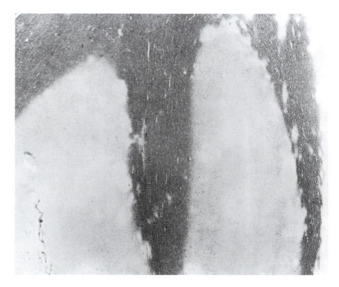

FIGURE 13.2   PML. Lower-power view of section of cerebral cortex and subcortical white matter stained for myelin. Multiple small foci of myelin pallor are present near the junction between cortex and white matter. Luxol fast blue stain.

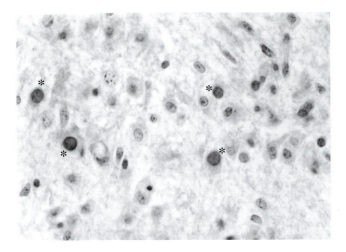

FIGURE 13.3 PML. Area at the margin of a demyelinated zone. Several oligodendrocyte nuclei are enlarged and hyperchromatic, with basophilic intranuclear inclusions (*). Hematoxylin and eosin stain.

some oligodendrocytes at the margins of lesions but is not usually detected in cells with inclusion-bearing nuclei (Morris et al., 1994) (Fig. 13.4).

A further characteristic finding within or closely adjacent to the demyelinated lesions is the presence of large astrocytes with bizarre, frequently multiple nuclei (see Fig. 1.8). These resemble some of the astrocytes seen in malignant astrocytomas, a resemblance that can lead to the mistaken diagnosis of an astrocytoma if a biopsy is examined. These abnormal astrocyte nuclei may also occasionally contain inclusion bodies. In the cerebellum, abnormal nuclei are sometimes found within the granule cell layer of the cortex, and there may be small foci of granule cell degeneration (Fig. 13.5). There may also be demyelinated foci in nearly cerebellar white matter. Immunohistology using antisera to JC polyomavirus has demonstrated viral antigen in nuclei of cells located near the demyelinated foci (Itoyama et al., 1982), presumed to be oligodendrocytes, and in situ hybridization using

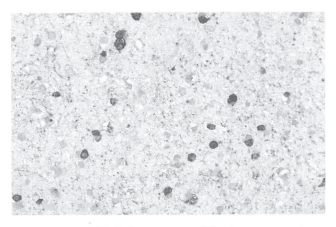

FIGURE 13.4 PML. Section stained for the enzyme carbonic anhydrase isoenzyme II, a marker of oligodendrocytes. Some oligodendrocytes show an intense reaction indicating a reactive state. Counterstained with hematoxylin.

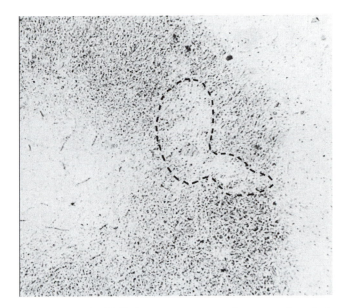

FIGURE 13.5 PML. Low-power view of section of cerebellar cortex showing patchy granule cell loss (outlined). Purkinje cells are also depleted. Hematoxylin and eosin stain.

JCV-specific nucleic acid probes demonstrates JCV DNA (see Fig. 1.5). Most of the abnormal astrocyte nuclei do not contain demonstrable viral antigen.

Electron Microscopy

Virus particles resembling polyomaviruses are detectable in nuclei corresponding to the hyperchromatic nuclei seen by light microscopy at the margins of the demyelinated foci. Such nuclei may, however, be scarce, and they are not seen near all lesions, particularly the ones that show evidence of chronicity. When present, viral particles are usually seen in the nuclei. They are numerous and tightly packed (Fig. 13.6). The particles are icosahedral in shape, moderately and uniformly electron dense, and have a diameter of about 33 nm. Filamentous forms of the virus are also seen.

Pathogenesis

JCV, the virus found in most cases of PML, is a ubiquitous virus that has not been associated with any other clinical disease. It must have a wide circulation in the population, for the majority of adults have antibodies to it. Its mode of spread is uncertain, but its only known route of excretion is through the kidney. JCV can be regularly detected by PCR in sewage, so infection by the oral route is possible (Bofill-Mas and Girones, 2001). Detection of the virus in human tonsil also supports this route of infection (Monaco et al., 1998). JC and BK polyomaviruses can also be detected in peripheral blood lymphocytes of healthy subjects and more frequently in those who are immunosuppressed (Tornatore et al., 1992; Degener et al., 1997). There can be little doubt that immune deficiency is the major factor enabling the virus to exert its damaging effects. The disorders associated with PML are noteworthy for the defects in cell-mediated immunity that accompany them. One study showed that cell-mediated immunity to JCV was deficient in six patients with PML, whereas normal responses were

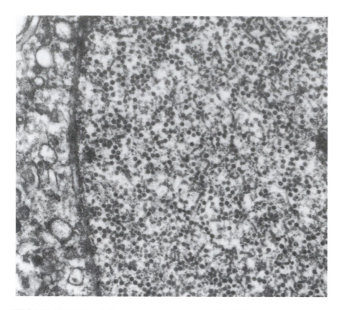

FIGURE 13.6 Electron micrograph of a biopsy from a case of PML showing a nucleus containing both spherical and filamentous polyomavirus particles. Uranyl acetate and lead citrate stain. Courtesy of A. M. Field.

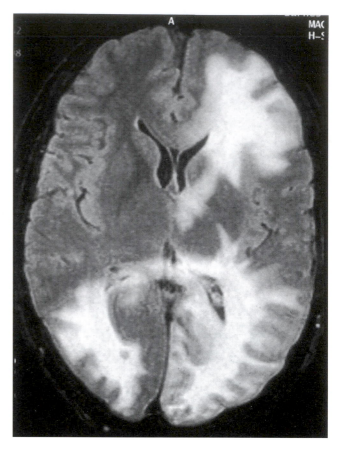

FIGURE 13.7 MRI of PML. Axial proton density image shows scattered areas of hyperintensity, predominantly in white matter but with some possible gray matter involvement. Mild mass effect is present. Courtesy of Judith Donovan Post, University of Miami School of Medicine.

present in all controls (Willoughby et al., 1980). It is not known whether the virus is harbored by the patient before the immune deficiency arises or whether PML develops in patients exposed to the virus for the first time when they are already immunocompromised. JCV has been isolated from normal human brain, so there is evidence that it is normally sequestered there (Greenlee, 1997; Gallia et al., 1997).

The widespread multifocal nature of the pathology suggests the possibility of blood-borne spread of virus to the brain; this is supported by the demonstration of JCV DNA in endothelial cells (Dorries et al., 1979). Lesions of differing size correspond to lesions of differing age, small ones being of recent origin. Foci of demyelination seem to enlarge by extension of infection to cells at the periphery of the lesions. It is not known how widely virus spreads within the CNS or whether fresh crops of lesions develop from virus spreading to the nervous system from outside. Virus can be detected in cerebrospinal fluid (CSF) by PCR in 85% of biopsy-proven cases in AIDS patients (Yiannoutsos et al., 1999). Lytic infection of oligodendrocytes provides a satisfactory explanation for the selectively demyelinating character of the lesions because death of an oligodendrocyte results in dissolution of the myelin sheath derived from its cell membrane.

The alteration in astrocyte form associated with the lesions of PML is of considerable interest. It is reminiscent of malignant change, and cerebral gliomas have been described in patients with PML (Sima et al., 1983; Gullotta et al., 1992). JCV and other polyomaviruses can induce malignant glioma formation in animals and malignant transformation of glial cells in vitro (Shein, 1967).

Diagnosis and Management

The diagnosis of PML in AIDS should be suspected in a patient with significant suppression of cell-mediated immunity, usually below 100 CD4 lymphocytes per mm^3, in whom

a subacute onset of multifocal neurological deficits is observed. In an early report of personal experience and a review of the literature, Berger et al. (1987) found extremity weakness, cognitive dysfunction, visual loss, and gait disturbance as common complaints. It should be noted that while multifocal abnormalities are often present, other presentations, such as diffuse impairment, or unifocal disorders, such as a pontocerebellar form, are observed. Computed tomography (CT) scanning may reveal hypodense areas in white matter, but CT is often unrevealing. Magnetic resonance imaging (MRI) is most useful, demonstrating focal and multifocal white matter lesions that can be confluent or discrete (Post et al., 1999) (Fig. 13.7). Minimal space-occupying characteristics and minimal contrast enhancement can be seen in a minority of cases. A useful configuration is the subcortical scalloped appearance of discrete lesions, reflecting involvement of the subcortical u-fibers. In our own experience, diagnostic confusion arises most commonly when confluent lesions are seen with features resembling HIV leukoencephalopathy. In contrast to two other chronic disorders, Creutzfeldt-Jakob disease and subacute sclerosing panleukoencephalitis (SSPE), the electroencephalogram (EEG) has no characteristic or suggestive features. Standard studies of CSF in non-HIV-associated

PML reveal only slightly elevated protein. In AIDS there may be a mild pleocytosis and oligoclonal bands in response to HIV, complicating the interpretation of the CSF formula in AIDS-associated PML. While brain biopsy had been the "gold standard" of diagnosis, a positive CSF PCR for JCV in combination with compatible clinical and MRI findings (Clifford et al., 1999) is diagnostically valid and less invasive. The presence of serum antibodies against JCV is of no diagnostic import because the majority of adults in the general population have such antibodies as the result of primary infection. The clinical features of the primary infection with JCV have not been identified.

Prior to the advent of HAART, the median survival time of AIDS-associated PML was 4 months (Gasnault et al., 1999), although occasional cases had been observed with markedly longer survival (Berger and Mucke, 1988). However, the use of HAART, more recently termed potent antiretroviral therapy, has resulted in a significant stabilization of neurological symptoms and prolongation of life in some patients (Clifford et al., 1999; Gasnault et al., 1999). Patients who were started on HAART before the CD4 lymphocyte count fell below 100 cells/μl had significantly better survival than those treated after the count fell below that value. However, as pointed out by Gasnault et al. (1999), early specific anti-JCV therapy would be of value because of the lack of significant improvement for patients whose PML progression had been stabilized. Thus far, no such therapy has been proven efficacious in a controlled propsective trial. The need for such trials is shown in the case of 1-β-D-arabinofuranosylcytosine (Ara-C), in which anecdotal reports suggested efficacy but a controlled clinical trial failed to show benefit (Hall et al., 1998). The importance of the study, while negative, was to spare subsequent patients the significant hematological toxicity of treatment and false hope of improvement. Recent practice has included cidofovir. The danger of nephrotoxicity, ocular hypotony, and the absence of parameters for duration of therapy in long-term survivors are the principal concerns. Observational studies suggested that a controlled randomized trial is needed (Gasnault et al., 2001; DeLuca et al., 2001). A pilot study by Marra et al. (2002) discovered no improvement at week 8 in neurological examination scores. Lower HIV viral load levels at entry portended better examination scores. A review of institutional experience with alpha interferon therapy, with or without HAART (Geschwind et al., 2001), demonstrated no improved survival benefit by adding alpha interferon to HAART.

CMV ENCEPHALITIS AND RADICULOMYELITIS

Prior to the AIDS epidemic, the principal human disease associated with cytomegalovirus (CMV) was cytomegalic inclusion disease of the newborn (Griffith and Booss, 1994). Congenital infection can be associated with microcephaly and periventricular calcifications in newborns. The subependymal region is a particular locus of congenital infection. Evidence for CMV in the brains of patients who had received renal allografts, notably microglial nodules, was presented by Schneck (1965), but no definite clinical syndrome was found to be associated.

The start of the AIDS epidemic brought with it the clinical recognition that some form of neurological disease was present in more than half of the patients with established AIDS (Harris, Dwyer, and Booss, unpublished). That observation has been sustained in recent neuropathological studies (Masliah et al., 2000). Prominent among the syndromes first recognized was a subacute encephalitis, variously also called subacute encephalopathy. There was early speculation that CMV might be the cause (Snider et al., 1983). However, Navia et al. (1986a, 1986b) demonstrated it to be due to HIV itself. Nonetheless, CMV is also a cause of subacute encephalopathy in AIDS patients that must be distinguished from the AIDS dementia complex (Holland et al., 1994). In a 1987 neuropathological report of Morgello and colleagues (1987), lesions were recognized in five categories: described neuropathological manifestations including inclusion-bearing cells in isolation, microglial nodules, focal parenchymal necrosis, necrotizing ventriculoencephalitis, and necrotizing radiculomyelitis. Of great importance has been the development of CSF PCR for rapid diagnosis of neurological disorders caused by CMV in AIDS (Cinque et al., 1992; Gozlan et al., 1992). PCR can also facilitate the rare diagnosis of CMV encephalitis in immunocompetent patients (Studahl et al., 1992). Fortunately, the advent of HAART has led to a very significant decline in CMV infections of the nervous system in AIDS (Clifford, 1999).

In a comprehensive review of the literature from 1965 to 1995 correlating clinical features and pathology, Arribas et al. (1996) found 676 published cases, of which 21 were in nonimmunocompromised patients, 77 were in organ transplant recipients, 574 were in HIV-infected individuals, and 4 were in patients with other causes of immunosuppression. Of the CNS forms of CMV infection, the most readily identifiable are those in advanced HIV disease in which significant tissue injury occurs. These include focal necrotizing encephalitis, ventriculoencephalitis, and necrotizing radiculomyelitis. Microglial nodule encephalitis is the most common manifestation, but clinical correlations are often difficult.

Pathology and Pathogenesis

CMV is the largest of the herpesviruses and takes its name from the characteristic cell enlargement with owl's eye intranuclear viral inclusions that it produces. The cell receptor for the virus is not yet known. The virus is occasionally acquired in utero or during breast-feeding from an infected mother, and this early infection can give rise to CNS disease (see below). Most primary infections occur later and are asymptomatic mononucleosis or are associated with an infectious type of illness. More than 80% of the population has acquired antibody by the age of 35 years (Love and Wiley, 2002). The virus spreads within the body via the bloodstream and can infect a wide variety of cell types including macrophages and their progenitor cells in bone marrow. These progenitors may act as a long-term source of the virus, which only rarely causes disease in immunocompetent individuals (Back et al., 1977) but can cause transverse myelitis (Miles et al., 1993; Giobbia et al., 1999), radiculomyelitis (Flood et al., 1997), or Guillain-Barré syndrome (Schmitz and Enders, 1977). In immunosuppressed subjects, particularly those with organ or bone marrow transplants and in AIDS patients, CMV causes a variety of pathological changes, most of them symptomatic.

Some understanding has derived from study of experimental models. In the murine model, CMV was itself found to be immunosuppressive, with the monocyte exerting an immunomodulating effect (Bixler and Booss, 1981). The guinea pig model of CMV infection of the CNS has demonstrated prominent microglial nodules and focal disruption of the ependyma, similar to findings in CMV-infected AIDS patients (Booss et al., 1988).

Neonatal and Congenital CMV Infection

Neurological involvement with CMV infection in neonates is almost always due to congenital infection, with the risk of clinical disease being great when maternal infection occurs during the first trimester of pregnancy. This can lead to disseminated CMV infection in which other organs such as the liver and eye as well as the brain are affected. The appearance of the brain in fatal affected cases is of severe microcephaly, sometimes with polymicrogyria (Fig. 13.8). Some cases show hydrocephalus or cerebellar hypoplasia. Foci of calcification in periventricular regions can impart a

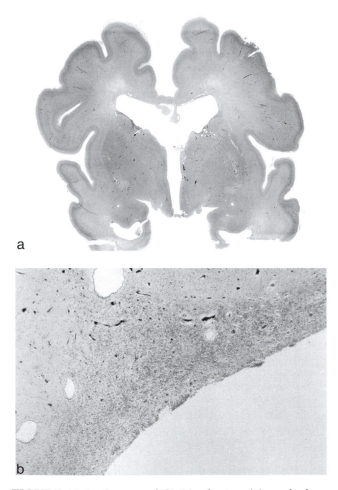

FIGURE 13.8 Congenital CMV infection: (a) cerebral section showing microcephaly and ventricular enlargement; (b) low-power view of ependymitis from the same case.

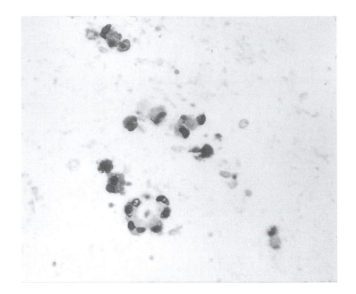

FIGURE 13.9 Congenital CMV. Demonstration of CMV antigen in inclusion-bearing cells in subependymal position.

grittiness on sectioning the brain. Cytomegalic cells are present and contain viral antigen in a widespread distribution but particularly in periventricular regions (Fig. 13.9). Infected cells can include neurons and glial cells. Inflammation may accompany these changes but is often not a prominent feature. Extensive infection and damage may be accompanied by cyst formation.

Adult CMV Infection

Adult CMV infection, usually in immunosuppressed subjects, can take a number of symptomatic forms with a correspondingly wide variety of pathologies. In AIDS sufferers, CMV is one of the most frequent opportunistic infections in the CNS, with a frequency from 10 to 30% (Bell, 1998; Zelman and Mossakowski, 1998; Setinek et al., 1995). Occult infection is detected with DNA amplification methods in a higher proportion, in some of whom it may be only latent. For example, after liver transplantation, DNA amplification detected CMV in the brain in 50% of cases, only 20% of which had microglial nodules and 11% of which had occasional positive cells with CMV-specific immunocytochemistry or in situ hybridization (Ribalta et al., 2002).

Parenchymal CNS disease takes three main forms: a multifocal low-grade encephalitis with microglial nodules that is quite frequently symptomless or gives rise to confusion or delirium (Grassi et al., 1998); a necrotizing encephalitis that often includes an ependymitis and ventriculitis; and a myelitis or myeloradiculitis. Low-grade encephalitis with microglial nodules was earlier recognized as a microglial nodule encephalitis (Booss and Esiri, 1986). CMV is the most common, though not the only, cause of this condition, in which there are scattered clusters of microglial cells and reactive astrocytes in gray matter in any part of the brain. The necrotizing encephalitis appears to spread from an ependymitis that is usually contiguous with the focus or foci of parenchymal necrosis. This sometimes involves the cerebellar dentate nuclei and white matter alongside a ventriculitis of the fourth ventricle (Fig. 13.10). There may

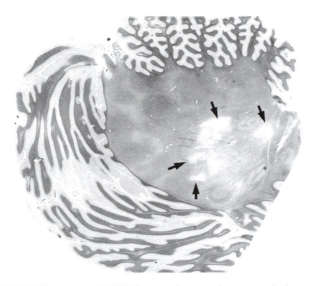

FIGURE 13.10 CMV. Ventriculo-ependymitis with foci of necrosis in nearby dentate nucleus of the cerebellum (arrows). Luxol fast blue-cresyl violet stain.

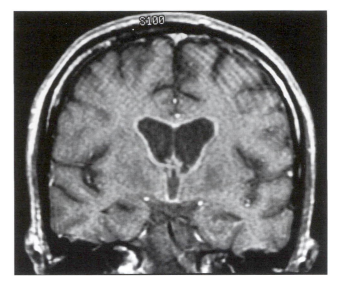

FIGURE 13.11 MRI of CMV ependymitis. T1-weighted coronal image with contrast demonstrating ependymal enhancement around the third and lateral ventricles. Courtesy of Gordon Sze, Yale University School of Medicine.

be little or no associated inflammation. Coinfection of CMV and other herpesviruses in AIDS patients appears to be more common than expected by chance (Chretien et al., 1997). In myeloradiculitis there are variable necrotizing or inflammatory foci, usually in the lumbosacral region of the spinal cord, and loss of myelin and, to a lesser extent, axons in lumbosacral nerve roots. Cytomegalic cells may be seen in cord lesions or in Schwann cells of affected nerve roots or sensory ganglia (Scaravilli and Gray, 1993). Ventriculoencephalitis and myeloradiculitis due to CMV are significantly associated, suggesting that the virus spreads via CSF in these conditions (Grassi et al., 1998).

Diagnosis and Management

CMV ventriculoencephalitis in adults was unknown prior to the HIV epidemic. It occurs with advanced immunosuppression (fewer than 50 CD4 lymphocytes per mm^3) and often in the presence of recent or current CMV infection such as retinitis, pneumonia, colitis, or radiculomyelitis. It can occur in the presence of CMV suppressive therapy (Kalayjian et al., 1993). Characteristically, lethargy, confusion, and disorientation develop subacutely over a median of 2 weeks, and oculomotor palsies and/or nystagmus, other cranial nerve abnormalities, and ataxia are recognizable clinical features of the syndrome (Kalayjian et al., 1993; Arribas et al., 1996). One or more focal features were reported in the review of Arribas et al. (1996) in half of the identified cases, but the other half presented without focal findings as an encephalopathic illness.

MRI and PCR of CSF are crucial to establishing the diagnosis and to providing specific antiviral therapy. The CSF can be markedly abnormal, with elevated numbers of white blood cells, including a significant component of neutrophils, raised protein, and reduced glucose levels if necrotizing radiculomyelitis coexists. Otherwise, the CSF pleocytosis may be only mildly abnormal, with protein elevation and no depression of glucose. The CT scan has been

relatively uninformative, often showing only cerebral atrophy, but the MRI is quite useful, demonstrating periventricular enhancement in half of the studied patients (Arribas et al., 1996) (Fig. 13.11). Based on a retrospective review of 100 AIDS cases with autopsy evidence of CMV, Mussini et al. (1997) concluded that a presumptive diagnosis of CMV encephalitis could be made based on a history of previous extraneural CMV disease, clinical findings, and neuroradiological features and that an etiologic diagnosis was dependent on a positive CSF PCR result. Arribas et al. (1996) found the CSF PCR to have sensitivity for CMV encephalitis of 79% and specificity of 95%. CMV ventriculoencephalitis is a subacute lethal disease, with mortality having a median course of 6 weeks (Arribas et al., 1996). Therapy should probably include both ganciclovir and foscarnet to offset the possibility of drug resistance. The marked drop-off in the incidence of serious infection of the CNS by CMV in the HAART era has precluded the controlled demonstration of the effectiveness of dual therapy (Clifford, 1999). However, an uncontrolled pilot study concluded that combination therapy could be safely used and that improvement or stabilization occurred in 74% (Anduze-Faris et al., 2000).

CMV radiculomyelopathy is a clinically recognizable syndrome that should be handled urgently. Progressive and necrotizing, the prognosis is poor unless therapeutic intervention is prompt (Cohen et al., 1993; Kim and Hollander, 1993; Cohen, 1996). This disease too was newly recognized in the AIDS epidemic. The disease is found in late-stage AIDS, often with evidence of other CMV complications. It is subacute in onset, often developing over a few days, with ascending flaccid paraparesis, pain, paresthesias and sensory loss in the lower extremities, often starting in the saddle area, and loss of bladder control commonly found. The key CSF finding is a pleocytosis with a prominent neutrophilic component. Protein elevation and low glucose are common components. MRI may demonstrate leptomeningeal enhancement and/or thickened nerve roots with enhancement. However, the role of MRI and myelography is principally to exclude a compressive lesion of the spinal cord. Electromyogram and nerve conduction studies are supportive investigations.

While the illness may start out resembling a conus medullaris or cauda equina syndrome and may evolve to require consideration of either the Guillain-Barré syndrome or a compressive spinal cord lesion, the combination of the characteristic clinical and CSF findings merits prompt empiric therapy. Other processes producing similar clinical features include herpes simplex virus type 2 (HSV-2), toxoplasmosis, syphilis, and metastatic disease (Cohen et al., 1993; So and Olney, 1994). In addition, a benign syndrome can occur in the absence of CMV with a slower onset, less severe deficits, probability of spontaneous improvement, and a CSF pleocytosis that is predominantly mononuclear (So and Olney, 1994). Even so, prompt therapy is urged because of the relentlessly progressive nature of the disease, poor reversibility of established deficits, and mortality. The etiologic diagnosis rests on the demonstration of CMV in the CSF by PCR, or less commonly, on isolation of the virus. Treatment with ganciclovir has resulted in stabilization in some cases but not all. Treatment regimens employing both foscarnet and ganciclovir have been recommended for study (Cohen, 1996). The fall-off in incidence of significant CMV disease of the nervous system in the HAART era has precluded prospective trials (Clifford et al., 1999). Nonetheless, a dual treatment regimen is advocated as reported by Anduze-Faris et al. (2000), in which report cases of CMV myelitis were included.

The clinical identification of other forms of CMV pathogenesis in the CNS, such as glial nodule or low-grade encephalitis, is more difficult than that of CMV ventriculoencephalitis or progressive CMV polyradiculomyelitis. Focal parenchymal necrosis, not including the subendymal area, is apparently rare (Arribas et al., 1996), but its presence can be suspected based on MRI findings and proven by biopsy demonstration of the virus (Masdeu et al., 1988).

ENTEROVIRAL CNS INFECTIONS IN PRIMARY HYPOGAMMAGLOBULINEMIA OR AGAMMAGLOBULINEMIA

Cell-mediated immunity plays the predominant role in control of many viral infections. AIDS is the clearest example, with the destruction of the helper-inducer subset of T cells. In contrast, disorders of immunoglobulin (Ig) production (Hermaszewski and Webster, 1993), including Bruton's X-linked agammaglobulinemia (Lederman and Winkelstein, 1985), common variable hypogammaglobulinemia (Cunningham-Rundles, 1989), and the more recently characterized X-linked hyper-IgM syndrome (Levy et al., 1997; Cunningham et al., 1999), bring recurrent bacterial infections in their wake, including bacterial meningitis. Children with primary hypogammaglobulinemia are at increased risk for chronic enterovirus encephalitis (Wilfert et al., 1977; McKinney et al., 1987; Rudge et al., 1996) and are at disproportionate risk of live virus oral vaccine-associated polio (Wyatt, 1973). The switch to the exclusive

use of inactivated polio vaccine in the United States in 2000 (Atkinson and Wolfe, 2002) reduces that risk.

Although the diagnosis of primary gammaglobulinemic disorders may be suspected within the first 2 years of life because of recurrent bacterial infections, the development of enterovirus meningoencephalitis may occur very early in life or later, including adult life. Manifestations in infants include an arrest and regression in milestone accomplishments. Seizures, impaired level of consciousness, and headache are common. Bilateral impaired hearing has also been commonly observed. Behavior problems and intellectual impairment are not uncommon. Motor signs include hemiparesis and quadraparesis. Evidence of a meningeal response such as nuchal rigidity combined with headache may be present, but not invariably so. Optic atrophy and ataxia have been recorded. Rudge et al. (1996) have described three clinical syndromes: progressive myelopathy, myelopathy with subsequent development of encephalopathy, and the more common encephalopathy alone. Associated findings included retinopathy, sensorineural hearing loss, and dermatomyositis.

Repeated lumbar punctures reveal a varied number of lymphocytes, from fewer than 10 to more than 1,000. The CSF protein is often somewhat elevated, and the glucose, while usually normal, may be somewhat depressed. The CSF pressure may occasionally be elevated. The EEG has varied from normal to abnormal without any specificity of findings to assist the diagnosis. MRI and CT have been normal at the start of neurological dysfunction but may proceed to atrophy and enlarged ventricles (Rudge et al., 1996). Several different types of enterovirus have been isolated from the CSF. In individual patients, repeated isolates have been reported for months and years (Wilfert et al., 1977). Virus may also be isolated from muscle biopsy in those patients who experience the dermatomyositis-like syndrome in combination with meningoencephalitis (Mease et al., 1981). CSF PCR can demonstrate enterovirus in culture-negative patients (Rotbart et al., 1990) and has been used to guide therapy (Quartier et al., 2000).

Other viral infections of CNS have been reported, including HSV and measles virus infections (both noted in Lederman and Winkelstein, 1985) and PML (Rudge et al., 1996).

Therapy is based on the delivery of IgG containing type-specific antibody so that it reaches the virus in the CNS. Since the 1980s, intravenous (i.v.) Ig has been the treatment of choice (Hermaszewski and Webster, 1993). Disagreement exists as to whether intrathecal Ig is beneficial (Rudge et al., 1996); it can be delivered through an Omaya reservoir (Erlendsson et al., 1985). The use of the antiviral agent pleconaril has been reported with some encouraging results (Pevear et al., 1999; Schmugge et al., 1999; Rotbart et al., 2001). Pleconaril is available on a compassionate-use basis from the manufacturer. Quartier et al. (2000) employed CSF PCR to guide intensive Ig therapy in two patients in whom pleconaril was also used. Allogeneic bone marrow transplantation has been used in the X-linked hyper-IgM syndrome to reverse the basic defect in this rare immunodeficiency disease, mutation of the CD40 ligand (Thomas et al., 1995).

IMMUNOSUPPRESSIVE MEASLES ENCEPHALITIS (IME)

Otherwise known as measles inclusion body encephalitis, immunosuppressive measles encephalitis (IME) differs from the acute immune-mediated encephalomyelitis following measles (chapters 7 and 8) and from SSPE (chapter 14). It is an infrequent complication of measles infection of immunosuppressed children, with 70% of the cases occurring in acute lymphocytic leukemia (ALL) (Mustafa et al., 1993). IME has been observed in HIV/AIDS (Budka et al., 1996).

Pathology

There are no characteristic macroscopic changes in the brain. It may appear normal or minimally atrophic, depending on the length of the illness. Microscopically, the most striking finding is of intranuclear eosinophilic inclusion bodies in neurons and oligodendrocytes. These resemble the inclusion bodies seen in SSPE. They react positively for measles antigen with the immunoperoxidase technique, and measles virus has been isolated from the brain in one case (Aicardi et al., 1977) and detected by immunocytochemistry, RNA studies, or electron microscopy in others (Mustafa et al., 1993; Budka et al., 1996). The inclusion bodies may need to be searched for carefully and in a number of locations, as they may be only focally abundant. Inflammation is conspicuous by its absence or sparsity. In one study there were occasional perivascular mononuclear cells, including a few IgM-containing plasma cells (Esiri et al., 1982). Multinucleate giant cells are sometimes present and may contain viral antigen (Fig. 13.12). They are probably formed by fusion of virus-containing glial cells. Hypertrophic astrocytes and microglial cells may be present, but there is little fibrillary gliosis or demyelination because the course of the disease is short. A few macrophages containing

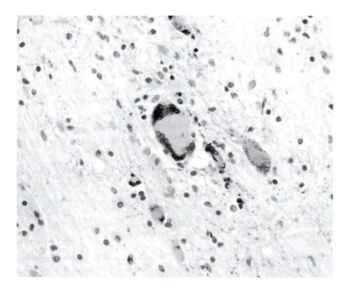

FIGURE 13.12 Multinucleate giant cell in the hypothalamus from a case of IME. Immunostain with measles antibody is immunopositive in the nuclei. Counterstained with hematoxylin.

neutral fat are usually present in the white matter and bear witness to the fact that some myelin breakdown has taken place.

Pathogenesis

There is generally a history of an attack of measles or of exposure to measles in the few months preceding the onset of neurological disease. IME seems to have the opportunity to develop when the virus is encountered for the first time when immunodeficiency is already present. The measles virus present in the brain in IME has been less intensively studied than the virus present in SSPE. The cases that have occurred have not been numerous, and the diagnosis has only rarely been made before the brain has been fixed at autopsy. As in SSPE, there has been report of a lack of detectable antibody to M protein (Roos et al., 1981) and of restricted measles virus gene expression in the brain in IME (Baczko et al., 1988; Suryanarayana et al., 1994). Measles virus antigen or RNA was detected in the CNS of 3 of 13 HIV-positive African children; most of the 13 died of a measles giant cell pneumonia, suggesting that in the setting of severe immunosuppression it is not uncommon for measles virus to gain access to the CNS (McQuaid et al., 1998). There are clear similarities between pathological changes present in SSPE and IME, and the differences are readily explicable on the basis of the immunosuppressed state of the patients and the shorter time course of the disease in IME.

Diagnosis and Management

Although cases in adults are on record (Wolinsky et al., 1977; Agamanolis et al., 1979; Chadwick et al., 1982), the mean age at encephalitis diagnosis was 6.1 years (Mustafa et al., 1993). Typically afflicting children with acute lymphocytic leukemia under regimens of antineoplastic therapy, other settings of immunosuppression, such as lymphoma, Hodgkin's disease, renal allograft, and AIDS, may create the necessary circumstances. It has occurred rarely in the absence of known immunosuppressive illness (Chadwick et al., 1982). There is nothing to indicate a more severe attack of measles itself. In fact, some cases may not be apparent, and in others the acute measles infection may not produce much of a rash. Furthermore, no obvious acute CNS sequelae are reported. In the period preceding the onset of the subacute encephalitis, no clinical signs appear to suggest what is to come. The interval between resolution of systemic measles and IME ranges from a few weeks to 7 months. The onset is well beyond the interval associated with the acute encephalomyelitis that follows systemic measles and well short of the interval associated with SSPE. The onset may be sudden, with the appearance of seizures followed by motor defects. Focal and generalized seizures that are difficult to control, including epilepsy partialis continua, occur (Mustafa et al., 1993). Myoclonus, aggravated by movement, has been noted (Wolinsky et al., 1977) but is rare. Focal motor signs are common, as are impairment of consciousness and confusion. Focal sensory defects and aphasia have been reported. Death may occur from the underlying illness or IME, with death attributed to IME in 76% of cases (Mustafa et al., 1993).

IME may be difficult to diagnose (Hughes et al., 1993). It should be suspected when a child with an immunosuppressive illness develops epilepsy partialis continua, which progresses to generalized seizures and coma over a matter of weeks. The initial differential includes extension of leukemia to the CNS with carcinomatous meningitis or parenchymal implants, hemorrhagic complications of leukemia and its therapy, and other parenchymal effects of chemotherapy and radiation therapy, as well as other opportunistic infections. The negative findings in some of the neurodiagnostic tests can be useful. CT studies do not demonstrate evidence of a mass or of bleeding and are often normal. MRI may be normal (cases of Mustafa et al., 1993) or abnormal with large patchy lesions (Bitnun et al., 1999) or small lesions (Budka et al., 1996). The lumbar puncture is usually normal, offering no support for carcinomatous meningitis or a chronic nonviral infection. Occasional cases with elevation of protein or a few cells have occurred. Oligoclonal bands in the CSF that are reduced when absorbed with measles virus have been reported (Roos et al., 1981) but are not usually present. In distinction to SSPE, characteristic EEG findings are not present. However, EEGs were found to be abnormal in all reported cases in Mustafa's 1993 review, with a spectrum of abnormalities.

The results of viral diagnostic studies have been variable. Serum measles antibodies have ranged from undetectable to more than 1:1,000, and those in the CSF have been undetected, low, or as high as 1:80 (Kipps et al., 1983; Chadwick et al., 1982). High serum levels of antibody to measles and/or local CNS synthesis of antimeasles antibody (Gazzola et al., 1999) may support the diagnosis of IME. The converse, however, does not hold; the absence of antibodies does not argue against the disease. Viral isolation has been achieved from brain tissue (for example, Aicardi et al., 1977); however, demonstration of the virus in the CNS is more usually achieved morphologically by immunohistology and by PCR. Eosinophilic intranuclear and cytoplasmic inclusions may be found on light microscopy, and paramyxovirus nucleocapsids may be found on electron microscopy. Immunohistological studies establish the specific agent (Drysdale et al., 1976; Esiri et al., 1982; Chadwick et al., 1982). Biopsy is usually required to make the diagnosis, particularly to exclude other treatable opportunistic infections. Treatment with ribavirin i.v. at 20 mg/kg daily for 15 weeks was associated with clinical recovery (Mustafa et al., 1993). However, ribavirin has not been successful in other cases (e.g., Bitnun et al., 1999), and there are insufficient data on which to make a recommendation.

Prevention by routine measles immunization of all children appears to be the principal strategy to reduce IME. Although the authors documented a case of vaccine-associated IME, Bitnun et al. (1999) note that measles vaccine can be used in many immunocompromised patients. Examples are given of children 2 years old or more following allogeneic bone marrow transplant, children with acute lymphocytic leukemia in remission, and HIV-infected children who are asymptomatic. Symptomatic HIV-infected children need to be evaluated for measles immunization on a case-by-case basis.

ENCEPHALITIS ASSOCIATED WITH ORGAN TRANSPLANTATION AND BONE MARROW ALLOGRAFTING

Organ transplantation has been applied with greater frequency as the surgical and immunological techniques have improved to facilitate their acceptance by the recipient. Renal, liver, cardiac, lung, and bone marrow transplants are widely employed; however, transplantation requires significant immunosuppressive therapy. In the case of solid-organ transplants, ongoing immunosuppressive therapy is directed at preventing graft rejection. After bone marrow grafting, graft-versus-host disease is a danger. In some cases, the diseases for which the transplant are required are themselves immunosuppressive. This is most clearly associated with bone marrow damage; however, it is also a feature of uremia. The combination of immunological suppression associated with the primary disease and medically induced immunosuppression to sustain the transplant results in a high incidence of opportunistic infections (Patel and Paya, 1997). Transplant recipients experience herpesvirus family infections associated with immunosuppression, including CMV, varicella-zoster virus (VZV), Epstein-Barr virus (EBV), and human herpesvirus 6 (HHV-6). Other viral infections occur on occasion, such as measles (Agamanolis et al., 1979) and mumps (Bakshi et al., 1996). Additionally, a leukoencephalitis associated with immunosuppressive therapy can cause profound neurological disability, which can be reversed (Singh et al., 2000).

While viral infections of the brain occur in transplanted/allografted patients, other types of neuropathology predominate. In an autopsy study of bone marrow transplant recipients, Mohrmann et al. (1990) found vascular disease including hematomas to be most common, followed by fungal and bacterial infections. More recently, Coley et al. (1999) reviewed 406 patients undergoing allogeneic bone marrow transplant and found 11 infections, most common of which was aspergillosis in 5 patients. CNS HHV-6, VZV, and PML were found in one patient each. Maschke et al. (1999) found CNS infections in 4% of 655 hematopoetic transplants, of which toxoplasmosis and aspergillosis were the most common. Bonham et al. (1998) performed a prospective study of 1,730 consecutive liver transplant patients to determine the nature of CNS lesions. Of 60 patients with neuroradiologically demonstrated lesions, 31 cases were due to vascular events including hemorrhage, 11 were due to abscesses, all of which were fungal, 7 were due to leukoencephalopathy associated with immunosuppressive therapy, 5 were due to central pontine myelinolysis, and 2 were due to malignancy. Thus, while opportunistic viral infections of the brain occur, they are by no means the predominant pathology or the predominant infection.

Leukoencephalopathy Syndromes following Transplantation

Characterized by subacute or abrupt onset of seizures, mental status changes, cortical visual loss, or motor abnormalities, immunosuppressive therapy-associated leukoencephalopathy is a syndrome that relates to the use of cyclosporin or tacrolimus for immunosuppression. White matter lesions that can be seen on CT scan are more frequently observed on MRI and tend to involve the posterior lobes of the brain. Singh et al. (2000) reviewed 50 cases in association with organ transplantation reported in the literature. More than 80% experienced the onset within 90 days of transplantation, with a median onset of 28 days. The clinical syndrome and the neuroimaging abnormalities reversed on reduction or cessation of cyclosporin or tacrolimus in about 95% of cases. Neurological improvement started first at a median of 4 days, while neuroimaging improved at a median of 20 days. More than 60% of cases occurred in liver transplants, but cases also occurred in transplants of kidney, lung, and heart. Associations with low serum cholesterol and also with elevated diastolic and systolic blood pressures were noted. CSF was generally unremarkable except that CSF protein could be elevated. The histopathology was characterized by myelin pallor.

Radiographically, the principal differential diagnostic consideration is PML. Clinically, however, rapid or abrupt onset of signs and symptoms and neuroimaging findings after institution of cyclospirin or tacrolimus, followed by the prompt resolution of the abnormalities on withdrawal or reduction of these agents, distinguishes it from PML. Aksamit et al. (1995) have published an instructive case in which immunosuppressive leukoencephalopathy and cerebellar hemorrhage developed sequentially. At autopsy, white matter lesions of cyclosporin encephalopathy revealed myelin pallor but not myelin absence, whereas small and clinically unsuspected lesions of PML were observed with an absence of myelin at the center of the lesions. In situ hybridization demonstrated JCV in abnormal oligodendrocyte nuclei. It was speculated that the removal of cyclosporin may have resulted in the attenuation of the PML so that it remained subclinical.

Other leukoencephalopathy syndromes to be considered in transplant recipients include PML and multifocal VZV leukoencephalopathy. Prior to 1984, Brooks and Walker found that slightly more than 6% of cases of PML occurred in renal transplant recipients. Subsequent development of AIDS-associated cases of PML overshadowed the occurrence of PML in transplant patients. Of note, however, in the transplant population is that reduction of immunosuppression with or without antiviral therapy may reduce the aggressiveness of the disease (Aksamit et al., 1995; Boulton-Jones et al., 2001). Multifocal VZV leukoencephalopathy, while first recognized over two decades ago (Horton et al., 1981), has gained increasing recognition as a complication in AIDS. However, in light of its potential reversal by antiviral agents, it should be aggressively sought in the differential diagnostic evaluation of the transplant patient with leukoencephalopathy. Findings on MRI may be sufficient to initiate empiric therapy with i.v. acyclovir (Weaver et al., 1999) (see chapter 9 and Fig. 9.3a and 9.3b).

Encephalitic Syndromes following Transplantation

With rare exceptions, most of the encephalitic syndromes, in distinction to the leukoencephalitic syndromes, reflect reactivation of viruses in the herpesvirus family. They have been dealt with elsewhere in this volume but will be briefly summarized here. Herpes simplex encephalitis can occur (Hirst et al., 1983), but it is an uncommon event in this population (Patel and Paya, 1997). There is concern, however, that antiviral prophylaxis for HSV in stem cell allograft recipients has produced resistant virus (Chen et al., 2000). Whether this will affect the incidence of herpes simplex encephalitis is not known.

CMV

CMV can cause systemic disease and attack the transplanted organ. Additionally, CMV pneumonitis, liver dysfunction, and gastrointestinal disease are important complications in the transplant patient. As reviewed by Sia and Patel (2000), the link between CMV and allograft dysfunction and rejection has been scrutinized but remains unresolved.

Although CNS infection by CMV is less frequent, it is important because of the availability of antiviral therapy (Maschke et al., 2002). The range of presentations of CMV in the nervous system in immunosuppressed patients is broad, including encephalopathy, radiculomyelitis, encephalitis, and ventriculoencephalitis. Hence, a very high level of suspicion must be maintained, and CSF PCR must be obtained promptly for CMV DNA. Depending on tolerance and previous antiviral therapy for CMV, ganciclovir and/or foscarnet is recommended for induction therapy by Maschke et al. (2002). Maintenance therapy will depend in part on the clinical response and reduction in viral titer, as determined by quantitative PCR (Sia and Patel, 2000).

Glial Nodule Encephalitis

In 1965, Schneck reported observations on brains of 34 patients who had expired following renal transplantation. In 12, there was evidence for viral encephalitis. Of these, 11 had glial nodules in the absence of other significant signs of inflammation. In two of these, intranuclear inclusions were found, and eight of the cases had evidence of CMV infection of the lungs. A review of the literature resulted in the conclusion that the pattern of glial nodule distribution was unlikely to result from uremia; hence, it was suggested that the findings were the result of CMV infection. More recently, Power et al. (1990) reported that in situ hybridization often demonstrated CMV DNA in the presence of microglial nodules in the brains of autopsied liver transplant cases. These observations suggest that CMV may be commonly found in the brains of transplant recipients, but the clinical relevance is not always clear.

VZV

Zoster (chapter 9) reactivates in a significant proportion of solid organ and bone marrow allografted patients, even in the face of acyclovir prophylaxis against HSV. The risk of primary VZV infection on exposure to VZV in transplant or bone marrow allograft recipients is cause for urgent treatment with zoster immune globulin within 72 h (Patel and Paya, 1997). Life-threatening disseminated primary varicella in this population can include encephalitis. Attempts to protect the VZV-naive population include vaccination (Hata et al., 2002).

Much has been learned about VZV infection of the CNS in HIV/AIDS-infected individuals. Note has been made above of VZV multifocal leukoencephalopathy and the need for prompt therapy. Meningoencephalitis successfully treated by acyclovir followed by the addition of foscarnet has been reported in an allo-bone marrow transplant recipient (Tauro et al., 2000). Because of the possibility of CNS zoster without vesicles or temporally remote from cutaneous lesions, a search for CSF antibody as well as CSF PCR for VZV should be undertaken in the transplant-allografted population with unexplained inflammatory disease of the CNS. Treatment with i.v. acyclovir at 10 to 15 mg/kg for 14 to 21 days is indicated. As in the case of Tauro et al. (2000), addition of a second antiviral compound and/or modification of the duration of therapy may be indicated in recalcitrant infections.

EBV

EBV (chapter 5) can cause nonspecific symptoms in transplant recipients, such as fever, malaise, sore throat, and headache, and also a range of lymphocytic proliferations subsumed under the term posttransplantation lymphoproliferative disease (Patel and Paya, 1997). The latter can involve the nervous system in the form of lymphoma. As pointed out by MacGinley et al. (2001), the diagnosis of EBV encephalitis in allograft recipients may be difficult to suspect. There are no particular clinical stigmata, neurological signs, or neuroimaging abnormalities that point directly to EBV. Furthermore, serological testing may be compromised because of immunosuppression. Hence, CSF PCR for EBV DNA is of particular importance. The renal allograft recipient reported by MacGinley et al. (2001) developed confusion without focal neurological signs followed by obtundation and a normal cerebral MRI. CSF revealed a pleocytosis and was positive for EBV DNA by PCR. Improvement was associated with i.v. ganciclovir treatment for 3 weeks followed by oral valacylovir for 3 months. There are insufficient data to know whether antiviral treatment should have a regular role in the treatment of EBV-associated encephalitis in the transplant recipient.

HHV-6

There are rare reports of HHV-6 encephalitis (chapter 5) in transplant or allograft recipients. Bollen et al. (2001) reported a 56-year-old male bilateral lung transplant recipient who developed a retrograde and anterograde amnesic syndrome followed by a generalized tonic-clonic seizure. The CSF revealed only an elevated protein, but MRI showed medial lesions in both temporal lobes. PCR done with blood and CSF was negative for other viruses, including HSV, but positive for HHV-6. The patient was treated successively with ganciclovir and foscarnet. Improvement ensued, but he was left with some memory impairment. Drobyski et al. (1994) described a complex case of a 37-year-old female who received a bone marrow allograft for Hodgkin's disease and had recurrent CMV viremia and positive HHV-6 blood cultures. Following death from an encephalitis associated with progressive impairment of mental status and amnesic symptoms, HHV-6-bearing cells were demonstrated in two regions of the brain by immunohistochemistry. As discussed in chapter 5, the pathogenic role of HHV-6 in certain instances remains controversial. Nonetheless, antiviral therapy appears merited in apparent CNS infection, particularly in the face of immunosuppression. As in the case of Bollen et al. (2001), ganciclovir and/or foscarnet should be used rather than acyclovir.

REFERENCES

Agamanolis, D. P., J. S. Tan, and D. L. Parker. 1979. Immunosuppressive measles encephalitis in a patient with a renal transplant. *Arch. Neurol.* **36:**686–690.

Aicardi, J., F. Goutieres, M.-L. Arsenio-Nunes, and P. Lebon. 1977. Acute measles encephalitis in children with immunosuppression. *Pediatrics* **59:**232–239.

Aksamit, A. J., Jr., and P. C. de Groen. 1995. Cyclosporine-related leukoencephalopathy and PML in a liver transplant recipient. *Transplantation* **60:**874–876.

Anduze-Faris, B. M., A.-M. Fillet, J. Gozlan, R. Lancar, N. Boukli, J. Gasnault, E. Caumes, J. Livartowsky, S. Matheron, C. Leport, D. Salmon, D. Costagliota, and C. Katlama. 2000. Induction and maintenance therapy of cytomegalovirus central nervous system infection in HIV-infected patients. *AIDS* **14:**517–524.

Arribas, J. R., G. A. Storch, D. B. Clifford, and A. C. Tselis. 1996. Cytomegalovirus encephalitis. *Ann. Intern. Med.* **125:**577–587.

Astrom, K.-E., E. L. Mancall, and E. P. Richardson Jr. 1958. Progressive multifocal leukoencephalopathy. A hitherto unrecognized complication of chronic lymphatic leukemia and Hodgkin's disease. *Brain* **81:**93–111, with 14 plates.

Atkinson, W., and C. S. Wolfe (ed.). 2002. Poliomyelitis, p. 71–82. *In Epidemiology and Prevention of Vaccine-Preventable Disease,* 7th ed. U.S. Dept. of Health and Human Services, Centers for Disease Control and Prevention, Atlanta, Ga.

Back, E., C. Hoglund, and H. O. Malmulund. 1977. Cytomegalovirus infection associated with severe encephalitis. *Scand. J. Infect. Dis.* **9:**141–143.

Baczko, K., U. G. Liebert, R. Cattaneo, M. A. Billeter, R. P. Roos, and V. ter Meulen. 1988. Restriction of measles virus gene expression in measles inclusion body encephalitis. *J. Infect. Dis.* **158:**144–150.

Bakshi, N., J. Lawson, R. Hanson, C. Ames, and H. V. Vinters. 1996. Fatal mumps meningoencephalitis in a child with severe combined immunodeficiency after bone marrow transplantation. *J. Child. Neurol.* **11:**159–162.

Bell, J. E. 1998. The neuropathology of adult HIV infection. *Rev. Neurol.* (Paris) **154:**816–829.

Berger, J. R., and E. O. Major. 1999. Progressive multifocal leucoencephalopathy. *Semin. Neurol.* **19:**193–200.

Berger, J. R., and L. Mucke. 1988. Prolonged survival and partial recovery in AIDS-associated progressive multifocal leukoencephalopathy. *Neurology* **38:**1060–1065.

Berger, J. R., B. Kaszovitz, J. D. Post, and G. Dickinson. 1987. Progressive multifocal leukoencephalopathy associated with human immunodeficiency virus infection. A review of the literature with a report of sixteen cases. *Ann. Intern. Med.* **107:**78–87.

Bitnun, A., P. Shannon, A. Durward, P. A. Rota, W. J. Bellini, C. Graham, E. Wang, E. L. Ford-Jones, P. Cox, L. Becker, M. Fearon, M. Petric, and R. Tellier. 1999. Measles inclusion-body encephalitis caused by the vaccine strain of measles virus. *Clin. Infect. Dis.* **29:**855–861.

Bixler, G. S., Jr., and J. Booss. 1981. Adherent spleen cells from mice acutely infected with cytomegalovirus suppress the primary antibody response *in vitro. J. Immunol.* **127:**1294–1299.

Bofill-Mas, S., and R. Girones. 2001. Excretion and transmission of JCV in human populations. *J. Neurovirol.* **7:**345–349.

Bollen, A. E., H. Haaxma-Reiche, A. N. Wartan, and A. P. Krikke. 2001. Amnestic syndrome after lung transplantation by human herpes virus-6 encephalitis. *J. Neurol.* **248:**619–620.

Bonham, C. A., E. A. Dominguez, M. B. Fukui, D. L. Paterson, G. A. Pankey, M. M. Wagener, J. J. Fung, and N. Singh. 1998. Central nervous system lesions in liver transplant recipients. *Transplantation* **66:**1596–1604.

Booss, J., and M. M. Esiri. 1986. *Viral Encephalitis: Pathology, Diagnosis and Management.* Blackwell Scientific Publications, Oxford, United Kingdom.

Booss, J., P. R. Dann, B. P. Griffith, and J. H. Kim. 1988. Glial nodule encephalitis in the guinea pig: serial observations following cytomegalovirus infection. *Acta Neuropathol.* **75:**465–473.

Boulton-Jones, J. R., C. Fraser-Moodie, and S. D. Ryder. 2001. Long term survival from progressive multifocal leukoencephalopathy after liver transplantation. *J. Hepatol.* **35:**828–829.

Brooks, B. R., and D. L. Walker. 1984. Progressive multifocal leukoencephalopathy. *Neurol. Clin.* **2:**299–313.

Budka, H., S. Urbanits, P. P. Liberski, S. Eichinger, and T. Papow-Kraupp. 1996. Subacute measles virus encephalitis: a new and fatal opportunistic infection in a patient with AIDS. *Neurology* **46:**586–587.

Chadwick, D. W., S. Martin, P. H. Buxton, and A. H. Tomlinson. 1982. Measles virus and subacute neurological disease: an unusual presentation of measles inclusion body encephalitis. *J. Neurol. Neurosurg. Psychiatr.* **45:**680–684.

Chen, Y., C. Scieux, V. Garrait, G. Socié, V. Rocha, J.-M. Molina, D. Thouvenot, F. Morfin, L. Hocqueloux, L. Garderet, H. Esperou, F. Sélimi, A. Devergie, G. Leleu, M. Aymard, F. Morinet, E. Gluckman, and P. Ribaud. 2000. Resistant herpes-simplex virus type 1 infection: an emerging concern after allogenic stem cell transplantation. *Clin. Infect. Dis.* **31:**927–935.

Ch'ien, L. T., R. A. Price, K. G. Murti, and J. Ochs. 1983. Fatal subacute immunosuppressive measles encephalitis (SIME) in children with acute lymphocytic leukemia—clinical, electroencephalographic, and computerized tomographic scan features. *Clin. Electroenceph.* **14:**214–220.

Chretien, F., L. Belec, L. Wingerstmann, P. de Truchis, M. Baudrimont, C. Perronne, and F. Gray. 1997. [Central nervous system infection due to Herpes simplex virus in AIDS.] *Arch. Anat. Cytol. Pathol.* **45:**153–158.

Cinque, P., L. Vago, M. Brytting, A. Castagna, A. Accordini, V.-A. Sundquist, N. Zanchetta, A. D. Monteforts, B. Wahren, A. Lazzarin, and A. Linde. 1992. Cytomegalovirus infection of the central nervous system in patients with AIDS: diagnosis by DNA amplification from cerebrospinal fluid. *J. Infect. Dis.* **166:**1408–1411.

Clifford, D. B. 1999. Opportunistic viral infections in setting of human immunodeficiency virus. *Semin. Neurol.* **19:**185–192.

Clifford, D. B., C. Yiannoutsos, M. Glicksman, D. M. Simpson, E. J. Singer, P. J. Piliero, C. M. Marra, G. S. Francis, J. C. McArthur, K. L. Tyler, A. C. Tselis, and N. E. Hyslop. 1999. HAART improves prognosis in HIV-associated progressive multifocal leucoencephalopathy. *Neurology* **52:**623–625.

Cohen, B. A. 1996. Prognosis and response to therapy of cytomegalovirus encephalitis and meningomyelitis in AIDS. *Neurology* **46:**444–450.

Cohen, B. A., J. C. McArthur, S. Grohman, B. Patterson, and J. D. Glass. 1993. Neurologic prognosis of cytomegalovirus polyradiculomyelopathy in AIDS. *Neurology* **43:**493–499.

Coley, S. C., H. R. Jager, R. M. Szydlo, and J. M. Goldman. 1999. CT and MRI manifestations of central nervous system infection following allogenic bone marrow transplantation. *Clin. Radiol.* **54:**390–397.

Cunningham, C. K., C. A. Bonville, H. D. Ochs, K. Seyama, P. A. John, H. A. Rotbart, and L. B. Weiner. 1999. Enteroviral meningoencephalitis as a complication of x-linked hyper IgM syndrome. *J. Pediatr.* **134:**584–588.

Cunningham-Rundles, C. 1989. Clinical and immunologic analyses of 103 patients with common variable immunodeficiency. *J. Clin. Immunol.* **9:**22–33.

Davies, J. A., J. T. Hughes, and J. R. Oppenheimer. 1973. Richardson's disease (progressive multifocal leukoencephalopathy). *Q. J. Med.* **42:**481–501.

Degener, A. M., V. Pietropaolo, C. Di Taranto, V. Rizzuti, F. Ameglio, P. Cordiali Fei, F. Caprilli, B. Capitanio, L. Sinibaldi, and N. Orsi. 1997. Detection of JC and BK viral genome in specimens of HIV-1 infected subjects. *New Microbiol.* **20:**115–122.

De Luca, A., M. L. Giancola, A. Ammassari, S. Grisetti, A. Cingolani, D. Larussa, L. Alba, R. Murri, G. Ippolito, R. Cauda, A. Monforte, and A. Antinori. 2001. Potent antiretroviral therapy with or without cidofovir for AIDS-associated progressive multifocal leukoencephalopathy: extended follow-up of an observational study. *J. Neurovirol.* **7:**364–368.

Dorries, K., R. T. Johnson, and V. ter Meulen. 1979. Detection of polyoma virus DNA in PML-brain tissue by (in situ) hybridization. *J. Gen. Virol.* **42:**49–57.

Drobyski, W. R., K. K. Knox, D. Majewski, and D. R. Carrigan. 1994. Brief report: fatal encephalitis due to variant B human herpesvirus-6 infection in a bone marrow transplant recipient. *N. Engl. J. Med.* **330:**1336–1360.

Drysdale, H. C., L. F. Jones, D. R. Oppenheimer, and A. H. Tomlinson. 1976. Measles inclusion-body encephalitis in a child with treated acute lymphoblastic leukaemia. *J. Clin. Pathol.* **29:**865–872.

Erlendsson, K., T. Swartz, and J. M. Dwyer. 1985. Successful reversal of echovirus encephalitis in X-linked hypogammaglobulinemia by the intraventricular administration of immunoglobulin. *N. Engl. J. Med.* **312:**351–353.

Esiri, M. M., D. R. Oppenheimer, B. Brownell, and M. Haire. 1982. Distribution of measles antigen and immunoglobulin-containing cells in the CNS in subacute sclerosing panencephalitis and atypical measles encephalitis. *J. Neurol. Sci.* **53:**29–43.

Flood, J., W. L. Drew, R. Miner, D. Jekic-McMullen, L. P. Shen, J. Kolberg, J. Garvey, S. Follansbee, and M. Poscher. 1997. Diagnosis of cytomegalovirus (CMV) polyradiculopathy and documentation of in vivo anti-CMV activity in cerebrospinal fluid by using branched DNA signal amplification and antigen assays. *J. Infect. Dis.* **176:**348–352.

Gallia, G. L., S. A. Houff, E. O. Major, and K. Khalili. 1997. Review: JC virus infection of lymphocytes–revisited. *J. Infect. Dis.* **176:**1603–1609.

Gasnault, J., Y. Taoufik, C. Goujard, P. Kousignian, K. Abbed, F. Boue, E. Dussaix, and J. F. Delfraissy. 1999. Prolonged survival without neurological improvement with AIDS-related progressive multifocal leukoencephalopathy on potent combined antiretroviral therapy. *J. Neurovirol.* **7:**421–429.

Gasnault, J., P. Kousignian, M. Kahraman, J. Rahoiljaon, S. Matheron, J. F. Delfraissy, and Y. Taoufik. 2001. Cidofovir in AIDS-associated progressive multifocal leukoencephalopathy: a monocenter observational study with clinical and JC virus load monitoring. *J. Neurovirol.* **7:**375–381.

Gazzola, P., L. Cocito, E. Capello, L. Roccatagliata, M. Canepa, and G. L. Mancardi. 1999. Subacute measles encephalitis in a young man immunosuppressed for ankylosing spondylitis. *Neurology* **52:**1074–1077.

Geschwind, M. D., R. I. Skolasky, W. S. Royal, and J. C. McArthur. 2001. The relative contributions of HAART and alpha-interferon for therapy of progressive multifocal leukoencephalopathy in AIDS. *J. Neurovirol.* **7:**353–357.

Giobbia, M., A. Carniato, P. G. Scotton, G. C. Marchiori, and A. Vaglia. 1999. Cytomegalovirus-associated transverse myelitis in a non-immunocompromised patient. *Infection* **27:**228–230.

Gozlan, J. J., M. Salord, E. Roullet, M. Baudrimont, F. Caburet, O. Picard, M. C. Meyohas, C. Duvivier, C. Jacomet, and J. C. Petit. 1992. Rapid detection of cytomegalovirus DNA in cerebrospinal fluid of AIDS patients with neurologic disorders. *J. Infect. Dis.* **166:**1416–1421.

Grassi, M. P., F. Clerici, C. Perin, A. D'Arminio Monforte, L. Vago, M. Borella, R. Boldorini, and A. Mangoni. 1998. Microglial nodular encephalitis and ventriculoencephalitis due to cytomegalovirus infection in patients with AIDS: two distinct clinical patterns. *Clin. Infect. Dis.* **27:**504–508.

Greenlee, J. E. 1997. Polyomaviruses, p. 549–567. *In* D. D. Richman, R. J. Whitley, and F. G. Hayden (ed.), *Clinical Virology*. Churchill Livingstone, New York, N.Y.

Griffith, B. P., and J. Booss. 1994. Neurologic infections of the fetus and newborn. *Neurol. Clin.* **12:**541–564.

Gullotta, F., T. Masini, G. Scarlato, and K. Kuchelmeister. 1992. Progressive multifocal leukoencephalopathy and gliomas in a HIV-negative patient. *Pathol. Res. Pract.* **188:**964–972.

Hall, C. D., U. Dafni, D. Simpson, D. Clifford, P. E. Wetherill, B. Cohen, J. McArthur, H. Hollander, C. Yainnoutsos, E. Major, L. Millar, J. Timpone, and the AIDS Clinical Trials Group 243 Team. 1998. Failure of cytarabine in progressive multifocal leukoencephalopathy associated with human immunodeficiency virus infection. *N. Engl. J. Med.* **338:** 1345–1351.

Hata, A., H. Asanuma, M. Rinki, M. Sharp, R. M. Wong, K. Blume, and A. M. Arvin. 2002. Use of an inactivated varicella vaccine in recipients of hematopoietic-cell transplants. *N. Engl. J. Med.* **347:**26–34.

Hermaszewski, R. A., and A. D. B. Webster. 1993. Primary hypogammaglobulinaemia: a survey of clinical manifestations and complications. *Q. J. Med.* **86:**31–42.

Hirst, L. W., A. W. Clark, J. S. Wolinsky, D. S. Zee, H. Kaizer, N. R. Miller, P. J. Tutschka, and G. W. Santos. 1983. Downbeat nystagmus. A case report of herpetic brain stem encephalitis. *J. Clin. Neuro-ophthalmol.* **3:**245–249.

Holland, N. R., C. Power, V. P. Matthews, J. D. Glass, M. Forman, and J. C. McArthur. 1994. Cytomegalovirus encephalitis in acquired immunodeficiency syndrome (AIDS). *Neurology* **44:**507–514.

Hon, J., P. N. Jensen, and E. O. Major. 2000. The biology and clinical consequence of JC virus infection in the human brain-progressive multifocal leucoencephalopathy, p. 205–222. *In* P. K. Peterson and J. S. Remington (ed.), *New Concepts in the Immunopathogenesis of CNS Infections*. Blackwell Science, Oxford, United Kingdom.

Horton, B., R. W. Price, and D. Jimenez. 1981. Multifocal varicella-zoster virus leukoencephalitis temporally remote from herpes zoster. *Ann. Neurol.* **9:**251–266.

Hughes, I., M. E. M. Jenney, R. W. Newton, D. J. Morris, and P. E. Klapper. 1993. Measles encephalitis during

immunosuppressive treatment for acute lymphoblastic leukemia. *Arch. Dis. Child.* **68:**775–778.

Itoyama, Y., H. D. Webster, N. H. Sternberger, E. P. Richardson Jr., D. L. Walker, R. H. Quarles, and B. L. Padgett. 1982. Distribution of papovavirus, myelin-associated glycoprotein, and myelin basic protein in progressive multifocal leukoencephalopathy lesions. *Ann. Neurol.* **11:**396–407.

Johnson, R. 1998. *Viral Infections of the Nervous System*, 2nd ed. Lippincott-Raven Press, Philadelphia, Pa.

Kalayjian, R. C., M. L. Cohen, R. A. Bonomo, and T. P. Flanigan. 1993. Cytomegalovirus ventriculoencephalitis in AIDS. A syndrome with distinct clinical and pathological features. *Medicine* **72:**67–77.

Kim, Y. S., and H. Hollander. 1993. Polyradiculopathy due to cytomegalovirus: report of two cases in which improvement occurred after prolonged therapy and review of the literature. *Clin. Infect. Dis.* **17:**32–37.

Kipps, A., G. Dick, and J. W. Moodie. 1983. Measles and the central nervous system. *Lancet* **ii:**1406–1410.

Lederman, H. M., and J. A. Winkelstein. 1985. X-linked agammaglobulinemia: an analysis of 96 patients. *Medicine* **64:**145–156.

Levy, J., T. Espanol-Boren, C. Thomas, A. Fischer, P. Tova, P. Bordigoni, I. Resnick, A. Faath, M. Baer, L. Gomez, E. A. M. Sanders, M.-D. Tabone, D. Plantaz, A. Etzioni, V. Monafo, M. Abinun, L. Hammarstrom, T. Abrahamsen, A. Jones, A. Finn, T. Klemola, E. DeVries, O. Sanal, M. C. Peitsch, and L. D. Notarangelo. 1997. Clinical spectrum of x-linked hyper IgM syndrome. *J. Pediatr.* **131:**47–54.

Love, S., and C. A. Wiley. 2002. Viral diseases, p. 1–105. *In* D. I. Graham and P. L. Lantos (ed.), *Greenfield's Neuropathology*. Arnold, London, United Kingdom.

MacGinley, R., P. B. Bartley, T. Sloots, and D. W. Johnson. 2001. Epstein-Barr virus encephalitis in a renal allograft recipient diagnosed by polymerase chain reaction on cerebrospinal fluid and successfully treated with ganciclovir. *Nephrol. Dial. Transplant.* **16:**197–198.

Marra, C. M., N. Rajicic, D. E. Barker, B. Cohen, D. Clifford, M. J. D. Post, A. Ruiz, B. C. Bowen, M.-L. Huang, J. Queen-Baker, J. Anderson, S. Kelly, S. Shriver, and the Adult AIDS Clinical Trials Group 363. 2002. A pilot study of Cidofovir for progressive multifocal leukoencephalopathy in AIDS. *AIDS* **16:**1791–1797.

Maschke, M., U. Dietrich, M. Prumbaum, O. Kastrup, B. Turowski, U. W. Schaefer, and H. C. Diener. 1999. Opportunistic CNS infection after bone marrow transplantation. *Bone Marrow Transplant.* **23:**1167–1176.

Maschke, M., O. Kastrup, and H.-C. Diener. 2002. CNS manifestations of cytomegalovirus infections. Diagnosis and treatment. *CNS Drugs* **16:**303–315.

Masdeu, J. C., C. B. Small, L. Weiss, C. M. Elkin, J. Liena, and R. Mesa-Tejada. 1988. Multifocal cytomegalovirus encephalitis in AIDS. *Ann. Neurol.* **23:**97–99.

Masliah, E., R. M. DeTeresa, M. E. Mallory, and L. A. Hansen. 2000. Changes in pathological findings at autopsy in AIDS cases for the last 15 years. *AIDS* **14:**69–74.

McKinney, R. E., Jr., S. L. Katz, and C. M. Wilfert. 1987. Chronic enteroviral meningoencephalitis in agammaglobulinemic patients. *Rev. Infect. Dis.* **9:**334–356.

McQuaid, S., S. L. Cosby, K. Koffi, M. Honde, J. Kirk, and S. B. Lucas. 1998. Distribution of measles virus in the central nervous system of HIV-seropositive children. *Acta Neuropathol.* (Berlin) **96:**637–642.

Mease, P. J., H. D. Ochs, and R. J. Wedgwood. 1981. Successful treatment of echovirus meningoencephalitis and myositis-fasciitis with intravenous immune globulin therapy in a patient with X-linked agammaglobulinemia. *N. Engl. J. Med.* **304:**1278–1281.

Miles, C., W. Hoffman, C. W. Lai, and J. W. Freeman. 1993. Cytomegalovirus-associated transverse myelitis. *Neurology* **43:**2143–2145.

Miller, J. R., R. E. Barrett, C. B. Britton, M. L. Tapper, G. S. Bahr, P. J. Bruno, M. D. Marquart, A. P. Hays, J. G. McMurtry III, J. B. Weissman, and M. S. Bruno. 1982. Progressive multifocal leukoencephalopathy in a male homosexual with T-cell immune deficiency. *N. Engl. J. Med.* **307:**1436–1438.

Mohrmann, R. L., V. Mah, and H. V. Vinters. 1990. Neuropathologic findings after bone marrow transplantation. An autopsy study. *Hum. Pathol.* **21:**630–639.

Monaco, M. C., P. N. Jensen, J. Hou, L. C. Durham, and E. O. Major. 1998. Detection of JC virus DNA in human tonsil tissue: evidence for site of initial viral infection. *J. Virol.* **72:**9918–9923.

Morgello, S., E.-S. Cho, S. Nielsen, O. Devinsky, and C. K. Petito. 1987. Cytomegalovirus encephalitis in patients with acquired immunodeficiency syndrome: an autopsy study of 30 cases and a review of the literature. *Hum. Pathol.* **18:**289–297.

Morris, C. S., M. M. Esiri, T. J. Sprinkle, and N. Gregson. 1994. Oligodendrocyte reactions and cell proliferation markers in human demyelinating diseases. *Neuropathol. Appl. Neurobiol.* **20:**272–281.

Mussini, C., N. Mongiardo, G. Manicardi, F. Trenti, A. Alessandri, F. Paolillo, A. Catania, M. Portolani, M. Pecorari, V. Borghi, G. Ficarra, A. Cossarizza, and B. DeRienzo. 1997. Relevance of clinical and laboratory findings in the diagnosis of cytomegalovirus encephalitis in patients with AIDS. *Eur. J. Clin. Microbiol. Infect. Dis.* **16:**437–444.

Mustafa, M. M., S. D. Weitman, N. J. Winick, W. J. Bellini, C. F. Timmons, and J. D. Siegel. 1993. Subacute measles encephalitis in the young immunocompromised host: report of the cases diagnosed by polymerase chain reaction and treated with ribavirin and review of the literature. *Clin. Infect. Dis.* **16:**654–660.

Navia, B. A., E.-S. Cho, C. K. Petito, and R. W. Price. 1986a. The AIDS dementia complex: I. Clinical features. *Ann. Neurol.* **19:**517–524.

Navia, B. A., E.-S. Cho, C. K. Petito, and R. W. Price. 1986b. The AIDS dementia complex: II. Neuropathology. *Ann. Neurol.* **19:**525–535.

Padgett, B. L., D. L. Walker, G. M. Zu Rhein, R. J. Eckroade, and G. H. Dessell. 1971. Cultivation of papova-like virus from human brain with progressive multifocal leukoencephalopathy. *Lancet* **i:**1257–1260.

Patel, R., and C. V. Paya. 1997. Infections in solid-organ transplant recipients. *Clin. Microbiol. Rev.* **10:**86–124.

Pevear, D. C., T. M. Tull, M. E. Seipel, and J. M. Groarke. 1999. Activity of pleconaril against enteroviruses. *Antimicrob. Agents Chemother.* **43:**2109–2115.

Post, M. J. D., C. Yiannoutsos, D. Simpson, J. Booss, D. B. Clifford, B. Cohen, J. K. McArthur, C. D. Hall, and the AIDS Clinical Trials Group, 243 Team. 1999. Progressive multifocal leukoencephalopathy in AIDS: are there any MR findings useful to patient management and predictive of patient survival? *Am. J. Neuroradiol.* **20:**1896–1906.

Power, C., S. D. Poland, K. H. Kassim, J. C. E. Kaufmann, and G. P. A. Rice. 1990. Encephalopathy in liver transplantation: neuropathology and CMV infection. *Can. J. Neurol. Sci.* **17:**378–381.

Quartier, P., S. Foray, J.-L. Casanova, I. H. Rainsard, S. Blanche, and A. Fischer. 2000. Enteroviral meningoencephalitis in x-linked agammaglobulinemia: intensive immunoglobulin therapy and sequential viral detection in cerebrospinal fluid by polymerase chain reaction. *Pediatr. Infect. Dis. J.* **19:**1106–1108.

Ribalta, T., A. J. Martinez, P. Jares, J. Muntane, R. Miquel, X. Claramonte, and A. Cardesa. 2002. Presence of occult cytomegalovirus infection in the brain after orthotopic liver transplantation. An autopsy study of 83 cases. *Virchows Arch.* **440:**166–171.

Roos, R. P., M. C. Graves, R. L. Wollman, R. R. Chilcote, and J. Nixon. 1981. Immunologic and virologic studies of measles inclusion body encephalitis in an immunocompromised host: the relationship to subacute sclerosing panencephalitis. *Neurology* **31:**1263–1270.

Rotbart, H. A., J. P. Kinsella, and R. L. Wasserman. 1990. Persistent enterovirus infection in culture negative meningoencephalitis: demonstration by enzymatic RNA amplification. *J. Infect. Dis.* **161:**787–791.

Rotbart, H. A., and A. B. D. Webster for the Pleconaril Treatment Registry Group. 2001. Treatment of potentially life threatening enterovirus infection with pleconaril. *Clin. Infect. Dis.* **32:**228–235.

Rudge, P., A. D. B. Webster, T. Revesz, T. Warner, T. Espanol, C. Cunningham-Rundles, and N. Hyman. 1996. Encephalomyelitis in primary hypogammaglobulinaemia. *Brain* **119:**1–15.

Scaravilli, F., and F. Gray. 1993. Opportunistic infections, p. 49–120. *In* F. Gray (ed.), *Atlas of the Neuropathology of HIV Infection.* Oxford University Press, Oxford, United Kingdom.

Schmitz, H., and G. Enders. 1977. Cytomegalovirus as a frequent cause of Guillain-Barre syndrome. *J. Med. Virol.* **1:**21–27.

Schmugge, M., R. Lauener, W. Bossart, R. A. Seger, and T. Gungor. 1999. Chronic enteroviral meningoencephalitis in x-linked agammaglobulinaemia: favorable response to anti-enteroviral treatment. *Eur. J. Pediatr.* **158:**1010–1011.

Schneck, S. A. 1965. Neuropathological features of human organ transplantation. I. Probable cytomegalovirus infection. *J. Neuropathol. Exp. Neurol.* **24:**415–429.

Setinek, U., E. Wondrusch, K. Jellinger, A. Steuer, M. Drlicek, W. Grisold, and F. Lintner. 1995. Cytomegalovirus infection of the brain in AIDS: a clinicopathological study. *Acta Neuropathol.* **90:**511–515.

Shein, H. M. 1967. Neoplastic transformation induced by simian virus 40 in Syrian hamster neuroglial and meningeal cell cultures. *Arch. Gesamte Virusforsch.* **22:**122–142.

Sia, I. G., and R. Patel. 2000. New strategies for prevention and therapy of cytomegalovirus infection and disease in solid-organ transplant recipients. *Clin. Microbiol. Rev.* **13:**83–121.

Sima, A. A., S. D. Finkelstein, and D. R. McLachlan. 1983. Multiple malignant astrocytomas in a patient with spontaneous progressive multifocal leukoencephalopathy. *Ann. Neurol.* **14:**183–188.

Singh, N., A. Bonham, and M. Fukui. 2000. Immunosuppressive-associated leukoencephalopathy in organ transplant recipients. *Transplantation* **69:**467–472.

Snider, W. D., D. M. Simpson, S. Nielsen, J. W. Gold, C. E. Metroka, and J. B. Posner. 1983. Neurological complications of acquired immune deficiency syndrome. Analysis of fifty patients. *Ann. Neurol.* **14:**403–418.

So, Y. T., and R. K. Olney. 1994. Acute lumbosacral polyradiculopathy in acquired immunodeficiency syndrome: experience in 23 patients. *Ann. Neurol.* **135:**53–58.

Studahl, M., A. Ricksten, T. Sandberg, and T. Bergstrom. 1992. Cytomegalovirus encephalitis in four immunocompetent patients. *Lancet* **340:**1045–1046.

Suryanarayana, K., K. Baczko, V. ter Meulen, and R. R. Wagner. 1994. Transcription inhibition and other properties of matrix proteins expressed by M genes cloned from measles viruses and diseased human brain tissue. *J. Virol.* **68:**1532–1543.

Tauro, S., V. Toh, H. Osman, and P. Mahendra. 2000. Varicella zoster meningoencephalitis following treatment for dermatomal zoster in an allo BMT patient. *Bone Marrow Transplant.* **26:**795–796.

Thomas, C., G. DeSaint Basile, F. LeDeist, D. Theophile, M. Benkerrou, E. Haddad, S. Blanche, and A. Fischer. 1995. Brief Report: correction of x-linked hyper IgM syndrome by allogenic bone marrow transplantation. *N. Engl. J. Med.* **333:**426–429.

Tornatore, C., J. R. Berger, S. A. Houff, B. Curfman, K. Meyers, D. Winfield, and E. O. Major. 1992. Detection of JC virus DNA in peripheral lymphocytes from patients with and without progressive multifocal leukoencephalopathy. *Ann. Neurol.* **31:**454–462.

Weaver, S., M. K. Rosenblum, and L. M. DeAngelis. 1999. Herpes varicella zoster encephalitis in immunocompromised patients. *Neurology* **52:**193–195.

Wilfert, C. M., R. H. Buckley, T. Mohanakumar, J. F. Griffith, S. L. Katz, J. K. Whisnant, P. A. Egglesto, M. Moore, E. Treadwell, M. N. Oxman, and F. S. Rosen. 1977. Persistent and fatal central nervous system echovirus infections in patients with agammaglobulinemia. *N. Engl. J. Med.* **296:**1485–1489.

Willoughby, E., R. W. Price, B. L. Padgett, D. L. Walker, and B. Dupont. 1980. Progressive multifocal leukoencephalopathy (PML): in vitro cell-mediated immune responses to mitogens and JC virus. *Neurology* **30:**256–262.

Wolinsky, J. S., P. Swoveland, K. P. Johnson, and K. P. Baringer. 1977. Subacute measles encephalitis complicating Hodgkin's disease in an adult. *Ann. Neurol.* **1:**452–457.

Wyatt, H. V. 1973. Poliomyelitis in hypogammaglobulinemics. *J. Infect. Dis.* **128:**802–806.

Yiannoutsos, C. T., E. O. Major, B. Curfman, P. N. Jensen, M. Gravell, J. Hou, D. B. Clifford, and C. D. Hall. 1999. Relation of JC virus DNA in the cerebrospinal fluid to survival in acquired immunodeficiency syndrome patients with biopsy-proven progressive multifocal leukoencephalopathy. *Ann. Neurol.* **45:**816–821.

Zelman, I. B., and M. J. Mossakowski. 1998. Opportunistic infections of the central nervous system in the course of acquired immune deficiency syndrome (AIDS). Morphological analysis of 172 cases. *Folia Neuropathol.* **36:**129–144.

Zu Rhein, G. M., and S.-M. Chou. 1965. Particles resembling papovaviruses in human cerebral demyelinating disease. *Science* **148:**1477–1479.

Encephalitis in Immunocompetent Patients

This chapter considers viruses that cause subacute and chronic encephalitis in immunocompetent persons. A number of viruses discussed earlier in this book are also associated with chronic encephalitis in immunocompetent patients. Russian spring-summer encephalitis (Far Eastern subtype of tick-borne encephalitis) has been associated with Kozhevnikov's epilepsy (epilepsy partialis continuans), and with a chronic progressive encephalitis (Ogawa et al., 1973). Although a common cause of acute meningoencephalitis, mumps virus is not usually associated with a chronic or recurrent encephalitis. However, Vaheri et al. (1982) reported a case of acute encephalomyelitis followed 8 years later by relapse, with another relapse 5 years after that. Mumps antibodies were found in the serum and cerebrospinal fluid (CSF) with evidence of intrathecal production of immunoglobulin G (IgG). Acute disseminated encephalomyelitis can assume a progressive subacute form, and brain stem encephalitis can have subacute and chronic presentations. Nipah virus has been demonstrated to produce delayed and recurrent encephalitis (Tan et al., 2002). However, each of the episodes was usually acute in nature.

SSPE

Subacute sclerosing panencephalitis (SSPE) is a rare late manifestation of measles virus infection, developing years after natural measles infection. Measles virus is a member of the morbillivirus group of the paramyxovirus family, along with canine distemper and rinderpest viruses. Measles virions are composed of a nucleocapsid containing single-stranded RNA and viral proteins surrounded by an envelope composed of lipid and glycoprotein, which is in part derived from the host cell membrane. Virus particles may be spherical or filamentous, 100 to 300 nm across, and up to 1,000 nm in length. The receptor for measles virus that enables it to enter cells is the CD46 complement receptor, to which the viral hemagglutin protein binds (Buchholz et al., 1997; Dorig et al., 1993; Naniche et al., 1993).

During the first half of the 20th century several papers were written describing the clinical and pathological features of SSPE, but different pathological variants were described as if they were different diseases. In one of these variants the brunt of the pathology was borne by the gray matter and was associated with the presence of intranuclear inclusion bodies. This disease was called Dawson's inclusion body encephalitis, after the person who first described the pathology in 1933. A second pathological variant was described by van Bogaert (1945) under the name of "leuco-encéphalite scléronsante subaigüe." This disease was a subacute encephalitis with prominent sclerosis of the white matter as its chief distinguishing feature. Subsequently, it was realized that similarities existed between these two forms of encephalitis and that cases frequently combined some of the features of both (Greenfield, 1950). The unifying term "SSPE" was introduced and proved generally acceptable.

Progress in understanding the etiology of the disease was held up until 1965, when Bouteille et al. described electron microscopic observations that suggested the presence in nuclei of tubular inclusions resembling those of measles virus. This led to the demonstration of very high measles antibody titers in the serum and observation of measles antigen by immunofluorescence in the brain (Connolly et al., 1967). Difficulties were experienced when attempts were made to culture measles virus from the brain, however, and success was achieved only when brain cells from patients were cocultivated with cells that were permissive for measles virus growth and replication (Horta Barbosa et al., 1969; Payne et al., 1969; Chen et al., 1969). Even since then, the majority of attempts to recover measles virus from the brain in SSPE have been unsuccessful (Wechsler and Meissner, 1982) because the virus produced in SSPE is incomplete (see below).

Pathology

Reviews of the pathology and pathogenesis of SSPE can be found in articles by Schneider-Schaulies and ter Meulen (1999) and Griffin and Bellini (1996). The appearances of the brain, both macroscopic and microscopic, depend to a large extent on the length of survival in any individual case, and this can range from 1 to 2 months to many years. Most patients die within 1 to 3 years of the onset. Macroscopically, there may be nothing abnormal to note if the disease has been in progress for only a few months. With longer survival, and more characteristically, there is evidence of white matter gliosis—the white matter feels firmer and more rubbery or granular in texture than normal (Fig. 14.1)—and atrophy, with compensatory enlargement of the third and lateral ventricles. The cortical ribbon may also appear thin and gyri may be narrowed, with widened sulci. This atrophy of gray and white matter becomes even more prominent in patients that have survived many years (Fig. 14.2).

Microscopic Appearance of the Brain

Microscopically, pathological changes are present throughout the parenchyma of cerebral gray and white matter. Cerebral involvement is diffuse, but in the majority of cases the areas most severely affected are the parietal, occipital, and temporal lobes. The deep gray matter of the thalamus, caudate nucleus, putamen, and globus pallidus can all be affected. Involvement of the brain stem and cerebellum is generally milder than that of the cerebrum, and the spinal cord shows only slight changes, often confined to the cervical region.

The microscopic pathology consists of five features: (i) inflammation, with lymphocytes, macrophages, and plasma cells in perivascular cuffs and parenchyma of both gray and white matter (Fig. 14.3); (ii) foci of neuronophagia in gray matter; (iii) diffuse myelin loss with relative but not complete sparing of axons; (iv) prominent reactive gliosis in gray

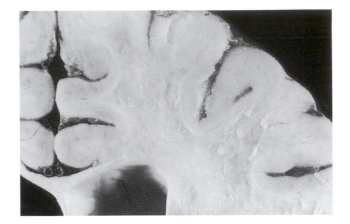

FIGURE 14.1   Close-up of fixed, sliced brain from a case of longstanding SSPE. The granular, rubbery consistency and discoloration of the white matter are evident.

and white matter; and (v) presence of inclusion bodies in nuclei of neurons and oligodendrocytes.

The relative preponderance of these various features depends on the stage of the disease. Inflammation tends to be more intense and accompanied by edema in cases with short survival, and more sparse in many cases with prolonged survival. Many of the inflammatory cells are T lymphocytes and major histocompatibility complex class II-immunoreactive macrophages and microglial cells (Kreth et al., 1982; Nagano et al., 1991). Plasma cells are plentiful and contain predominantly IgG. They are the source of the very high levels of oligoclonal IgG that accumulate in the CSF, much of which is directed against measles virus antigens (Link et al., 1973; Vandvik et al., 1974). Myelin loss and white matter gliosis are more extensive with prolonged survival than with short survival. In some cases the severity of the gliosis seems out of proportion to the relatively mild myelin loss. Inclusion bodies, which are intranuclear in position and eosinophilic and round in appearance, are variable in number but tend to be more numerous with short survival, when they are often focally abundant.

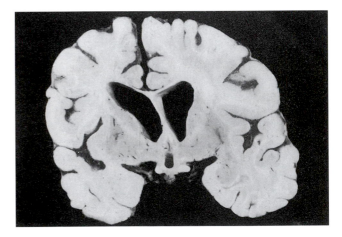

FIGURE 14.2   Sliced cerebrum from the case in Fig. 14.1. There is loss of white and gray matter, ventricular dilatation, and narrowed corpus callosum.

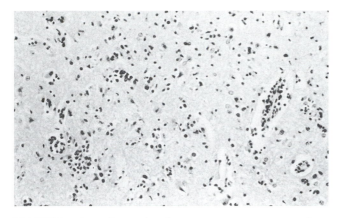

FIGURE 14.3 Cortical inflammation consisting predominantly of lymphocytes and macrophages in a case of SSPE of 3 months' duration. Hematoxylin and eosin stain.

After prolonged survival they may be difficult or impossible to find. The immunoperoxidase technique displays measles virus antigen in inclusion bodies in neurons and oligodendrocytes (Fig. 14.4) but not in astrocytes, at least where these are in a readily recognizable hypertrophied form. Measles antigen is also present in some neuron and oligodendrocyte nuclei that lack well-defined inclusion bodies and in the cytoplasm of the same types of cells. In neurons, antigen can be seen in dendritic cell processes (Fig. 14.4a). In oligodendrocytes, in which cytoplasm is not readily visible with routine stains, antigen-containing cells often appear to have ragged, degenerate cytoplasm and pyknotic nuclei. Viral antigen is more abundant in cases of short or intermediate duration than in very long-standing cases (Esiri et al., 1982). Some long-standing cases may contain no inclusion bodies but retain demonstrable viral RNA (Allen et al., 1996).

Neuron cell loss is usually obvious in the late stages of the disease but may be difficult to detect early on. Wallerian degeneration secondary to neuronal loss is also present in the late stages, although it is difficult to distinguish from the axonal loss accompanying demyelination that occurs in

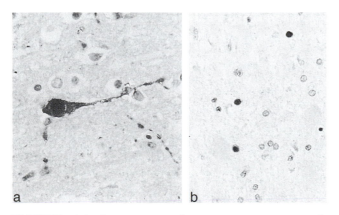

FIGURE 14.4 Immunoperoxidase staining using antimeasles antibody to demonstrate measles virus antigen in (a) neuron cytoplasm, processes, and nucleus and (b) oligodendrocyte nuclei in a case of SSPE of 9 months' duration. Counterstained with hematoxylin.

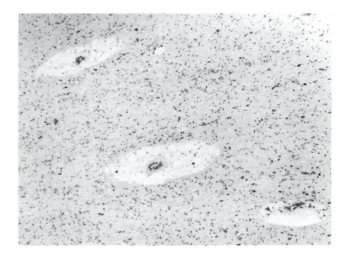

FIGURE 14.5 White matter from a case of long-standing SSPE. There is an increase in glial nuclei and widened perivascular spaces containing reticulin fibers, but little inflammation. Hematoxylin and eosin stain.

white matter as a result of the widespread oligodendrocyte infection and degeneration. In late cases there are also secondary changes around blood vessels, particularly veins, with widening of perivascular spaces and deposition of excess reticulin (Fig. 14.5). Another interesting feature in late cases is the presence in scattered remaining cortical neurons of neurofibrillary tangles similar to those seen in the cerebral cortex and hippocampus in Alzheimer's disease (Malamud et al., 1950; Corsellis, 1951; Gutewa and Osetowska, 1961; Mandybur et al., 1977; Paula-Barbosa et al., 1979; Bancher et al., 1996). These are not always colocalized with neurons containing measles virus antigen (Bancher et al., 1996; McQuaid et al., 1994) and can occur in oligodendroglia (Ikeda et al., 1995). Leptomeninges frequently show lymphocytic infiltration, particularly in the cases with short survival. Later, they show slight, diffuse thickening with collagen deposition.

Electron Microscopy

The intranuclear inclusion bodies consist ultrastructurally of multiple microtubules resembling the nucleocapsids of paramyxovirus or myxovirus particles (Bouteille et al., 1965; Tellez-Nagel and Harter, 1966; Shaw et al., 1967; Perier et al., 1968; Herndon and Rubinstein, 1968; Toga et al., 1969; Oyanagi et al., 1971). Nucleocapsids have been found in endothelial cells as well as in neurons and oligodendrocytes (Kirk et al., 1991). The tubules are of varying length (Fig. 14.6). Interspersed among the tubules are accumulations of electron-dense granular material. Similar collections of tubules and granular material may be present in the cytoplasm, although they display a notable failure to line up adjacent to the cell membrane. In culture, many of the nucleocapsids derived from SSPE brain have a smooth appearance that differs from the fuzzy outline of particles that are produced in acute measles isolates (Dubois-Dalcq et al., 1974).

The pathological picture in SSPE must be distinguished from other conditions that may superficially resemble its various stages. Thus, early cases, in which inflammation is

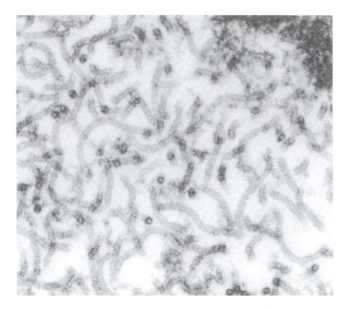

FIGURE 14.6   Electron micrograph of intranuclear paramyxovirus tubules from the temporal lobe at autopsy from a case of SSPE. ×125,000. Courtesy of J. E. Richmond.

severe and widespread, must be distinguished from other causes of encephalitis, most of which affect the gray matter predominantly and which, apart from herpes simplex encephalitis, lack intranuclear inclusion bodies. Herpes simplex encephalitis does not normally give rise to confusion because, if inclusion bodies are present, the course of the disease is more acute than SSPE and the topographical distribution of the lesions is characteristic. In geographic regions in which it occurs, trypanosomiasis can give rise to changes confusingly similar to those of SSPE, but inclusion bodies are, of course, absent. The perivascular demyelination of perivenous encephalitis has quite a different distribution from the diffuse demyelination of SSPE. Prolonged cases of SSPE are distinguished from other causes of diffuse myelin damage, such as the leukodystrophies, on the basis of the additional gray matter damage and the presence of inclusion bodies in neuron and oligodendrocyte nuclei in SSPE.

Pathogenesis

The precise sequence of events that results in the development of SSPE in a tiny portion of the population is not known. The great majority of children who develop SSPE are known to have had an attack of classical measles, usually many years before. More than 50% of cases have had the disease at the unusually early age of less than 2 years. This suggests that immaturity of either the immune system or the nervous system or both may be a factor of importance in pathogenesis. When SSPE has developed, there is no overwhelming evidence of immune deficiency either in a general sense or with regard to humoral and immune responses to measles virus (Agnarsdottir, 1977), although the results of such studies have not been unanimous (Valdimarsson et al., 1979; Ueda et al., 1982). An unusual variant of the complement C4 protein, C4AQO, is overrepresented among people with SSPE (Rittner et al., 1984). Antibody levels to measles virus are exceptionally high in most cases, but

because the disease has been described in children with hypogammaglobulinemia, it seems unlikely that the high antibody levels themselves are of primary importance (Hanissian et al., 1972; White et al., 1972). However, it has been shown that in experimental animals and in tissue culture the presence of specific antibody can promote persistent infection with measles virus. It is generally presumed that measles virus survives in a nonlytic state between the initial attack of measles and the development of SSPE. Once SSPE has developed, measles virus can be detected in blood lymphocytes (Fournier et al., 1985), lymphoid tissue, and other organs (Brown et al., 1989).

Are host factors or viral mutations of major importance for the development of SSPE? Most of the recent evidence about the molecular biology of the virus suggests that SSPE is caused by a mutated virus that can spread insidiously from cell to cell in the nervous system without the need for the cells to express the CD46 receptor, through which it normally gains entry to cells (Lawrence et al., 2000). Patients with SSPE lack antibody to the matrix (M) protein while at the same time possessing high titers of antibody to the other measles virus proteins (Hall et al., 1979; Wechsler et al., 1979). The M protein becomes aligned along the inner surface of the host cell membrane in normal measles virus assembly and appears to be important for virus assembly. The probable reason for the lack of M-protein antibody became apparent when it was shown that brain cells cultured from a case of SSPE failed to synthesize M protein, although other measles virus proteins were produced (Hall and Choppin, 1981; Lin and Thormar, 1980). Mutations affecting the M protein and other proteins have been described in SSPE (Cattaneo et al., 1988; Billeter et al., 1994; Schmid et al., 1992; Hall and Choppin, 1981). Other studies have documented molecular changes in the cytoplasmic tail of the fusion protein (Ning et al., 2002). Failure of viral assembly, related to partial or complete failure of M-protein synthesis, is present in the brain in most cases of SSPE.

Under the influence of a strong humoral response to viral proteins other than the M protein, clonal expansion of mutated virus in the brain succeeds in spreading from cell to cell by means of cell fusion. Measles virus lacking the M protein has been shown to propagate and spread in an experimental model of SSPE (Cathomen et al., 1998). It is uncertain whether the damage to the infected neurons and oligodendrocytes results from direct viral effects or from a cell-mediated immune attack on infected cells that have incorporated measles virus antigens in the cell membrane. Either way, apoptotic mechanisms are thought to be involved (Anlar et al., 1999). Immune complexes containing viral antigen have been described in brain, serum, and CSF (Jenis et al., 1973; Perrin and Oldstone, 1977; Sotrel et al., 1983) in patients with SSPE, but their contribution to the damage produced is not certain.

Diagnosis and Management

With widespread implementation of measles immunization, complications of measles infection, including SSPE, have declined markedly in the industrialized world. In the developing world, however, measles and its complications, including SSPE, remain significant public health problems (Saha et al., 1990). Earlier epidemiological analysis of cases in the United States demonstrated several consistent features (Jabbour et al., 1972; Modlin et al., 1979; Halsey et al., 1980; Sever, 1983). Approximately half of the cases in the prevaccine era were associated with natural measles infection at or before 2 years of age. Cases in males were two to three times more frequent than in females, and a marked preponderance of incidence in whites compared to blacks was found. Children in rural habitats, those in the southeast region of the United States, and those in the Ohio River valley were at greater risk. Concurrent with use of the vaccine, the mean age of onset has risen from about 7 years of age to almost 11 years. Where known, adult onset of SSPE is associated with an interval of 14 to 22 years between measles and SSPE (Singer et al., 1997). Although SSPE may occur in vaccinated children, the risk appears to be between 5 and 50 times lower than the risk following natural measles (Graves, 1984). The peak number of cases reported to the National SSPE Registry in the United States was 53 cases in both 1967 and 1968. Fifteen years later, following widespread immunization, the average incidence of cases from 1982 to 1986 in the United States was 4.2 per year (Dyken, 1989).

The onset of the illness is characteristically insidious and without clinical signs of systemic or central nervous system (CNS) infection. Clinical disability most commonly manifests itself as a falling off of school performance or in changes of personality and behavior (Freeman, 1969; Huttenlocher and Mattson, 1979). Not infrequently, a psychological cause will be sought. Disobedience, emotional lability, distractability, and terrifying hallucinations suggest a psychological basis. However, impaired memory and failing school performance denote an evolving dementia. On intelligence testing, the nonverbal tests are most severely affected. Visual agnosia and apraxia can often be demonstrated. The psychological and intellectual defects constitute what many have considered as the first stage of the illness. Visual system abnormalities with ophthalmoscopic findings such as retinitis and chorioretinitis can be found early in the course of the illness (Green and Wirtschafter, 1973; Case Records, 1998). Visual symptomatology is particularly common in adult-onset SSPE. Singer et al. (1997) found that 8 of 13 cases had presentation with ophthalmological symptoms.

Evolution of the illness is frequently described in terms of the four-stage system of Jabbour et al. (1969). Progression of the illness varies greatly from patient to patient and the appearance of any given disability also varies. The first stage, just described, will often have a duration of 1 or 2 months. In the second stage, evidence of motor disability and paroxysmal disorders emerges. Repeated myoclonus, convulsive seizures, incoordination, pyramidal signs, extrapyramidal movements, and disorders of tone all occur. Most characteristic are the myoclonic jerks that at first may appear as clumsiness. When developed, they are sudden flexion movements of head, trunk, and extremities that are followed by a slower relaxation phase of 1 to 2 s. They may occur several times a minute during waking hours, do not themselves interfere with consciousness, and disappear during sleep. The myoclonus is synchronized with paroxysmal, high-amplitude, slow-wave electroencephalogram (EEG) activity. However,

the EEG paroxysms continue during sleep even though the myoclonus abates. In addition to the myoclonic attacks, grand mal and akinetic seizures may occur.

As the neurological condition worsens in stage 2, several pyramidal and extrapyramidal motor disorders and ataxia may evolve. Hemiparesis, hyperreflexia, upgoing plantar responses, and generalized spasticity may occur. Tremor, rigidity, and masklike facies contribute to a parkinsonian appearance. However, dyskinesias such as chorea, ballismus, athetosis, or dystonia may be seen in other patients. In addition, swallowing difficulties and poverty of speech manifest themselves. Vision may be impaired by choreoretinitis, optic neuritis, or cortical blindness. On occasion, papilledema may be found.

Development of coma and decerebrate rigidity characterize stage 3, which may come about from one to several months after the start of the illness. Absence of conscious responses, reflex posturing, and irregular, noisy breathing constitute the desperate picture. Episodes of autonomic dysfunction produce diaphoresis, hyperthermia, vasomotor instability with pallor and flushing, and instability of pulse and blood pressure. Much of the activity noted in stage 3 abates after one to several months with progress to stage 4. However, these stages may be difficult to differentiate even by experienced observers.

In stage 4, the myoclonus often subsides, the hypertonia gives way to hypotonia, random eye movements may occur, and pathological crying and laughing may be stimulated by handling (Jabbour et al., 1969). The duration of illness to death can be as short as 6 weeks or as long as 10 years or more, although the great majority of patients succumb by 9 months to 3 years. PeBenito et al. (1997) found nine cases in the literature in which the duration of illness was 2 months or less. Long-term survival has been reported, and up to 5% of patients may experience spontaneous long-term improvement (Risk et al., 1978). Apparent improvement or a plateau in disease activity can also occur at any point (Risk and Haddad, 1979), making the assessment of treatment difficult.

Of the laboratory studies the lumbar puncture (LP), EEG, and viral antibody studies are crucial. The LP reveals fluid with normal or minimally elevated cells and total protein. The important determination is the Ig level, which is elevated in most patients (Jabbour et al., 1969). The CSF contains oligoclonal bands of Ig, which can be demonstrated to consist of antibody against components of measles virus. The characteristic EEG finding is a repetitive complex of high-voltage slow waves (Cobb and Hill, 1950). The complexes may be followed by relative absence of activity, termed burst suppression. The periodicity may result in complexes every 4 to 20 s. Yaqub (1996) identified three types of periodic complexes on EEG: giant delta waves; giant delta waves mixed with rapid spikes or fast activity; and spike wave discharges extended but broken up by giant deltal waves. With computerized tomography (CT), areas of low attenuation, atrophy, and ventricular enlargement are seen. Periventricular and subcortical white matter lesions of high intensity are found on T2-weighted magnetic resonance imaging (MRI) images, as is cerebral atrophy (Brismar et al., 1996; Anlar et al., 1996; Ozturk et al., 2002). However, pathognomic findings and clear correlation of neuroimaging findings with disease course are not found.

The key virological study is determination of measles antibody levels in the serum and CSF. Although the hemagglutination inhibition antibody level is usually highest years after natural measles, in SSPE the complement fixation antibody level is usually highest (Sever, 1983). Thus, while serum titers of complement fixation antibody were 8 to 16 in healthy children years after measles, Jabbour et al. (1969) found patients with SSPE to have serum levels from 64 to 4,096. Furthermore, complement fixation antibody to measles is not normally found in the CSF; therefore, its documentation is a very useful diagnostic point in SSPE. Brain biopsy was previously frequently obtained to seek evidence of measles virus in brain tissue. Nucleocapsids can be seen on electron microscopy, viral antigens can be identified by immunofluorescence studies, and virus can be isolated on occasion by cocultivation techniques. PCR can be applied to brain tissue to identify measles genome (Godec et al., 1990). However, biopsy is not recommended except in cases in which an alternative, treatable disease is also being considered. PCR on CSF or biopsy has been suggested by Baram et al. (1994) in cases with atypical antibody findings.

Much of the therapy in SSPE is symptom based. Treatment of the myoclonus involves clonazepam or valproate. Convulsive seizures should be treated with standard anticonvulsant medication. Evaluation of therapy directed toward the underlying measles infection remains problematic because of the inherent variability of the disease course (Risk and Haddad, 1979). In 1974, Mattson (R. H. Mattson, Abstr., *Neurology* **24**:383, 1974) reported a dramatic remission of deterioration following the administration of inosiplex (isoprinosine) to a patient with SSPE. Jones et al. (1982) reported a study of 98 treated patients compared with historical controls and reached the conclusion that inosiplex prolonged life. Current practice suggests that combined therapy of intraventricular alpha-2b interferon and oral inosiplex carries the best short-term outcome (Case Records, 1998). Alpha interferon is administered through an Ommaya reservoir in courses of 5 days per week, repeated at 2- to 6-month intervals for up to six courses. More recently, the combination of intrathecal alpha interferon and intravenous (i.v.) ribavirin has been advocated (Tomoda et al., 2001).

PROGRESSIVE RUBELLA PANENCEPHALITIS (PRP)

Progressive rubella panencephalitis (PRP) is a slowly progressive fatal disease of insidious onset whose key features are dementia, ataxia, and elevated antirubella antibody titers in the serum and CSF. First observed in Paris (P. Lebon and G. Lyon, Letter, *Lancet* ii:468, 1974), it is an exceedingly rare disease, with fewer than 20 cases known by the late 1990s (Asher, 1997). It can follow congenital rubella or childhood rubella. The absence of recent reports suggests that PRP may have essentially disappeared. The reasons for its appearance and disappearance are mysterious. It shares certain features with SSPE. These include a slowly progressive dementia in children with an abnormally high antiviral serological response and elevated CSF IgG. However, it differs not only with regard to the causative virus but also in a more prolonged course, lack of prominence of myoclonic jerks, infrequency of viral antigen in the brain, and evidence of disease of cerebral vessels. In contrast to SSPE, reports on PRP are not emerging from underdeveloped nations with incomplete immunization coverage, supporting the notion of its disappearance.

Pathology

The pathology in two cases was described by Townsend et al. (1982). There was a widespread subacute encephalitis of the cerebrum, mainly affecting white matter, with perivascular cuffing by lymphocytes and plasma cells, microglial nodules, and astrocytosis. Some diffuse myelin loss was evident in the centrum semiovale. No inclusion bodies were seen, and no rubella antigen was demonstrable. Mild neuronal loss was seen in the cerebral cortex and basal ganglia. The cerebellum, pons, and medulla were shrunken and covered with brown, thickened leptomeninges, and ependymal surfaces appeared granular. The cerebellum was severely atrophied, with Purkinje cell and granule cell loss in the cortex, but no inclusion bodies. A noteworthy feature was the presence of widespread amorphous basophilic deposits, sometimes with calcification in the parenchyma and in the walls of small blood vessels, mainly in the cerebral and cerebellar cortex. The vascular changes, but not the inflammation, are reminiscent of the appearance of the brain in congenital rubella infection without progressive neurological deterioration. The CSF from a case was reported to contain rubella-specific oligoclonal IgG and free light chains (Vandvik et al., 1978). Immunological studies of affected children have failed to show why a progressive encephalitis occurred in a minority of children with congenital rubella infection (Wolinsky et al., 1979).

The absence of inclusion bodies, presence of basophilic deposits, and severe cerebellar damage distinguish this condition from SSPE due to measles virus.

Diagnosis and Management

The age at initial infection with rubella of the first described case (Lebon and Lyon, Letter) was not known. However, four subsequent cases described from California developed 11 to 14 years following the congenital rubella syndrome (Townsend et al., 1975; Weil et al., 1975). It has since also been observed following childhood rubella infection (Townsend et al., 1982). No particular features of the congenital or childhood rubella infections which predisposed patients to PRP have been identified. Although there was concern that the 1964 rubella epidemic in the United States, in which more than 20,000 cases were likely to have occurred, would be followed years later by significant numbers of cases of PRP, that did not happen. All known cases have occurred in males, and the age of onset has varied from 8 to 19 years (Wolinsky, 1989). Some of the cases following congenital rubella carried congenital disabilities, including cataracts, cardiac murmurs, microcephaly, and mental retardation.

The onset was insidious, with impairment of school performance and clumsiness. Over several years, the intellectual impairment progressed to global amnesia. The clumsiness often resulted from ataxia. Ultimately, gait, trunk, and all four limbs could be affected. Although myoclonus was seen (Abe et al., 1983), it was not usually the consistent problem that it is in SSPE. Convulsive seizures were, however, a common problem. Patients typically became chair- or wheelchair-bound as spastic quadraparesis evolved. Other findings included dysarthria, facial weakness, and impairment of extraocular movement. Optic atrophy could occur and resulted from demyelination and gliosis (Townsend et al., 1982). The course was one of steady deterioration over 8 to 10 years, with dementia and spasticity progressively reducing the patient's activity.

The most useful laboratory studies were examination of the CSF and antiviral antibody determinations. The CSF often contained a mild mononuclear pleocytosis and moderate elevation of protein. However, there was a marked increase of IgG. Oligoclonal bands were found in the CSF, and these contained antirubella antibody (Vandvik et al., 1978). The EEG could demonstrate slowing of background rhythms without focal features. However, the periodic paroxysms of high-amplitude slow-wave activity so characteristic of SSPE were not a prominent part of the EEG records in PRP. Pneumoencephalography and CT examination revealed enlarged ventricles, particularly enlargement of the fourth ventricle and atrophy of the cerebellar cortex.

The key virological studies were antibody determinations. There was usually a marked elevation of serum antibody against rubella virus, and antibody could also be demonstrated in the CSF. Further, examination of brain tissue following autopsy demonstrated a high level of antirubella antibody in brain parenchyma (Townsend et al., 1982). Virus was isolated from the brain by Cremer et al. (1975); however, attempts at isolation from brain and searches for viral antigens in brain samples have been generally unsuccessful in other cases. There would be little diagnostic reason to perform biopsy should cases reappear that were characterized by the appropriate clinical features and elevated antibody titers. Virus has been isolated from lymphocytes (Wolinsky et al., 1979), and viral antigen has been identified in CSF cells (Abe et al., 1983). Molecular diagnostic viral assays for viral protein and RNA could be employed should future cases emerge (Wolinsky and McCarthy, 1995). Immune complexes in PRP were demonstrated to contain both rubella virus antigens and rubella-specific antibody (Coyle and Wolinsky, 1981). In light of the evidence for significant cerebral vasculitis in PRP (Townsend et al., 1982), such immune complexes may have been of pathogenetic significance.

Therapy has been symptom based and similar to that described for SSPE. Convulsive seizures were treated with standard anticonvulsant medication. Myoclonic jerks were treated with clonazepam and valproate (Abe et al., 1983). However, no therapy has been reported to interrupt the basic disease process. Based on the example of SSPE, isoprinosine has been used, but without success (Wolinsky et al., 1979; Jan et al., 1979), nor was amantadine successful (Wolinsky, 1989). In light of the demonstrated cerebral vasculitis (Townsend et al., 1982) and circulating immune complexes (Coyle and Wolinsky, 1981), the use of plasmapheresis might be considered.

HAM/TSP

Human T-cell leukemia virus type 1 (HTLV-1) is a retrovirus that was initially identified as the agent responsible for human T-cell leukemia. It is an endemic infection in the Caribbean, South America, and parts of Africa and southwest Japan. Antibodies to HTLV-1 were present in the serum of 57% of patients on the Caribbean island of Martinique having the chronic myelopathy known as tropical spastic paraparesis (TSP) (Gessain et al., 1985). Similar findings were also reported from Jamaica and Colombia. A similar syndrome in Japan was associated with the antibodies to the virus and with atypical lymphocytes in CSF (Osame et al., 1987). This condition is known as HTLV-1-associated myelopathy (HAM). The great majority of cases of HAM/TSP are now known to be caused by HTLV-1, with occasional cases caused by a related retrovirus, HTLV-2 (Black et al., 1996; Jacobson et al., 1993; Murphy et al., 1997).

Pathology and Pathogenesis

Like human immunodeficiency virus (HIV), HTLV-1 is an enveloped retrovirus containing single-stranded positive-sense RNA, which, once inside a cell, synthesizes a double-stranded DNA provirus that becomes integrated in host cell DNA. The cell receptor has not been identified. The virus is transmitted through sexual intercourse, blood transfusion, breast milk, or blood contamination in injection drug abusers. Less than 5% of those who are carriers of HTLV-1 develop leukemia, and even fewer develop HAM/TSP. High virus load is a risk factor for development of HAM/TSP (Jeffery et al., 1999), but the exact mechanism of its development is unclear.

The pathology of HAM/TSP consists of myelin loss and a lesser degree of axon loss in the white matter of the spinal cord, particularly the corticospinal tracts in lateral column white matter (Fig. 14.7). The low thoracic and lumbar levels are those most affected. There is variable

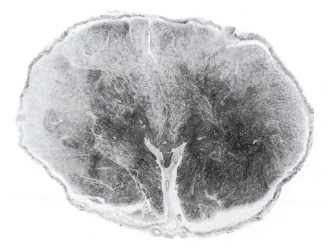

FIGURE 14.7 Low-power view of myelin-stained section of the spinal cord in HAM/TSP. Note pallor of staining in the lateral corticospinal tracts and posterior columns.

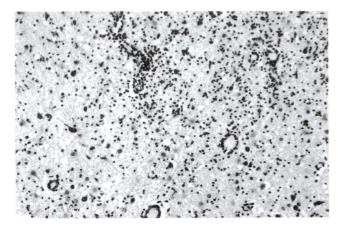

FIGURE 14.8 Inflammation in the spinal cord in HAM/TSP with small veins and cord parenchyma infiltrated with mononuclear inflammatory cells.

mononuclear cell inflammation, which is most marked in cases of relatively short duration. These cells occupy perivenous and perivenular spaces of gray and white matter (Fig. 14.8). Some cases show inflammation in brain stem, optic nerves, and cerebrum. In situ hybridization or immunocytochemistry has demonstrated sparse HTLV-1 DNA or protein within lesions in lymphocytes (Hara et al., 1994; Moore et al., 1989). In addition to the myelitis, there is a local meningitis or, in chronic cases, meningeal thickening and radiculitis (Fig. 14.9).

Development of HAM/TSP requires the presence of HTLV-1-infected CD4 T lymphocytes in the CNS. These cells are targets of a brisk immune response, which may have the capacity to damage CNS parenchyma locally by a "bystander mechanism." Activated CD8 lymphocytes specific for the viral Tax 11-19 peptide can be demonstrated in blood and CSF in HAM/TSP (Greten et al., 1998). An autoimmune reaction to neuronal antigens has also been postulated to have a role in mediating damage to axons in HAM/TSP (Levin et al., 2002).

A minority of patients with HAM/TSP develop the complication of myositis (Smadja et al., 1995), which in some

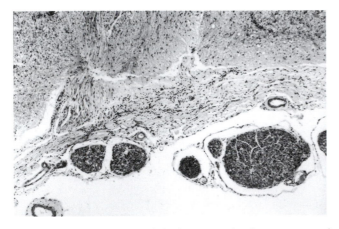

FIGURE 14.9 Meningeal thickening and inflammation and slight perivascular and meningeal inflammation in HAM/TSP.

cases has features of inclusion body myositis (Cupler et al., 1996).

Diagnosis and Management

HAM/TSP usually presents in an insidious manner as a slowly progressive, often asymmetric, spastic paraparesis (Osame and McArthur, 1992). Onset can be more rapid, as can be progression, for example when acquired by transfusion (Gout et al., 1990). While sometimes found in childhood, onset is most common in adult life, with illness in women more frequent than in men. Bladder dysfunction may occur early in the course, and impotence is a common feature (Osame and McArthur, 1992). Variable sensory symptoms such as tingling and burning have been found, lower lumbar radiating pain has been reported, and evidence of impaired vibratory sensation has been observed on exam. Motor weakness in the lower extremities, most prominent proximally, and reflex findings of hyperreflexia, clonus, and pathological reflexes such as Babinski signs are characteristic.

The differential diagnosis of HAM/TSP includes the spinal cord form of chronic progressive multiple sclerosis (MS). Rudge et al. (1991) reported that of Afro-Caribbean-origin patients living in the United Kingdom with myelopathy of unknown cause, those with HTLV-1 antibodies were classified as having TSP. None of the patients in whom antibody was tested and who satisfied criteria for MS had HTLV-1 antibodies. Clinical features supporting the diagnosis of MS included more frequent evidence of cranial nerve dysfunction, including asymmetry of the visual evoked response and more extensive evidence of demyelination on brain and cervical spinal cord studies by MRI. In contrast, the dorsal spinal cord was found to be atrophic on MRI in 60% of patients with TSP. Other patients in whom the diagnosis may be clinically perplexing are those coinfected with HIV as well as HTLV-1 (McArthur et al., 1990; Berger et al., 1991). While evidence for both viruses may be present in CSF, if studies of the CD4 T-cell subset are within normal limits, HTLV-1 may be the pathogenic virus. In such cases, treatment with steroids such as prednisone may be associated with improvement (McArthur et al., 1990; Berger et al., 1991). Berger et al. (1991) also reported an HIV/HTLV-2 dually infected patient whose myelopathy improved spontaneously. Other intrinsic and extrinsic spinal cord disorders must be considered in any HTLV-1-positive patient with spinal cord findings. Conversely, an epidemic form of TSP in HTLV-1-negative patients has been associated with ingestion of the cassava bean.

The spectrum of disease associated with HTLV-1 has expanded considerably beyond adult T-cell leukemia/lymphoma and HAM/TSP. Inflammatory nerve (Said et al., 1988) and muscle (Leon-Monzon et al., 1994; Ozden et al., 2001) diseases are each recognized. Other HTLV-1-associated illnesses include infective dermatitis, uveitis, infiltrative pneumonitis, and polyarthropathy (Blattner, 1997; Manns et al., 1999). MRI studies reveal cerebral white matter lesions, which can be found to progress on longitudinal study (Kira et al., 1991); however, cerebral signs clearly distinct from those resulting from the myelopathy are rare. For a brief period there was interest in the possibility of HTLV-1 as a cause of MS. However, confirmation has not been forthcoming (summarized in Booss and Kim, 1990).

The diagnosis is suspected in a patient with a chronic progressive myelopathy whose origins are in an HTLV-I endemic area or who has been breast-fed by an HTLV-1-positive woman. Others may have been exposed through unscreened blood products, i.v. drug abuse, or sexual relations with an HTLV-1-infected partner. Some cases have been identified by blood screening for blood donation (Centers for Disease Control and Prevention, 1993). The World Health Organization diagnostic criteria of 1989 note the presence of HTLV-1 antigens or antibodies in blood and spinal fluid and virus isolation from serum and/or CSF "when possible." It is noted that the CSF may contain a mild lymphocytic pleocytosis and a mild to moderate increase of protein. Lobulated lymphocytes ("flower cells") can be found in blood or CSF. McKendall et al. (1991) demonstrated serum and CSF antibodies to HTLV-1 and positive PCR of cultured CSF lymphocytes and circulating mononuclear cells in three patients from Texas. More recently, Puccioni-Sohler et al. (2001) recommended CSF PCR for proviral DNA and the specific antibody index for intrathecal antibody production in CSF to make the diagnosis of HAM/TSP. Oligoclonal bands were found in CSF in about 90% of the HAM/TSP patients examined.

Short-term therapeutic benefit has accrued from treatment with prednisone or other steroids (Osame and McArthur, 1992). However, the effect has been variable, being most evident in cases acquired by blood transfusion and/or in which there was a rapid evolution. Steroids have been unsuccessful in more chronic cases (Gout et al., 1990). Other immunomodulating or immunosuppressive therapies, including the anabolic steroid danazol (Harrington et al., 1991), plasmapheresis, i.v. Ig, and azathioprine, have been tried in uncontrolled studies (summarized in Osame and McArthur, 1992; Lehky et al., 1998). Initial treatment trials with the antiretroviral reverse transcriptase inhibitor zidovudine failed to produce a favorable clinical response (Gout et al., 1991).

However, as presently understood, the pathogenesis of HAM/TSP would suggest that a two-pronged therapy, antiretroviral and immunomodulating, should be attempted. Three studies lend some support to the strategy. Izumo et al. (1996), in a double-blind, multicenter randomized trial, demonstrated therapeutic benefit of human lymphoblastoid alpha interferon. Two-thirds of patients treated with 10^6 IU had a good to excellent clinical response. Lehky et al. (1998), in an open-label trial of humanized anti-Tac antibody, were able to down-regulate activated T cells and reduce viral load by about 50% in peripheral blood lymphocytes as measured by HTLV-1 DNA PCR. Taylor et al. (1999) also demonstrated a reduction in viral DNA following treatment with lamivudine, a reverse transcriptase inhibitor.

At present, a short-term treatment strategy, particularly in acutely evolving cases and/or cases related to blood transfusion, is steroid therapy. Long-term interventions could employ combination therapies of antiretroviral treatment and immunomodulatory treatment that explicitly target lymphocytes activated by HTLV-1 infection (Nakamura, 2000).

Recommendations for counseling of persons found to be seropositive for HTLV-1 or -2 start with informing the patient of the infection (Centers for Disease Control and Prevention, 1993). People should also be counseled that they should share the information with their physicians, refrain from cell or tissue donations, refrain from sharing needles or syringes, refrain from breast-feeding infants, and use latex condoms in sexual relations with HTLV-seronegative partners.

RASMUSSEN'S ENCEPHALITIS

Rasmussen's encephalitis is a condition of chronic intractable epilepsy in children that is associated with signs of progressive hemispheral dysfunction and unilateral brain atrophy. Resected brain tissue can demonstrate perivascular infiltrates and glial nodules, usually in the absence of clinical features of encephalitis, i.e., an acellular spinal fluid and an afebrile state. Describing the syndrome in 1958, Rasmussen et al. commented, "We call this an encephalitis on histologic grounds, recognizing that we have no indication as to the etiology of this condition." Evidence for an antibody response against the glutamate receptor Glu R3 has been found in some patients (Rogers et al., 1994), and evidence of virus in cerebral tissue, most commonly cytomegalovirus (CMV), has been found in others (Power et al., 1990). However, the etiology and pathogenesis of the syndrome remain matters of investigation.

Most patients are children, with a median age of onset of 5 years in the Montreal Neurologic Institute series (Oguni et al., 1992); however, cases in adults have been reported (McLachlan et al., 1993). The first and a defining feature is intractable epilepsy. Simple partial motor seizures were most common in the Montreal Neurologic Institute series, but complex partial seizures and status epilepticus were observed and epilepsia partialis continua developed in more than half. Rasmussen's syndrome is one of the principal causes of chronic progressive epilepsia partialis continua of childhood, otherwise known as Kojewnikow's syndrome (Commission on Classification and Terminology of the International League Against Epilepsy, 1989). Signs of hemispheral dysfunction emerge, including hemiparesis and cognitive and behavioral abnormalities. Clinically, Oguni et al. (1992) divided the course into three stages: (1) before the development of fixed hemiparesis; (2) development of hemiparesis to completion of disability; and (3) a stable but ongoing state without further progression. The time of deterioration ranged from 3 months to 20 years, with a median of 4 years (Oguni et al., 1992).

Bien et al. (2002b) reported that the first findings on MRI (Fig. 14.10) are a focal area of swollen cortex with a hyperintense T2 fluid-attenuated inversion recovery signal, followed by evidence for progressive atrophy. The neuroimaging findings were correlated with histopathological evidence of inflammation with T cells and microglial nodules at the earliest stages, which diminished over time. The CSF, as noted, is often bland. The EEG may provide a clue to the diagnosis early in the course, with focal theta activity and multifocal interictal epileptiform discharges developing (Carney, 2001). As the disease advances, positron-emission tomography and MRI reveal hypometabolism and hemispheral atrophy (Tien et al., 1992).

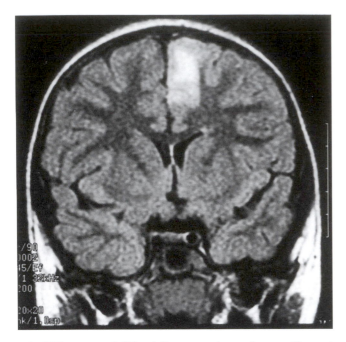

FIGURE 14.10 MRI of Rasmussen's syndrome. Coronal FLAIR image demonstrates hyperintensity in the cortical and subcortical regions of the medial superior frontal lobe. Courtesy of Dennis Spencer, Yale University School of Medicine.

Rasmussen et al. (1958) suggested in the first description of the syndrome that the cause might be viral. However, in contrast to progressive multifocal leukoencephalopathy, SSPE, and PRP, no virus has emerged as the clear etiology of Rasmussen's encephalitis. The most commonly identified virus in brain tissue has been CMV. Power et al. (1990) demonstrated CMV by in situ hybridization in 7 of 10 patients and 2 of 46 controls. McLachlan et al. (1993) found CMV by in situ hybridization in three adult patients with Rasmussen's encephalitis. These findings led McLachlan et al. to recommend treatment with ganciclovir in a later report (1996). They reported a reduction of seizures in two of three patients treated. Vinters et al. (1993) challenged the significance of the evidence for the herpes family of viruses in Rasmussen's encephalitis, including CMV. They suggested that the small amounts of CMV and Epstein-Barr virus genome material found in patients with and without encephalitis argued against these viruses as a direct cause. Later studies by Jay et al. (1995) yielded evidence for the presence of CMV in 6 of 10 chronic encephalitis cases and for the presence of herpes simplex virus type 1 in two cases. Suffice it to say that the role of viral infection remains a matter of investigation.

Following observations made in experimental rabbits immunized with recombinant glutamate receptors, Rogers et al. (1994) reported the presence of serum antibodies to a component of the receptor Glu R3 in patients with Rasmussen's encephalitis. Subsequently, it was reported that plasmapheresis produced dramatic, although transient, reduction in frequency of seizures and improvement of neurological function (Andrews et al., 1996). Not all patients with Rasmussen's encephalitis have antiglutamate receptor

antibodies, and conversely, patients with focal epilepsy of other types may have antibodies to portions of the glutamate receptor (Wiendl et al., 2001). Wiendl et al. (2001) concluded that these antibodies were not specific to Rasmussen's encephalitis, but that they could contribute to or perpetuate the seizure state in antibody-positive patients. More recently, Bien et al. (2002a) presented immunohistochemical evidence for a pathogenic role of cytotoxic T cells. Taken together, there is evidence suggesting that inflammatory and immune-mediated mechanisms play a role in the disease.

Hence, there does appear to be a rationale for immune-based therapy (Greenlee and Rose, 2000), particularly in the early stages of the illness before resorting to hemispherectomy. In addition to plasmaphoresis, high-dose steroids and/or i.v. Ig have been employed (Hart et al., 1994). Leach et al. (1999) found in two adult patients that improvement following i.v. Ig was delayed until after two to four monthly cycles of high-dose i.v. Ig. Single-photon emission tomography (SPECT) demonstrated improvement of cerebral perfusion and was recommended as an additional outcome measure. Antiviral therapy decisions must be made on a case-by-case basis. If the presence of viral genome is demonstrated on biopsy, it would be reasonable to initiate antiviral therapy. If immunologically based therapy fails, the decision of if and when to undertake hemispherectomy is clearly important. Arguments can be advanced for early or late surgical intervention (Oguni et al., 1992). Considerations include the possibility of shifting functions to the intact hemisphere and the risk of further neurological decline.

VILYUISK ENCEPHALITIS—BOKHOROR

Vilyuisk encephalitis is a remarkable disease affecting the Iakut people in the Vilyuisk region and neighboring areas in Russian Siberia (Petrov, 1970; Goldfarb and Gajdusek, 1992). Although the region of involvement has gradually enlarged over the past several decades, it remains a geographically isolated disease. Subacute, slowly progressive, and chronic forms are recognized (McLean et al., 1997). Though it is suspected to be an infectious disease, the agent has not been established.

Neuropathological findings in patients who expired after subacute disease demonstrated changes in the meninges and in the CNS (McLean et al., 1997; Goldfarb and Gajdusek, 1992). The meninges demonstrated thickening and cellular infiltrates, predominantly mononuclear. In the CNS itself, changes were found at many levels from the cortex to the spinal cord, including conspicuous changes in the basal ganglia. Multiple small foci of necrosis surrounded by mononuclear cells, microglia, and astrocytes were the principal finding. Findings were similar in the slowly progressive form but with less frequent necrotic foci. Confluence of lesions was seen in some patients, resulting in extensive tissue damage. In the chronic form, in which death supervened after up to 13 years of the illness, gliotic lytic lesions were found and active lesions were absent. Atrophy, microcysts, and gliosis could be found in the cortex. Intranuclear inclusions have not been found. Virus has not been isolated in tissue culture or experimental animals by using a variety of samples, including brain tissue, as reported by Goldfarb and Gajdusek (1992), nor has a serological response to known viruses been found. Reported isolates by other investigators have not been confirmed. Hence, while the neuropathological changes appear to be those of a chronic encephalitis, an immune-mediated process is not excluded.

Known as Bokhoror (stiffness), Vilyuisk encephalitis occurs in Iakut peoples, among whom it has a significant prevalence. Found in small rural settlements, spread of the illness has been associated with migration of the Iakut people. Although most cases occur from May to July, cases occur all year round and do not appear to be dependent on an insect vector. The incubation period has been variously calculated from cases with common exposure, and an average of 15.7 years has been found (Goldfarb and Gajdusek, 1992). Why an illness with an apparent incubation period measured in years should have an onset predominantly at one time of year merits reflection. The average age of onset is between 35 and 40 years.

The subacute (rapid) disease is often preceded by a prodromal stage of 2 to 3 days of malaise, weakness, nausea, and vomiting. This is followed by severe headache, fever, and chills. Neurological findings include ptosis, ophthalmoplegia, bradykinesia, extrapyramidal rigidity, spastic weakness, and ataxia. Psychiatric symptoms include delirium and depression. The CSF demonstrates a moderate pleocytosis of 5 to 30 mononuclear cells and an elevation of protein. The acute or subacute phase is reported to last between a few days and 4 months or more. Exacerbations occasionally occur. Death can occur 2 to 3 months into the illness (Goldfarb and Gajdusek, 1992).

Slowly progressive encephalitis can follow the subacute form after a period of partial recovery. This form lasts 2 to 5 years and is characterized by apathy, stiffness, clumsiness, weakness, bradykinesia, and dysarthria. Global dementia and pyramidal tract findings develop. Special forms include involvement of lower motor neurons, producing an amyotrophic form. Seizures occur in a minority of patients. Hypothalmic symptoms have been seen in some patients, and sexual dysfunction has been prominent, particularly among males. Terminally, global dementia, incontinence, and profound disability are found.

The chronic form may or may not be initiated by a mild subacute phase. It is characterized by slow progression of clinical abnormalities followed by stabilization. Death ultimately supervenes up to 20 years later (McLean et al., 1997).

A mononuclear CSF pleocytosis and protein elevation can be seen in the subacute (rapid) and slowly progressive forms of the illness. No pathognomic features have characterized the EEG, and neuroimaging studies have not been reported. No diagnostic clinical virology studies are positive. Viral studies are performed to exclude other causes of encephalitis.

Considerable international scientific interest in Vilyuisk encephalitis has emerged (Stone, 2002). The contribution of genetic stock to a potentially infectious disease of long incubation has drawn attention. Similar to encephalitis lethargica, the disease has an acute phase in which the upper brain stem is heavily involved and a later chronic phase in which extrapyramidal signs are prominent. In contrast to encephalitis lethargica, however, Vilyuisk encephalitis appears to be an endemic disease, and the chronic phase has more widespread CNS destruction.

BORNA DISEASE

Borna disease is a meningoencephalitis of horses, sheep, and other farm animals found principally in Germany. It is named after a town in the German state of Saxony where, between 1894 and 1896, an epidemic occurred among cavalry horses (Staeheli et al., 2000). Remarkably, despite international trade of horses and the free movement of farm animals, the disease endemic area has remained relatively stable. Whether there is a more broad global distribution of viral infection and whether other species serve as reservoirs of the virus is unknown, as is the mode of transmission (Lipkin et al., 2001). Pathologically, in horses, lymphocytic infiltrates are found in the hippocampus, brain stem, and cerebral cortex (Gosztonyi and Ludwig, 1984). Virus isolation sometimes proves to be difficult, and Joest-Degen inclusion bodies, when found, are diagnostically useful. The virus is enveloped, contains negative-strand RNA, and constitutes the prototype of the virus family *Bornaviridae*. Experimental models have been useful to examine the pathogenesis of neurodevelopmental abnormalities and also behavioral defects, the role of immune-mediated damage, and the development of chronic Borna disease (Carbone, 2001; Narayan et al., 1983).

In 1985, Rott et al. reported positive indirect immunofluorescent antibodies in the serum of 16 out of 979 patients with psychiatric disorders. The original group consisted mainly of persons with cyclic affective disorders. Since that time, the relationship of Borna virus or closely related viruses and human psychiatric disease, including mood disorders and schizophrenia, has remained frustratingly unresolved (Lipkin et al., 2001; Staeheli et al., 2000; Carbone, 2001). Much of the controversy arises from variability in findings from various laboratories, for example, those using reverse transcriptase PCR (Lipkin et al., 2001). Carbone (2001) reviewed the several assays used to establish the diagnosis of human Borna virus infection and their pitfalls. Bode et al. (2001) reported data on circulating immune complexes, free antibodies, and plasma p40/p24 antigens to explain the variable detectability of Borna virus infection in human psychiatric illness. The results of a multi-institution controlled study using standardized methodology on blinded samples will be awaited with interest (Lipkin et al., 2001).

REFERENCES

Abe, T., T. Nukada, H. Hatanaka, M. Tajima, M. Hiraiwa, and H. Ushijima. 1983. Myoclonus in a case of suspected progressive rubella panencephalitis. *Arch. Neurol.* **40**:98–100.

Agnarsdottir, G. 1977. Subacute sclerosing panencephalitis, p. 22–29. *In* A. P. Waterson (ed.), *Recent Advances in Clinical Virology.* Churchill Livingstone, London, United Kingdom.

Allen, I. V., S. McQuaid, J. McMahon, J. Kirk, and R. McConnell. 1996. The significance of measles virus antigen and genome distribution in the CNS in SSPE for mechanisms of viral spread and demyelination. *J. Neuropathol. Exp. Neurol.* **55**:471–480.

Andrews, P. I., M. A. Dichter, S. F. Berkovic, M. R. Newton, and J. O. McNamara. 1996. Plasmapheresis in Rasmussen's encephalitis. *Neurology* **46:**242–246.

Anlar, B., I. Saatci, G. Kose, and K. Yalaz. 1996. MRI findings in subacute sclerosing panencephalitis. *Neurology* **47:**1278–1283.

Anlar, B., K. Yalaz, F. Oktem, and G. Kose. 1997. Long-term follow-up of patients with subacute sclerosing panencephalitis treated with intraventricular α-interferon. *Neurology* **48:**526–528.

Anlar, B., F. Soylemezoglu, B. Elibol, T. Dalkara, S. Aysun, G. Kose, D. Belen, and K. Yalaz. 1999. Apoptosis in brain biopsies of subacute sclerosing panencephalitis patients. *Neuropediatrics* **30:**239–242.

Asher, D. M. 1997. Slow viral infection, p. 199–221. *In* W. M. Scheld, R. J. Whitley, and D. T. Durack (ed.), *Infections of the Central Nervous System.* Lippincott-Raven, Philadelphia, Pa.

Bancher, C., H. Leitner, K. Jellinger, H. Eder, U. Setinek, P. Fischer, J. Wegiewl, and H. M. Wisneiwski. 1996. On the relationship between measles virus and Alzheimer neurofibrillary tangles in subacute sclerosing panencephalitis. *Neurobiol. Aging* **17:**527–533.

Baram, T. Z., I. Gonzalez-Gomez, Z.-D. Xie, D. Yao, F. H. Gilles, M. D. Nelson, Jr., H. T. Nguyen, and J. Peters. 1994. Subacute sclerosing panencephalitis in an infant: diagnostic role of viral genome analysis. *Ann. Neurol.* **36:**103–108.

Berger, J. R., S. Raffanti, A. Svenningsson, M. McCarthy, S. Snodgrass, and L. Resnick. 1991. The role of HTLV in HIV-I neurologic disease. *Neurology* **41:**197–202.

Bien, C. G., J. Bauer, T. L. Deckwerth, H. Wiendl, M. Deckert, O. D. Wiestler, J. Schramm, C. E. Elger, and H. Lassman. 2002a. Destruction of neurons by cytotoxic T cells: a new pathogenic mechanism in Rasmussen's encephalitis. *Ann. Neurol.* **51:**311–318.

Bien, C. G., H. Urbach, M. Deckert, J. Schramm, O. D. Wiestler, H. Lassman, and C. E. Elger. 2002b. Diagnosis and staging of Rasmussen's encephalitis by serial MRI and histopathology. *Neurology* **58:**250–257.

Billeter, M. A., R. Cattaneo, P. Spielhofer, K. Kaelin, M. Huber, A. Schmid, K. Baczko, and V. ter Meulen. 1994. Generation and properties of measles virus mutations typically associated with subacute sclerosing panencephalitis. *Ann. N.Y. Acad. Sci.* **724:**367–377.

Black, F. L., R. J. Biggar, R. B. Lal, A. A. Baggai, and J. P. Filho. 1996. Twenty-five years of HTLV type II follow-up with a possible case of tropical spastic paraparesis in the Kayapo, a Brazilian Indian tribe. *AIDS Res. Hum. Retrovir.* **12:**1623–1627.

Blattner, W. A. 1997. Human lymphotropic viruses: HTLV-I and HTLV-II, p. 683–705. *In* D. D. Richman, R. J. Whitle, and F. G. Hayden (ed.), *Clinical Virology.* Churchill Livingstone, New York, N.Y.

Bode, L., P. Reckwald, W. E. Severus, R. Stoyloff, R. Ferszt, D. E. Dietrich, and H. Ludwig. 2001. Borna disease virus-specific circulating immune complexes, antigenemia, and free antibodies—the key marker triplet determining infection and prevailing in severe mood disorders. *Mol. Psychiatry* **6:**481–491.

Booss, J., and J. H. Kim. 1990. Evidence for a viral etiology of multiple sclerosis, p. 41–61. *In* S. D. Cook (ed.), *Handbook of Multiple Sclerosis.* Marcel Dekker, New York, N.Y.

Bouteille, M., C. Fontaine, C. Vedrenne, and J. Delarue. 1965. Sur un cas d'encéphalite subaigüe à inclusions: étude anatomo-clinique et ultrastructurale. *Rev. Neurol.* **113:**454–458.

Brismar, J., G. G. Gascon, K. V. von Steyem, and S. Bohlega. 1996. Subacute sclerosing panencephalitis: evaluation with CT and MR. *Am. J. Neuroradiol.* **17:**761–772.

Brown, H. R., N. L. Goller, R. D. Rudelli, J. Dymecki, and H. M. Wisniewski. 1989. Postmortem detection of measles virus in non-neural tissues in subacute sclerosing panencephalitis. *Ann. Neurol.* **26:**263–268.

Buchholz, C. J., D. Koller, P. Devaux, C. Mumenthaler, J. Schneider-Schaulies, W. Braun, D. Gerlier, and R. Cattaneo. 1997. Mapping of the primary binding site of measles virus to its receptor CD46. *J. Biol. Chem.* **272:**22072–22079.

Carbone, K. M. 2001. Borna disease virus and human disease. *Clin. Microbiol. Rev.* **14:**513–527.

Carney, P. R. 2001. Rasmussen's syndrome: intractable epilepsy and progressive neurological deterioration from a unilateral central nervous system disease. *CNS Spectr.* **6:**398, 409–416.

Case Records of the Massachusetts General Hospital. 1998. Case 15-1998. *N. Engl. J. Med.* **338:**1448–1456.

Cathomen, T., B. Mrkic, D. Spehner, R. Drillien, R. Naef, J. Pavlovic, A. Aguzzi, M. A. Billeter, and R. Cattaneo. 1998. A matrix-less measles virus is infectious and elicits extensive cell fusion: consequences for propagation in the brain. *EMBO J.* **17:**3899–3908.

Cattaneo, R., A. Schmid, M. A. Billeter, R. D. Sheppard, and S. A. Udem. 1988. Multiple viral mutations rather than host factors cause defective measles virus gene expression in a subacute sclerosing panencephalitis cell line. *J. Virol.* **62:**1388–1397.

Centers for Disease Control and Prevention. 1993. Recommendations for counseling persons infected with human T-lymphotrophic diseases, types I and II. *Morb. Mortal. Wkly. Rep.* **42**(RR-9)**:**1–13.

Chen, T. T., I. Watanabe, W. Zeman, and J. Mealey. 1969. Subacute sclerosing panencephalitis: propagation of measles virus from brain biopsy in tissue culture. *Science* **163:**1193–1194.

Cobb, W., and D. Hill. 1950. Electroencephalogram in subacute progressive encephalitis. *Brain* **73:**392–404.

Commission on Classification and Terminology of the International League Against Epilepsy. 1989. Proposal for revised classification of epilepsies and epileptic syndromes. *Epilepsia* **30:**389–399.

Connolly, J. H., I. V. Allen, L. J. Hurwitz, and J. H. D. Millar. 1967. Measles-virus antibody and antigen in subacute sclerosing panencephalitis. *Lancet* **i:**542–544.

Corsellis, J. 1951. Subacute sclerosing panencephalitis: clinical and pathological report of 2 cases. *J. Ment. Sci.* **97:**570–583.

Coyle, P. K., and J. S. Wolinsky. 1981. Characterization of immune complexes in progressive rubella panencephalitis. *Ann. Neurol.* **9:**557–562.

Cremer, N. E., L. S. Oshiro, M. L. Wei, E. H. Lennette, H. H. Itabashi, and L. Carnay. 1975. Isolation of rubella virus from brain in chronic progressive panencephalitis. *J. Gen. Virol.* **29:**143–153.

Cupler, E. J., M. Leon-Monzon, J. Miller, C. Semino-Mora, T. L. Anderson, and M. C. Dalakas. 1996. Inclusion body myositis in HIV-1 and HTLV-1 infected patients. *Brain* **119:**1887–1893.

Cutewa, J., and E. Osetowska. 1961. A chronic form of subacute sclerosing panencephalitis (a case with a history of 5 years): clinical and pathological study, p. 386–404. *In* L. van Bogaert, J. Radermecker, J. Hozay, and A. Lowenthal (ed.), *Encephalitides.* Elsevier, Amsterdam, The Netherlands.

Dorig, R. E., A. Marcil, A. Chopra, and C. D. Richardson. 1993. The human CD46 molecule is a receptor for measles virus (Edmonston strain). *Cell* **75:**295–305.

Dubois-Dalcq, M., L. H. Barbosa, and J. L. Sever. 1974. Comparison between productive and latent subacute sclerosing panencephalitis viral infection in vitro. An electron microscopic and immunoperoxidase study. *Lab. Investig.* **30:**241–250.

Dyken, P. R. 1985. Subacute sclerosing panencephalitis: current status. *Neurol. Clin.* **3:**179–196.

Dyken, P. R. 1989. Changing character of subacute sclerosing panencephalitis in the United States. *Pediatr. Neurol.* **5:**L339–341.

Esiri, M. M., D. R. Oppenheimer, B. Brownell, and M. Haire. 1982. Distribution of measles antigen and immunoglobulin-containing cells in the CNS in subacute sclerosing panencephalitis (SSPE) and atypical measles encephalitis. *J. Neurol. Sci.* **53:**29–43.

Fournier, J. G., M. Tardieu, P. Lebon, O. Robain, G. Ponsot, S. Rozenblatt, and M. Bouteille. 1985. Detection of measles virus RNA in lymphocytes from peripheral-blood and brain perivascular infiltrates of patients with subacute sclerosing panencephalitis. *N. Engl. J. Med.* **313:**910–915.

Freeman, J. F. 1969. The clinical spectrum and early diagnosis of Dawson's encephalitis. With preliminary notes on treatment. *J. Pediatr.* **75:**590–603.

Gessain, A., F. Barin, J. C. Vernant, O. Gout, L. Maurs, A. Calender, and G. de Thé. 1985. Antibodies to human T-lymphotropic virus type-I in patients with tropical spastic paraparesis. *Lancet* **ii:**407–410.

Godec, M. S., D. M. Asher, P. T. Swoveland, Z. A. Eldah, S. M. Feinstone, L. G. Goldfarb, C. J. Gibbs, Jr., and D. C. Gajdusek. 1990. Detection of measles virus genomic sequences in SSPE brain tissue by polymerase chain reaction. *J. Med. Virol.* **30:**237–244.

Gokcil, Z., Z. Odbasi, S. Demirkaya, E. Eroglu, and O. Vural. 1999. α-Interferon and isoprinisine in adult-onset subacute sclerosing panencephalitis. *J. Neurol. Sci.* **162:**62–64.

Goldfarb, L. G., and D. C. Gajdusek. 1992. Viliusk encephalomyelitis in the Iakut people of Siberia. *Brain* **115:**961–978.

Gosztonyi, G., and H. Ludwig. 1984. Borna disease of horses. An immunohistological and virological study of naturally infected animals. *Acta Neuropathol.* **64:**213–221.

Gout, O., M. Baulac, A. Gessain, F. Semah, F. Saal, J. Pèries, C. Cabrol, C. Foucault-Fretz, D. Laplane, F. Sigaux, and G. de Thé. 1990. Rapid development of myelopathy after HTLV-I infection acquired by transfusion during cardiac transplantation. *N. Engl. J. Med.* **322:**383–388.

Gout, O., A. Gassain, M. Iba-Zizen, S. Kouzan, F. Bolgert, G. de Thé, and O. Lyon-Caen. 1991. The effect of zidovudine on chronic myelopathy associated with HTLV-I. *J. Neurol.* **238:**108–110.

Graves, M. C. 1984. Subacute sclerosing panencephalitis. *Neurol. Clin.* **2:**267–280.

Green, S. H., and J. D. Wirtschafter. 1973. Ophthalmoscopic findings in subacute sclerosing panencephalitis. *Br. J. Ophthalmol.* **57:**780–787.

Greenfield, J. 1950. Encephalitis and encephalomyelitis in England and Wales during the last decade. *Brain* **73:**141–166.

Greenlee, J. E., and J. W. Rose. 2000. Controversies in neurological infectious diseases. *Semin. Neurol.* **20:**375–386.

Greten, T. F., J. E. Slansky, R. Kubota, S. S. Soldan, E. M. Jaffee, T. P. Leist, D. M. Pardoll, S. Jacobson, and J. P. Schneck. 1998. Direct visualization of antigen-specific T cells: HTLV-1 Tax 11-19-specific CD8(+) T cells are activated in peripheral blood and accumulate in cerebrospinal fluid from HAM-TSP patients. *Proc. Natl. Acad. Sci. USA* **95:**7568–7573.

Griffin, D. E., and W. J. Bellini. 1996. Measles virus, p. 1267–1312. *In* B. N. Fields, D. M. Knipe, and P. M. Howley (ed.), *Fields Virology.* Raven, Philadelphia, Pa.

Gutewa, J., and E. Osetowska. 1961. A chronic form of subacute sclerosing panencephalitis (a case with a history of

5 years), clinical and pathological study, p. 386–404. *In* L. Bogaert, J. Radermecker, J. Hozay, and A. Lowenthal (ed.), *Encephalitides.* Elsevier, Amsterdam, The Netherlands.

Hall, W. W., and P. W. Choppin. 1981. Measles-virus proteins in the brain tissue of patients with subacute sclerosing panencephalitis: absence of the M protein. *N. Engl. J. Med.* **304:**1152–1155.

Hall, W. W., R. A. Lamb, and P. W. Choppin. 1979. Measles and subacute sclerosing panencephalitis virus proteins: lack of antibodies to the M protein in patients with subacute sclerosing panencephalitis. *Proc. Natl. Acad. Sci. USA* **76:**2047–2051.

Halsey, N. A., J. F. Modlin, J. T. Jabbour, L. Dubey, D. L. Eddins, and D. D. Ludwig. 1980. Risk factors in subacute sclerosing panencephalitis: a case-control study. *Am. J. Epidemiol.* **111:**415–424.

Hanissian, A. S., J. T. Jabbour, S. de Lamerens, J. H. Garcia, and L. Horta-Barbosa. 1972. Subacute encephalitis and hypogammaglobulinemia. *Am. J. Dis. Child.* **123:**151–155.

Hara, H., M. Morita, T. Iwaki, T. Hatae, Y. Itoyama, T. Kitamoto, S. Akizuki, I. Goto, and T. Watanabe. 1994. Detection of human T lymphotrophic virus type I (HTLV-I) proviral DNA and analysis of T cell receptor V beta CDR3 sequences in spinal cord lesions of HTLV-I-associated myelopathy-tropical spastic paraparesis. *J. Exp. Med.* **180:**831–839.

Harrington, W. J., Jr., W. A. Sheremata, S. R. Snodgrass, S. Emerson, S. Phillips, and J. R. Berger. 1991. Tropical spastic paraparesis/HTLV-I-associated myelopathy (TSP/HAM): treatment with an anabolic steroid danazol. *AIDS Res. Hum. Retrovir.* **7:**1031–1034.

Hart, Y. M., M. Cortez, F. Andermann, P. Hwang, D. R. Fish, O. Dulac, K. Silver, N. Fejerman, H. Cross, A. Sherwin, and R. Caraballo. 1994. Medical treatment of Rasmussen's syndrome (chronic encephalitis and epilepsy): effect of high-dose steroids or immunoglobulins in 19 patients. *Neurology* **44:**1030–1036.

Herndon, R. M., and L. J. Rubinstein. 1968. Light and electron microscopy observations on the development of viral particles in the inclusions of Dawson's encephalitis (subacute sclerosing panencephalitis). *Neurology* **18:**8–20.

Hollsberg, P., and D. A. Hafler. 1993. Pathogenesis of diseases induced by human lymphotropic virus Type I infection. *N. Engl. J. Med.* **328:**1173–1182.

Horta-Barbosa, L., D. A. Fuccillo, J. L. Sever, and W. Zeman. 1969. Subacute sclerosing panencephalitis: isolation of measles virus from a brain biopsy. *Nature* **221:**974.

Huttenlocher, P. R., and R. H. Mattson. 1979. Isoprinosine in subacute sclerosing panencephalitis. *Neurology* **29:**763–771.

Ichiyama, T., S. Houdou, T. Kisa, K. Ohno, and K. Takeshita. 1990. Varicella with delayed hemiplegia. *Pediatr. Neurol.* **6:**279–281.

Ikeda, K., H. Akiyama, H. Kondo, T. Arai, N. Arai, and S. Yagishita. 1995. Numerous glial fibrillary tangles in oligodendroglia in cases of subacute sclerosing panencephalitis with neurofibrillary tangles. *Neurosci. Lett.* **194:**133–135.

Izumo, S., I. Goto, Y. Itoyama, T. Okajma, S. Watanabe, Y. Kuroda, S. Araki, M. Mori, S. Nagataki, S. Matsukura, T. Akamine, M. Nakagawa, I. Yamamoto, and M. Osame. 1996. Interferon-alpha is effective in HTLV-I myelopathy: a multicenter, randomized, double-blind, controlled trial. *Neurology* **46:**1016–1021.

Jabbour, J. T., D. A. Duenas, J. L. Sever, H. M. Krebs, and L. Horta-Barbosa. 1972. Epidemiology of subacute sclerosing panencephalitis (SSPE). A report of the SSPE registry. *JAMA* **220:**959–962.

Jabbour, J. T., J. H. Garcia, H. Lemmi, J. Ragland, D. A. Duenas, and J. L. Sever. 1969. Subacute sclerosing panencephalitis. A multidisciplinary study of eight cases. *JAMA* **207**:2248–2254.

Jacobson, S., T. Lehky, M. Nishimura, S. Robinson, D. E. McFarlin, and S. Dhib-Jalbut. 1993. Isolation of HTLV-II from a patient with chronic, progressive neurological disease clinically indistinguishable from HTLV-I-associated myelopathy/tropical spastic paraparesis. *Ann. Neurol.* **33**:392–396.

Jan, J. E., A. J. Tingle, G. Donald, M. Kettyls, W. St. J. Buckler, and C. L. Dolman. 1979. Progressive rubella panencephalitis: clinical course and response to isoprinosine. *Dev. Med. Child Neurol.* **21**:648–652.

Jay, V., L. E. Becker, H. Otsubo, M. Cortez, P. Hwang, H. J. Hoffman, and M. Zielenska. 1995. Chronic encephalitis and epilepsy (Rasmussen's encephalitis): detection of cytomegalovirus and herpes simplex virus 1 by the polymerase chain reaction and in situ hybridization. *Neurology* **45**:108–117.

Jeffery, K. J., K. Usuku, S. E. Hall, W. Matsumoto, G. P. Taylor, J. Procter, M. Bunce, G. S. Ogg, K. I. Welsh, J. N. Weber, A. L. Lloyd, M. A. Nowak, M. Nagai, D. Kodama, S. Izumo, M. Osame, and C. R. Bangham. 1999. HLA alleles determine human T-lymphotropic virus-I (HTLV-I) proviral load and the risk of HTLV-I-associated myelopathy. *Proc. Natl. Acad. Sci. USA* **96**:3848–3853.

Jenis, E. J., M. R. Kneiser, P. A. Rothanse, G. E. Jensen, and R. M. Scott. 1973. Subacute sclerosing panencephalitis—immunostructural localization of measles virus antigen. *Arch. Pathol.* **95**:81–89.

Jones, C. E., P. R. Dyken, P. R. Huttenlocher, J. T. Jabbour, and K. W. Maxwell. 1982. Inosiplex therapy in subacute sclerosing panencephalitis. A multicentre, nonrandomised study in 98 patients. *Lancet* **i**:1034–1037.

Kira, J.-I., K. Fujihara, Y. Itoyama, I. Goto, and K. Hasuo. 1991. Leukoencephalopathy in HTLV-I-associated myelopathy/ tropical spastic paraparesis: MRI analysis and a two year follow-up study after corticosteroid therapy. *J. Neurol. Sci.* **106**:41–49.

Kirk, J., A. L. Zhou, S. McQuaid, S. L. Cosby, and I. V. Allen. 1991. Cerebral endothelial cell infection by measles virus in subacute sclerosing panencephalitis: ultrastructural and in situ hybridization evidence. *Neuropathol. Appl. Neurobiol.* **17**:289–297.

Kreth, H. W., R. Dunker, H. Rodt, and R. Meyermann. 1982. Immunohistochemical identification of T-lymphocytes in the central nervous system of patients with multiple sclerosis and subacute sclerosing panencephalitis. *J. Neuroimmunol.* **2**:177–183.

Lawrence, D. M., C. E. Patterson, T. L. Gales, J. L. D'Orazio, M. M. Vaughn, and G. F. Rall. 2000. Measles virus spread between neurons requires cell contact but not CD46 expression, syncytium formation, or extracellular virus production. *J. Virol.* **74**:1908–1918.

Leach, J. P., D. W. Chadwick, J. B. Miles, and I. K. Hart. 1999. Improvement in adult-onset Rasmussen's encephalitis with long-term immunomodulatory therapy. *Neurology* **52**:738–742.

Lehky, T. J., M. C. Levin, R. Kubota, R. N. Bamford, A. N. Flerage, S. S. Soldan, T. A. Fleisher, L. E. Top, S. Light, H. F. McFarland, T. A. Waldmann, and S. Jacobson. 1998. Reduction in HTLV-I proviral load and spontaneous lymphoproliferation in HTLV-I-associated myelopathy/tropical spastic paraparesis patients treated with humanized anti-tac. *Ann. Neurol.* **44**:942–947.

Leon-Monzon, M., I. Illa, and M. C. Dalakas. 1994. Polymyositis in patients infected with human T-cell leukemia virus type I.

The role of the virus in cause of disease. *Ann. Neurol.* **36**:643–649.

Levin, M. C., S. M. Lee, F. Kalume, Y. Morcos, F. C. Dohan, Jr., K. A. Hasty, J. C. Callaway, J. Zunt, D. Desiderio, and J. M. Stuart. 2002. Autoimmunity due to molecular mimicry as a cause of neurological disease. *Nat. Med.* **8**:509–513.

Lin, F. H., and H. Thormar. 1980. Absence of M protein in a cell-associated subacute sclerosing panencephalitis virus. *Nature* **285**:490–492.

Link, H., M. Panelius, and A. A. Salmi. 1973. Immunoglobulins and measles antibodies in subacute sclerosing panencephalitis. *Arch. Neurol.* **28**:23–30.

Lipkin, W. I., M. Hornig, and T. Briese. 2001. Borna disease virus and neuropsychiatric disease—a reappraisal. *Trends Microbiol.* **9**:295–298.

Malamud, N., W. Haymaker, and H. Pinkerton. 1950. Inclusion encephalitis with clinicopathologic report of 3 cases. *Am. J. Pathol.* **26**:133–153.

Mandybur, T. I., A. S. Nagpaul, Z. Pappas, and W. J. Niklowitz. 1977. Alzheimer neurofibrillary change in subacute sclerosing panencephalitis. *Ann. Neurol.* **1**:103–107.

Manns, A., M. Hisada, and L. LaGrenade. 1999. Human T-lymphotropic virus type I infection. *Lancet* **353**:1951–1958.

McArthur, J. C., J. W. Griffin, D. R. Cornblath, D. E. Griffin, T. Tesoriero, R. Kunel, C. J. Gibbs, H. Farzadegan, and R. T. Johnson. 1990. Steroid-responsive myeloneuropathy in a man dually infected with HIV-I and HTLV-I. *Neurology* **40**:938–944.

McKendall, R. R., J. Oas, and M. D. Lairmore. 1991. HTLV-1 associated myelopathy endemic in Texas-born residents and isolation of virus from CSF cells. *Neurology* **41**:831–836.

McLachlan, R.S., J. P. Girvin, W. T. Blume, and H. Reichman. 1993. Rasmussen's chronic encephalitis in adults. *Arch. Neurol.* **50**:269–274.

McLachlan, R. S., S. Levin, and W. T. Blume. 1996. Treatment of Rasmussen's syndrome with ganciclovir. *Neurology* **47**:925–928.

McLean, C. A., C. L. Masters, V. A. Vladimirtsev, I. A. Prokhorova, L. G. Goldfarb, D. M. Asher, A. I. Vladimirtsev, V. P. Alekseev, and D. C. Gajdusek. 1997. Viliuisk encephalomyelitis—review of the spectrum of pathological changes. *Neuropathol. Appl. Neurobiol.* **23**:212–217.

McQuaid, S., I. V. Allen, J. McMahon, and J. Kirk. 1994. Association of measles virus with neurofibrillary tangles in subacute sclerosing panencephalitis: a combined in situ hybridization and immunocytochemical investigation. *Neuropathol. Appl. Neurobiol.* **20**:103–110.

Modlin, J. F., N. A. Halsey, D. L. Eddins, J. L. Conrad, J. T. Jabbour, L. Chien, and H. Robinson. 1979. Epidemiology of subacute sclerosing panencephalitis. *J. Pediatr.* **94**:231–236.

Moore, G. R., U. Traugott, L. C. Scheinberg, and C. S. Raine. 1989. Tropical spastic paraparesis: a model of virus-induced, cytotoxic T-cell-mediated demyelination? *Ann. Neurol.* **26**:523–530.

Murphy, E. L., J. Fridey, J. W. Smith, J. Engstrom, R. A. Sacher, K. Miller, J. Gibble, J. Stevens, R. Thomson, D. Hansma, J. Kaplan, R. Khabbaz, and G. Nemo. 1997. HTLV-associated myelopathy in a cohort of HTLV-I and HTLV-II-infected blood donors. The REDS investigators. *Neurology* **48**:315–320.

Nagano, I., S. Nakamura, M. Yoshioka, and K. Kogure. 1991. Immunocytochemical analysis of the cellular infiltrate in brain lesions in subacute sclerosing panencephalitis. *Neurology* **41**:1639–1642.

Nakamura, T. 2000. Immunopathogenesis of HTLV-I-associated myelopathy/tropical spastic paraparesis. *Ann. Med.* **32**:600–607.

Naniche, D., G. Varior-Krishnan, F. Cervoni, T. F. Wild, B. Rossi, C. Rabourdin-Combe, and D. Gerlier. 1993. Human membrane cofactor protein (CD46) acts as a cellular receptor for measles virus. *J. Virol.* **67:**6025–6032.

Narayan, O., S. Herzog, K. Frese, H. Scheefers, and R. Rott. 1983. Behavioral disease in rats caused by immunopathological responses to persistent borna virus in the brain. *Science* **220:**1401–1403.

Ning, X., M. Ayata, M. Kimura, K. Komase, K. Furukawa, T. Seto, N. Ito, M. Shingai, I. Matsunaga, T. Yamano, and H. Ogura. 2002. Alterations and diversity in the cytoplasmic tail of the fusion protein of subacute sclerosing panencephalitis virus strains isolated in Osaka, Japan. *Virus Res.* **86:**123–131.

Ogawa, M., H. Okubo, Y. Tsuji, N. Yasui, and K. Someda. 1973. Chronic progressive encephalitis occurring 13 years after Russian spring-summer encephalitis. *Neurol. Sci.* **19:**363–373.

Oguni, H., F. Andermann, and T. B. Rasmussen. 1992. The syndrome of chronic encephalitis and epilepsy. A study based on the MNI series of 48 cases. *Adv. Neurol.* **57:**419–433.

Osame, M., and J. C. McArthur. 1992. Neurologic manifestations of infection with human T cell lymphotropic virus type I, p. 1331–1339. *In* A. K. Asbury, G. M. McKhann, and W. I. McDonald (ed.), *Diseases of the Nervous System. Clinical Neurobiology,* 2nd ed. W.B. Saunders, Philadelphia, Pa.

Osame, M., M. Matsumoto, K. Usuku, S. Izumo, N. Ijichi, H. Amitani, M. Tara, and A. Igata. 1987. Chronic progressive myelopathy associated with elevated antibodies to human T-lymphotropic virus type I and adult T-cell leukemialike cells. *Ann. Neurol.* **21:**117–122.

Oyanagi, S., V. ter Meulen, M. Katz, and H. Koprowski. 1971. Comparison of subacute sclerosing panencephalitis and measles viruses: an electron microscope study. *J. Virol.* **7:**176–187.

Ozden, S., A. Gessain, O. Gout, and J. Mikol. 2001. Sporadic inclusion body myositis in a patient with human T cell leukemia virus type I-associated myelopathy. *Clin. Infect. Dis.* **32:**510–514.

Ozturk, A., C. Gurses, B. Baykan, A. Gokyigit, and M. Eraksoy. 2002. Subacute sclerosing panencephalitis: clinical and magnetic resonance imaging evaluation of 35 patients. *J. Child. Neurol.* **17:**25–29.

Paula-Barbosa, M. M., R. Brito, C. A. Silva, R. Faria, and C. Cruz. 1979. Neurofibrillary changes in the cerebral cortex of a patient with subacute sclerosing panencephalitis (SSPE). *Acta Neuropathol.* **48:**157–160.

Payne, F. E., J. V. Baublis, and H. H. Itabashi. 1969. Isolation of measles virus from cell cultures of brain from a patient with subacute sclerosing panencephalitis. *N. Engl. J. Med.* **281:**585–589.

PeBenito, R., S. H. Naqvi, M. M. Arca, and R. Schubert. 1997. Fulminating subacute sclerosing panencephalitis: case report and literature review. *Clin. Pediatr.* **36:**149–154.

Perier, O., L. Thiry, J. J. Vanderhaegen, and S. Pelc. 1968. Attempts at experimental transmission and electron microscopic observations in subacute sclerosing panencephalitis. *Neurology* **18:**138–143.

Perrin, L. H., and M. B. A. Oldstone. 1977. The formation and fate of virus antigen-antibody complexes. *J. Immunol.* **118:**316–322.

Petrov, P. A. 1970. V. Vilyuisk encephalitis in the Yakut Republic (USSR). *Am. J. Trop. Med. Hyg.* **19:**146–150.

Power, C., S. D. Poland, W. T. Blume, J. P. Girvin, and G. P. A. Rice. 1990. Cytomegalovirus and Rasmussen's encephalitis. *Lancet* **336:**1282–1284.

Puccioni-Sohler, M., M. Rios, S. M. F. Carvalho, R. R. Goncalves, C. Oliveira, R. B. Correa, S. Novis, P. De Oliveira, and C. Bianco. 2001. Diagnosis of HAM-TSP based on CSF proviral DNA and HTLV-I antibody index. *Neurology* **57:**725–727.

Rasmussen, T., J. Olszewski, and J. Lloyd-Smith. 1958. Focal seizures due to chronic localized encephalitis. *Neurology* **8:**435–445.

Reyes, M. G., R. Fresco, S. Chokroverty, and E. Q. Salud. 1976. Viruslike particles in granulomatous angiitis of the central nervous system. *Neurology* **26:**797–799.

Risk, W. S., and F. S. Haddad. 1979. The variable natural history of subacute sclerosing encephalitis. A study of 118 cases from the Middle East. *Arch. Neurol.* **36:**610–614.

Risk, W. S., F. S. Haddad, and R. Chemali. 1978. Substantial long-term improvement in subacute sclerosing panencephalitis. Six cases from the Middle East and a review of the literature. *Arch. Neurol.* **35:**494–502.

Rittner, C., E. M. Meier, B. Stradmann, C. M. Giles, R. Kochling, E. Mollenhauer, and H. W. Kreth. 1984. Partial C4 deficiency in subacute sclerosing panencephalitis. *Immunogenetics* **20:**407–415.

Rogers, S. W., P. I. Andrews, L. C. Gahring, T. Whisenand, K. Cauley, B. Crain, T. E. Hughes, S. F. Heinemann, and J. O. McNamara. 1994. Autoantibodies to glutamate receptor Glu R3 in Rasmussen's encephalitis. *Science* **265:**648–651.

Rott, R., S. Herzog, B. Fleischer, A. Winokur, J. Amsterdam, W. Dyson, and H. Koprowski. 1985. Detection of serum antibodies to Borna disease virus in patients with psychiatric disorders. *Science* **228:**755–756.

Rudge, P., A. Ali, and J. K. Cruickshank. 1991. Multiple sclerosis, tropical spastic paraparesis and HTLV-I infection in Afro-Carribbean patients in the United Kingdom. *J. Neurol. Neurosurg. Psychiatr.* **54:**689–694.

Saha, V., T. J. John, P. Mukundan, C. Gnanamuthu, S. Prabhakar, G. Arjundas, Z. A. Sayeed, G. Kumaresan, and K. Srinivas. 1990. High incidence of subacute sclerosing panencephalitis in South India. *Epidemiol. Infect.* **104:**151–156.

Said, G., C. Goulon-Goeau, C. Lacroix, A. Fève, H. Descamps, and M. Fouchard. 1988. Inflammatory lesions of peripheral nerve in a patient with human T lymphotropic virus type I-associated myelopathy. *Ann. Neurol.* **24:**275–277.

Scaravilli, F., and F. Gray. 1993. Opportunistic infections, p. 49–120. *In* F. Gray (ed.), *Atlas of the Neuropathology of HIV Infection.* Oxford University Press, Oxford, United Kingdom.

Schmid, A., P. Spielhofer, R. Cattaneo, K. Baczko, V. ter Meulen, and M. A. Billeter. 1992. Subacute sclerosing panencephalitis is typically characterized by alterations in the fusion protein cytoplasmic domain of the persisting measles virus. *Virology* **188:**910–915.

Schneider-Schaulies, S., and V. ter Meulen. 1999. Pathogenic aspects of measles virus infections. *Arch. Virol. Suppl.* **15:**139–158.

Sebire, G., L. Meyer, and S. Chabrier. 1999. Varicella as a risk factor for cerebral infarction in childhood: a case-control study. *Ann. Neurol.* **45:**679–680.

Sever, J. L. 1983. Persistent measles infection of the central nervous system: subacute sclerosing panencephalitis. *Rev. Infect. Dis.* **5:**467–473.

Shaw, C. M., G. C. Buchan, and C. B. Carlson. 1967. Myxovirus as a possible etiologic agent in subacute inclusion body encephalitis. *N. Engl. J. Med.* **277:**511–515.

Singer, K. C., A. E. Lang, and O. Suchowersky. 1997. Adult-onset subacute sclerosing panencephalitis: case reports and review of the literature. *Mov. Disord.* **12:**342–353.

Smadja, D., R. Bellance, P. Cabre, S. Arfi, and J. C. Vernanat. 1995. Clinical characteristics of HTLV-1 associated dermato-polymyositis. Seven cases from Martinique. *Acta Neurol. Scand.* **92:**206–212.

Sotrel, A., S. Rosen, M. Ronthal, and D. B. Ross. 1983. Subacute sclerosing panencephalitis: an immune complex disease? *Neurology* **33:**885–890.

Staeheli, P., C. Dauder, J. Hausmann, F. Ehrensperger, and M. Schwemmie. 2000. Epidemiology of Borna disease virus. *J. Gen. Virol.* **81:**2123–2135.

Stone, R. 2002. Siberia's deadly stalker emerges from the shadows. *Science* **296:**642–645.

Tan, C. T., K. J. Goh, K. T. Wong, S. A. Sarji, K. B. Chua, N. K. Chew, P. Murugasu, Y. L. Toh, H. T. Chong, K. S. Tan, T. Thayaparan, S. Kumar, and M. R. Jusoh. 2002. Relapsed and late-onset Nipah encephalitis. *Ann. Neurol.* **51:**703–708.

Taylor, G. P., S. E. Hall, S. Navarrete, C. A. Michie, R. Davis, A. D. Witkover, M. Rossor, M. A. Nowak, P. Rudge, E. Matutes, C. R. Bangham, and J. N. Weber. 1999. Effect of lamivudine on human T-cell leukemia virus type 1 (HTLV-1) DNA copy number, T-cell phenotype, and anti-*tax* cytotoxic T-cell frequency in patients with HTLV-1-associated myelopathy. *J. Virol.* **73:**10289–10295.

Tellez-Nagel, I., and D. H. Harter. 1966. Subacute sclerosing leukoencephalitis. I. Clinico-pathological, electron microscopic and virological observations. *J. Neuropathol. Exp. Neurol.* **25:**560–581.

Tien, R. D., B. C. Ashdown, D. V. Lewis, Jr., M. R. Atkins, and P. C. Burger. 1992. Rasmussen's encephalitis: neuroimaging findings in four patients. *Am. J. Radiol.* **158:**1329–1332.

Toga, M., D. Dubois, M. Berard, M. F. Tripier, J. P. Cesorini, and R. Choux. 1969. [Ultrastructural study of 4 cases of subacute sclerosing leukoencephalitis.] *Acta Neuropathol.* **14:**1–13.

Tomoda, A., S. Shiraishi, M. Hosoya, A. Hamada, and T. Miike. 2001. Combined treatment with interferon-alpha and ribavirin for subacute sclerosing panencephalitis. *Pediatr. Neurol.* **24:**54–59.

Townsend, J. J., J. R. Baringer, J. S. Wolinsky, N. Malamud, J. P. Mednick, H. S. Panitch, R. A. T. Scott, L. S. Oshiro, and N. E. Cremer. 1975. Progressive rubella panencephalitis. Late onset after congenital rubella. *N. Engl. J. Med.* **292:**990–993.

Townsend, J. J., W. G. Stroop, J. R. Baringer, J. S. Wolinsky, J. H. McKerrow, and B. O. Berg. 1982. Neuropathology of progressive rubella panencephalitis after childhood rubella. *Neurology* **32:**185–190.

Ueda, K., T. Imamura, T. Kawaguchi, H. Tamari, and T. Kambara. 1982. Subacute sclerosing panencephalitis. An autopsy case with impaired cellular immunity. *Acta Pathol. Jpn.* **32:**1103–1110.

Vaheri, A., I. Julkunen, and M.-L. Koskiniemi. 1982. Chronic encephalomyelitis with specific increase in intrathecal mumps antibodies. *Lancet* **ii:**685–688.

Valdimarsson, H., G. Agnarsdottir, and P. J. Lachmann. 1979. Subacute sclerosing panencephalitis, p. 406–418. *In* F. Rose (ed.), *Clinical Neuroimmunology.* Blackwell Scientific Publications, Oxford, United Kingdom.

Van Bogaert, L. 1945. Une leuco-encéphalite scléronsante subaigüe. *J. Neurol. Neurosurg. Psychiatr.* **8:**101–120.

Vandvik, B., J. Natvig, and E. Norrby. 1974. Immunopathological studies in subacute sclerorising panencephalitis and multiple sclerosis with special reference to evidence for homogeneous antibody responses to measles virus within the central nervous system, p. 448–463. *In* A. Nowoslawski (ed.), *Schering Symposium on Immunopathology.* Pergamon Press, Oxford, United Kingdom.

Vandvik, B., M. L. Weil, M. Grandien, and E. Norrby. 1978. Progressive rubella virus panencephalitis: synthesis of oligoclonal virus-specific IgG antibodies and homogeneous free fight chains in the central nervous system. *Acta Neurol. Scand.* **57:**53–64.

Vinters, H. V., R. Wang, and C. A. Wiley. 1993. Herpesviruses in chronic encephalitis associated with intractable childhood epilepsy. *Hum. Pathol.* **24:**871–879.

Wechsler, S., and H. Meissner. 1982. Measles and SSPE viruses: similarities and differences. *Prog. Med. Virol.* **28:**65–95.

Wechsler, S. L., H. L. Weiner, and B. N. Fields. 1979. Immune response in subacute sclerosing panencephalitis: reduced antibody response to the matrix protein of measles virus. *J. Immunol.* **123:**884–889.

Weil, M. L., H. H. Itabashi, N. E. Cremer, L. S. Oshiro, E. H. Lennette, and L. Carnay. 1975. Chronic progressive panencephalitis due to rubella virus simulating subacute sclerosing panencephalitis. *N. Engl. J. Med.* **292:**994–998.

White, H. H., J. H. Kepes, C. H. Kirkpatrick, and R. N. Schimke. 1972. Subacute encephalitis and congenital hypogammaglobulinemia. *Arch. Neurol.* **26:**359–365.

Wiendl, H., C. G. Bien, P. Bernasconi, B. Fleckenstein, C. E. Elger, J. Dichgans, R. Mantegazza, and A. Melms. 2001. Glu R3 antibodies: prevalence in focal epilepsy but no specificity for Rasmussen's encephalitis. *Neurology* **57:**1511–1514.

Wolinsky, J. S., P. C. Dau, E. Buimovici-Klein, J. Mednick, B. O. Berg, P. B. Lang, and L. Z. Cooper. 1979. Progressive rubella panencephalitis: immunovirological studies and results of isoprinosine therapy. *Clin. Exp. Immunol.* **3S:**397–404.

Wolinsky, J. S. 1989. Progressive rubella encephalitis, p. 405–416. *In* R. R. McKendall (ed.), *Handbook of Clinical Neurology,* vol. 12, of Revised Series, vol. 56. Elsevier Science, B.V., Amsterdam, The Netherlands.

Wolinsky, J. S., and M. McCarthy. 1995. Rubella, p. 19–45. *In* J. S. Porterfield (ed.), *Exotic Viral Infections.* Chapman and Hall, London, United Kingdom.

World Health Organization. 1989. Virus diseases: human T lymphotropic virus type I, HTLV-I. *Wkly. Epidem. Rec.* **64:**382–383.

Yaqub, B. A. 1996. Subacute sclerosing panencephalitis (SSPE): early diagnosis, prognostic factors, and natural history. *J. Neurol. Sci.* **139:**227–234.

15

Creutzfeldt-Jakob Disease and Other Prion Disorders

Creutzfeldt-Jakob disease (CJD) is not an inflammatory disease of the brain. It might therefore be argued that a discussion of it does not belong in a consideration of encephalitis. We have included it here because it has been shown to be associated with a transmissible agent. This agent, the prion (proteinaceous infectious particles) (Prusiner, 1982), is unique as a pathogen in being a protein whose abnormal configuration can act as a template for conversion of host protein of the same amino acid structure to a more pathogenic form and in this way transmitting disease. Because a host protein is involved, the disease fails to evoke an immune response. This property helps to explain the absence of any inflammation in the disease. Before transmission of CJD to animals was demonstrated, the disease was considered to be one of several degenerative diseases of the central nervous system (CNS) in which progressive degeneration and disappearance of neurons occurred in the absence of a known cause.

CJD is a rare, progressive, fatal, degenerative disease of the CNS with the pathological features of multifocal neuronal loss, gliosis, and parenchymal spongy change. It occurs throughout the world with an incidence of 0.5 to 1 cases per million per year. It has been recognized since the early 1920s (Jakob, 1921 and 1923, quoted by Masters and Gajdusek, 1982). The cerebral cortex is a major site of pathology in typical cases, but variants of the disease in which the emphasis of the pathology lies in different parts of the CNS have been described, for example, a cerebellar variant (Brownell and Oppenheimer, 1965). Most cases seem to arise spontaneously, but some are now recognized to occur following transmission, although none are contagious.

In the 1950s attention was drawn to the occurrence of a degenerative disease of the CNS that affected people of the Fore tribe in New Guinea (Gajdusek and Zigas, 1957). This disease had a remarkably high incidence of about 1% per year at that time, although it has declined dramatically since. Women and children were affected to a greater extent than men. The disease was known as "kuru," and the main clinical feature was ataxia. The disorder started with very slight impairment of gait and progressed to conspicuous incoordination, with a variety of involuntary movements. Tremors of the extremities and truncal ataxia were prominent. Dementia and weakness appeared later. Excessive emotionality was seen, but seizures and sensory loss were not found (Hornabrook, 1978). The majority of cases succumbed in 9 months to 2 years, and there was no evidence of arrest of disease or recovery.

TABLE 15.1   Spongiform encephalopathies of humans and animals[a]

Disease	Species affected
sCJD	Human
Inherited CJD	Human
GSS	Human
Iatrogenic CJD	Human
Kuru	Human
vCJD	Human
FFI	Human
Scrapie	Sheep, goat
Transmissible mink encephalopathy	Mink
CWD	Deer, elk
BSE	Cattle
Feline spongiform encephalopathy[b]	Cat, cheetah, puma, ocelot
Spongiform encephalopathy of captive exotic ungulates[b]	Kudu, nyala, oryx, gemsbok, eland

[a] Adapted from de Silva and Will, 2000.
[b] Related to BSE.

When first described, kuru was thought to be an inherited disease, but the evidence was subsequently thought to favor its spread by ritual cannibalism that involved consumption of brain tissue from affected victims by their relatives. The decline in its incidence in the second half of the 20th century paralleled the elimination of the practice of cannibalism. The pathology of kuru is closely similar to that of CJD (Klatzo et al., 1959).

Hadlow (1959) pointed out the similarities of the pathology of kuru to that of scrapie, a degenerative disease of sheep that had been shown to be associated with a transmissible agent (Cuille and Chelle, 1936). Following this lead, successful attempts were made to transmit kuru and CJD to chimpanzees (Gajdusek et al., 1966; Gibbs et al., 1968) and later to small laboratory animals (Manuelidis et al., 1978). Together with scrapie, the novel disease of cattle known as bovine spongiform encephalopathy (BSE), and a number of other animal diseases of similar type (Table 15.1), kuru and CJD form the group of spongiform encephalopathies. These share the properties of being transmissible nervous system diseases with unusually long incubation periods, measured in years or even decades, associated with prions and demonstrating a relatively similar pathology. There are, in addition, inherited forms of human prion diseases (see below).

Prion diseases of humans and animals are associated with the accumulation in the brain of an abnormal aggregated and unusually protease-resistant form of a normal glycoprotein, prion protein, which is coded for in humans by a gene, *PRNP*, on the short arm of chromosome 20. The disease-related form of the protein differs only conformationally from its normal counterpart (PrP^c) in that it is rich in β sheets while the normal protein contains alpha helices and very little β sheet. The β-sheet-rich form, designated PrP^{sc}, accumulates in lysosomes in an insoluble form. When injected into a normal animal host brain, it gains entry to nerve cells, alters the host PrP^c to PrP^{sc}, and in this way transmits disease. Exactly how the conformational change

occurs is not fully understood. The PrP^c is a highly conserved protein whose function is not fully known, but it is thought to have a role in modulating cellular responses to oxidative stress (Brown et al., 1997). Genetically modified mice that lack the gene for this protein develop normally and show no deficits in learning but do show some alteration in circadian rhythm and sleep pattern (Tobler et al., 1996). Such mice are resistant to transmission of prion diseases. However, if they have a PrP gene restored by insertion of the gene from another species, they then become susceptible to transmission of prion disease from that species (Weissmann et al., 1999).

Prion diseases can be transmitted less readily from one species to another than within a species. Nevertheless, there is now strong evidence that the novel disease variant CJD (vCJD), which was first described in the United Kingdom in 1996 (Will et al., 1996a), is acquired from the cattle prion disease BSE (Collinge and Rossor, 1996; Collinge et al., 1996; Bruce et al., 1997; Hill et al., 1997). BSE itself appeared as a new disease of cattle in 1975 (Wells et al., 1987) and then became a devastating epidemic in the United Kingdom affecting more than 177,000 cattle over the succeeding 15 years. Much smaller numbers of affected cattle have been detected in continental Europe (Dormont, 1999). The mechanism of spread of BSE was via ruminant-derived feed supplements that may have acquired disease prions from an unrecognized spontaneously arising case of prion disease in a cow or sheep, although most forms of sheep scrapie differ from BSE in their strain characteristics when transmitted to mice. Alterations to manufacturing processes in the conversion of ruminant carcasses into feed supplements may have hampered inactivation of the agent, which is very resistant to heating (Ernst and Race, 1993).

PATHOLOGY

In most cases of CJD the naked-eye appearance of the brain is unremarkable. The sole noteworthy feature in such cases is a mild degree of cerebral atrophy (Fig. 15.1). Extensive cerebral atrophy has been described in a few cases with a prolonged clinical course, but this is distinctly unusual (Ohta et al., 1978; Park et al., 1980; Kitagawa et al., 1983). In

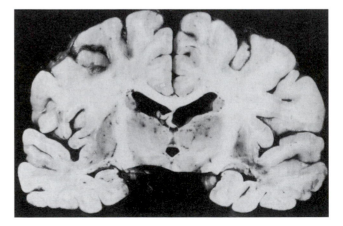

FIGURE 15.1   Coronal slice through fixed brain from a case of CJD. There is only minimal cerebral atrophy with ventricular dilation and prominent sulci.

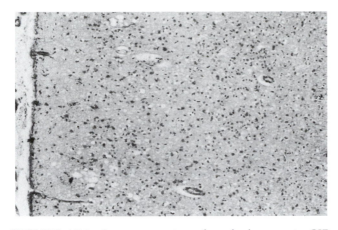

FIGURE 15.2 Low-power view of cerebral cortex in CJD showing mild patchy spongiform change, mainly in layers 2 and 3. Hematoxylin and eosin stain.

cerebellar forms of the disease the cerebellar folia, in particular those of the vermis, may appear shrunken. In kuru, cerebellar atrophy with a relatively well-preserved cerebrum was the rule.

Microscopic Appearance

The main abnormalities in CJD occur in the gray matter of the CNS. Changes in the white matter, if present, are due mainly to Wallerian degeneration. Gray matter frequently involved in CJD includes the cerebral cortex, basal ganglia, thalamus, and cerebellar cortex. The cerebral cortex may show variation in the extent of the pathology from lobe to lobe. In affected areas there are four main abnormalities. First and most characteristic is spongy change consisting of vacuoles of sizes varying from about 5 to 50 μm and occupying the neuropil (Fig. 15.2 and 15.3). The extent of the spongy change is very variable, ranging from a few clusters of small rounded spaces to a very extensive lacy network of larger coalescing microcysts pervading the whole region. Mild forms of spongy change need to be distinguished from artefactual vacuoles and should not be accepted as evidence of CJD without supporting evidence of gliosis (Masters and Richardson, 1978) and immunostaining for protease-resistant PrP. More severe forms of spongy

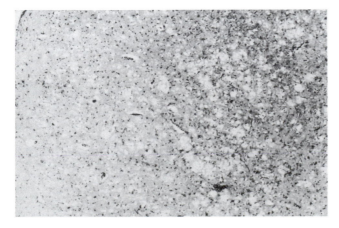

FIGURE 15.3 Low-power view of cerebral cortex showing more extensive spongiform change. PTAH stain.

change due to CJD need to be distinguished from the loose sponginess that develops in gray matter as a secondary consequence of severe neuronal loss, for example, following severe hypoxia or in advanced cases of Pick's disease. Distinction from such conditions can be difficult on the basis of the character of the vacuoles alone and may depend also on finding other evidence favoring another process. In the cerebellum, spongy change is most frequently apparent in the molecular layer of the cortex. There is no clear relation between the duration of the disease and the extent of the spongy change, although some authorities have noted a tendency for it to be more severe early on in the disease. In kuru, spongy change was less constant than in CJD and tended to be most frequently found in limbic structures.

The second change seen in CJD is loss of neurons in affected parts of the brain. This also varies in extent. Mild degrees are difficult to detect by ordinary inspection of stained sections, but in most cases of CJD, cell loss is readily apparent and may be so severe that few identifiable neurons remain. The overall cellularity in such an area is not invariably reduced because of the concurrent increase in glial cells. The overall effect in a Nissl-stained section of cerebral cortex is of a loss of the normal cytoarchitectonic pattern due to replacement of large neurons by haphazardly arranged smaller glial cells (Fig. 15.4). The neuron cell loss affects all cortical layers but does so in a patchy fashion. Beck and Daniel (1979) considered that small- and medium-sized neurons were principally affected. In the basal ganglia and thalamus the loss may involve both large and small neurons, but again the extent of the loss is variable. Thalamic neuron loss and gliosis are particularly severe in fatal familial insomnia (FFI). Remaining neurons appear shrunken, chromatolytic, or rarely, vacuolated. In kuru, vacuolation of neuronal perikarya was common. Golgi studies have identified morphological changes in neurons with loss of dendritic spines and axonal processes (Ferrer et al., 1981; Landis et al., 1981). Brain stem nuclei are less frequently affected by the neuronal fallout than the cortex, basal ganglia, and thalamus in CJD but were regularly affected in kuru. In the cerebellum, neuron cell loss can occur in both the deep nuclei and the cortex. Granule cells are more severely affected than the Purkinje cells in the cortex. Neuronal fallout in CJD is not usually accompanied by neuronophagia, in contrast to conventional forms of encephalitis. Microglial cells show variable proliferation in affected regions.

The third pathological feature in CJD is reactive gliosis (Fig. 15.5). This is an almost universal finding in any disease of the CNS parenchyma, but astrocytic hyperplasia and hypertrophy tend to be particularly widespread and severe in comparison to the manifest neuronal loss in CJD. Several early writers about the disease speculated over whether the reactive gliosis was a primary change in CJD. This is no longer generally considered likely, one reason being the greater recognition that mild degrees of neuron loss are easy to overlook. Another reason, pointed out by Oppenheimer (1975), is that astrocytic hyperplasia occurs not only at sites where neuron cell bodies have been lost but also at sites where axonal terminations have degenerated. It may, therefore, be seen in regions where neuron cell bodies are largely preserved. Degeneration of axon terminals is difficult to detect using routine neuropathological techniques.

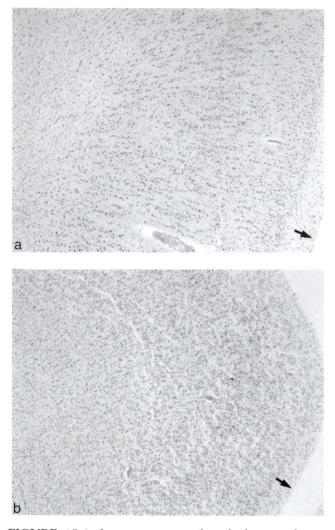

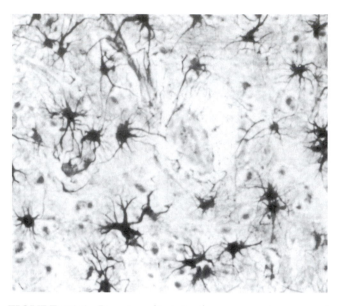

FIGURE 15.5   Reactive gliosis in the putamen in a case of CJD. Cajal's stain.

FIGURE 15.4   Low-power view of cerebral cortex from a healthy control (a) and a case of CJD (b). In CJD, neurons are lost and the cortical organization is haphazard. Small nuclei are those of glial cells. Arrows in (a) and (b) indicate the pial surface. Nissl stain.

White matter lesions in CJD are usually absent or trivial compared to those affecting gray matter. However, a few cases have been described in which the white matter damage has been too extensive to be attributed solely to Wallerian degeneration. The majority of these cases have been described from Japan (Ohta et al., 1978; Mizutani et al., 1981; Kitagawa et al., 1983). In one case, transmission experiments resulted in spongy change of white matter as well as of gray matter of inoculated mice (Tateishi et al., 1980). In most such cases the total brain weight is reduced below 1,000 g, and there is conspicuous atrophy of the cerebrum and cerebellum with compensatory ventricular dilatation. Spongy change occurs in the cerebral cortex with neuronal depletion and reactive gliosis. In the centrum ovale and subcortical white matter, patchy and diffuse myelin pallor is found, together with microcystic cavitation. Neutral fat-containing macrophages and hypertrophic astrocytes are abundant in affected white matter. Kuru plaques (see below) have occurred

in some of these cases. This presentation appears to be a separate and distinctive subgroup of CJD and illustrates a variability in pathology among prion diseases that forms the basis of what were initially described as "strain differences," manifested first in different isolates of the scrapie agent (Dickinson and Meikle, 1969, 1971; Fraser, 1973). These strain differences have been considered in the past to suggest that there must be some nucleic acid component to the transmissible agent of prion diseases, but more recently it has been thought likely that they can be explained by differences in glycosylation and conformation of prion proteins. The discovery that prions can also be found in fungi and yeasts and that these also manifest strain differences that are not dependent on nucleic acid for their generation has provided greater confidence that prion diseases are "protein only" in origin (Derkatch et al., 1996).

A further pathological feature seen occasionally in sporadic CJD (sCJD), more commonly in scrapie and kuru, and invariably in some inherited forms of prion disease and vCJD is the presence of microscopic plaques of amyloidlike material (Masters et al., 1981). Cerebellar ataxia is prominent in the clinical presentation of most inherited prion diseases, and pathologically they often show spino-cerebellar tract degeneration and loss of Clarke's column cells as well as cerebellar pathology. These cases are identical clinically and pathologically to cases of Gerstmann-Sträussler-Scheinker syndrome (GSS) (Seitelberger, 1962; Boellard and Scholte, 1980). Some but not all cases show spongy change, and transmission experiments have been successful in such cases (Masters et al., 1981). The amyloid plaques consist of small round masses of granular or finely fibrillary material that stains positively with the periodic acid-Schiff stain and silver stains and for amyloid (Fig. 15.6). The plaques occur in small clusters, most commonly in the cerebellar cortex, and less commonly in the cerebral cortex in GSS. In vCJD they are very common in cerebral cortex, deep gray matter, and

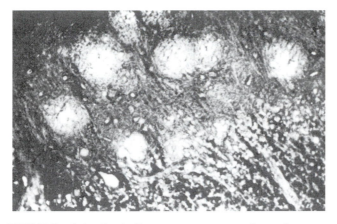

FIGURE 15.6 Cerebellar cortex containing kuru plaques in the molecular layer (above). Thioflavine T stain photographed under fluorescent light.

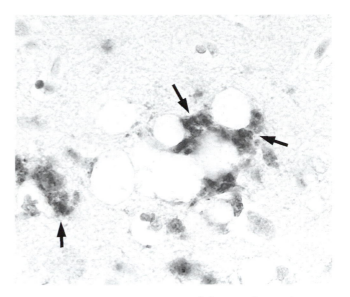

FIGURE 15.8 PrP immunostained deposits (arrows) in cortex in sCJD.

cerebellum, and in this variant they are often surrounded by a cluster of spongiform vacuoles and are referred to as "florid" plaques (Fig. 15.7). The material present in the plaques is now known to be aggregated protease-resistant prion protein (Bockman et al., 1985; Ironside and Bell, 1997). The amyloid plaques differ from the argyrophilic plaques seen in the cerebral cortex in Alzheimer's disease in their more widespread distribution and in their clustering.

The fourth characteristic microscopic feature of prion diseases is the presence of immunocytochemically stainable, proteinase K-resistant prion protein (Bell and Ironside, 1993; Ironside and Bell, 1997). Although there are prion diseases in experimental animals that lack detectable PrP^{sc} (Hsiao et al., 1990; Collinge et al., 1995), the natural human forms of prion disease all show demonstrable PrP^{sc}, although the amounts detectable are very variable and can be readily missed in a small biopsy sample. Ironside and Bell (1997) refer to two main patterns of PrP immunostaining: perivacuolar and plaque. The perivacuolar deposits are seen around the vacuoles of spongiform change, most characteristically in the cerebral cortex in sCJD (Fig. 15.8). Immunostained plaques are most commonly seen in the cerebellum, particularly the granule cell layer, in inherited and ataxic cases of

CJD (Fig. 15.9). They are also abundant in all locations in vCJD (Fig. 15.10). Other patterns of PrP staining include perineuronal, in which their distribution may be synaptic, colocalizing with synaptophysin in one study (Kitamoto et al., 1992), and peridendritic (Fig. 15.11). Despite the frequent localization of perivacuolar immunostaining of PrP in foci of spongiform change, there is not always precise correspondence of spongiform change and PrP immunostaining.

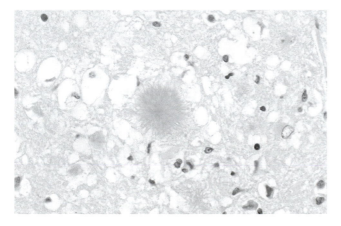

FIGURE 15.7 "Florid" plaque in vCJD surrounded by spongiform vacuoles.

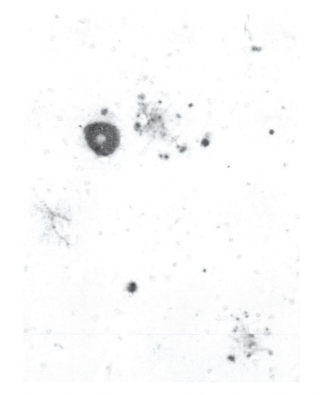

FIGURE 15.9 PrP immunostained plaques in cerebellum in inherited ataxic form of CJD.

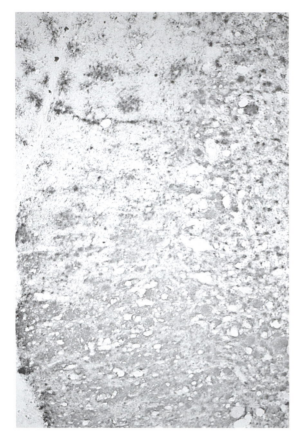

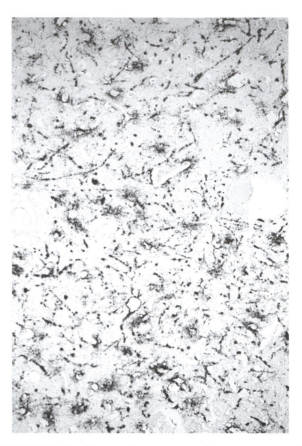

FIGURE 15.10   PrP immunostaining of vCJD cerebellar cortex.

FIGURE 15.11   Peridendritic pattern of immunostaining for PrP in the basal ganglia from a case of vCJD.

Amounts of PrP detectable in the brain tend to be greatest in cases with relatively prolonged clinical histories, including cases of vCJD.

Electron Microscopy

Most ultrastructural studies have been carried out on tissues from animals that have developed spongiform encephalopathy following inoculation of kuru or CJD brain homogenates. Spongiform change here and in biopsies from patients with CJD has been shown to consist of swollen, vacuolated dendrites and, to a lesser extent, neuronal perikarya and astrocyte processes (Lampert et al., 1971, 1975; Landis et al., 1981; Kim and Manuelidis, 1983) (Fig. 15.12). The affected areas are devoid of organelles but may contain granular material. Surface membranes show interruptions with formation of separate curled membrane fragments. Repeated attempts to identify the transmissible agent in affected brains in humans and animals have failed to identify viruslike particles.

PATHOGENESIS OF CJD

As already mentioned, CJD has many features in common with the transmissible disease of sheep known as scrapie. Many of the shared properties were first defined in experimental work on scrapie after it had been shown that scrapie could be transmitted to mice and other small laboratory

animals. Recognition of the proteinaceous nature of the transmissible agent, devoid of nucleic acid, was a major step in developing understanding of the prion diseases and was initially based on the resistance of the scrapie agent to factors that normally damage nucleic acid, such as UV and other irradiation, heat, alkylating agents, and formalin (Alper et al., 1967; Griffiths, 1967). Prusiner (1982) demonstrated that

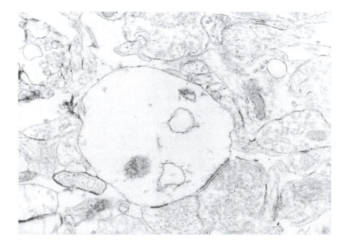

FIGURE 15.12   Electron micrograph of cerebral cortex in CJD. Vacuolar distension of a postsynaptic neuritic process is seen. Courtesy of I. Janota.

the infective fraction of scrapie brain homogenate contained a protein of 27 to 30 kDa. It was subsequently demonstrated that PrP-null mice did not develop scrapie when intracerebrally inoculated with scrapie brain homogenate, indicating that disease transmission is dependent on a source of host PrP (Büeler et al., 1993). Transgenic mice carrying a mutation in the *PRNP* gene were found to spontaneously develop a spongiform encephalopathy that could be transmitted (Hsiao et al., 1990). Investigation of inherited forms of human prion diseases showed that these are caused by mutations in the *PRNP* gene (Hsiao et al., 1989; DeArmond et al., 2002) that enhance the chance of the PrP^c-to-PrP^{sc} conversion. These investigations strengthened the evidence in favor of the prion theory of the spongiform encephalopathies.

In general, then, there are two recognized mechanisms by which prion diseases arise. The first is by transmission, particularly parenteral transmission, from a source of prion disease. This has accounted for several recognized forms of iatrogenically acquired CJD in humans—by contaminated neurosurgical instruments, cadaver-derived growth hormone, corneal transplants, and dura mater grafts. vCJD is attributed to oral transmission of BSE, although epidemiologic studies have failed to explain exactly how this has occurred, and the extent of the risk to humans has yet to be discovered (Cousens et al., 1997; Ghani et al., 1999). The risk of acquiring transmitted CJD and the length of the incubation period for the disease are to some extent related to possession of common *PRNP* polymorphisms at codon 129, where the gene codes for either a methionine or a valine amino acid residue. Those who are heterozygous at this codon (50% of the population) are relatively resistant to transmitted CJD or sCJD, whereas an excess of valine homozygotes (present in 11% of the normal population) has been found in growth hormone recipients with CJD and exclusively methionine homozygotes (found in 39% of the normal population) have been found in vCJD (Alperovitch et al., 1999; Collinge et al., 1991). It is not known how this polymorphism exerts this effect.

The second mechanism by which prion diseases arise is spontaneous conversion of the normal PrP^c to PrP^{sc} in the brain. This occurs more readily in those who have disease-associated mutations in *PRNP* that cause familial CJD, GSS, or FFI. Even in these cases the delay in symptom onset until late middle age in most cases suggests that aging processes may also play a part. In the absence of such mutations, conversion of PrP^c to PrP^{sc} occurs very rarely to give rise to classical sCJD. In these manifestations of prion disease, the codon 129 polymorphism again plays a part: in an inherited mutation at codon 178, the disease that is manifested clinically is CJD if valine is coded for at codon 129, and FFI if methionine is coded for at codon 129 (Goldfarb et al., 1992). In sCJD, methionine homozygotes at this codon are overrepresented (Palmer et al., 1991). Although sCJD is presently considered to be a spontaneously arising disease, there is evidence that a variety of surgical procedures constitute risk factors for this condition, which raises the possibility that unrecognized transmission events might be responsible for at least some cases (Collinge, 1999; Collins et al., 1999; Ward et al., 2002).

Prion diseases are unusual for the prolonged incubation period that elapses before pathological changes or clinical disease is manifest in infected animals. The reason for this is not clear. Natural scrapie in affected sheep does not become clinically apparent until the sheep reach the age of at least 2 years. BSE in cattle has a mean incubation period of 5 to 6 years (Dormont, 1999). For kuru the incubation period has been estimated to be more than 4 and as long as 40 years (Collinge, 1999), and for human CJD, in cases in which it has been produced by iatrogenic means, there has been an incubation period ranging from 18 months to 30 years. In experimental scrapie the length of the incubation period is determined mainly by the similarity in genotype between donor and host *PRNP* as well as by dose and route of prions received by the host.

There remain some other aspects of prion disease that are not yet entirely accounted for. Although conversion of PrP^c to PrP^{sc} has been demonstrated in a cell-free system (Kocisko et al., 1994; Hill et al., 1999b), the PrP^{sc} produced in this way has not yet transmitted disease. The involvement of the reticuloendothelial system in the pathogenesis of prion diseases, which has long been recognized in scrapie (Fraser et al., 1992), is not well understood. PrP^{sc} is detectable in lymphoreticular tissue during the incubation period of scrapie, before it is detectable in the brain, even when scrapie material is inoculated into the brain (Kimberlin and Walker, 1986). Yet there is no evidence that the immune system is damaged. PrP^{sc} can be detected in follicular dendritic cells in lymphoid tissue, and transmission of disease to the CNS seems to require the presence of B cells (Klein et al., 1997). In vCJD but not in other human prion diseases, abundant PrP^{sc} is detectable in tonsil, appendix, and other lymphoid tissues before and during the clinical phase of the disease (Hilton et al., 1998; Hill et al., 1999a), raising concerns about the risk of spreading this form of the disease via surgical instruments or blood products but also providing a method of diagnosing the disease. Once within the CNS, abnormal prions can spread along synaptically linked pathways, provided the neurons along those pathways contain PrP^c (Kimberlin and Walker, 1986; Brandner et al., 1996).

The mechanism by which PrP^{sc} causes neurons to die is another aspect of these diseases that remains obscure. Two potential mechanisms would seem possible, or there may be a combination of the two effects: conversion of PrP^c to PrP^{sc} deprives neurons of the function of PrP^c, or PrP^{sc} itself may exert toxic effects. The normal growth and development of PrP^c-null mice seem to suggest that loss of PrP^c function on its own is unlikely to explain the rapid neuron death that occurs. However, the recent evidence that PrP^c may modulate cellular responses to oxidative stress (Brown et al., 1997; White et al., 1999; Milhavet et al., 2000) may indicate that neurons are left vulnerable to excitotoxic and other processes that generate such stress. Neural cell lines infected with scrapie prions show little cytopathology, except for mouse hypothalamic neurons that have been immortalized; these show some tendency to undergo apoptosis (Schatzl et al., 1997). This could reflect either the effects of PrP^c depletion or PrP^{sc} toxicity. Muramoto and colleagues (1997) have reported that certain *PRNP* deletion mutants accumulated cytoplasmic deposits of PrP and developed fatal CNS disease resembling neuronal storage diseases, suggesting a possible toxic effect of PrP on normal lysosomal function.

A further point of uncertainty is whether entry of PrP^{sc} or PrP^c into cells involves interaction with a receptor. Clathrin-coated pits and vesicles are the site of endocytic uptake of PrP^c (Shyng et al., 1994), and the laminin receptor precursor protein is thought to act as a receptor that can interact with PrP^c (Rieger et al., 1997). Whether such a putative receptor is also involved in PrP^{sc} entry or in conversion of PrP^c to PrP^{sc} is a matter of considerable interest because interaction with a receptor might provide a means to intervene therapeutically in these diseases.

DIAGNOSIS AND MANAGEMENT

Confronted with a patient in his or her 50s or 60s with a rapidly evolving dementia, myoclonus, and periodic sharp-wave complexes on electroencephalogram (EEG), most neurological clinicians would suspect CJD as the most likely diagnosis. However, the spectrum of symptoms and signs presented by CJD is wide, and the rapidity of evolution can range from a few months to more than 2 years. The variety of forms is reflected in the clinical-pathological literature in which various features are emphasized such as visual loss (Heidenhein variant), ataxia (Brownell and Oppenheimer variant), and a disputed amyotrophic form (Salazar et al., 1983). The challenge is made more complex for the clinician by the presence of familial forms, in which insomnia and dysautonomia (FFI) or ataxia (GSS) predominate, and iatrogenic forms, which may present principally as clumsiness and incoordination (from autopsy-derived growth hormone) or dementia (from autopsy-derived dura mater grafts). Finally, the emergence of a new variant form characterized by a young age of onset, longer duration, and presentation with psychiatric or sensory symptoms further complicates the clinical diagnostic issue.

To a certain extent the wide range of clinical presentations reflects an evolution of understanding of the disease process from transmissibility of spongiform pathology to molecular characterization of the prion protein. Recently, for example, the attempt has been made to characterize clinical forms of sCJD based on the electrophoretic mobility of the prion protein and the genotype at codon 129 (Parchi et al., 1999; Zerr et al., 2000b). However, absent a highly sensitive specific or surrogate blood-based assay, the clinician may be sorely challenged. The diagnostic issue is made more difficult because, absent an alternative treatable disease, brain biopsy is discouraged because of concerns for contamination of operating instruments.

Perhaps the best clinical approach for the clinician is to consider the range of signs and symptoms that trigger a concern for human prion disease, the diagnoses for which prion disorders are included in the differential diagnosis, and information from the clinical and epidemiologic history that would help in the differentiation of the various prion disorders. Following a general consideration of signs and symptoms, alternative diagnoses, clinical-epidemiologic history features, and laboratory studies, we will consider the various categories of human prion disorders by mode of pathogenesis.

What types of symptoms and signs should raise a consideration of prion disorders? sCJD represents 85% or so of human prion disease. Will and Matthews (1984) found that dementia, ataxia, behavioral disturbance, dizziness, and visual disturbance were the most common symptoms at presentation. Poser et al. (1999) found dementia of less than 2 years' duration, myoclonus, gait ataxia, and rigidity/other extrapyramidal signs to be most common. However, visual disturbances, akinetic mutism, and weakness/spasticity were each found in approximately half of the patients studied. In familial CJD, Brown et al. (1994) found that the types of signs and symptoms were similar to those of sCJD. These included memory loss, behavioral abnormalities, and cerebellar and visual/oculomotor disturbances.

The differential diagnostic workup for dementia should be systematic. While Alzheimer's disease and multi-infarct dementia are most commonly found, other causes, particularly reversible causes, must be sought. Depression as a cause of pseudodementia and chronic encephalopathy from numerous types of toxi-metabolic states and chronic organ failures are among the first distinctions to be made. Laboratory studies to uncover metabolic and endocrine causes, including vitamin B$_{12}$ deficiency and hypothyroidism, are undertaken. Chronic infections such as neurosyphilis, human immunodeficiency virus/AIDS-related cognitive-motor complex, and chronic meningitic infections are to be considered. Space-occupying lesions such as chronic subdural hematoma and slow-growing tumors, benign or malignant, can present as dementia. A thorough consideration of the diagnostic workup for dementia is outside the scope of this chapter. The interested reader is referred to current textbooks of neurology for the organization of the workup and to the practice parameter of the American Academy of Neurology for an assessment of the various diagnostic tests and definitions (Knopman et al., 2001).

Abnormalities in the eponymic forms of inherited CJD, FFI and GSS, include sleep disturbance and dysautonomia for FFI and ataxia and dementia for GSS. Iatrogenic forms that have sufficient numbers of cases to review include patients who have received cadaveric growth hormone or cadaveric dura mater. Ataxia and imbalance have been the most common presentations of cases related to cadaveric growth hormone (Fradkin et al., 1991), and cerebellar signs have been the most common presentation associated with cadaveric dura mater, with visual and mental presentations being less common (Brown et al., 2000). vCJD, first described in the United Kingdom in 1996 by Will et al. (1996a), differs from sCJD in a number of features, not the least of which is the onset of the illness. In a subsequent publication, Will et al. (2000) reported that psychiatric symptoms were significantly more common at the outset than forgetfulness, and sensory symptoms were slightly more common. A consolidated table of clinical features found across the several forms of human prion disease is presented (Table 15.2) and provides a basis for the descriptions of the specific types of prion disorders. The table reflects a long list of symptoms the clinician will encounter on first presentation of the patient with one of the prion disorders. However,

TABLE 15.2 Initial clinical features found across the spectrum of human prion disorders

Subacute dementia
Ataxia/imbalance
Psychiatric and behavioral disturbances
Myoclonus/extrapyramidal symptoms
Visual disturbances
Sleep disturbances
Dysautonomia
Sensory disturbances
Weakness/spasticity

TABLE 15.4 Diagnoses in which CJD has been suspected[a]

Alzheimer's disease
Multi-infarct dementia
Lewy body dementia
Unclassified dementia
Psychiatric disorders
Amyotrophic lateral sclerosis
Encephalitis of undetermined etiology
Olivopontocerebellar atrophy
Degenerative CNS disease
Hashimoto's encephalitis

[a] De Silva and Will, 2000; Poser et al., 1999; Will et al., 2000; Kuzuhara et al., 1983.

across all types of prion disorders, subacute dementia, ataxia, and psychiatric disorders are the triad of most common clinical features. Specific features such as sleep disturbance and dysautonomia or visual disturbances reflect particular syndromes.

What clinical and epidemiologic features are particularly important in the evaluation of a potential human prion disorder case? Another way of considering the question is to ask about the risk factors for human prion disease (Table 15.3). Family history should be sought. The familial forms of human prion disease have an autosomal dominant pattern of inheritance. Medical interventions that include exposure to human materials such as growth hormone, gonadotropin, dura mater grafts, or corneal transplants (Brown et al., 2000) are potential risk factors. Intracranial surgery and placement of reusable intracranial electrodes have been risk factors. A history of other surgery has been found to be associated with the risk for sCJD (Ward et al., 2002). Prior to the emergence of vCJD, considerable attention had been given to the potential for transmission by blood transfusion without unambiguous demonstration of actual transmission to humans (Ricketts et al., 1997). Concern that vCJD could be transmitted in blood led to a change in regulations for the blood supply. Place of residence, in relation to the epizootic of BSE, a.k.a. "mad cow disease," is considered a risk factor because of the consumption of beef products. The epizootic developed in the United Kingdom in the late 1980s, peaked in 1992, and declined rapidly as a result of the ban on ruminant-derived protein feed. While no transmission to humans has been demonstrated, the expanding epizootic of chronic wasting disease (CWD) in North American deer

and Rocky Mountain elk has led to concern that prion disease might be transmitted to hunters or others who consume venison (Belay et al., 2001). Ritual cannibalism as a risk factor for kuru must be noted.

The most common illnesses in which human prion diseases are considered are shown in Table 15.4. Most prominent among these is Alzheimer's disease. This is particularly the case in rapidly progressive Alzheimer's disease, in which myoclonic jerks are observed. Other types of dementia, including multi-infarct dementia, and neurodegenerative disease, including amyotrophic lateral sclerosis, have raised concern about CJD. On the other hand, behavioral abnormalities and personality change have led to consideration of psychiatric disorders, particularly in vCJD. Multiple-system atrophy has been considered in the ataxic forms of prion diseases. Thus, olivopontocerebellar degeneration has been suspected in GSS disease.

While there can be considerable clinical variation in the presentation of human prion disorders, laboratory studies (Table 15.5) can provide assistance, if not a definitive diagnosis, in supporting the nature of the disease process. Brain biopsy to make a diagnosis of CJD is discouraged unless there is an alternative diagnosis for which treatment exists (World Health Organization [WHO], 1998), because of concern for contamination of operating instruments. Tissue examination, when available, can establish a definite diagnosis based on the presence of characteristic histopathology and immunohistochemical demonstration of the pathological form of the prion protein. The finding of periodic sharp-wave complexes has been a diagnostic feature in CJD

TABLE 15.3 Risk factors for human prion disease

Family history
  Familial CJD
  FFI
  GSS
Medical-surgical interventions
  Corneal transplant
  Neurosurgery, reusable intracranial electrodes
  Cadaveric dura mater graft
  Other surgery
  Cadaveric growth hormone or gonadotropin
Residence
  Consumption of beef products in United Kingdom from the late 1980s to the early 1990s
Ritual cannibalism
  Kuru—Fore highlanders of Papua New Guinea

TABLE 15.5 Laboratory investigations for human prion disease

EEG
  Periodic sharp-wave complexes
CSF
  14-3-3 protein
MRI
  CJD—bilateral increased signal in caudate and putamen
  vCJD—pulvinar sign
PrP^{sc}—prion protein studies
  Brain
  Tonsil in vCJD only
Molecular genetic analysis
  Mutational analysis of the prion protein gene (*PRNP*) in suspected familial or iatrogenic cases

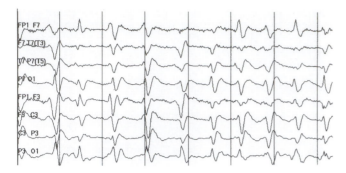

FIGURE 15.13　EEG in sCJD: a 72-year-old woman with a history of progressive dementia and myoclonus. EEG shows periodic complexes predominantly over the left hemisphere. Courtesy of Huned Patwa, Yale University School of Medicine.

(Fig. 15.13). A blinded study showed this finding to have a sensitivity of 67% and a specificity of 86% for CJD (Steinhoff et al., 1996). However, sharp wave complexes may appear late in the course of disease.

The presence of 14-3-3 protein in cerebrospinal fluid (CSF) has been particularly useful in helping to distinguish CJD from other causes of dementia. Aksamit et al. (2001) combined the examination of CSF 14-3-3 protein and neuron-specific enolase to improve the diagnosis. While CSF 14-3-3 protein can be positive in stroke, CNS infection, malignancy, and encephalopathy, its use in the appropriate clinical context is highly effective (Lemstra et al., 2000). Zerr et al. (2000b) found the sensitivity and specificity of CSF 14-3-3 protein to be higher than those of periodic sharp-wave complexes on EEG and recommended its incorporation into the diagnostic criteria for CJD. There has been disagreement, however, with Kenney et al. (K. L. Kenney, G. Hsieh, C. Brechtel, and C. J. Gibbs, Abstr., *Neurology* **58**[Suppl. 3]:A250, 2002) supporting its use and Geschwind et al. (M. D. Geschwind, D. Miller, J. L. Martindale, S. J. Armond, N. M. Barbaro, D. A. Gashkin, S. Prusiner, and B. L. Miller, Abstr., *Neurology* **58**[Suppl. 3]: A250, 2002) concluding that its diagnostic usefulness is "gravely limited."

Careful evaluation of magnetic resonance imaging (MRI) has revealed increased signal intensity in putamen and caudate nuclei on T2- and proton density-weighted images in 79% of patients with sCJD (Finkenstaedt et al., 1996). Hyperintensity of the pulvinar on MRI has been found to be highly sensitive for vCJD and has been referred to as the "pulvinar sign" on MRI (Zeidler et al., 2000; Collie et al., 2001) (Fig. 15.14). A special protocol has been developed for MRI imaging of patients with suspected vCJD (Collie et al., 2001).

As pointed out by a WHO consultation, genetic analysis for PrP mutations raises ethical concerns, and written consent is mandatory in countries where genetic analysis is culturally acceptable (WHO, 1998). Genetic analysis of PrP is recommended in cases in which a family history is positive and in cases suspected of being vCJD. We would add suspected iatrogenic cases for such testing. Consultation services concerning the prion diseases are available through the National Prion Disease Surveillance Center at Case Western Reserve University in Cleveland, Ohio. The National CJD

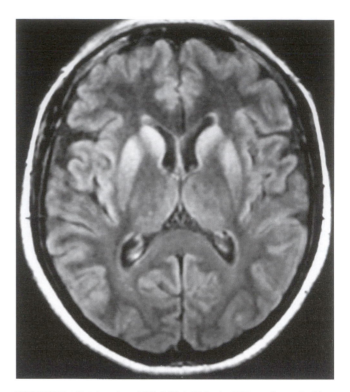

FIGURE 15.14　Axial FLAIR MRI of sCJD with graded hyperintensity more marked in the anterior putamen relative to the posterior half of the nucleus. No significant pulvinar or dorsal thalamic hyperintensity. There is also some cortical hyperintensity in the right insula. Courtesy of David Summers, U.K. National CJD Surveillance Unit, Edinburgh, Scotland.

Surveillance Unit in the United Kingdom is at the Western General Hospital in Edinburgh, Scotland. Reference centers for vCJD are listed in Annex VII of the report of the WHO consultation on the revision of the surveillance case definition for vCJD (WHO, 2002).

sCJD

Overview

sCJD, attributed to somatic mutation or spontaneous conversion to the pathogenic form of the protein, accounts for about 85% of human prion diseases. While the overall incidence is 1 case per million population annually, it is almost 5 cases per million annually in the age range from 60 to 74 years (Prusiner, 2001). The definition of the prion disorders has evolved considerably from clinical-pathological description, to transmissibility to animals of spongiform encephalopathy, and most recently to abnormalities of the prion protein (Richardson and Masters, 1995).

Parchi et al. (1999) analyzed the molecular characteristics of the prion protein and the zygosity of codon 129 of the prion protein gene and correlated these characteristics with clinical phenotypes. The clinical abnormalities included dementia, ataxia, myoclonus, visual abnormalities, insomnia, agitation, hallucinations, and specific EEG findings. The presence of six clinical phenotypes was demonstrated, which the investigators concluded were determined by the properties of the prion protein and the genotype at codon 129 and which would allow molecular classification of the clinical variations. Seventy percent of the study group had the "typical CJD triad" of dementia, myoclonus, and characteristic EEG. This group was found to be associated with two molecular groups. Visual signs preceded severe dementia in 30% of cases. A clinical ataxic variant was associated with a single molecular group in 16% of patients. Most of these patients did not show a characteristic EEG, and one-third did not have prominent myoclonus. Another variant was associated with kuru-type plaques, dementia, and long duration. A rare variant, a thalamic form, was similar to FFI.

As is true of most cases of dementia, the initial complaints in CJD are apt to be vague and ill-defined, with elements of both somatic and psychological dysfunction. Kirschbaum (1968) described CJD as occurring in three stages and characterized the start of the illness as "an organically tainted depressive mental reaction." The alert physician may recognize a variety of diffuse complaints as heralding an incipient dementia.

However, little can be said for certain until the second stage, when cortical, pyramidal, and extrapyramidal dysfunctions are clearly demonstrable. Matthews (1978) pointed out that although the prodromal period may be prolonged, it is more common for clear signs of neurological dysfunction to occur within weeks. In addition to dementia and myoclonus, cortical visual loss, focal limb weakness, aphasia, ataxia, and other evidence of regional brain dysfunction may occur. The coincidence of dementia and lower motor dysfunction has presented a diagnostic problem. Salazar et al. (1983) concluded that cases of dementia associated early in the course with signs of lower motor neuron dysfunction were more likely to be related to amyotrophic lateral sclerosis rather than representing transmissible CJD. Another type of CJD is that with occipito-parietal predominance, the Heidenhein variant. In this presentation, visual abnormalities, agnosias, and dyskinetic symptoms were noted to be prominent. In certain cases the cerebellum appears to be the special target of the disease. It should be noted that the cerebellum is the principal site of disease in kuru (Hornabrook, 1978). Brownell and Oppenheimer (1965) identified an ataxic form of CJD in four of their own cases and six from the literature. Clinically, the cases were characterized by ataxia, dysarthria, nystagmus, dementia, and involuntary movements. Pathologically, Brownell and Oppenheimer (1965) found severe depletion of the granule cells in the cerebellum. Despite the diversity of presentation, each of these variants reflects dysfunction of gray matter. Only on rare occasions is white matter involved in cases in the western hemisphere (Park et al., 1980). In Japan, however, a panencephalitic type has been observed in which the white matter suffers primary involvement as well as the gray matter. Mizutani et al. (1981) described eight cases clinically characterized by mental deterioration, paraplegia or tetraplegia, rigidity, myoclonus, and EEGs with synchronous periodic discharges.

CJD may become devastating within 1 to 2 months into the middle stage. The final stage is often characterized by mutism, rigidity, and depressed levels of consciousness leading to coma. Patients may persist in this vegetative state for weeks or months. Masters et al. (1979) found that the average total duration of the disease was 7.3 months. However, the median survival time was about 4 months. Less than 10% of cases will survive for 2 years or more. Using histopathological criteria for diagnosis, Brown et al. (1984) found that 9% of 357 cases survived for greater than 2 years. The longest survival in which documentation was supported by transmission to primates was 13 years. As a group, the cases of longer duration were characterized by a higher familial incidence, lower average age of onset, and lower incidence of myoclonus and periodic EEG activity. The long-duration cases were difficult to distinguish clinically from other dementias such as Alzheimer's disease. CJD is virtually always lethal, and no successful therapy has been demonstrated under controlled study. However, therapies that have reduced accumulation in vitro (e.g., Korth et al., 2001) may be under investigation in local protocols.

Diagnostic Criteria

Masters et al. (1979) established case inclusion criteria for their comprehensive review of the worldwide occurrence of CJD. Probable cases included progressive dementia and at least one of the following: myoclonus, pyramidal characteristic EEG, cerebellar signs, and extrapyramidal signs. A definite diagnosis added histopathological demonstration of spongiform encephalopathy. Refinement of the criteria has evolved, including the addition of the 14-3-3 assay. The WHO consultation criteria are listed in Table 15.6. The WHO consultation noted that high-intensity signal in the basal ganglia on T2- and proton density-weighted MRI supported the diagnosis of sCJD (WHO, 1998). That report discouraged the use of cerebral biopsy except to make a diagnosis of an alternative treatable disease. Olfactory biopsy as a means of making the diagnosis of sCJD merits further study (Zanusso et al., 2003).

Seipelt et al. (1999) drew attention to the close similarity of clinical abnormalities in Hashimoto's encephalitis and those in sCJD. Similarities included dementia, myoclonus, and personality changes, among other characteristics. However, Hashimoto's encephalitis was much more likely to include seizures and reduced consciousness and did not have periodic sharp-wave complexes on EEG or 14-3-3 protein in the CSF.

There are presently no disease-reversing therapies. Based on in vitro studies of inhibition of formation of pathological forms of the prion protein, quinacrine and chlorpromazine

TABLE 15.6 Diagnostic criteria for probable sCJD[a]

Progressive dementia

and

At least two of the following four features:
   Myoclonus
   Visual or cerebellar disturbance
   Pyramidal/extrapyramidal dysfunction
   Akinetic mutism

and

A typical EEG during an illness of any duration
A positive 14-3-3 CSF assay and a clinical duration to death of
   less than 2 years
Routine studies fail to suggest an alternative diagnosis

[a]WHO, 1998.

have been suggested as candidates for treatment of CJD (Korth et al., 2001). While quinacrine did not prolong survival in a murine model of experimental CJD, it was noted that clinical trials were awaited with great interest (Collins et al., 2002). In vitro studies have also suggested that antiprion protein antibodies might serve to inhibit pathogenic prion proteins (Enari et al., 2001; Peretz et al., 2001). Symptomatic management of progressive dementia requires expert input concerning environmental, behavioral, and possible pharmacological management of symptoms distressing to the patient. Valproate or clonazepam has been recommended for myoclonus. In vitro studies have shown an increase of prion proteins in the presence of valproic acid (Shaked et al., 2002). However, significant effects on an experimental model were not found, and the clinical relevance has not been determined.

Other Forms of Human Prion Disease Including vCJD

While human prion disease is rarely seen, the clinician must be alert to its occurrence with specific mechanisms of transmission (Table 15.7). These include familial forms in which there are mutations in the germ line of the PrP gene (Prusiner, 2001). Familial CJD, FFI, and GSS will be considered next, followed by transmission associated with ingestion of contaminated proteins which includes cannibalism and consumption of BSE-contaminated beef. Finally, several types of iatrogenic transmission will be described.

Familial Presentations

Three inherited human prion disorders are distinguished. Familial CJD can appear to be much like sCJD in its symptom complex (Brown et al., 1994). In general, the age of onset is earlier by about a decade, and the duration of illness is twice as long as for sCJD (de Silva and Will, 2000). Familial CJD has been transmitted to experimental animals (Masters et al., 1979). There appears to be overlap between familial CJD and GSS in that both presentations can be found in the same family (Prusiner et al., 1989).

GSS Disease. Characterized by the prominence of gait ataxia and cerebellar incoordination, GSS is vertically transmitted as an autosomal dominant disorder. It is more slowly progressive than CJD, and the onset occurs at a younger age. The average age of appearance is 43 years, with a

TABLE 15.7 Types of human prion disease by type of transmission

sCJD
Familial
  CJD
  FFI
  GSS
Ingestion
  Kuru—ritual cannibalism
  vCJD—consumption of BSE-contaminated beef
Iatrogenic
  Intracerebral procedures and electrodes
  Dura mater grafts
  Corneal grafts
  Cadaveric growth hormone or gonadotropin

mean duration of 5 years (Prusiner et al., 1989). Dementia and/or pyramidal tract signs can occur in some forms of the illness. Periodic complexes on EEG are usually not found. The histopathology is remarkable for multicentric, PrP-positive, argyrophilic plaques. System atrophies such as in the spinocerebellar and corticospinal tracts and dorsal columns are found. As a consequence, the differential diagnosis may include olivopontocerebellar atrophy, spinocerebellar degeneration, or multiple sclerosis (Kuzuhara et al., 1983; Prusiner et al., 1989). Hsiao et al. (1989) first demonstrated the association of mutations in the gene coding for the prion protein. Kretzschmar et al. (1991) found the same mutation described by Hsiao et al. (1989) at codon 102 in a member of the family in which the disease was originally described. As of 1991, that family had been traced through nine generations back to the late 18th century (H. Budka, F. Seitelberger, M. Feucht, P. Wessely, and H. A. Kretzschmar, Abstr., *Clin. Neuropathol.* **10**:99,1991). Interestingly enough, while GSS is a genetically transmitted disease, it can be transmitted to experimental animals and bears some clinical and histopathological resemblance to kuru, a horizontally transmitted disorder (Prusiner et al., 1989).

FFI. FFI, first reported by Lugaresi et al. (1986), is characterized by progressive insomnia and dysautonomia. In 1992, a report by Medori et al. placed it in the inherited prion disorder group by identifying a mutation at codon 178 of the prion protein gene. Subsequent work has also implicated codon 129 (Montagna et al., 1998). Symptoms related to the sleep disorder include insomnia, oneiric states, confusional periods, and complex hallucinations. Autonomic disturbances include diaphoresis, meiosis, sphincter dysfunction, hypertension, and hyperthermia, among a plenitude of manifestations. Endocrine abnormalities studied by Montagna et al. (1998) indicated overactive sympathetic activity. Myoclonus, dysarthria, ataxia, and spasticity can be found. Montagna et al. (1998) argue that FFI should not be defined as a dementing illness because they found normal intellective tests and behavior. Rather, they emphasize the confusion and dreamlike states and alterations in vigilance. The mean age of onset is about 51 years, with a variable mean duration of illness of 9 or 31 months, depending on zygosity at codon 129, according to Montagna et al. (1998). The histopathology is principally one of atrophy of the thalamus and inferior olives. Transmission to experimental animals has been reported (Tateishi et al., 1995).

Ingestion

Vertical transmission by germ line mutation of the prion protein genome in familial forms of CJD (Prusiner, 2001) and lateral transmission by "infectious" means, as has occurred by a number of iatrogenic mechanisms such as reuse of stereotactic brain electrodes (Brown et al., 2000), are readily apparent mechanisms of CJD transfer. In the case of vCJD, the data are convincing that the human disease derived from the prion protein of BSE (Scott et al., 1999). The mechanism appears to be consumption of contaminated beef, a mechanism that may have a parallel in the transmission of kuru by ritual cannibalism.

Kuru. While the origins of kuru are a mystery (e.g., whether a species barrier was crossed), it is clear that it was sustained in the Fore peoples of Papua New Guinea by ritual cannibalism. Its disappearance has followed the cessation of cannibalism (Prusiner et al., 1989). Following an incubation period of years to decades, a prodromal period of 6 to 12 weeks occurred in which joint pains and headache were experienced before difficulty in walking. Tremor, limb and truncal ataxia, rigidity, and cogwheeling were found in addition. Prusiner et al. (1989) reported finding signs of dementia at advanced stages of the illness. They found the average duration of illness to death to be 16 months.

vCJD. vCJD appears to have arisen as a result of consumption of beef contaminated with the prion of BSE. BSE itself appears to have arisen as the result of transmission of a scrapielike agent to cattle by ruminant-derived meat and bone meal (Wilesmith et al., 1988). Thus two species barriers may have been crossed in the derivation of vCJD from a scrapielike agent passed through cattle. BSE was first recognized in cattle in April 1985 as behavioral change, gait ataxia, and recumbency (Wells et al., 1987). Marked reduction in the incidence of BSE followed an order in 1988 to ban ruminant-derived animal protein in ruminant foodstuffs. The results of an extensive inquiry into BSE and vCJD in the United Kingdom are available at www.bse.org.uk.

New variant CJD, now called vCJD, was recognized as a result of the reinstitution of CJD surveillance in the United Kingdom following concerns about the BSE epizootic (Will et al., 1996a). The surveillance had originally been established years earlier in the United Kingdom by W. B. Matthews. Ten cases of vCJD were recognized with disease onsets from February 1994 to October 1995. In relation to the BSE epizootic, an incubation period of 5 to 10 years was suggested. The cases were clinically unique in the young age at death, with a median of 29 years; prolonged clinical course, with a median of 12 months; and a clinical picture characterized by early behavioral changes, dysesthesia, and ataxia. Dementia and myoclonus developed later in the course of the illness, and none of the cases was found to have the characteristic EEG changes of sCJD. The most striking unique and consistent histological feature was the presence of large kurulike PrP-positive plaques (florid plaques) on neuropathological examination.

In 2000, Will et al. reviewed the experiences of 35 fatal cases, of which 33 had autopsy evaluation, and proposed diagnostic criteria. These have subsequently been refined in a case definition document based on further diagnostic experience (WHO, 2002) (Table 15.8). Psychiatric symptoms were found early in the illness. The common psychiatric symptoms were depression, anxiety, and withdrawal. Forgetfulness and persistent sensory symptoms such as dysesthesia and paresthesia, including frank pain, were seen in a number of patients from the start. Ataxia was found in all cases, and involuntary movements including myoclonus, chorea, and dystonia were found in all from whom adequate data was obtained. Periodic sharp-wave complexes were not found, and 50 to 60% of patients had a positive 14-3-3 assay. Mutations were not found in the gene encoding the prion protein. The most useful noninvasive test finding was bilateral high signal in the pulvinar on MRI (Fig. 15.15). Tonsil biopsy for PrP is reserved for cases suspicious for vCJD but negative for the pulvinar sign (WHO, 2002). The differential diagnoses include sCJD, idiopathic encephalopathy, Alzheimer's

TABLE 15.8 Case definition for vCJD[a]

Definite vCJD requires IA and neuropathological confirmation

Probable vCJD requires I and four out of five of II plus IIIA and IIIB, or I and IVA

Possible vCJD requires I and four out of five of II plus IIIA

  I. A. Progressive neuropsychiatric disorder
        B. Duration of illness more than 6 months
        C. No alternative diagnosis
        D. No iatrogenic exposure
        E. No evidence of a familial form of transmissible spongiform encephalopathy
 II. A. Early psychiatric signs (depression, anxiety, apathy, withdrawal, delusions)
        B. Persistent painful sensory symptoms (frank pain and/or unpleasant dysesthesia)
        C. Ataxia
        D. Myoclonus or chorea or dystonia
        E. Dementia
III. A. EEG not done or does not show the typical appearance of sCJD of generalized triphasic periodic complexes at approximately one per second
        B. Bilateral pulvinar high signal on MRI, relative to the signal intensity of other deep gray matter nuclei and cortical gray matter
IV. A. Positive tonsil biopsy
          Routine biopsy is not recommended, not in cases with EEG typical of sCJD. It can be useful in cases compatible with vCJD in which MRI does not reveal bilateral high signal in pulvinar.

[a] WHO, 2002.

disease, and cerebral vasculitis, among a variety of conditions.

It is recommended that blood and blood products from persons with strongly suspected vCJD should be withdrawn from the blood supply.

CWD. Originally reported in captive mule deer in Colorado and Wyoming, CWD was first observed in 1967 (Williams and Young, 1980). It was subsequently reported in free-ranging deer and Rocky Mountain elk (Miller et al., 2000). More recently, there has been concern that commercial distribution of farmed elk has resulted in a much more widespread distribution in the United States (Enserink, 2001). The clinical signs in affected animals include behavioral changes, listlessness, depression, weight loss, and excessive salivation. Widespread spongiform changes are found in the brain and spinal cord (Williams and Young, 1980). There has been worry about the potential risk to humans of transmission by the consumption of contaminated venison, analogous to the apparent transmission mechanism of BSE/vCJD. Thus far, evidence of such transmission of CWD to humans has not been found (Belay et al., 2001).

Iatrogenic Transmission

Brown et al. (2000) provided a valuable compilation of iatrogenic cases of CJD to mid-2000 (Table 15.9). The two most numerous causes were growth hormone preparations from cadaveric pooled pituitary glands and cadaveric dura mater grafts. The first reported associations, in the 1970s, were caused by a corneal graft and intracerebral EEG needles.

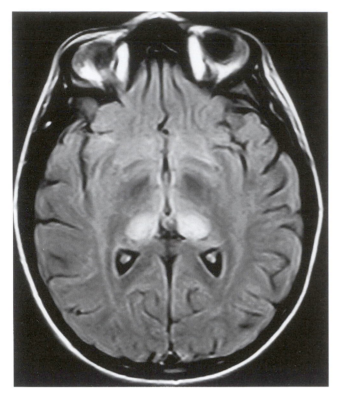

FIGURE 15.15   Axial FLAIR MRI of vCJD demonstrating symmetrical hyperintensity of the pulvinar nuclei of the thalamus relative to the caudate head and other gray matter. Courtesy of David Summers, U.K. National CJD Surveillance Unit, Edinburgh, Scotland.

Young age has often been a factor against suspecting the true nature of the disease at first but paradoxically provided a clue that an unusual mechanism of transmission may have been at work. The first reported dura-grafted patient with CJD, for example, was 28 years old and had received a dura mater graft following removal of a cholesteatoma (Thadani et al., 1988). The patient was confused and disoriented and had myoclonus, and an EEG revealed periodic sharp waves. Biopsy established the diagnosis of CJD. It is reassuring that blood transfusion and administration of pooled blood products have not been found to be associated with CJD. No cases of CJD have been identified in hemophilia patients from U.S. centers (Ricketts et al., 1997). Homozygosity at codon 129 of the prion-coding gene appears to be a risk factor for iatrogenic transmission; it is found in 80% of iatrogenic cases tested (Brown et al., 2000).

TABLE 15.9   Iatrogenic cases of CJD to mid-2000[a]

Source	No. of cases
Cadaveric growth hormone	139
Cadaveric dura mater grafting	114
Neurosurgical instruments	5
Cadaveric gonadotropin	4
Corneal transplant	3
Stereotactic EEG	2

[a] Brown et al., 2000.

Clinically, there has been a disproportionate presentation of ataxic-cerebellar forms of the illness among some causes of iatrogenic CJD. In growth hormone-related cases, for example, ataxia and incoordination were usually the initial presentations rather than impaired cognition (Fradkin et al., 1991). Laboratory studies have been useful. Examination for CSF protein 14-3-3 has been positive in 77% of iatrogenic cases (Brown et al., 2000). Periodic complexes may be present on EEG, and hyperlucency on MRI of the putamen can be positive but may not be present early in the disease process (Brown et al., 2000). We suspect that we have not seen the last of the unusual mechanisms of transmission of CJD and that diagnosis of future first cases of iatrogenic transmission will be aided by laboratory investigations.

INFECTION CONTROL

Related to the concern for iatrogenic causes of CJD are the efforts to prevent future transmissions through the use of infection control guidelines (WHO, 2000; Rutala and Weber, 2001; CJD Incidents Panel, 2001). The issue is made complex by the resistance of the prion protein to many disinfecting compounds that inactivate standard infectious agents (Rutala and Weber, 2001). There has been increased recent attention to prion infection control due to the publication of a WHO consultation (WHO, 2000), a report on the management of possible exposure to CJD or vCJD by an expert committee in the United Kingdom (CJD Incidents Panel, 2001), and development of an evidence-based guideline based on a critique of the literature (Rutala and Weber, 2001). Discussion of infectivity in tissues and fluids is often based on a report on experimentally transmitted disease from the U.S. National Institutes of Health (Brown et al., 1994). In addition to review of operating room procedures and instruments, these documents consider clinical diagnostic laboratories, hospitalization and nursing procedures, dental work, pathology, endoscopy, and waste disposal. Only general comments will be offered here. The reader is directed to the original documents cited above for explicit recommendations.

The WHO guidelines (2000) note that there is no risk in social and clinical contact or in noninvasive clinical investigations such as imaging procedures. Isolation of patients in health care settings is unnecessary, and standard precautions in nursing are recommended. Blood specimens, other body fluids (except CSF), secretions, and excretions do not require special handling. It is noted that CSF may be infectious and should be handled with care, including the recommendation that laboratory analysis should not be automated (WHO, 2000). The risk of infection from CSF is categorized as low (Rutala and Weber, 2001). Transmissibility of disease was achieved in 4 of 27 primates inoculated intracerebrally with CSF as reported by Brown et al. (1994). It should be noted that intracerebral inoculation maximizes transmissibility. Furthermore, exposure of intact skin is reported to pose negligible risk (WHO, 2000). Noting that "no case of human TSE (transmissible spongiform encephalopathy) is known to have occurred through occupational accident or injury," the WHO (2000) recommended common-sense actions following an exposure. These include washing with detergent and "abundant quantities" of warm water following contamination of unbroken skin. Maximum safety can be achieved with a 1-min exposure to 0.1 N NaOH or bleach diluted 1:10 (WHO, 2000).

Although the risk of transmissibility in most health care settings is negligible, comprehensive institutionwide evaluation for risk and implementation of infection control guidelines for the human prion disorders are necessary.

REFERENCES

Aksamit, A. J., C. M. Preissner, and H. A. Homburger. 2001. Quantitation of 14-3-3 and neuron specific enolase proteins in CSF in Creutzfeldt-Jakob disease. *Neurology* **57:**728–730.

Alper, T., W. A. Cramp, D. A. Haig, and M. C. Clarke. 1967. Does the agent of scrapie replicate without nucleic acid? *Nature* **214:**764–766.

Alperovitch, A., I. Zerr, M. Pocchiari, E. Mitrova, J. de P. Cuesta, I. Hegyi, S. Collins, H. Kretzschmar, C. Van Duijn, and R. G. Will. 1999. Codon 129 prion protein genotype and sporadic Creutzfeldt-Jakob disease. *Lancet* **353:**1673–1674.

Beck, E., and P. M. Daniel. 1979. Kuru and Creutzfeldt-Jakob disease: neuropathological lesions and their significance, p. 253–270. *In* S. B. Prusiner and W. J. Hadlow (ed.), *Slow Transmissible Diseases of the Nervous System.* Academic Press, New York, N.Y.

Belay, E. D., P. Gambetti, L. B. Schonberger, P. Parchi, D. R. Lyon, S. Capellari, J. H. McQuiston, K. Bradley, G. Dowdle, J. M. Crutcher, and C. R. Nichols. 2001. Creutzfeldt-Jakob disease in unusually young patients who consumed venison. *Arch. Neurol.* **58:**1673–1678.

Bell, J. E., and J. W. Ironside. 1993. How to tackle a possible Creutzfeldt-Jakob disease necropsy. *J. Clin. Pathol.* **46:**193–197.

Bockman, J. M., D. T. Kingsbury, M. P. McKinley, P. E. Bendheim, and S. B. Prusiner. 1985. Creutzfeldt-Jakob disease prion proteins in human brains. *N. Engl. J. Med.* **312:**73–78.

Boellard, W., and W. Scholte. 1980. Subacute spongiforme Encephalopathie mit multi-former Plaquebildung. *Acta Neuropathol.* **49:**205–212.

Brandner, S., A. Raeber, A. Sailer, T. Blaettler, M. Fischer, C. Weissmann, and A. Aguzzi. 1996. Normal host prion protein (PrPᶜ) required for scrapie spread within the central nervous system. *Proc. Natl. Acad. Sci. USA* **93:**13148–13151.

Brown, P., P. Rodgers-Johnson, F. Carthala, C. J. Gibbs Jr., and D. C. Gajdusek. 1984. Creutzfeldt-Jakob disease of long duration: clinicopathological characteristics, transmissibility, and differential diagnosis. *Ann. Neurol.* **16:**295–304.

Brown, D. R., W. J. Schulz-Schaeffer, B. Schmidt, and H. A. Kretzschmar. 1997. Prion protein-deficient cells show altered response to oxidative stress due to decreased SOD-1 activity. *Exp. Neurol.* **146:**104–112.

Brown, P., M. A. Preece, and R. G. Will. 1992. "Friendly fire" in medicine: hormones, homografts and Creutzfeldt-Jakob disease. *Lancet* **340:**24–27.

Brown, P., C. J. Gibbs Jr., P. Rodgers-Johnson, D. M. Asher, M. P. Sulima, A. Bacote, L. G. Goldfarb, and D. C. Gajdusek. 1994. Human spongiform encephalopathy: the National Institutes of Health series of 300 cases of experimentally transmitted disease. *Ann. Neurol.* **35:**513–529.

Brown, P., M. Preece, J.-P. Brandel, T. Sato, L. McShane, I. Zerr, A. Fletcher, R. G. Will, M. Pocchiari, N. R. Cashman, J. H. d'Aignaux, L. Cervenáková, J. Fradkin, L. B. Schonberger, and S. J. Collins. 2000. Iatrogenic Creutzfeldt-Jakob disease at the millennium. *Neurology* **55:**1075–1081.

Brownell, B., and D. R. Oppenheimer. 1965. An ataxic form

of subacute presenile polioencephalopathy (Creutzfeldt-Jakob Disease). *J. Neurol. Neurosurg. Psychiatr.* **28:**350–361.

Bruce, M. E., R. G. Will, J. W. Ironside, I. McDonell, D. Drummond, A. Suttie, L. McCardle, A. Chree, J. Hope, C. Birkett, S. Cousens, H. Fraser, and C. J. Bostock. 1997. Transmissions to mice indicate that 'new variant' CJD is caused by the BSE agent. *Nature* **389:**498–501.

Büeler, H., A. Aguzzi, A. Sailer, R. A. Greiner, P. Autenried, M. Aguet, and C. Weissman. 1993. Mice devoid of PrP are resistant to scrapie. *Cell* **73:**1339–1347.

CJD Incidents Panel. 2001. Management of possible exposure to CJD through medical procedures. [Online.] http://www.doh.gov.uk/cjdconsultation.

Collie, D. A., R. J. Sellar, M. Zeidler, A. C. F. Colchester, R. Knight, and R. G. Will. 2001. MRI of Creutzfeldt-Jakob disease: imaging features and recommended MRI protocol. *Clin. Radiol.* **56:**726–739.

Collinge, J. 1999. Variant Creutzfeldt-Jakob disease. *Lancet* **354:**317–323.

Collinge, J., and M. Rossor. 1996. A new variant of prion disease. *Lancet* **347:**916–917.

Collinge, J., M. S. Palmer, and A. J. Dryden. 1991. Genetic predisposition to iatrogenic Creutzfeldt-Jakob disease. *Lancet* **337:**1441–1442.

Collinge, J., M. S. Palmer, K. C. L. Sidle, I. Gowland, R. Medori, J. Ironside, and P. Lantos. 1995. Transmission of fatal familial insomnia to laboratory animals. *Lancet* **346:**569–570.

Collinge, J., K. C. L. Sidle, J. Meads, J. Ironside, and A. F. Hill. 1996. Molecular analysis of prion strain variation and the aetiology of "new variant" CJD. *Nature* **383:**685–690.

Collins, S., M. G. Law, A. Fletcher, A. Boyd, J. Kaldor, and C. L. Masters. 1999. Surgical treatment and risk of sporadic Creutzfeldt-Jakob disease: a case-control study. *Lancet* **353:**693–697.

Collins, S. J., V. Lewis, M. Brazier, A. F. Hill, A. Fletcher, and C. L. Masters. 2002. Quinacrine does not prolong survival in a murine Creutzfeldt-Jakob disease model. *Ann. Neurol.* **52:**503–506.

Cousens, S. N., E. Vynnycky, M. Zeidler, R. G. Will, and P. G. Smith. 1997. Predicting the CJD epidemic in humans. *Nature* **385:**197–198.

Cuille, J., and P. L. Chelle. 1936. Pathologie animale—la maladie dite trémblante du mouton est-elle inoculable. *C. R. Hebd. Séances Acad. Sci.* **203:**1552–1554.

DeArmond, S. J., H. A. Kretzschmar, and S. B. Prusiner. 2002. Prion diseases, p. 273–323. *In* D. I. Graham and P. Lantos (ed.), *Greenfield's Neuropathology.* Arnold, London, United Kingdom.

Derkatch, I. L., Y. O. Chernoff, V. V. Kushnirov, S. G. Inge-Vechtomov, and W. Leibman. 1996. Genesis and variability of [PSI] prion factors in *Saccharomyces cerevisiae. Genetics* **144:**1375–1386.

de Silva, R., and R. G. Will. 2000. Human prion diseases, p. 215–230. *In* L. E. Davis and P. G. E. Kennedy (ed.), *Infectious Diseases of the Nervous System.* Butterworth-Heinemann, Oxford, United Kingdom.

Dickinson, A. G., and V. M. H. Meikle. 1969. A comparison of some biological characteristics of the mouse-passed scrapie agents, 22A and ME7. *Genet. Res.* **13:**213–225.

Dickinson, A. G., and V. M. H. Meikle. 1971. Host-genotype and agent effects in scrapie incubation: change in allelic interaction with different strains of agent. *Mol. Gen. Genet.* **112:**73–79.

Dormont, D. 1999. Bovine spongiform encephalopathy and the new variant of Creutzfeldt-Jakob disease, p. 177–191. *In* D. A. Harris (ed.), *Prions: Molecular and Cellular Biology.* Horizon Scientific Press, Norfolk, United Kingdom.

Enari, M., E. Flechsig, and C. Weissmann. 2001. Scrapie prion protein accumulation by scrapie-infected neuroblastoma cells abrogated by exposure to a prion protein antibody. *Proc. Natl. Acad. Sci. USA* **98:**9295–9299.

Enserink, M. 2001. U.S. gets tough against chronic wasting disease. *Science* **294:**978–979.

Ernst, D. R., and R. E. Race. 1993. Comparative analysis of scrapie agent inactivation methods. *J. Virol. Methods* **41:**193–201.

Ferrer, I., F. Costa, and J. M. Grau Veciana. 1981. Creutzfeldt-Jacob disease: a Golgi study. *Neuropathol. Appl. Neurobiol.* **7:**237–242.

Finkenstaedt, M., A. Szudra, I. Zerr, S. Poser, J. H. Hise, J. M. Stoebner, and T. Weber. 1996. MR imaging of Creutzfeldt-Jakob disease. *Radiology* **199:**793–798.

Fradkin, J. E., L. B. Schonberger, J. L. Mills, W. J. Gunn, J. M. Piper, D. K. Wysowski, R. Thomson, S. Durako, and P. Brown. 1991. Creutzfeldt-Jakob disease in pituitary growth hormone recipients in the United States. *JAMA* **265:**880–884.

Fraser, H. 1973. Scrapie in mice: agent-strain differences in the distribution and intensity of grey matter vacuolation. *J. Comp. Pathol.* **83:**29–40.

Fraser, H., M. E. Bruce, D. Davies, C. F. Farguhar, and P. A. McBridge. 1992. The lymphoreticular system in the pathogenesis of scrapie, p. 308–317. *In* S. B. Prusiner, J. Collinge, J. Powell, and B. Anderton (ed.), *Prion Diseases of Humans and Animals.* Ellis Horwood, London, United Kingdom.

Gajdusek, D. C., and V. Zigas. 1957. Degenerative disease of the central nervous system in New Guinea. The endemic occurrence of 'kuru' in the native population. *N. Engl. J. Med.* **257:**974–978.

Gajdusek, D. C., C. J. Gibbs, and M. Alpers. 1966. Experimental transmission of a kuru-like syndrome to chimpanzees. *Nature* **209:**794–796.

Gambetti, P., and E. Jugaresi. 1998. Conclusions of the symposium. *Brain Pathol.* **8:**571–575.

Ghani, A. C., N. M. Ferguson, C. A. Donnelly, T. J. Hagenaars, and R. M. Anderson. 1999. Epidemiological determinants of the pattern and magnitude of the vCJD epidemic in Great Britain. *Proc. R. Soc. London Ser B. Biol. Sci.* **265:**2243–2252.

Gibbs, C. J., D. C. Gajdusek, D. M. Asher, M. P. Alpers, E. Beck, P. M. Daniel, and W. B. Matthews. 1968. Creutzfeldt-Jakob disease (spongiform encephalopathy): transmission to the chimpanzee. *Science* **161:**388–389.

Goldfarb, L. G., R. B. Petersen, M. Tabaton, P. Brown, A. C. Leblanc, P. Montagna, P. Cortelli, J. Julien, C. Vital, W. W. Pendelbury, M. Haltia, P. R. Wills, J. J. Hauw, P. E. McKeever, L. Monari, B. Schrank, G. D. Swergold, L. Autilio-Gambetti, D. C. Gajdusek, E. Lugaresi, and P. Gambetti. 1992. Fatal familial insomnia and familial Creutzfeldt-Jakob disease—disease phenotype determined by a DNA polymorphism. *Science* **258:**806–808.

Griffiths, J. 1967. Self-replication and scrapie. *Nature* **215:**1043–1044.

Hadlow, W. J. 1959. Scrapie and kuru. Lancet **ii:**289–290.

Hill, A. F., M. Desbrulais, S. Joiner, K. C. Sidle, I. Gowland, J. Collinge, L. J. Doey, and P. Lantos. 1997. The same prion strain causes vCJD and BSE. *Nature* **389:**448–450, 526.

Hill, A. F., R. J. Butterworth, S. Joiner, G. Jackson, M. N. Rossor, D. J. Thomas, A. Frosh, N. Folley, J. E. Bell, M. Spencer, A. King, S. Al-Sarraj, J. W. Ironside, P. L. Lantos, and J. Collinge. 1999a. Investigation of variant Creutzfeldt-Jakob disease and other human prion disease with tonsil biopsy samples. *Lancet* **353:**183–189.

Hill, A., M. Antoniou, and J. Collinge. 1999b. Protease-resistant prion protein produced in vitro lacks detectable infectivity. *J. Gen. Virol.* **80:**11–14.

Hilton, D. A., E. Fathers, P. Edwards, J. W. Ironside, and J. Zajicek. 1998. Prion immunoreactivity in appendix before clinical onset of variant Creutzfeldt-Jakob disease. *Lancet* **352:**703–704.

Hornabrook, R. W. 1978. Slow virus infections of the central nervous system, p. 275–290. *In* P. J. Vinken and G. W. Bruyn (ed.), in collaboration with H. L. Klawans, *Handbook of Clinical Neurology*, Part II, *Infections of the Nervous System*, vol. 34. North-Holland Publishing Co., Amsterdam, The Netherlands.

Hsiao, K., H. F. Baker, T. J. Crow, M. Poulter, F. Owen, J. Tewiliger, D. Westaway, J. Ott, and S. Prusiner. 1989. Linkage of a prion protein missense variant to Gerstmann-Sträussler syndrome. *Nature* **338:**342–345.

Hsiao, K. K., M. Scott, D. Foster, D. F. Groth, S. J. DeArmond, and S. B. Prusiner. 1990. Spontaneous neurodegeneration in transgenic mice with mutant prion protein. *Science* **250:**1587–1590.

Ironside, J. W., and J. E. Bell. 1997. Pathology of prion diseases, p. 57–88. *In* J. Collinge and M. S. Palmer (ed.), *Prion Diseases.* Oxford University Press, Oxford, United Kingdom.

Kim, J. H., and E. E. Manuelidis. 1983. Pathology of human and experimental Creutzfeldt-Jakob disease. *Pathol. Annu.* **18:**359–373.

Kimberlin, R. H., and C. A. Walker. 1986. Pathogenesis of scrapie (strain 263K) in hamsters infected intracerebrally, intraperitoneally or intraocularly. *J. Gen. Virol.* **67:**255–263.

Kirschbaum, W. R. 1968. *Jakob-Creutzfeldt Disease.* American Elsevier Publishing Co., New York, N.Y.

Kitagawa, Y., F. Gotoh, A. Koto, S. Ebihara, H. Okayasu, T. Ishii, and H. Matsuyama. 1983. Creutzfeldt-Jakob disease: a case with extensive white matter degeneration and optic atrophy. *J. Neurol.* **229:**97–101.

Kitamoto, T., R. W. Shin, K. Doh-ura, N. Tomokane, M. Miyazono, T. Muramoto, and J. Tateishi. 1992. Abnormal isoform of prion protein accumulates in synaptic structures of the central nervous system in patients with Creutzfeldt-Jakob disease. *Am. J. Pathol.* **140:**1285–1289.

Klatzo, I., D. C. Gajdusek, and V. Zigas. 1959. Pathology of kuru. *Lab. Investig.* **8:**799–847.

Klein, M. A., R. Frigg, E. Flechsig, A. J. Raeber, U. Kalinke, H. Bluethmann, F. Bootz, M. Suter, R. M. Zinkermagel, and A. Aguzzi. 1997. A crucial role for B cells in neuroinvasive scrapie. *Nature* **390:**687–690.

Knopman, D. S., S. T. DeKosky, J. L. Cummings, H. Chui, J. Corey-Bloom, N. Relkin, G. W. Small, B. Miller, and J. C. Stevens. 2001. Practice parameter: diagnosis of dementia (an evidence based review). Report of the Quality Standards Subcommittee of the American Academy of Neurology. *Neurology* **56:**1143–1153.

Kocisko, D. A., J. H. Come, S. A. Priola, B. Chesebro, G. J. Raymond, P. T. Lansbury, and B. Caughy. 1994. Cell-free formation of protease-resistant prion protein. *Nature* **370:**471–474.

Korth, C., B. C. H. May, F. E. Cohen, and S. B. Prusiner. 2001. Acridine and phenothiazine derivatives as pharmacotherapeutics for prion disease. *Proc. Natl. Acad. Sci. USA* **98:**9836–9841.

Kretzschmar, H. A., G. Honold, F. Seitelberger, M. Feucht, P. Wessely, P. Mehrain, and H. Budka. 1991. Prion protein mutation in family first reported by Gerstmann, Sträussler, and Scheinker. *Lancet* **337:**1160.

Kuzuhara, S., I. Kanazawa, H. Sasaki, T. Nakanishi, and

K. Shimamura. 1983. Gerstmann-Sträussler-Scheinker's disease. *Ann. Neurol.* **14**:216–225.

Lampert, P. W., D. C. Gajdusek, and C. J. Gibbs Jr. 1971. Experimental spongiform encephalopathy (Creutzfeldt-Jakob disease) in chimpanzees. Electron microscopic studies. *J. Neuropathol. Exp. Neurol.* **30**:20–32.

Lampert, P. W., D. C. Gajdusek, and C. J. Gibbs Jr. 1975. Pathology of dendrites in subacute spongiform virus encephalopathies. *Adv. Neurol.* **12**:465–470.

Landis, D. M., R. S. Williams, and C. L. Masters. 1981. Golgi and electron microscopic studies of spongiform encephalopathy. *Neurology* **31**:538–549.

Lemstra, A. W., M. T. van Meegen, J. P. Vreyling, P. H. S. Meijerink, G. H. Jansen, S. Bulk, F. Baas, and W. A. van Gool. 2000. 14-3-3 testing in diagnosing Creutzfeldt-Jakob disease. A prospective study. *Neurology* **55**:514–516.

Lugaresi, E., R. Medori, P. Montagna, A. Baruzzi, P. Cortelli, A. Lugaresi, P. Tinnper, M. Zucconi, and P. Gambetti. 1986. Fatal familial insomnia and dysautonomia with selective degeneration of thalamic nuclei. *N. Engl. J. Med.* **315**:997–1003.

Manuelidis, E. E., E. J. Gorgacz, and L. Manuelidis. 1978. Transmission of Creutzfeldt-Jakob disease with scrapie-like syndromes to mice. *Nature* **271**:778–779.

Masters, C. L., and E. P. Richardson Jr. 1978. Subacute spongiform encephalopathy (Creutzfeldt-Jakob disease). The nature and progression of spongiform change. *Brain* **101**:333–344.

Masters, C. L., and D. C. Gajdusek. 1982. The spectrum of Creutzfeldt-Jakob disease and the virus-induced subacute spongiform encephalopathies, p. 139–162. *In* W. T. Smith and J. B. Cavanagh (ed.), *Recent Advances in Neuropathology*. Churchill Livingstone, Edinburgh, Scotland.

Masters, C. L., J. O. Harris, C. Gajdusek, C. J. Gibbs Jr., C. Bernoulli, and D. M. Asher. 1979. Creutzfeldt-Jakob disease: patterns of worldwide occurrence and the significance of familial and sporadic clustering. *Ann. Neurol.* **5**:177–188.

Masters, C. L., D. C. Gajdusek, and C. J. Gibbs, Jr. 1981. Creutzfeldt-Jakob disease virus isolations from the Gerstmann-Sträussler syndrome with an analysis of the various forms of amyloid plaque deposition in the virus-induced spongiform encephalopathies. *Brain* **104**:559–588.

Matthews, W. B. 1978. Creutzfeldt-Jakob disease. *Postgrad. Med. J.* **54**:591–594.

Medori, R., H.-J. Tritschler, A. LeBlanc, F. Villare, V. Manetto, H. Y. Chen, R. Xue, S. Leal, P. Montagna, P. Cortelli, P. Tinuper, P. Avoni, M. Mochi, A. Baruzzi, J. J. Hauw, J. Ott, E. Lugaresi, L. Autilio-Gambetti, and P. Gambetti. 1992. Fatal familial insomnia, a prion disease with a mutation at codon 178 of the prion protein gene. *N. Engl. J. Med.* **326**:444–449.

Milhavet, O., M. E. M. McMahon, W. Rachidi, N. Nishida, S. Katamine, A. Mangé, M. Arlotto, D. Casanova, J. Riondel, A. Favier, and S. Lehmann. 2000. Prion infection impairs the cellular response to oxidative stress. *Proc. Natl. Acad. Sci. USA* **97**:13937–13942.

Miller, M. W., E. S. Williams, C. W. McCarty, T. R. Spraker, T. J. Kreeger, C. T. Larsen, and E. T. Thorne. 2000. Epizootiology of chronic wasting disease in free-ranging cervids in Colorado and Wyoming. *J. Wildlife Dis.* **36**:676–690.

Mitzutani, T., A. Okumura, M. Oda, and H. Shirki. 1981. Panencephalitic type of Creutzfeldt-Jakob disease: primary involvement of the cerebral white matter. *J. Neurol. Neurosurg. Psychiat.* **44**:103–115.

Montagna, P., P. Cortelli, P. Avoni, P. Tinuper, G. Plazzi, R. Galassi, F. Portaluppi, J. Julien, C. Vital, M. B. Delisle, P. Gambetti, and E. Lugaresi. 1998. Clinical features of fatal familial insomnia: phenotypic variability in relation to a polymorphism at codon 129 of the prion protein. *Brain Pathol.* **8**:515–520.

Muramoto, T., S. J. DeArmond, M. Scott, G. C. Telling, F. E. Cohen, and S. B. Prusiner. 1997. Heritable disorder resembling neuronal storage disease in mice expressing prion protein with deletion of an alpha-helix. *Nat. Med.* **3**:750–755.

Ohta, M., M. Koga, J. Tateishi, S. Motomara, and S. Yamashita. 1978. An autopsy report of spongiform encephalopathy associated with kuru plaques and leucomalacia. *Adv. Neurol. Sci.* **22**:487–496.

Oppenheimer, D. R. 1975. Pathology of transmissible and degenerative diseases of the nervous system, p. 161–174. *In* L. S. Illis (ed.), *Viral Diseases of the Nervous System*. Bailliére Tindall, London, United Kingdom.

Palmer, M. S., A. J. Dryden, J. T. Hughes, and J. Collinge. 1991. Homozygous prion protein genotype predisposes to sporadic Creutzfeldt-Jakob disease. *Nature* **352**:340–342.

Parchi, P., A. Giese, S. Capellari, P. Brown, W. Schulz-Schaeffer, O. Windl, I. Zerr, H. Budka, N. Kopp, P. Piccardo, S. Poser, A. Rojiani, N. Streichemberger, J. Julien, C. Vital, B. Ghetti, P. Gambetti, and H. Kretzschmar. 1999. Classification of sporadic Creutzfeldt-Jakob disease based on molecular and phenotypic analysis of 300 subjects. *Ann. Neurol.* **46**:224–233.

Park, T. S., G. M. Kleinman, and E. P. Richardson. 1980. Creutzfeldt-Jakob disease with extensive degeneration of white matter. *Acta Neuropathol.* **52**:239–242.

Peretz, D., R. A. Williamson, K. Kaneke, J. Vergara, E. Leclerc, G. Schmitt-Ulms, I. R. Mehlhorn, G. Legname, M. R. Wormald, P. M. Rudd, R. A. Dwek, D. R. Burton, and S. B. Prusiner. 2001. Antibodies inhibit prion propagation and clear cell cultures of prion infectivity. *Nature* **412**:739–743.

Poser, S., B. Mollenhauer, A. Krauss, I. Zerr, B. J. Steinhoff, A. Schroeter, M. Finkenstaedt, W. J. Schulz-Schaeffer, H. A. Kretzschmar, and K. Felgenhauer. 1999. How to improve the clinical diagnosis of Creutzfeldt-Jakob disease. *Brain* **122**:2345–2351.

Prusiner, S. B. 1982. Novel proteinaceous infectious particles cause scrapie. *Science* **216**:136–144.

Prusiner, S. B. 2001. Shattuck lecture—neurodegenerative diseases and prions. *N. Engl. J. Med.* **344**:1516–1526.

Prusiner, S. B., K. K. Hsiao, D. E. Bredesen, and S. J. DeArmond. 1989. Prion disease, p. 543–580. *In* R. R. McKendall (ed.), *Handbook of Clinical Neurology*, vol. 12(56): *Viral Disease*. Elsevier Science, Amsterdam, The Netherlands.

Richardson, E. P., Jr., and C. L. Masters. 1995. The nosology of Creutzfeldt-Jakob disease and conditions related to the accumulation of PrP^{CJD} in the nervous system. *Brain Pathol.* **5**:33–41.

Ricketts, M. N., N. R. Cashman, E. E. Stratton, and S. E. L. Saadany. 1997. Is Creutzfeldt-Jakob disease transmitted in blood. *Emerg. Infect. Dis.* **3**:155–163.

Rieger, R., F. Edenhofer, C. I. Lasmezas, and S. Weiss. 1997. The human 37-kDa laminin receptor precursor interacts with the prion protein in eukaryotic cells. *Nat. Med.* **3**:1383–1388.

Rutala, W. A., and D. J. Weber. 2001. Creutzfeldt-Jakob disease: recommendations for disinfection and sterilization. *Clin. Infect. Dis.* **32**:1348–1356.

Salazar, A. M., C. L. Masters, D. C. Gajdusek, and C. J. Gibbs. 1983. Syndromes of amyotrophic lateral sclerosis: relation to transmissible Creutzfeldt-Jakob disease. *Ann. Neurol.* **14**:17–26.

Schatzl, H. M., L. Laszlo, D. M. Holtzman, J. Tatzelt, S. J. DeArmond, R. I. Weiner, W. C. Mobley, and S. B. Prusiner. 1997. A hypothalamic neuronal cell line persistently infected with scrapie prions exhibits apoptosis. *J. Virol.* **71**:8821–8831.

Scott, M. R., R. Will, J. Ironside, H.-O. B. Nauyen, P. Tremblay, S. J. Armond, and S. B. Prusiner. 1999. Compelling transgenic evidence for transmission of bovine spongiform encephalopathy prions to humans. *Proc. Natl. Acad. Sci. USA* **96:**15137–15142.

Seipelt, M., I. Zerr, R. Nau, B. Mollenhauer, S. Kropp, B. J. Steinhoff, C. Wilhelm-Gossling, C. Bamberg, R. W. C. Janzen, P. Berlit, F. Manz, K. Felgienhauer, and S. Poser. 1999. Hashimoto's encephalitis as a differential diagnosis of Creutzfeldt-Jakob disease. *J. Neurol. Neurosurg. Psychiatr.* **66:**172–176.

Seitelberger, F. 1962. Eigenartige familiar-hereditare Krankheit des Zentralnerven-systems in einer niederosterreichen Sippe. *Wien Klin. Wschr.* **74:**687–691.

Shaked, G. M., R. Englstein, I. Auraham, H. Rosenmann, and R. Bagizon. 2002. Valproic acid treatment results in increased accumulation of prion proteins. *Ann. Neurol.* **52:**416–420.

Shyng, S. L., J. E. Heuser, and D. A. Harris. 1994. A glycolipid-anchored prion protein is endocytosed via clathrin-coated pits. *J. Cell Biol.* **125:**1239–1250.

Steinhoff, B. J., S. Racker, G. Herrendorf, S. Poser, S. Grosche, I. Zerr, H. Kretzschmar, and T. Weber. 1996. Accuracy and reliability of periodic sharp wave complexes in Creutzfeldt-Jakob disease. *Arch. Neurol.* **53:**162–166.

Tateishi, J., Y. Sato, M. Koga, H. Doi, and M. Ohta. 1980. Experimental transmission of human subacute spongiform encephalopathy to small rodents. I. Clinical and histological observations. *Acta Neuropathol.* **51:**127–134.

Tateishi, J., P. Brown, T. Kitamoto, Z. M. Hogue, R. Roos, R. Wollman, L. Cerevenáková, and D. C. Gajdusek. 1995. First experimental transmission of fatal familial insomnia. *Nature* **376:**434–435.

Thadani, V., P. L. Penar, J. Partington, R. Kalb, R. Janssen, L. B. Schonberger, C. S. Rabkin, and J. W. Prichard. 1988. Creutzfeldt-Jakob disease probably acquired from a cadaveric dura mater graft. *J. Neurosurg.* **53:**1197–1201.

Tobler, I., S. E. Gaus, T. Deboer, P. Achermann, M. Fischer, T. Rülicke, M. Moser, B. Oesch, P. A. McBridge, and J. C. Manson. 1996. Altered circadian activity rhythms and sleep in mice devoid of prion protein. *Nature* **380:**639–642.

Ward, H. J. T., D. Everington, E. A. Croes, A. Alperovitch, N. Delasnerie-Laupretre, I. Zerr, S. Poser, and C. M. van Duijn for the European Union (ED) Collaborative Study Group of Creutzfeldt-Jakob Disease (CJD). 2002. Sporadic Creutzfeldt-Jakob disease and surgery: a case-control study using community controls. *Neurology* **59:**543–548.

Weissmann, C., A. J. Raeber, D. Shmerling, A. Cozzio, E. Flechsig, and A. Aguzzi. 1999. The use of genetically modified mice in prion research, p. 87–106. *In* D. A. Harris (ed.), *Prions: Molecular and Cellular Biology.* Horizon Scientific Press, Norfolk, United Kingdom.

Wells, G. A. H., A. C. Scott, C. T. Johnson, R. F. Gunning, R. D. Hancock, M. Jeffrey, M. Dawson, and R. Bradley. 1987. A novel progressive spongiform encephalopathy in cattle. *Vet. Rec.* **121:**419–420.

White, A. R., S. J. Collins, F. Maher, M. F. Jobling, L. R. Stewart, J. M. Thyer, K. Beyreuther, C. L. Masters, and R. Cappai. 1999. Prion protein-deficient neurons reveal lower glutathione reductase activity and increased susceptibility to hydrogen peroxide toxicity. *Am. J. Pathol.* **155:**1723–1730.

Wilesmith, J. W., G. A. H. Wells, M. P. Cranwell, and J. B. M. Ryan. 1988. Bovine spongiform encephalopathy: epidemiological studies. *Vet. Rec.* **123:**638–644.

Will, R. G., and W. B. Matthews. 1984. A retrospective study of Creutzfeldt-Jakob disease in England and Wales 1970–79. I. Clinical features. *J. Neurol. Neurosurg. Psychiatr.* **47:**134–140.

Will, R. G., J. W. Ironside, M. Zeidler, S. N. Cousens, K. Estibeiro, A. Alperovitch, S. Poser, M. Pocchiari, A. Hofman, and P. G. Smith. 1996a. A new variant of Creutzfeldt-Jakob disease in the UK. *Lancet* **347:**921–925.

Will, R. G., M. Zeidler, P. Brown, M. Harrington, K. H. Lee, and K. L. Kenney. 1996b. Cerebrospinal-fluid test for new-variant Creutzfeldt-Jakob disease. *Lancet* **348:**955.

Will, R. G., M. Zeidler, G. E. Stewart, M. A. Macleod, J. W. Ironside, S. N. Cousens, D. M. Stat, J. Mackenzie, K. Estibeiro, A. J. E. Green, and R. S. G. Knight. 2000. Diagnosis of new variant Creutzfeldt-Jakob disease. *Ann. Neurol.* **47:**575–582.

Williams, E. S., and S. Young. 1980. Chronic wasting disease of captive mule deer: a spongiform encephalopathy. *J. Wildlife Dis.* **16:**89–98.

World Health Organization. 1998. Human transmissible spongiform encephalopathies. *Weekly Epidemiol. Rec.* **73:**361–365.

World Health Organization. 2000. WHO infection control guidelines for transmissible spongiform encephalopathies. (http://www.whoint/inf-fs/en/fact113.html).

World Health Organization. 2002. The revision of the surveillance case definition for variant Creutzfeldt-Jakob disease (vCJD). Report of a WHO consultation. World Health Organization, Edinburgh, United Kingdom.

Zanusso, G., S. Ferrari, F. Cardone, P. Zampieri, M. Gelati, M. Fiorini, A. Farinazzo, M. Gardiman, T. Cavallaro, M. Bentivoglio, P. G. Righetti, M. Pocchiari, N. Rizzuto, and S. Monaco. 2003. Detection of pathologic prion protein in the olfactory epithelium in sporadic Creutzfeldt-Jakob disease. *N. Engl. J. Med.* **348:**711–719.

Zeidler, M., R. J. Sehlar, D. A. Collie, R. Knight, G. Stewart, M.-A. Macleod, J. W. Ironside, S. Cousens, A. F. C. Colchester, D. M. Hadley, and R. G. Will. 2000. The pulvinar sign on magnetic resonance imaging in variant Creutzfeldt-Jakob disease. *Lancet* **355:**1412–1418.

Zerr, I., M. Pocchiari, S. Collins, J. P. Brandel, J. dePedro Cuesta, R. S. G. Knight, H. Bernheimer, F. Cardone, N. Delasnerie-Laupretre, N. C. Corrales, A. Ladogana, M. Bodemer, A. Fletcher, T. Awan, A. R. Bremon, H. Dubka, J. L. Laplanche, R. G. Will, and S. Poser. 2000a. Analysis of EEG and CSF 14-3-3 proteins as aids to the diagnosis of Creutzfeldt-Jakob disease. *Neurology* **55:**811–815.

Zerr, I., W. J. Schulz-Schaeffer, A. Giese, M. Bodemer, A. Schroter, K. Henke, H. J. Tschampa, O. Windl, A. Pfahlberg, B. J. Steinhoff, O. Gefeller, H. A. Kretzschmar, and S. Poser. 2000b. Current clinical diagnosis in Creutzfeldt-Jakob disease: identification of uncommon variants. *Ann. Neurol.* **48:**323–329.

Index